Yoder-Wise's
Leading *and* Managing
in Canadian Nursing

Evolve®

YOU'VE JUST PURCHASED
MORE THAN
A TEXTBOOK!

Enhance your learning with Evolve Student Resources.

These online study tools and exercises can help deepen your understanding of textbook content so you can be more prepared for class, perform better on exams, and succeed in your course.

Activate the complete learning experience that comes with each textbook purchase by registering at

http://evolve.elsevier.com/Canada/Yoder-Wise/leading/

REGISTER TODAY!

Yoder-Wise's
Leading *and* Managing
in Canadian Nursing

SECOND EDITION

Janice I. Waddell, RN, MA, PhD
Professor
Daphne Cockwell School of Nursing
Yeates School of Graduate Studies
Ryerson University
Toronto, Ontario

Nancy A. Walton, RN, PhD
Director and Associate Professor
Daphne Cockwell School of Nursing
Ryerson University
Toronto, Ontario

Chair, Research Ethics Board
Women's College Hospital
Toronto, Ontario

US Author
Patricia S. Yoder-Wise, RN, EdD, NEA-BC, ANEF, FAAN

Professor and Dean Emerita
Texas Tech University Health Sciences Center
Lubbock, Texas

ELSEVIER

YODER-WISE'S LEADING AND MANAGING IN CANADIAN NURSING,
SECOND EDITION

ISBN: 978-1-77172-167-7

Copyright © 2020 Elsevier Inc. All Rights Reserved.

Previous edition copyrighted 2015 by Elsevier Canada, a Division of Reed Elsevier Canada, Ltd.

Adapted from *Leading and Managing in Canadian Nursing*, 7th edition, by Patricia S. Yoder-Wise. Copyright © 2019 by Elsevier, Inc. Previous editons copyrighted 2015, 2011, 2007, 2003, 1999, 1995.

978-0-323-44913-7
(softcover)

Notice

Library of Congress Control Number: 2019944071

VP Education Content: Kevonne Holloway
Content Strategist (Canada Acquisitions): Roberta A. Spinosa-Millman
Director, Content Development: Laurie Gower
Content Development Specialist: Sandy Matos
Publishing Services Manager: Shereen Jameel
Project Manager: Umarani Natarajan

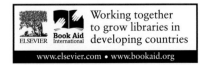

Working together to grow libraries in developing countries

www.elsevier.com • www.bookaid.org

Last digit is the print number: 9   8   7   6   5   4   3   2   1

This book is dedicated to the nursing students, faculty and nurses who are committed to the development and practice of excellence in nursing leadership and management. Through the process of editing this edition, we were inspired by the many nurses and nursing students who have exemplified moral courage and risk-taking in assuming leadership in diverse health systems and settings, in research and policy work, in direct patient care, and in nursing education across Canada.

Janice I. Waddell, Nancy A. Walton

ACKNOWLEDGEMENTS

We are delighted to present the second edition of *Yoder-Wise's Leading and Managing in Canadian Nursing*. The completed work is a culmination of the efforts of many. The contributors who worked with us were generous with their expertise, time, and commitment to producing what we believe is a comprehensive and relevant discussion of nursing leadership and management. We would like to take this opportunity to both express our gratitude and to acknowledge the work and dedication reflected in their significant contributions.

In developing the second edition, we aimed to ensure that the content reflects the realities of leadership and management in a Canadian context. We further directed our efforts to ensure that the discussions within and across all chapters are responsive to students at various stages during their nursing education.

We are honoured to have helped build on the first edition and continue to curate the wealth of knowledge all the authors bring to the text. The diversity in our authorship demonstrates to students the richness of perspectives available, and we hope the pool of talent gathered for this edition inspires students to find a role model and mentor with the goal of advancing their own unique ambitions for nursing leadership and management.

We extend our appreciation to Roberta Spinosa-Millman who invited us to come on board as co-editors of this rich resource for nursing students and faculty members and for her commitment to advancing nursing students' capacity in both leadership and management realms within their nursing education. We would also like to extend our gratitude to our Developmental Editor, Sandy Matos, who was highly responsive to our questions and suggestions as well as those of our many chapter authors. In addition to her strong expertise as an editor, Sandy also ensured that we, as editors, as well as all contributing authors were organized and on track with deadlines and content deliverables. We further wish to extend our thanks to the many 'behind the scenes' Elsevier staff who also supported the completion of this edition.

On behalf of all the editorial team and the contributors, we would like to acknowledge all reviewers who contributed their time and expertise to provide feedback and suggestions, all of which have informed the revisions and new additions included in this edition of *Yoder-Wise's Leading and Managing in Canadian Nursing*.

It is our hope that students at each stage of their nursing education program consider the knowledge and insights included in this textbook to be relevant and meaningful to their development as exceptional and influential nurse leaders and managers.

Janice I. Waddell, RN, MA, PhD
Nancy A. Walton, RN, PhD

CANADIAN CONTRIBUTORS

Genevieve Armstrong, RN, BScN, MN
Public Health Nurse
Tuberculosis Program
Toronto Public Health
Daphne Cockwell School of Nursing
Ryerson University
Toronto, Ontario

Lisa Ashley, RN, BScN, MEd, CCHN(C)
Senior Health Consultant
Lisa Ashley Consulting
Ottawa, Ontario

**Yolanda Babenko-Mould,
RN, BScN, MScN, PhD**
Associate Professor
Arthur Labatt Family School of Nursing
Faculty of Health Sciences
Western University
London, Ontario

Jocelyn Bennett, BScN, MScN
Nurse Consultant
Toronto, Ontario

Richard G. Booth, RN, PhD
Assistant Professor
Arthur Labatt Family School of Nursing
Western University
London, Ontario

Danielle Bourque, RN, BScN, MScN
School of Nursing
McMaster University
Hamilton, Ontario

Domonique Bourque, RN, BScN
School of Nursing
University of Alberta
Edmonton, Alberta

R. Lisa Bourque Bearskin, RN, BScN, MN, PhD
Associate Professor
School of Nursing
Thompson Rivers University
Kamloops, British Columbia

Judy Boychuk Duchscher, RN, BScN, MN, PhD
Associate Professor
Nursing
Thompson Rivers University
Kamloops, British Columbia

Krystal Buchanan, PN, RN, BScN, MScN
Coordinator PN & PSW
School of Health, Wellness, and Sciences
Georgian College
Orangeville, Ontario

Barbara Campbell, RN, BN, MN, PhD
Associate Professor
Faculty of Nursing
Director of International Relations Office
University of Prince Edward Island
Charlottetown, Prince Edward Island

Simon Carroll, PhD
Assistant Teaching Professor
Department of Sociology
University of Victoria
Victoria, British Columbia

Maureen Cava, RN, BScN, MN, FCCHL
Manager, Professional Development & Education
(retired)
Performance & Standards
Toronto Public Health
Toronto, Ontario

Nancy Clark, RN, PhD
Assistant Professor
Faculty of Human and Social Development
School of Nursing
University of Victoria
Victoria, British Columbia

Judy Costello, BN, MScN
Senior Clinical Director
Princess Margaret Cancer Centre
University Health Network
Adjunct Lecturer
Faculty of Nursing
University of Toronto
Toronto, Ontario

Shannon Dames, BN, MPH, EdD
Professor
Nursing
Vancouver Island University
Nanaimo, British Columbia

Wendy A. Gifford, RN, PhD
Associate Professor
Co-Director, Centre for Research on Health
  and Nursing
Faculty of Health Sciences
  School of Nursing
University of Ottawa
Ottawa, Ontario

Marcia Hills, RN, BScN, MA, PhD, FAAN,
Distinguished Scholar in Caring Science (WCSI)
Professor
School of Nursing
University of Victoria
Victoria, British Columbia

Andrea Kennedy, RN, PhD
Associate Professor
School of Nursing and Midwifery
Faculty of Health, Community and Education
Mount Royal University
Calgary, Alberta

Arden Krystal, BScN, MHA, CHE
President and CEO
Southlake Regional Health Centre
Newmarket, Ontario
Adjunct Professor
School of Nursing
University of British Columbia
Vancouver, British Columbia

Sara Lankshear, RN, PhD
Faculty
BScN Collaborative Program
Georgian College
Barrie, Ontario

Nancy Lefebre, RN, BScN, MScN, FCCHSE
Chief Clinical Executive and Senior Vice President,
  Knowledge and Practice
Saint Elizabeth Health Care
Markham, Ontario

Heather MacMillan, RN, BSc, MSc(A)
Regional Manager
Regional Perioperative Education Program (RPEP)
Vancouver Coastal Health, Clinical Education
Vancouver, British Columbia

Maura MacPhee, RN, PhD
Professor
School of Nursing
University of British Columbia
Vancouver, British Columbia

Janet McCabe, BScN, MEd, PhD
Associate Professor
Faculty of Health Sciences
University of Ontario Institute of Technology
Oshawa, Ontario

Colleen A. McKey, RN, BScN, MScHSA, PhD, CHE,
LFACHE
Associate Professor
School of Nursing
McMaster University
Hamilton, Ontario

Mallory McKey
BScN Student
Department of Nursing
Brock University
St. Catharines, Ontario

Christina Murray, BA, BScN, MN, PhD
Assistant Professor
Faculty of Nursing
University of Prince Edward Island
Charlottetown, Prince Edward Island

Bhavik B. Patel, RN, BScN
Professor
Practical Nursing
Loyalist College
Belleville, Ontario

Sandra Regan, RN, BScN, MScN, MA, PhD
Adjunct Associate Professor
Arthur Labatt Family School of Nursing
Western University
London, Ontario
Deputy Registrar, Education Program Review
British Columbia College of Nursing Professionals
Vancouver, British Columbia

Karen Spalding, RN, PhD
Associate Professor
School of Health Services Management
Ted Rogers School of Management
Ryerson University
Toronto, Ontario

Gillian Strudwick, RN, PhD
Independent Scientist
Information Management Group
Centre for Addiction and Mental Health
Toronto, Ontario

Terri Stuart-McEwan, RN, BScN, MHS
Executive Director
Princess Margaret Cancer Centre
University Health Network
Adjunct Professor
Bloomberg School of Nursing
University of Toronto
Toronto, Ontario

James H. Tiessen, MSc, BSc, PhD
Associate Professor & Director
School of Health Services Management
Ted Rogers School of Management
Ryerson University
Toronto, Ontario

Annita Velasque Moreira, BA, BScN
Daphne Cockwell School of Nursing
Ryerson University
Toronto, Ontario

Mary M. Wheeler, RN, MEd
Certified Coach
Partner, donnerwheeler
Brampton, Ontario

Erin Wilson, BN, MScN, PhD
Assistant Professor and Family
    Nurse Practitioner
School of Nursing
University of Northern British Columbia
Prince George, British Columbia

US CONTRIBUTOR

Susan Sportsman, RN, PhD
Dean
College of Health Sciences
    and Human Services
Midwestern State University
Wichita Falls, Texas

REVIEWERS LIST

CANADIAN REVIEWERS

Peer review is critical to the quality and utility of scholarly and practice informing publications. Through the efforts of expert peers, knowledge is tested for its veracity and completeness and questions are asked that improve and refine our thinking and writing. Peer review is also important to the development of best practices, best evidence, and continuous development of the nursing profession, so it is welcomed and appreciated. Our peer reviewers provided insightful comments and suggestions that helped refine the presentation of the material in this textbook. The end result of their efforts, as in any peer review process, is a stronger presentation of information for the readership. We are grateful to the reviewers of this publication. Thank you!

Dr. Sally Dampier, RN, BScN, MMedSc, DNP
Professor
School of Health and Community Studies
Confederation College
Thunder Bay, Ontario

Pamela Farthing, RN, BA, MSc, PhD(C)
Research Chair
Diabetes Care Faculty
Saskatchewan Collaborative Bachelor of Science in Nursing
School of Nursing
Saskatchewan Polytechnic
Saskatoon, Saskatchewan
Undergraduate Adjunct Professor
University of Regina
Regina, Saskatchewan

Dr. Tracy Hoot, RN, BScN, MSN, DHEd
Associate Dean
School of Nursing
Thompson Rivers University
Kamloops, British Columbia

Tania Killian, MEd, BEd, BScN, CCN
School of Health Sciences, Nursing
Seneca College
Toronto, Ontario

Francine Laurencelle, RN, MEd, DHA
Senior Instructor
College of Nursing
University of Manitoba
Winnipeg, Manitoba

Bhavik Patel, RN, BScN
Professor
Practical Nursing
Loyalist College
Belleville, Ontario

Jennifer Siemens, BScN, MScN
Nurse Educator
College of the Rockies
Cranbrook, British Columbia

Judith T. Strickland, RN, BN, MN, CON (C)
Nurse Educator
Western Regional School of Nursing
Corner Brook, Newfoundland

Karen Tautz, RN, BSN, MN
Nursing Instructor
British Columbia Institute of Technology
Burnaby, British Columbia

Kari Ubels, CD, HBScN, RN
Associate Chair of Practical Nurse Curriculum
NorQuest College
Edmonton, Alberta

Wendy Wheeler, RN, MN
Instructor, Faculty of Nursing
School of Health Sciences
Red Deer College
Red Deer, Alberta

PREFACE TO THE INSTRUCTOR

Effective leadership and management are two important obligations of all professional nurses, and in today's dynamic health care systems they are more important than ever. Along with leadership knowledge and competencies, nurse leaders and managers need opportunities to explore important leadership and management concepts within complex health care systems, challenging contexts and a variety of nursing settings with diverse colleagues and stakeholders.

Nursing scholarship and literature in areas of leadership and management offer a variety of perspectives on optimal leadership and management across diverse health care settings and contexts. Building on this existing expertise in nursing, the second edition of *Yoder-Wise's Leading and Managing in Canadian Nursing* offers students the opportunity to reflect upon learning activities that help them to apply theoretical concepts to "real life" practice scenarios. By engaging in both individual and group reflective exercises and case studies provided in each chapter and by using resources available on Evolve, nursing students can bring important leadership and management concepts to life. In this edition, we have included three new chapters with content and concepts that are highly relevant to the current realities of nursing practice and education in Canada. Chapter 31, entitled *Leading and Managing Your Career* provides nursing students and faculty with a career planning and development model to help them use this text and their nursing education to actively and meaningfully develop the knowledge and competencies to grow as leaders and managers. Also included in this chapter is a link to an online career planning and development program that students can use throughout their nursing education and career. This text also includes a new chapter (Chapter 32, *Nursing Students as Leaders*) written by recent alumni. It provides a student-focused and novel approach to developing as leaders and managers. This chapter explores student leadership within the academic community, engagement in scholarly projects, and participation in professional practice initiatives. The authors present case scenarios of three nursing students who enhanced their leadership capacity within and across years of their academic program. Exercises are provided to help students reflect on their own leadership knowledge and competencies, and how they can enhance and enrich these attributes at each phase of their academic trajectory.

This book reflects our commitment to approaching nursing leadership and management from a perspective that is both student-focused and reflective of the current realities of nursing practice. In this second edition, we have further acknowledged the diversity of settings in which nurses practice and learn, and the diversity of our nursing workforce. As such, the text is an important and timely resource for learners as they focus on the understanding and development of leadership and management across the career continuum. A highlight of the second edition is the inclusion of Chapter 4, *Nursing Leadership in Indigenous Health*. This chapter focuses on nursing leadership when working with Indigenous populations across Canada and is unique in that it speaks to the importance of our experiences, language, and culture as touchstones to uncovering truth and developing nursing leadership styles and approaches when working in diverse First Nations, Inuit, and Métis communities.

DIVERSITY OF PERSPECTIVES

Contributors and authors represent diverse settings, roles, and geographic areas and offer a diversity of perspectives on the critical elements of nursing leadership and management. To help reflect the integration of nursing education and practice, contributors were recruited from both practice and academic settings across Canada and from a variety of points across the nursing career continuum.

This book is written for undergraduate learners in nursing leadership and management courses at all stages of education. Nurses in practice who are considering taking on leadership or management roles, may find this text useful to help reflect upon their own professional experiences to enhance their understanding about nursing leadership and management.

ORGANIZATION

We have organized this text around concepts that are relevant to nurses in today's dynamic health care environments.

First, it is important for learners to situate themselves as developing nurse leaders and managers within their educational programs and professional contexts. To support learners' efforts to do so, the text provides them with a model they can use throughout their professional practice career. In the first section of the book, learners are provided with an in-depth introduction to key concepts as they relate to nursing leadership and management. But nurses do not engage in leadership and management in a vacuum. Across a multitude of health care settings, nurses are faced with ethical, legal, sociopolitical and other contexts of practice. Nurse leaders and managers are also faced with diverse approaches and sets of values within the context of leading teams and across all collegial and professional interactions. The first section of the text (*Core Concepts*) aims to explore many of these important and diverse contexts and provide an opportunity for learners to develop a strong foundational knowledge of important leadership concepts. In the second section of the text (*Managing Resources*), we delve into everyday types of challenges that nurse leaders and managers face—the allocation of resources and setting of priorities, care delivery and planning and the integration of communication technology into nursing practice and management. For this edition, we have moved two key chapters to the Evolve website (Chapter 16, *Staffing and Scheduling* and Chapter 17, *Selecting, Developing, and Evaluating*) for easy access for both students and educators.

The third section of the text (*Changing the Status Quo*) allows learners to move beyond key foundational and contextual considerations to examine the realities in which they engage in nursing leadership and management. Learners are provided with discussions of how to question, inquire, and plan as well as for ways to advocate and to challenge the status quo—always within a nursing leadership and management context. Working in teams, advocating, building strategy, and leading through changes are each explored as ways to build capacity and advocate as nurse leaders and managers. The last section (*Interpersonal and Personal Skills*) focuses on the interpersonal relationships that are a key part of nursing professional practice and how, within the context of these relationships, we provide leadership and manage both people and complex situations. Leading and managing through conflict and through challenges and problems are common experiences for nurses at every stage of their careers. Understanding roles and obligations and enhancing our problem-solving and conflict-resolution skills are parts of building capacity and developing leadership skills and competencies.

In this book, no one chapter stands alone. Because none of these foci exist in isolation from one another, key concepts and themes are integrated throughout the chapters to allow the learner to understand the dynamic interplay of leadership and management. We have also made an effort to express a variety of different perspectives on many topics, as is reflected in the profession and in the diverse professional contexts in which nurses practice.

DESIGN

The functional full-colour design is used to emphasize and identify the text's teaching and learning strategies. Full-colour photographs add visual interest and also provide visual reinforcement of concepts. Figures elucidate and depict concepts and activities that are described in the text.

TEACHING AND LEARNING STRATEGIES

Diverse teaching and learning strategies are featured in this text to both stimulate learners' interest and active engagement with the material and the concepts. Current nursing scholarship and research is integrated throughout every chapter to ensure that learners are introduced to and can apply key concepts using an evidence-informed approach.

CHAPTER OPENER ELEMENTS

- The introductory paragraph briefly describes the purpose and scope of the chapter.
- *Objectives* articulate the chapter's learning goals, typically at the application level or higher.
- *A Challenge* presents a complex nursing practice scenario, related to the chapter's focus.

ELEMENTS WITHIN THE CHAPTERS

Glossary Terms appear in colour type in each chapter. Definitions appear in the Glossary at the end of the text.

Exercises stimulate learners to think critically about how to apply concepts to nursing practice. They help to reinforce key leadership and management concepts and competencies. Exercises are highlighted within a full-colour box and are numbered sequentially within each chapter.

Research Perspectives and *Literature Perspectives* illustrate the relevance and applicability of current nursing scholarship to practice.

Theory Boxes provide a brief description of relevant theory and key concepts.

Numbered boxes contain lists, tools such as forms and work sheets, and other information relevant to chapter content that learners will find useful and interesting.

END-OF-CHAPTER ELEMENTS

A Solution provides a perspective on and a response to the situation presented at the beginning of the chapter in *A Challenge*.

The Evidence describes scholarship of relevance to the topic.

Need to Know Now summarizes critical key points for both nursing students and new graduates as they transition into the profession.

Chapter Checklists summarize key concepts from the chapter.

Tips offer practical guidelines for learners to follow in applying concepts presented in each chapter.

The *Glossary*, found at the end of the text, is a comprehensive list of definitions of all boldfaced terms used in the chapters.

COMPLETE TEACHING AND LEARNING PACKAGE

In addition to the text *Yoder-Wise's Leading and Managing in Canadian Nursing,* Instructor Resources are provided online through *Evolve* (http://evolve.elsevier.com/Canada/Yoder-Wise/leading/). These resources are designed to help instructors present the material in this text. They include the following assets:

- **PowerPoint Slides** for each chapter with lecture notes where applicable (over 600 slides total)
- **ExamView Test Bank** with over 750 multiple-choice questions. Rationales are based on NCLEX Competencies. Answers are also provided.
- **TEACH RN and TEACH PN** are instructor manuals for registered nursing and practical nursing students.
  - Chapter Objectives
    Nursing Curriculum Standards
  - Key Terms
  - Teaching Suggestions with Learning Activities
  - Skills Checklist
- **Application Activities and Answers** for each chapter
- **Case Studies** for each chapter
- **Questions to Consider** for each chapter
- **Exercise Answers** for each chapter
- **Image Collection** (over 50 images)

Student Resources can also be found online through *Evolve* (http://evolve.elsevier.com/Canada/Yoder-Wise/leading/). These resources provide students with additional tools for learning and include the following assets:

- **Sample Cover Letters and Resumés**
- **Suggested Readings and Internet Resources**

LEARNER'S GUIDE

As a professional nurse in today's changing health care system, you will need strong leadership and management skills more than ever, regardless of your specific role. You will also need to be an independent, dependable follower. The second edition of *Yoder-Wise's Leading and Managing in Canadian Nursing* not only provides the conceptual knowledge you will need but also offers practical strategies to help you hone the various skills so vital to your success as a leader and manager.

Because repetition is a key strategy in learning and retaining new information, you will find many topics discussed in more than one chapter. In addition, as in the real world of nursing, you will often find several different views expressed on a single topic. This repetition reinforces ideas and illustrates how one concept has multiple applications. Rather than referring you to another portion of the text, the key information is provided within the specific chapter, but perhaps in less depth. Because leading and managing are skills that require specific situation considerations, you can see why such a diversity of views exists.

To help you make the most of your learning experience, try the following strategy. Read the opening paragraph of each chapter. This preview should create a context for your reading. The *Objectives* suggest what your accomplishments should be by the time you conclude the chapter. Look at the end of the chapter for the checklist of the key points. *A Challenge* allows you to "hear" a real-life situation and always asks what you think you would do if you were the nurse (*A Solution*, at the end of the chapter, examines what the nurse did in the situation and asks you to think about how that fits for you and why). The introduction and subsequent content, like any text, provide critical information. For some learners, it is useful to skim those headings and the box content to gain an overall sense of the concepts inherent in the chapter. For others, reading and reflecting from the beginning of the chapter to the end might be useful. The material in boxes (boxes, tables, *Research Perspectives*, *Literature Perspectives*, and *Theory Boxes*)

is designed to augment understanding of the content in the text narrative. *The Evidence* at the end of the chapters highlights what we know in at least one case about the topic. The checklist at the end of each chapter highlights the key points the chapter presented, and tips illustrate ways to apply the content just studied. After you complete each chapter, stop and think about what the chapter conveyed. What does it mean for you as a leader, follower, and manager? How do the chapter's content and your interaction with it relate to the other chapters you have already completed? How might you briefly synthesize the content for a nonnurse friend? Reading the chapter, restating its key points in your own words, and completing the text exercises and online activities will go far to help you make the content truly your own.

We think you will find leading and managing to be an exciting, challenging field of study, and we have made every attempt to reflect that belief in the design and approach of this edition.

LEARNING AIDS

Yoder-Wise's Leading and Managing in Canadian Nursing incorporates important tools to help you learn about leading and managing and apply your new knowledge to the real world. The next few pages graphically point out how to use these study aids to your best advantage.

The vivid full-colour chapter opener *photographs* and other photographs throughout the text help convey each chapter's key message while providing a glimpse into the real world of leading and managing in nursing.

The *introductory paragraph* tells you what you can expect to find in the chapter. To help set the stage for your study of the chapter, read it first and then summarize in your own words what you expect to gain from the chapter.

The list of *Objectives* helps you focus on the key information you should be able to apply after having studied the chapter.

In *A Challenge*, practising nurse leaders or managers offer their real-world views of a concern related to the chapter. Has a nurse you know had similar or dissimilar challenges?

A CHALLENGE

After Terry graduated from her nursing program, she was hired for a full-time position on a medical-surgical unit. Terry had completed the final clinical practicum on this unit, and the management there felt it was important to start Terry's career on a unit where she knew about the patients and the unit policies and procedures. In her interview, Terry liked the nurse manager; she also liked the nurse preceptor who worked with her during her practicum. Terry, however, focused on her clinical skills during her practicum, and she did not do a thorough evaluation of the presence (or absence) of important leadership and followership behaviours. Was the clinical nurse leader available and supportive? Were the nurses and leader positive and supportive of each other? In addition, Terry did not inquire about transition-to-practice opportunities at this hospital or the possibility of having a nurse act as a preceptor and/or mentor to her during her transition period.

Unfortunately, Terry received a very short orientation and little mentorship support from the staff. Although the clinical nurse leader and staff were welcoming on her first day on the unit, they were busy with their own work, and Terry realized that as a staff person, it was "business as usual." She particularly had trouble keeping up with the workload, and no one was available to answer her questions. The nurse leader, in particular, was seldom available because of her own responsibilities. Terry began to develop different perceptions of her workplace. She began to wonder if this was the right start to her nursing career.

During her clinical practicum, Terry had an opportunity to observe interactions between the clinical nurse leader and staff. What positive leader and follower behaviours should Terry have watched for? During her interview with the manager, what questions could Terry have asked to gain an understanding of leadership within the context of the unit?

Most chapters contain a *Theory Box* to highlight and summarize pertinent theoretical concepts.

THEORY BOX
Kramer's Reality Shock/Duchscher's Transition Shock

Theory/Contributor	Key Ideas	Application to Practice
Kramer (1974) is credited with establishing the knowledge behind "reality shock" in her seminal publication "*Reality Shock: Why Nurses Leave Nursing*". *Reality shock* was coined as the alarming experience of new nursing graduates leaving the safety of a known and relatively protected context (nursing education) and entering the unknown realm of accountable, professional nursing practice. Duchscher (2008, 2009) followed Kramer's work some 4 decades later with a robust theoretical construct that built on Kramer's work, outlining the *Stages of Transition* (Table 29.1) for the newly graduated nurse, along with an experience she coined "*Transition Shock*" (Fig. 29.1), representing the intensity, depth and breadth of the initial interface between the new practitioner with their professional practice context.	Role change precedes role stress, which can be a precursor to role strain. Role stress is associated with low productivity and performance. Role stress and role strain can lead a person to withdraw psychologically from the role. Knowledge of the impending role change, its ramifications and implications, along with clear, realistic role expectations can decrease the role stress (and even prevent role strain, which speaks to stress over time) for someone in a new role (e.g., a new nurse graduate, a nurse moving from direct care to an educator or manager role).	Knowledge of the Stages of Transition and Transition Shock during the preparatory (undergraduate education or BEFORE the role change), accompanied by clear and realistic expectations of the change, significantly reduce stress, avoid strain and increase both productivity and role fulfillment.

Every chapter contains numbered *Exercises* that challenge you to think critically about concepts in the text and apply them to real-life situations.

EXERCISE 3.2 In your current area of work, speak to a nurse manager and staff nurse and identify the type of health care informatics being used. How is the data being collected? How is the data being used within the clinical area? Brainstorm how data might be used more effectively to improve person-centred care.

Key terms appear in boldface type throughout the chapter. (A list of all key terms used in the chapter appears at the start of the chapter and the *Glossary* at the end of the text contains a list of their definitions.)

The *boxes* in every chapter highlight key information, such as lists, and contain forms, work sheets, and self-assessments to help reinforce chapter content.

BOX 13.2 Potential Benefits of Open Notes in Patient Portals

1 Demonstrating respect and reducing stigma
2 Empowering patients
3 Organizing care and tracking progress
4 Providing a tool for behaviour change
5 Enhancing trust and the therapeutic relationship
6 Make care safer
5 Potential for reducing workload

The *tables* that appear throughout the text provide convenient capsules of information for your reference.

TABLE 4.1 Respectful Practice

R Reflect deeply on your own cultural values and beliefs.
E Examine and question assumptions and biases in practice.
S Share and recognize ethical space of nurse-patient relationship.
P Participate and celebrate cultural uniqueness.
E Engage in relationship building.
C Create open and trusting environments.
T Treat people with dignity and compassion.

Most chapters contain at least one *Research Perspective* or *Literature Perspective* box. These boxes summarize articles of interest and point out their relevance and applicability to practice. Check the journal that the article came from to find a list of indexing terms to help you locate additional and even more recent articles on the same topic.

RESEARCH PERSPECTIVE

Resource: Doey, T., Hines, P., Myslik, B., et al. (2008). Creating primary care access for mental health care clients in a community mental health setting. *Canadian Journal of Community Mental Health*, 27(2): 129–138.

The authors described how a strategic planning exercise conducted by the Canadian Mental Health Association was used as a point of advocacy to address the unique primary care needs of people with mental illness in Windsor-Essex County in Ontario. A Primary Care Working Group was established to explore options to provide mental health care within a primary care model. The working group reports on the process that led to the establishment of City Centre Health Centre,

an interdisciplinary mental and primary care facility, and the patient-focused evaluation of the services provided.

In 2018, 10 years after publishing this research paper, the City Centre Health Centre continues to provide services in the community. They have updated their Strategic Plan—Vision 2020—as a means of planning future directions and ensuring they meet their mandate. See https://windsor-essex.cmha.ca/about-cmha/strategic-plan.

Implications for Practice
Strategic planning processes can be used to identify gaps in service delivery and to advocate for patient-focused strategies.

The numerous full-colour *illustrations* visually reinforce key concepts.

LITERATURE PERSPECTIVE

Resource: Bishop, A., & Macdonald, M. (2017). Patient involvement in patient safety: A qualitative study of nursing staff and patient perceptions. *Journal of Patient Safety*, 13(2), 82–87.

How can health care organizations improve their culture of patient safety? The authors conducted focus groups with nursing staff and patients in two hospitals in Eastern Canada to understand perceptions of safety. Their analysis identified four themes:
1. Wanting control: Both patients and nurses described patients as knowing enough about their health care.
2. Feeling connected: Both patients and nurses need to connect with one another. This occurs through respect and sharing information.

3. Encountering roadblock: Patients perceived that nursing staff were too busy to answer questions or spend time with them while nurses reported that their workload prevented them from interacting with patients in a meaningful way.
4. Sharing responsibility for safety: Both patients and nurses identified their roles in improving safety. For patients, these roles included asking questions and advocating for their well-being. Nurses considered their role in improving safety as engaging in teamwork and improving communication.

Implications for Practice
Nurses can contribute to patient safety by sharing information, showing respect, and involving patients in their care.

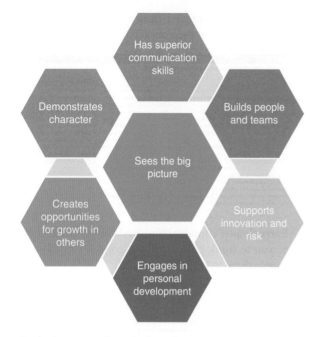

The *Chapter Checklist* provides a quick summary of key points in the chapter. To help you keep in mind the broad themes of the chapter, read it immediately *before* you start reading the chapter. Reading it afterward reinforces the key points.

CHAPTER CHECKLIST

The role of the nurse manager is multi-faceted and complex. Integrating clinical concerns with management functions, synthesizing leadership abilities with management requirements, and addressing human concerns while maintaining efficiency, are the challenges facing the nurse manager. Thus, the nurse manager's role is to ensure effective operation of a defined area, contribute to the overall mission of the organization, and create an environment that supports quality of care for persons and their families.

The basic functions of a manager are as follows:
• Establishes and communicates goals and objectives.

• Organizes, analyzes, and divides work into tasks.
• Motivates and communicates.
• Analyzes, appraises, and interprets performance and measurements.
• Develops people, including self.

A nurse manager is responsible for the following:
• Relationships with those above themselves, peers, and staff for whom they are accountable.
• Professionalism.
• Management of resources.
• Application of evidence-informed decision-making.
• Role-modelling.

The *Tips* offer guidelines to follow for each chapter before applying the information presented in the chapter.

TIPS FOR IMPLEMENTING THE ROLE OF NURSE MANAGER

Aspects of the role of the nurse manager include being a leader as well as a follower. To be effective in the role, the nurse manager must be dedicated to the following:
• A management philosophy that values people.

• A commitment to person-focused quality of care outcomes that include evidence-informed processes and health outcomes of the client.
• The desire for ongoing learning about health care change and its effect on the nurse manager's role and functions.

The *Glossary* at the end of the text lists in alphabetical order all the terms that are boldfaced blue in the text.

GLOSSARY

A
absenteeism The rate at which an individual misses work on an unplanned basis. (Ch. 25)
academic community The body of people who compose the community at your university or school, including students, faculty, and supporting staff. (Ch. 32)

availability bias The tendency for people to base their judgement on a preceding and memorable event that is readily recalled rather than complete information on the present situation. (Ch. 8)
average daily census (ADC) Average number of patients cared for per day in the unit for the reporting period. (Ch. 16)

bureaucracy Characterized by formality, low autonomy, a hierarchy of authority, an environment of rules, division of labour, specialization, centralization, and control. (Ch. 10)
burnout A prolonged response to chronic emotional and interpersonal stressors on the job. (Ch. 29)

Each chapter ends with these features:

A Solution provides an effective method to handle the situation presented in *A Challenge*.

A SOLUTION

In Canada, the US, and many other countries, having a mix of different staff is a reality. Care and due process in introducing these changes can help make the transition easier. Supporting nursing care that is patient focused and patient centred helps ensure that staffing conflicts and tensions do not adversely affect the care the public receives. Patient-centred care helps direct staff energy in productive ways, and patient-centred care, combined with appreciative inquiry, helps shift the focus on abilities and away from deficits. This situation clearly requires manager involvement. Team building is required. Asking staff to express their concerns using reference to *the pa-* *tient* rather than *I* is one means of shifting the focus. Asking individuals to "walk in another's shoes" and consider what it is like to be the other health care provider and to identify what skills and abilities the other person brings to the unit is another technique. Jack and his staff should look for ways to modify the culture of care in the medical unit to foster patient centredness, collaborative practice, and a culture of safety.

What other techniques might you suggest for improving patient focus and a culture of care in this work environment? What is the role and responsibility of student nurses in contributing to improving patient-focused care?

Each of these sections is designed to help learners transfer the words of the text into a personal understanding about what leading, managing, and following mean. Achieving success in those roles helps nurses be effective team members and contribute to positive patient care outcomes.

The Evidence identifies and discusses evidence-based research or best practices related to material in the chapter.

THE EVIDENCE

Nurses have an integral role in promoting patient safety. In 2007, the symposium 'Advancing Nursing Leadership for a Safer Healthcare System' was held in Toronto. Jeffs et al. (2009) summarized the themes emerging from the research presented at this symposium. They identified four future directions for nursing, including focusing on the patient in patient safety, broadening the knowledge base on patient safety beyond acute care, linking healthy work environments and a culture of patient safety, and bridging evidence-informed research and practice. Nurses continue to lead the way for patient safety in direct care, education, research, and leadership.

Need to Know Now is designed to summarize what the authors think is expected of most new graduates in their first professional positions.

CONTENTS

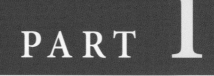

PART 1

Core Concepts

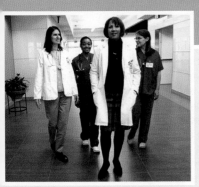

Leading, Managing, and Following

Maura MacPhee

Leading, managing, and following are integral to professional nursing practice. By engaging in constructive behaviours associated with these concepts, nurses can positively influence patient care and organizational outcomes, regardless of their position title. By understanding the competencies related to leading, managing, and following, the professional nurse can positively influence the quality of health care delivery.

OBJECTIVES

- Link leadership, management, and followership to key theories from a variety of disciplines, including psychology, sociology, management science, and organizational development.
- Identify key competencies associated with effective leadership, management, and followership.
- Examine practical applications associated with leadership, management, and followership.
- Relate personal attributes, such as emotional intelligence and appreciative inquiry, to the capacity of professional nurses to lead, manage, and follow.
- Recognize the challenges associated with leading, managing, and following in complex health care environments.

TERMS TO KNOW

appreciative inquiry (AI)
authentic leadership
Canada Health Act
complexity science
emotional intelligence (EI)

followership
leadership
management
mindfulness
resilience

social determinants of health
strengths-based leadership
transactional leadership
transformational leadership

❓ A CHALLENGE

After Terry graduated from her nursing program, she was hired for a full-time position on a medical-surgical unit. Terry had completed the final clinical practicum on this unit, and the management there felt it was important to start Terry's career on a unit where she knew about the patients and the unit policies and procedures. In her interview, Terry liked the nurse manager; she also liked the nurse preceptor who worked with them during her practicum. Terry, however, focused on her clinical skills during her practicum, and she did not do a thorough evaluation of the presence (or absence) of important leadership and followership behaviours. Was the clinical nurse leader available and supportive? Were the nurses and leader positive and supportive of each other? In addition, Terry did not inquire about transition-to-practice opportunities at this hospital or the possibility of having a nurse act as a preceptor and/or mentor to her during her transition period.

Unfortunately, Terry received a very short orientation and little mentorship support from the staff. Although the clinical nurse leader and staff were welcoming on her first day on the unit, they were busy with their own work, and Terry realized that as a staff person, it was "business as usual." She particularly had trouble keeping up with the workload, and no one was available to answer her questions. The nurse leader, in particular, was seldom available because of her own responsibilities. Terry began to develop different perceptions of her workplace. She began to wonder if this was the right start to her nursing career.

During her clinical practicum, Terry had an opportunity to observe interactions between the clinical nurse leader and staff. What positive leader and follower behaviours should Terry have watched for? During her interview with the manager, what questions could Terry have asked to gain an understanding of leadership within the context of the unit?

INTRODUCTION

The Canadian Health Care System

The Canadian health care system is a publicly funded system known as Medicare. Each province and territory has a medical services plan (MSP) that ensures that all Canadian residents have reasonable access to primary health care in the community and medically necessary hospital care. The provincial and territorial governments oversee the delivery of health care services for their residents, and the federal government provides funding for health services and sets national standards for the delivery of these services. The Canada Health Act, passed by Parliament in 1984, sets out five criteria or standards of health services delivery: public administration, comprehensiveness, universality, portability, and accessibility. Canadians are proud of their public Medicare system; in fact, the values underlying our single-payer health care system have become a symbol of our society's strong belief in universal access for all—regardless of ability to pay (Government of Canada, Canada's Health Care System website, 2017). According to the Government of Canada website, primary health care services should be every Canadian resident's first point of contact with our publicly funded health care system. Primary health care providers also coordinate patients' health services from diagnosis to recovery and access to specialized services and hospitalization. Chapter 7 provides more background on the basic framework of publicly funded health care services.

> **EXERCISE 1.1** Explore the Government of Canada website: *Canada's Health Care System* at https://www.canada.ca/en/health-canada/services/canada-health-care-system.html
> 1. Provide a brief description of each of the five criteria in the Canada Health Act that must be met by provinces and territories to receive funding for health services delivery from the federal government.
> 2. What other health-related functions are carried out by the federal government?

Another important aspect of Canada's approach to health care is our recognition that social determinants of health (such as education, justice, housing, and transit) influence quality of life. Canadians' desire to support social services, such as public housing, is perhaps a barometer of how we define quality of life. Lack of food and housing, for instance, is strongly associated with health inequalities. Health is also influenced by social exclusion, a form of alienation experienced by particular groups (such as Indigenous peoples). Nurses play an important role in helping people, particularly members of socially excluded groups, access the social determinants of health. Through advocacy, policy analysis, and political activities, all Canadian nurses can make a positive difference in the health of Canadians (Falk-Rafael & Becker, 2012). Refer to Chapter 21 for further discussion of nursing advocacy.

The Government of Canada hosts a website entitled: *What Makes Canadians Healthy or Unhealthy?* On this website, each of the social determinants of health is described, and evidence is provided that links each key determinant to the health and well-being of Canadians.

EXERCISE 1.2 Go to the Government of Canada website *What Makes Canadians Healthy or Unhealthy?* Read through Jason's story. This story illustrates how superficially, we see that Jason is in the hospital because of a leg infection. But, as we delve deeper, we appreciate the influence of the social determinants of health.

1. What underlying determinants of health have influenced Jason's need for hospitalization?
2. Provide a brief description, based on the evidence, of links between two determinants of health (education and literacy and employment/working conditions) and health outcomes.
3. Direct care nurses are informal leaders. As informal leaders, what can direct care nurses do to advocate for Jason and his family?

The Organization for Economic Cooperation and Development (OECD) maintains a health database of health and health systems statistics across more than 35 member countries, including Canada. As we become more globalized, it's important to know how we are doing in Canada. The OECD website, *Health at a Glance 2017: OECD Indicators for Canada,* provides an overview of Canada's global rankings with respect to quality of life, health care delivery and health spending. The good news is that Canadians' access to care and our quality of life are above the OECD average, and our health spending is not much higher than the OECD average. Where are we failing? Our obesity rates are above the OECD average, and our health care system needs to make improvements with respect to unnecessary tests and treatments performed each year. As informal nurse leaders, direct care nurses need to know where our health care system is failing, and we need to know how to advocate for practices and policies that support healthy living. We can also play a role in efficaciously managing scarce health resources. Part 1 of this book introduces core concepts related to nursing and our health care system; Part 2 introduces you to the tools you'll need to manage health care resources responsibly; Part 3 delves further into strategic change and advocacy; and Part 4 is an invitation to personally and professionally

contribute to a healthy lifestyle for yourself and for the health and well-being of others in our Canadian society and globally.

EXERCISE 1.3 Read through the "Health at a Glance 2017: OECD Indicators for Canada."

1. Under "selected policy issues," what are some health services delivery practices and policies in place that have controlled health care spending?
2. Why does Canada have high cancer survival rates?
3. What are some policies under consideration to curb obesity in Canada? They already exist in other countries, such as Finland and Mexico.
4. As informal nurse leaders, how can direct care nurses use best evidence to address Canada's obesity problem?

Nursing in Canada

After a brief exploration of our Canadian health care system and how Canada ranks globally with respect to population health indicators, let's look more closely at our nurse profession in Canada. Nursing constitutes the backbone of the health care system, both in numbers and in its span of influence across the clinical spectrum. Nurses bear the responsibility of providing safe, quality care to patients in acute care settings; clients in community settings; and residents in long-term care settings. Nurses are also at the forefront of health systems transformation and innovation—engaging with other health care professionals and the public to support healthier communities. The Canadian Nurses Association published a report in 2012 entitled: *A Nursing Call to Action: The health of our nation, the future of our health care system.* This report was prepared by an independent, expert commission of nurses, other health care professionals and decision makers. Here is an excerpt from the report's preface: "Through their sheer numbers and collective knowledge, nurses are a mighty force for change. Canadians expect nurses to harness that power and act. We present this report to bolster their actions going forward and to support nurses so they are equipped to do their part in shaping Canada's health-care delivery system in the decade ahead." Revisit this report and its recommendations for nurse leadership and health systems transformation when you study Part 3 of this textbook: Changing the Status Quo. As one example, our population is aging, and many seniors occupy acute care beds. Senior care is more effective and less costly when nurses provide home care services in communities where seniors live. Nurse-delivered hospice services also promise to shift end-of-life care away from hospitals to homes. How will nurses lead the shift in care from institutions to community and home?

Nurses as Leaders, Managers, and Followers

Advocating and leading change requires strengths-based leadership (Gottlieb et al., 2012). The strengths-based movement and the field of positive psychology are relatively new, beginning when researchers discovered that effective leaders build on their own and others' strengths (Donaldson et al., 2015). Strengths-based approaches have better outcomes than approaches that focus on people's deficits (Wong & Laschinger, 2013). Negative criticism, for instance, makes us fearful and anxious and shuts down our capacity to think creatively. Reflect on how you feel when you receive positive feedback versus negative criticism. What energizes you the most?

Strengths-based nurse leaders are essential change agents, but in today's complex health care environments, nurses also need to know how to be strengths-based managers and followers.

What does strengths-based nursing look like? A central tenet of twenty-first-century nursing is that nurses must apply critical thinking to critical actions in complex health care settings to achieve positive patient and organizational outcomes. The core work of nurses is making decisions and taking corresponding actions on behalf of their patients. This core work demands that nurses be strengths-based leaders, managers, and followers at the point-of-care, unit, institutional, and even societal levels (Gottlieb et al., 2012).

Too often, nurses new to the profession believe their ability to perform clinical procedures is what makes them appear professional to those receiving care, to their peers, or to the public. They might also believe that leadership is only for those holding formal management positions or that following means blindly adhering to the direction of others. New nurses may fail to realize that their professional nursing image and success depend equally on their independent decision making as well as their ability to engage and collaborate with others. These professional behaviours, evidence of strengths-based nursing, are the first lens through which patients, families, supervisors, and other health care providers gain confidence in our nursing abilities.

The way nurses lead, manage, and follow has changed over time. Formerly, nurses took direction unquestioningly from physicians or senior nurses (such as "head" or "charge" nurses). Today, the expectation has shifted from nurses being told what to do to a model of autonomous practice and shared decision making and action in collaboration with others. The complexity of health care delivery has grown beyond what a command-and-control model can accommodate in traditional hierarchical organizations. Moreover, patient acuity requires immediate and autonomous, self-directed responses that are often different from responses that can be preassigned. Twenty-first-century nurses must know how to make independent decisions and how to work collaboratively in teams comprised of nurses (i.e., intraprofessional) and with other health care providers (i.e., interprofessional). Direct care nurses therefore have much more control over practice. Instead of micromanaging what nurses do with their patients, nurse leaders and managers have other accountabilities that we will discuss later in this chapter and in Chapters 2 and 3. In this twenty-first century, we also have greater access to technology. Technology provides nurses with more information and tools for making critical decisions, and technology enables us to reach beyond the confines of our physical settings to connect with nurses and other health care professionals globally. Access to information and communications technologies is one means for nurses to create a common voice and engage in collective action related to their areas of interest, such as oncology nurses or maternity nurses. The field of informatics is also becoming a new career avenue for nurses (see Chapter 13).

The study of leadership, management, and followership behaviours has never been more important to the nursing profession and the public during this time of ongoing health care reforms, including the introduction of new technologies. Each nurse, from direct care nurses to leaders and managers with formal positions, is accountable for making the best use of scarce nursing resources, including each other's knowledge and expertise. Professional nurses are expected to meet their organization's mission and goals, efficiently manage limited health care resources, avoid making mistakes (e.g., medication errors), achieve patient satisfaction, and ensure positive patient outcomes. In addition, organizations expect nurses to contain costs when delivering patient care, contribute to quality improvement and change initiatives, and interact with other health care team members to resolve clinical and organizational problems. These expectations mean that each nurse must engage in strengths-based leading, managing, and following.

- This chapter presents various perspectives on the concepts of leading (leadership), managing (management), and following (followership). These concepts are integrated, which means that nurses lead, manage, and follow concurrently. Leading, managing, and following are not activities that are bound to certain types of nursing roles only—all nurses lead, manage, and follow. Before we examine each concept more closely to highlight their differences, we begin with the operational definitions for leadership, management, and followership.

- **Leadership** is the process of engaging and influencing others (Yukl, 2006). Strengths-based leaders are associated with words such as visionary, energetic, inspirational, and innovative: they go beyond the status quo to make a difference for others. Any nurse can be a nurse leader, no matter the personality type, gender, ethnicity, or age.

- **Management** is about getting the job done and ensuring that people have the necessary resources to get the job done (Yukl, 2006). Effective managers are able to set goals and objectives and ensure that they are met within established timelines and budgets. Management is traditionally associated with formal authority positions within organizations, and key management competencies, such as deciding how to allocate scarce resources, is important for all levels of nursing.

- **Followership** involves engaging with others who are leading or managing by contributing to the work that needs to be done (Yukl, 2006). Followers can promote team effectiveness, for instance, by maintaining collaborative work relationships, offering constructive criticism, and sharing leadership and management responsibilities. Effective followers know how to manage themselves (self-management), and they work well with others, particularly in today's complex health care environments where the emphasis is on interdisciplinary teamwork. According to Yukl (2006), important followership guidelines include the following: "Find out what you are expected to do; take the initiative to deal with problems; show appreciation and provide recognition when appropriate; and challenge flawed plans and proposals" (p. 138).

The collective behaviours that reflect strengths-based leading, managing, and following enhance one another. All health care providers, including nurses, experience situations each day in which they must lead, manage, and follow. Some formal nursing positions, such as nurse managers and directors, require an advanced set of leading and managing know-how to establish organizational goals and objectives, oversee human resources, provide staff with performance feedback, facilitate change, and manage conflict to meet patient-care and organizational requirements. Other nursing positions, such as direct care nurses and front-line or clinical nurse leaders, must shift between leading, managing, and following, sometimes on a moment-by-moment basis. For instance, clinical nurse leaders lead, manage, and follow in daily clinical practice through assignment making, patient and family problem solving, discharge planning, patient education, and coaching and mentoring staff. Having a positive and open approach is what strengths-based nursing is all about.

PERSONAL ATTRIBUTES AND BEHAVIOURS NEEDED TO LEAD, MANAGE, AND FOLLOW

Strengths-based leadership, management, and followership are associated with certain key personal attributes and behaviours, such as a sense of ethical responsibility and the capacity to role model and reinforce ethical, professional behaviour. A Canadian code of ethics document for registered nurses (CNA, 2017) articulates nursing values and the ethical responsibilities that apply to nurse interactions with patients and their families, the public, and other health care providers. *Ethical individuals* are not coercive or manipulative, and they collaborate with others. Nurses need to value fundamental ethical principles, such as beneficence, autonomy, truthfulness, confidentiality, justice, and integrity. The 2017 edition of the Canadian Nurses Association code of ethics covers contemporary topics such as medical assistance in dying, bullying in the workplace, and nurse advocacy. An important ethical attribute is how the nurse is in a relationship with the patient. Although members of health care organizations must always consider clinical and organizational goals and priorities, the underlying philosophy associated with excellent health care delivery is patient-centred/focused or person-centred/focused care (Feo et al., 2016). This type of care includes patients and their family members in the design and delivery of their health care. Ethical leadership is based on a willingness to identify and act on complex problems in an ethical manner (Storch et al., 2013). Leadership can be misused when coercive relationships form and information and true goals are withheld. See Chapter 5 for a discussion of patient-focused-centred/person-focused/centred) care and Chapter 6 for an in-depth discussion on ethics.

Emotional intelligence (EI) is a key attribute closely aligned with individuals' capacity to know themselves and others. Emotionally intelligent individuals are aware of their own emotions and can regulate and control their emotions, particularly in response to stressful or challenging situations. Individuals with EI are also aware of others' emotions and can assist others with understanding and controlling their emotions (Walton, 2012). Nursing is considered a stressful profession because of nurses' regular exposure to emotionally charged situations where they are expected to respond to the emotional needs of their patients and families (Gorgens-Ekermans & Brand, 2012). Some evidence suggests that EI can be a buffer against stressful workplace demands and mitigate workplace bullying (Bennett & Sawatsky, 2013). High levels of EI as associated with more effective nurse leadership, because EI leaders are able to build positive and constructive relationships with their staff (Tyczkowski et al., 2015). One Canadian study, however, demonstrated that even high-EI leaders cannot offset detrimental effects from challenging work conditions when they have too great a span of control. Span of control refers to the number of staff that directly reports to a leader. A large span of control impairs a leader's capacity to form close working relationships with staff (Lucas et al., 2008).

In two studies in the United States, nursing students with higher EI scores had better communications and interpersonal skills than students with lower EI scores on a validated emotional quotient (EQ) questionnaire. Students with higher EI scores also reported greater well-being and enhanced perceptions of competency (Beauvais et al., 2011; Por et al., 2011). Given positive outcomes associated with EI and nursing students, many nurse educators believe that nursing students should receive EI training during their education programs (Orak et al., 2016).

Another key attribute for effective leadership, management and followership is **appreciative inquiry (AI)**, which is associated with how we question and problem solve. Appreciative inquiry is a strengths-based strategy from positive psychology (Lewis, 2011). AI is used at all levels (e.g., individual, group, and organizational) to engage people in identifying and accentuating positives within a context, such as a practice environment. Specifically, instead of focusing on the negative (i.e., seeing the glass as half empty), AI emphasizes the positive (i.e., seeing the glass as half full) (Watkins et al., 2016). Australian neonatal nurses and parents used an AI approach to collaboratively develop family-centred care approaches for one neonatal intensive care unit (Trajkovski et al., 2013). In an earlier US study, AI was used to improve the patient hand-off process (Shendell-Falik et al., 2007). Hand-offs occur between nurses when patients are transferred from one practice setting to another. Communication breakdowns during transfer reports or hand-offs have been associated with adverse events. In this US nursing study, the researchers transformed the hand-off process using five steps in one version of AI known as the 5-D cycle: (1) definition, (2) discovery, (3) dream, (4) design, and (5) destiny. The AI cycle engaged direct care nurses in finding the best possible approach to hand-offs. "Using a strengths-based improvement process enabled nursing leaders to leverage the staff's ideas. Patient safety was enhanced and an empowered, exceptional work environment was created" (p. 103).

Resilience is an attribute associated with surviving or thriving in the aftermath of an adverse or tragic event. Resilient individuals are able to bounce back after crisis and adversity (Turner, 2014). Resilience has been linked to other characteristics such as self-efficacy (i.e., the belief you can succeed), optimism, and hope. Two areas of resilience research are physiological and psychological coping and adaptation. Some positive, psychological coping strategies include support seeking, problem solving and work-life balance. Jackson et al., (2007) identified a number of strategies associated with personal resilience-building in nurses: establishing positive professional support networks, maintaining a positive attitude (e.g., using AI strategies to approach problems in the workplace), and using reflection (e.g., journaling). In one literature review of resilience in nurses, contributing factors to workplace adversity for new nurses included feelings of ambiguity and anxiety and dissonance between academic preparation and workplace reality. As stated by the reviewers: "The development of resilient behaviour by nurses in response to an overwhelming workplace has been associated with increased quality of life, better health, and effective use of adaptive coping strategies" (Hart et al., 2014, p. 728).

The latest addition of attributes and behaviours that support effective leadership, management and followership is **mindfulness**. A mindful person has increased awareness of what is happening in the present. Our attention often drifts to past or future events over which we have no current control. Mindfulness buffers against mental drift and it can also guard against knee-jerk reactions. Rather than immediately evaluating and labeling emotions in a situation, the mindful person creates a neutral space for reflection. In a leadership study by Roche and colleagues (2014), mindfulness practice enhanced positive and authentic thinking (see authentic leadership) and dampened negative feelings. The Institute for Healthcare Improvement (IHI) Open School for health care students and faculty recently introduced a mindfulness series for clinical practice that includes several interviews with nurses and other health care professionals, discussing the importance of mindfulness in the workplace (IHI, 2018).

A related concept from positive psychology, reflected best self (RBS), is similar to mindfulness practice. RBS prompts individuals to stop and reflect before responding to a situation. Before you do or say anything, ask yourself: "Are my words and actions going to be the best reflection of my core values and beliefs?" A short reflective pause for deeper processing can result in more genuine, authentic responses to others' words and actions—versus a reactive, potentially damaging response (Roberts et al., 2005).

EXERCISE 1.4

1. Gather together a small group of your student peers, perhaps your clinical group. Sit in a circle facing each other. This arrangement promotes EI (self-awareness, other-awareness), because everyone can make eye contact and read each other's nonverbal cues. If you feel comfortable including clinical faculty members, please invite them to join your circle. Go around the circle in an open and honest fashion. Everybody should have a turn to speak. Appoint a student to record notes on a white board or flip chart. Ask the following AI questions:
   a. What does a supportive clinical learning environment look like to you?
   b. What is working well for us in our clinical learning environments?
   c. What can each of us do better to contribute to an excellent clinical learning environment?
   d. What can we do together to contribute to an excellent clinical learning environment?

Based on the conversation and the circle's answers to the questions, summarize key recommendations to share with your other student peers and School of Nursing faculty members. This exercise can be a stepping stone for making learning improvements that will benefit you, your student peers, and the nursing faculty.

THEORY DEVELOPMENT IN LEADING, MANAGING, AND FOLLOWING

Theories have several important functions for the nursing profession. They propose relationships among concepts that can be scientifically tested. They also serve as analytic tools for understanding, explaining, and predicting phenomena of importance to professional nursing. They can add to our body of professional nursing knowledge and contribute to evidence-informed practices as well (Chinn & Kramer, 2007). Although leadership, management, and followership are intertwined concepts, distinct theories are associated with each of them. Our knowledge of these concepts is continuously evolving as the complexity of health care organizations grows. Many of the theories associated with these concepts originated from other disciplines, such as psychology, sociology, management science, and organizational development. Earlier theory-based research was often classified by its theoretical emphasis on either leader and manager characteristics, follower characteristics, or environmental and situational characteristics. More sophisticated research designs and methods are helping researchers better determine how leadership, management, and followership are connected and how they influence each other. Leadership, management, and followership theories can also be classified based on interactional levels (e.g., dyadic, team, organizational) and power dynamics (e.g., empowerment theories). Chapters 9 and 10 discuss organizational structures within health care settings and team characteristics. Chapter 12 provides an overview of types of power and empowerment strategies of importance to nurses.

Leadership Theories

The Theory Box provides an overview of key leadership theories: from trait theories of the early 1900s to current transformational leadership theories and authentic leadership. Transformational leadership theories and authentic leadership represent a shift in thinking about leadership, management, and followership; from a task focus to a relationship focus (Cummings et al., 2010; Mortier et al., 2016). Health care settings are complex, demanding, and constantly undergoing change to meet population demands. Stressors from work-related demands plague nurses and other health care professionals. Leadership styles can be categorized as either relational or task focused. Both types of leaders need to achieve workplace goals, but their focus is either on the

LITERATURE PERSPECTIVE

Resource: Laschinger H, Wong C, Regan S, Young-Ritchie C, Bushell P. Workplace incivility and new graduate nurses' mental health: the protective role of resiliency. *Journal of Nursing Administration*, 2013; 43(7/8): 415-421.

The purpose of this survey study was to examine relationships between new nurses' mental health, the protective role of resiliency, and workplace incivility. New graduates transition easier to practice within work environments that promote positive workplace relationships. Workplace incivility is a form of negative treatment that includes dismissing someone's ideas; making demeaning, disparaging remarks about someone; or excluding individuals from a social gathering or function. Incivility is typically a subtler, more indirect form of mistreatment than bullying. "Workplace incivility is stressful for nurses and can threaten their mental health" (p. 415). New graduate nurses are particularly susceptible to incivility because they are the newcomers trying to fit in. Individual responses to incivility may depend on personal resiliency and the capacity to develop effective coping mechanisms. As defined in the text, resilience is the capacity to bounce back from adversity. "Resilient individuals tend to develop strong beliefs, perceive life as meaningful, and be flexible in adapting to change" (p. 416). Nurse resiliency has been linked to greater job satisfaction and better job performance. Alternatively, ineffective coping often leads to depression, anxiety, and turnover intentions (i.e., a desire to leave). Previous health services researchers found that frequencies for incivility were highest among coworkers, followed by incivility from physicians, and lastly frequencies of supervisor incivility.

For this study, over 800 new graduate nurses on a nurse registry list in Ontario were sent an e-survey with questions about their mental health, incivility (supervisor, coworker, physician), and resiliency. The study participants were mostly females (88%) with an average age of 27 years and less than one year's work experience. Some 63% of new nurses were working full time on medical-surgical units.

New graduates reported low levels of incivility (<2 on a 5-point scale). Similar to other research findings, the source of most uncivil behaviour was from coworkers (12% daily), followed by physicians (7%), and then supervisors (4.8%). In addition, new graduate nurses had average low levels of negative mental health symptoms (2.48 on a 6-point scale), and they reported average high levels of resiliency (4.4 on a 6-point scale). Using a statistical technique known as multiple regression analysis, the researchers found that the presence of coworker incivility and lack of personal resiliency were predictive of poor mental health. They also found that personal resiliency helps decrease the negative effects of coworker incivility on new nurses' mental health.

Implications for Practice

Although levels of uncivil behaviour were low in new nurses' workplaces, over time, incivility can take a toll. This study and other research found that coworkers were the biggest source of incivility, and new nurses' socialization in the workplace often depends on the presence of welcoming and supportive colleagues. Strengths-based approaches from leaders, managers, and followers include role modeling positive, supportive behaviour and ensuring new graduates feel included and valued in their workplaces. The article mentions civility/incivility training programs that have had positive results.

---

quality of relationships among their followers (relational leadership) or on specific tasks that must be completed (task-focused leadership) (Wong at al., 2013). The full range theory includes transformational, transactional, and laissez faire styles of leadership (Antonakis & House, 2013). Transformational leaders are relationship-focused, and they possess four specific characteristics. Two characteristics, idealized influence and motivational inspiration, are associated with charisma or the capacity to mobilize large groups of followers. These leaders are able to share their vision and ideals in inspirational ways. The other two characteristics, individualized consideration and intellectual stimulation, are more commonly employed by transformational leaders when they are with individuals or small groups of followers. In these instances, they are attentive and respectful listeners, and they engage with their followers to examine problems and find solutions together. Nurse researchers have shown that transformational leaders are trusted and admired, and their followers will go above and beyond typical work expectations. Transformational nurse leaders are associated with greater job satisfaction and autonomy among nurses (Fischer, 2016), and these leaders are also associated with better patient outcomes, including lower morbidity and mortality rates and greater patient satisfaction (Wong et al., 2013). Researchers in the United States found positive associations between nurse leaders with transformational leadership styles and their levels of EI, indicating how emotional self and other awareness and regulation of emotions are important attributes for building and sustaining positive workplace relationships with followers (Spano-Szekely et al., 2016).

Some leadership theorists believe that EI is the foundation for all relationally focused leadership styles, and they describe EI leaders as resonant leaders (Boyatzis & McKee, 2005). In one study with Canadian nurses, resonant leadership was strongly, positively related to nurse reports of workplace empowerment, and this style of leadership was strongly negatively related to workplace incivility. This means that nurse followers felt more empowered by leaders who used resonant styles of interacting with them, and in the presence of these leaders they reported less incivility (Laschinger et al., 2014).

Another leadership style associated with full range theory is transactional leadership.

Research has shown that effective managers have characteristics similar to transactional leaders (also known as *contingent reward leaders*). Although this is a task-oriented leadership style, followers know what is expected of them by their leaders. Followers have clearly defined roles and accountabilities, they receive necessary resources and support to do their work, and they know they will be rewarded for work done. Transactional leaders must be present to recognize if their followers have work-related needs, and to monitor work accomplishments. There are three other leadership styles within full range theory—management by exception active, management by exception passive, and laissez-faire leadership. In all three instances, leaders are not visible or attentive to follower needs, and they typically intervene when a problem has arisen or where failures have occurred. Transactional leadership, in contrast to these nonleadership styles, is a proactive approach to monitoring performance and intervening with resources and supports as needed (Antonakis & House, 2013). Relational and task-oriented nurse leadership styles have been associated with increased patient satisfaction. In complex health care environments, both approaches (e.g., transformational and transactional leadership) may be needed to ensure quality, safe patient care delivery (Wong et al., 2013).

A recent addition to the family of relational leadership styles is authentic leadership (Wong & Laschinger, 2013). Authentic leaders have heightened awareness of themselves in relation to others around them; they have an internalized moral perspective, and they align their words and actions to match their underlying values and beliefs—they are not swayed by external pressures; they apply balanced processing or the thoughtful consideration of all the evidence available to them; and they are transparent and open to others (i.e., relational transparency). Canadian nurse researchers found that authentic leadership was positively associated with nurses' job satisfaction and self-rated performance (Wong & Laschinger, 2013). Other research by Laschinger and colleagues found that turnover intentions among new nurse graduates were reduced in work environments with authentic leaders (Laschinger at al., 2012). A recent study with Belgian nurses found that authentic nurse leaders express more empathy towards their followers, resulting in nurses who were more invigorated and more engaged in job-related learning. These Belgian researchers concluded that authentic leadership best supports thriving at work (Mortier et al., 2016). Thriving at work is a positive psychology concept associated with "a sense of vitality and a sense of learning at work" (Spreitzer et al., 2005, p. 538).

THEORY BOX
Key Leadership Theories

Theory/Contributor	Key Idea	Application to Practice
Trait Theories Trait theories were studied from 1900 to 1950. These theories are sometimes referred to as the *Great Man Theory*, from Aristotle's philosophy extolling the virtue of being "born" with leadership traits. Stogdill (1948) is usually credited as the pioneer of this school of thought.	Leaders have a certain set of physical and emotional characteristics that are crucial for inspiring others toward a common goal. Some theorists believe that traits are innate and cannot be learned; others believe that leadership traits can be developed in each individual.	Self-awareness of traits is useful for assessing personal strengths (such as drive, motivation, integrity, confidence, cognitive ability) and matching those strengths to types of employment.

THEORY BOX—cont'd
Key Leadership Theories

Theory/Contributor	Key Idea	Application to Practice
Style Theories Instead of focusing on traits, style theories consider how leaders behave. Three main lines of research were the Ohio State University and University of Michigan studies in the 1950s, and the Blake and Mouton managerial grid (Blake et al., 1964).	All style theories are based on two types of behaviour: task and relationship behaviours. The combination of these two types of behaviours has been extensively studied to determine the most effective leadership styles. The assumption is that styles can be learned and cultivated.	According to the Blake and Mouton managerial grid (Blake et al., 1964), "high-high" leaders are ideal leaders—they have high concern for accomplishing task objectives and high concern for building and maintaining collaborative relationships. Leaders need to develop both types of competencies.
Situational-Contingency Theories Situational-contingency theory emerged in the 1960s and 1970s. It proposed that leadership effectiveness depends on any given situation. Situational variables are research-tested variables related to leadership effectiveness in different situations. Outcomes are contingent on situational factors. Examples of this type of theory include Fiedler's (1967) contingency model, Vroom and Yetton's (1973) normative decision-making model, House and Mitchell's (1974) path-goal theory, and Hersey and Blanchard's situational leadership theory (1977).	Path-goal theory: There are four types of leader behaviours: supportive, directive, participative, and achievement oriented. Leader behaviour should be contingent on task and follower characteristics. Stressful tasks, for instance, require supportive leaders to lower follower anxiety. Situational leadership theory: The level of follower maturity influences the appropriate mix of task characteristics and leader behaviour. With novice followers (those who are new at a task), leaders should be directive.	Nurses and leaders must assess each situation as unique and determine appropriate actions accordingly. Leaders must adapt their styles to complement the specific issue faced.
Transformational Theories Burns (1978) originally introduced the concepts of transformational and transactional leadership. Transactional leadership is based on a leader–follower exchange, where the follower expects rewards in exchange for effort. Transactional leaders are similar to managers: they manage the status quo or day-to-day operations. Transformational leadership is a process whereby leaders and followers set higher goals and work together to achieve them. Burns felt that this style of leadership was connected with higher moral values. Avolio & Bass (1991) developed a full-range leadership theory with three typologies: transformational, transactional, and laissez-faire. They also developed an accompanying assessment tool, the Multifactor Leadership Questionnaire (MLQ), which has been used extensively in research. See Antonakis & House (2013) for an update on research related to the original full-range theory.	Transformational leaders are known for the four *I*s: idealized influence, intellectual stimulation, individualized consideration, and inspirational motivation. There are three types of transactional leaders: contingent reward leaders focus on role clarification and ensuring followers receive appropriate supports to do their work; management-by-exception active leaders are vigilant and only intervene when a problem starts to arise; management-by-exception passive leaders only intervene after mistakes have occurred. Laissez-faire leaders avoid making decisions and abdicate responsibility.	Cummings et al. (2010) examined relationships between types of nurse leaders and follower outcomes. Transformational nurse leaders were associated with positive outcomes such as nurse retention, group cohesion, role clarity, and effectiveness. Wong et al. (2013) conducted a systematic review of the nursing literature and found significant positive associations between relational leadership styles, such as transformational leadership, and patient outcomes, such as lower morbidity and mortality rates and greater patient satisfaction reports.

THEORY BOX—cont'd

Key Leadership Theories

Theory/Contributor	Key Idea	Application to Practice
Authentic Leadership Authentic leadership arises from the positive psychology tradition (Avolio & Gardner, 2005). Authentic leaders are aware of their own values and moral convictions and are constantly realigning their actions to match their values.	Authentic leaders are characterized by balanced processing (objectively weighing the evidence); an internalized moral perspective or internal moral compass; genuine, open transparency about one's feelings and thoughts; heightened awareness of self, others, and the context.	Authentic leadership is strongly, positively associated with followers' trust in their leaders and with followers' positive emotions. Some evidence suggests that authentic leaders' values-based moral perspective has the biggest influence on followers' emotions. Followers are inspired by these leaders and trust them based on perceived congruence between their values and the leaders' values (Agote et al., 2016).

Management Theories

A plethora of undergraduate, graduate, and doctoral management programs exist across Canada and internationally. A quick online search of prominent management programs reveals that new course offerings incorporate modern technology, such as computer simulation modelling of health care systems and operations, and management information systems (see Chapter 13). Management science has come a long way from the early 1900s when Taylor (1947) became the founder of "scientific management" and the "efficiency movement." Taylor introduced concepts such as labour division and specialization; systematic analysis of the relationship between workers and their assigned tasks; written, standardized procedures; close supervision; rewards for output; worker selection based on the right skills for the right task at the right time; shared manager–worker responsibility for goal achievement; and quality control. Many concepts associated with contemporary leadership, management, and followership are embedded in Taylor's early management theory (Anderson et al., 2012).

Henry Mintzberg, a Canadian academic in business and management, wrote extensively on organizational structures and processes, contributing to our knowledge of early management theory (Mintzberg, 1990). He proposed coordination mechanisms to accomplish complex tasks, including the standardization of work processes,

outputs, worker skills and knowledge, and organizational norms (or beliefs about the nature of work within the organization). Mintzberg also defined ten management roles that fall within three categories: informational, interpersonal, and decisional. For example, the leader role, which falls in the interpersonal category, involves directing, motivating, training, advising, and influencing followers. LEAN, from Toyota automobile manufacturing, is the latest management tool devoted to productivity and efficiencies. The Saskatchewan Ministry of Health committed millions of dollars to LEAN integration within the province's health care settings (Kinsman et al., 2014).

Followership Theories

Our understanding of followership is evolving along with our understanding of leadership and management. In the literature, the trend has been to replace follower terms with team terms because of the importance of effective teamwork within complex health care environments. However, a small body of followership theory literature exists, distinct from the leadership and management theory literature. According to Baker (2007), social sciences research on followership began in the 1950s, although most research concentrated on leaders and managers. The field of followership enjoyed a renaissance in the 1980s. At that time, Steger, Manners, and Zimmerer (1982) proposed a followership theory based on followers' desire for self-enhancement and self-protection or both. They proposed nine follower-ship styles based on high, medium, or low combinations of these dimensions. Steger et al. (1982) were also interested in the influence of power on follower behaviours. The publication of Kelley's (1988) article, "In Praise of Followers," in the *Harvard Business Review* also drew attention to how followers actively contribute to organizational success. In their more recent review of follow-ership theory, Uhl-Bien and colleagues (2014) provided excellent summaries of follower roles with respect to many of the major leadership theories in this chapter's Theory Box (e.g., leadership trait theories, contingency theories, transformational leadership). Many leadership theories are leader-centric, focusing on leader characteristics rather than follower characteristics. For example, transformational leader characteristics, such as idealized influence and inspirational motivation, are necessary leadership qualities for building relationships and obtaining commitment from followers. As stated by Uhl-Bien et al., "This theory (transformational leadership) does not particularly recognize the characteristics or initiatives of followers. There is a focus on improving the quality of the leader-follower relationship, but it is still leader-centric in that it falls short of viewing followers in a broader manner" (2014, p. 86).

Key conclusions drawn from followership research are as follows: a follower is a role rather than a person with inherent characteristics; effective followers are active, not passive; effective followers share the same goals and purpose as leaders; and an effective relationship between followers and leaders is based on interdependency, mutual trust, and respect. A promising area of leadership–followership research is investigating how leaders and followers interact with each other. What patterns of leading and following work well together? Another area of investigation is nonfollowing. There are many occasions when leaders fail because no one responds to their calls for action. In these instances, outcomes are attributed to ineffective leaders or low-quality leader–member relationships. But what about follower attributes and behaviours that contribute to leader failure?

THE PROMISE OF COMPLEXITY SCIENCE

New theories are continually being created, tested, and put into practice—a function carried out by nurse researchers and others. This chapter has included an overview of leadership, management, and followership theories with an emphasis on strengths-based, positive approaches. Leaders, managers, and followers do not interact in a vacuum: they are significantly influenced by their work environments. One of the most important branches of new science that is devoted to complex systems is complexity science. Complexity science began with chaos theory and the physical and mathematical sciences. Since then, the social sciences and health care have adopted complexity science principles to better understand the nature of relationships in complex social systems, such as complex health care environments.

Classic science developed theories that used reductionist approaches to understand systems; for example, the study of machines and the human body focused mainly on the parts. Complexity science views systems holistically; it considers the whole to be greater than the sum of its parts. The world is full of systems within systems that interact and adapt through relationships. The interactions may appear to be random, but patterns emerge over time. Complexity science offers nurses a new way of understanding complex patient and family dynamics, teamwork within organizations, and even health and well-being (Sturmberg & Martin, 2013).

An important premise of complexity science is that human systems can adapt well to complex situations, often finding their own creative solutions to problems when controls are relaxed. Health care organizations are complex adaptive systems (CAS) where the individuals interacting within them are interconnected, always changing and unpredictable. Over time, patterns of interactions occur among individuals who find the best ways of doing work and solving problems together. These patterns are observable and can be used by leaders to get a "good enough" appreciation of what's working or not within their practice environments (Hast et al., 2013). Porter-O'Grady and Malloch (2009) used the term *quantum leadership* to describe leaders who function effectively in complex systems: "Leaders play a central role in reading the 'signposts of change' and guiding others to respond in a manner that promotes sound organizational response" (p. 46). Complexity science thinking stands in sharp contrast to traditional systems thinking, which focuses on developing elaborate plans and specific details on what must be done at every level of an organization. In organizations that follow a complexity science approach, traditional organizational hierarchy is replaced with decision making distributed across the organization. At the practice level, for instance, complexity science encourages health care providers to loosen their control over patients and families. Every voice counts, and every encounter between and among patients and staff contributes to effective decision making (Sturmberg & Martin, 2013). In nursing education, problem-based learning is typically based on complexity science principles. Faculty and students engage in real-time health concerns of patients and their families, recognizing that patients and families are CAS, always changing and adapting on their own. This educational approach can be frustrating to students who expect straightforward solutions to health care issues. Instead, students are provided with a few basic directions for problem-solving, and they are expected to create knowledge versus passively accepting information (Kong et al., 2014). As a student, how comfortable are you with a complexity science approach to education? And why?

Complexity science has borrowed a number of terms from other disciplines, including sociology, psychology, ecology, physics, and chemistry. The following complexity concepts are described in relation to nursing. (For more on complexity science, see Uhl-Bien et al., 2008; Weberg, 2012).

Networking

A network is any related group with common involvement in an area of focus or concern. Social networks are found within organizations but also beyond organizational boundaries. For example, nurses can network within their organizations or with professional groups and associations outside their workplace, such as with nurses at a Canadian Nurses Association conference or nursing students at a Canadian Nursing Student Association Conference.

Attractors

Attractors are values-based characteristics that give an organization its personality. Although the performance of nursing procedures and functions may be similar in health care settings, an intangible caring attractor may exemplify the quality of care delivery in one organization, whereas cost efficiencies may be the attractor of another organization.

Emergence

The concept of emergence addresses how individuals in positions of responsibility engage with and discover, through active organizational involvement, those networks that are best suited to respond to problems in creative, surprising, and artful ways—or thinking outside the box. Nurse staff meetings can be organized to encourage participative decision making, tapping into everyone's creative energy.

Systems Thinking

To have a broader sense of an issue, it's important to think of how systems are interconnected. Nurses use systems thinking when they realize how their unit is one component of a hospital system, and the hospital is part of the public health care system. Similarly, it is important for nurses to recognize that their patients are really emotional, mental, physical, and spiritual systems who belong to family systems, nested within communities. Understanding how systems interact and influence each other can help us appreciate how nursing decisions at the bedside can have ripple effects throughout many systems.

The Butterfly Effect: Nonlinear Dynamics

One small change can lead to an unpredictable, nonlinear chain of events. The expression *butterfly effect* refers to this phenomenon. Based on mathematical complexity principles, a butterfly beating its wings in a South American jungle can trigger changes in the air resulting in hurricane-like weather patterns on the east coast of Canada. A very small change therefore can have disproportionate, seemingly disconnected outcomes. It is important that nurses recognize that making too many changes to a patient's regimen at the very beginning may lead to unexpected and unwanted outcomes. Instead, identify one small, useful change that a patient can implement and allow time for the patient and family to determine if the change is working for them or not.

How has complexity science influenced our understanding of leadership, management, and followership? Leaders and managers do not need to have hypervigilant control over their work environments and followers; instead, they need to allow time and space for followers to network with each other. Emergence of new, innovative solutions arises through CAS/followers' interactions.

EXERCISE 1.5 As a student nurse, think of how you can apply each of the following complexity concepts. Give an example of how you will use each concept during your clinical practicums.

Complexity concepts: Networking, attractors, emergence, systems thinking, butterfly effect.

EXERCISE 1.6 Read the article in the following Research Perspective, which includes a discussion of multiple patient/simultaneity complexity (MP/SC) situations. Now think of an MP/SC situation you have experienced as a student nurse. Write down a description of the situation. How did you feel in this situation? Who helped you prioritize and make decisions? If you could go back to this situation and do it all over again, who would you engage in creative problem solving? Remember that the patients and families should be engaged as partners in decision making whenever possible.

LEADING, FOLLOWING, AND MANAGING COMPETENCIES

When dealing with theories and concepts, it is easy to lose sight of how to put these ideas into practice. The following sections review important competencies for leaders, managers, and followers. Competencies comprise knowledge, skills, and attitudes, and they are often arranged in checklists or frameworks for self-assessment. Competencies are influenced by the practice setting and the formal level of authority (e.g., front-line nurse leader, departmental manager, and executive director) (Jennings et al., 2007).

RESEARCH PERSPECTIVE

Resource: Kramer M, Brewer B, Halfer D, et al. Changing our lens: seeing the chaos of professional practice as complexity. *Journal of Nursing Management*, 2013; 21(4): 690–704.

In an interview study conducted with newly licensed registered nurses (RNs), experienced RNs, and managers and educators from 20 Magnet hospitals in the United States, the chaos of the work environment was most often cited as the major adaptation difficulty for new graduates transitioning into practice. "Getting work done" was a particular concern for new RNs. The purpose of this study was to identify barriers to work effectiveness for new RNs and to identify management practices to best support new RNs' capacity to safely and effectively complete their work.

A major barrier for new RNs was their inability to coordinate care for multiple patients with multiple simultaneous needs—what the authors call "multiple patient/simultaneity complexity" or MP/SC. To assist new RNs with a safe transition to MP/SC care provision, a complexity science education intervention was piloted with nine volunteer hospitals. New RNs were given MP/SC cases to study before their class. Participants were asked to anonymously describe what they would do in each situation, and to indicate comfort or discomfort with the decision. After completing their preassessments of MP/SC dilemmas, the new RNs attended an interactive class with educators and peers to discuss alternative, valid solutions. Complex systems principles were reinforced throughout the class discussion. For example, in a complex system, the many elements or agents in a system can interact in multiple ways, leading to myriad possible courses of action and outcomes. Best solutions for patients

often emerge through careful observation and continuous assessment of the patient and system. After participating in this class, new RNs shifted their thinking from a one-solution approach to an appreciation for thoughtful RN surveillance and the possibility of multiple, potential right answers. The class discussions also helped new RNs feel more at ease with the unpredictability of MP/SC work environments.

Implications for Practice
This study took place in US Magnet hospitals. Magnet hospitals are considered the gold standard for nursing work environments, and they act as a magnet to recruit and retain nurses. Hospitals must undergo a rigorous accreditation process to receive Magnet certification. Magnet hospitals typically offer new graduate internships and orientation programs to ease the transition process. This study found that even new RNs in Magnet hospitals require extra learning supports to help them gain comfort with MP/SC situations.

Kramer et al. (2013) found that MP/SC case-based learning and peer discussion were important strategies for nurses to learn from one another. In CAS, individuals adapt and learn together. Another example of CAS, mentioned in the Kramer et al. article, was *interassignment rounding* between nurses and physicians. This rounding format is ideal for facilitating collaboration, problem solving, and more effective, efficient development of joint plans of care. Porter O'Grady, Clark, and Wiggins (2010) contend that complexity science education should be included in pregraduate nursing education programs and postgraduate continuing education opportunities.

Leading and Managing

Leadership and management are so closely intertwined that the American Organization of Nurse Executives and the American Association of Critical Care Nurses developed a Nurse Manager Leadership Partnership Learning Domain Framework that emphasizes how leadership-management domains influence each other (Baxter & Warshawsky, 2014). Fig. 1.1 demonstrates overlaps among three competency domains: leading within, leading people, and managing the business.

Leadership development always receives the most attention in the literature: the reason is related to the critical importance of beginning with your own leadership development. Leading from within is something each of us can do at any point along the nursing career trajectory. More complex competencies related to leading people and managing the business take time, practice, and effort (Ulrich et al., 2014).

Strengths-based leadership therefore begins with knowing yourself—your core values and ethics. This domain requires self-reflection practice and development of emotional intelligence (i.e., self-awareness, emotional self-regulation, other-awareness, and interpersonal skills). Each of us can be a successful leader through conscious efforts to be our authentic, best self.

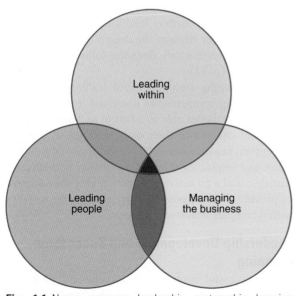

Fig. 1.1 Nurse manager leadership partnership learning framework.

Managing the business includes the following core competencies: human resource management, financial accountability, critical thinking, clinical practice knowledge, performance management, strategic planning, and technology use. Human resource management entails having the right numbers and types of staff available to meet patient needs. Clinical practice knowledge is a related competency, because managers must know their patient populations to make effective staffing decisions. Other competencies include critical thinking skills associated with the constant monitoring of patients' status, including patient discharges, transfers, and admissions. In addition, managers need to understand the big picture of patient movement within their hospital or facility—not just what is happening in their unit or department. Managers attend meetings daily to plan strategies for patient management throughout their hospital or facility. Managers are also responsible for overseeing staff performance and providing constructive feedback and supports, particularly for newer nurses. With the advent of technology for communications and documentation, managers must know how to use data, generated by technology, to inform their critical decisions. An over-arching concern for managers is safe, quality care that is cost effective. When scheduling staff and ordering supplies, managers are held financially accountable for their decisions. The Triple Aim movement in Canada is an example of complexity principles at work: networks of health care organizations and providers work together to ensure adoption of evidence-based practices associated with Triple Aim: better population health, improved patient experiences, and cost effectiveness. At their organizational levels, managers are charged with implementing and evaluating Triple Aim practices (Farmanova et al., 2016).

The third domain of leading people includes relationship-building and use of influence tactics to promote best practices. A key competency is knowing how to engage others in solving problems and making decisions. Promoting collaboration is particularly important for ensuring effective teamwork (Baxter & Warshawsky, 2014). This US-based framework clearly articulates the interconnected nature of leadership and management. In Canada, an excellent leadership resource that includes management competencies is the Registered Nurses Association of Ontario (RNAO) Best Practice Guidelines for Developing and Sustaining Nursing Leadership (2013).

Following

Typically, followers are considered to be passive, uninspired, and waiting for direction. However, just the opposite is true. Followership is an understudied area in the leadership literature, but interest is growing in the ways in which members of a group or team organize themselves into leader–follower relationships that synergize outcomes for the group or team. In effective leader–follower relationships, followers play an important role in sharing and discussing relevant information that informs the leader's decisions. Proactive followers versus passive followers are associated with better leader–follower communications and outcomes when leaders acknowledge and support followers' efforts to speak up and engage in finding collaborative solutions (Uhl-Bien et al., 2014). Proactive or strengths-based follower competencies include rational, positive influence tactics and constructive feedback seeking. One positive influence tactic is rational persuasion where the follower shares their evidence-based observations and concerns with a leader to avert problems and contribute to a better outcome. Rational evidence-based influence tactics are more effective than negative tactics, such as complaining and pressuring. Constructive feedback-seeking is another, positive way for followers to establish effective working relationships between leaders and followers, particularly when using an approach such as appreciative inquiry (Uhl-Bien et al., 2014). Rather than waiting for a leader's response, a follower can ask: What went well of us? How can we do better next time?

LEADING, MANAGING, AND FOLLOWING DURING COMPLEX TIMES

The twenty-first-century health care industry is going through unparalleled change, often away from the traditional industrial models that reigned throughout the twentieth century. Most health care organizations today have ethnically diverse staff with educations that range from non–high school graduates to clinicians with PhDs. There are multiple generations of workers with varying values and expectations of the workplace that are held accountable for Triple Aim care. The complexity of the health care system includes vast amounts of information and data that often leads to worker fatigue from trying to keep up with everything related to quality, safe, cost-effective care. These problems and other variables make leading, managing, and following increasingly challenging. Burns (2000) states, "It would seem so simple at first glance—that leaders lead and followers follow. When the leader dreams the dream or takes the initiative or issues the call, does the follower even hear the leader?" (p. 11).

By developing strengths-based leading, managing, and following competencies discussed in this chapter, nurses will be better able to adapt to and accept differences and changes in their daily work life as positive rather than negative forces. It is rewarding to be an innovative and inspirational leader, an efficient and effective manager, and a proactive follower—taking the initiative to provide the best possible safe, quality care delivery within complex health care systems.

Leadership Development and Succession Planning

Many successful professional development programs include a mentorship component and hands-on, relevant leadership and management experiences within health care settings (MacPhee et al., 2014).

EXERCISE 1.7 In your clinical setting, arrange a shadow experience with the front-line nurse leader.

1. Observe and document what the leader does during your time together. Afterwards, categorize their behaviours under leading, managing, and follower competencies.
2. Observe staff interactions with the leader. Document examples of proactive leadership/follower competencies.
   a. Share and discuss your notes in class. Are your responses to the above questions similar to those of your colleagues?

EXERCISE 1.8 While you are in a unit during your clinical practicum or rotation, observe leader-follower interactions during change of shift. Change of shift is a time when the clinical nurse leader and staff will often negotiate assignments based on patient needs and nurse competencies.

Are there discussions between the leader and staff about patient needs? Is the leader soliciting staff ideas? Is the staff offering information and advice?

The change-of-shift observation is an example of just one leader–follower exchange. Based on what you know about leaders and followers from this chapter, critique the quality of leader–follower relationship. Would you want to work on this unit? Why or why not?

In addition to educational opportunities and supports for current staff, health care leadership needs to systematically plan for the future. Succession planning includes the identification of nurses with leadership interests and potential. Based on a projected nurse shortage, by 2022 Canada could be short of over 4 000 nurse managers (Wong et al., 2013). Recruiting nurses into management roles is challenging because of the perceived challenges associated with these roles. A Canadian qualitative study was conducted with nurses from four regions of the country (i.e., West, Ontario, Quebec and Atlantic) (Wong et al. 2013). The purpose of the study was to ask staff nurses about their interest in pursuing managerial roles. Interviewees felt that they would need more education to be effective managers. More experienced nurses did not want to commit to more education because of other life commitments. Younger and less experienced nurses were interested in going on for further education and career advancement, but they wanted to become more clinically competent before considering a management position. Interviewees often felt confident that they could be leaders, based on their clinical abilities and interpersonal skills, but they were concerned about their capacity to manage budgets and human resources.

When asked about skills they associated with the management role, nurses said: "interpersonal skills (e.g., conflict management, giving feedback, listening and communication skills), intergenerational understanding, mentoring skills, leadership skills, such as the ability to empower staff, and technical skills such as dealing with budgets and technology" (p. 235). Do you see similarities between nurses' perceptions of what managers do and the leading and managing competencies described previously?

In this qualitative study (Wong et al., 2013), interviewees felt that organizations should be engaged in succession planning, identifying and recruiting nurses to participate in internal or external leadership programmes. In addition, nurses recognized the importance of having experienced nurse leaders available to them as mentors and coaches. Unfortunately, the majority of nurses came from organizations where such leadership development opportunities were not in place. Interviewees also gave their own suggestions for ways to develop management skills, such as acting in temporary charge roles, working on projects, and serving on committees. Overall, only 19% of study participants were interested in pursuing management roles. Although nurse interviewees recognized formal management roles as an opportunity to make positive differences in their work environments, they were more influenced by their negative perceptions of these roles, particularly lack of organizational support for leadership development, heavy workloads, and human resource and financial accountabilities (Wong et al., 2013).

Exposure to positive role models allows student and registered nurses to develop an appreciation for the importance of effective nurse leaders in formal positions of authority within health care organizations. Nurses often consider that few rewards are associated with formal leadership and management positions (Merrill et al., 2013). In nursing, many units or facilities have first-line or clinical nurse leaders who oversee day-to-day operations and act as liaisons between direct care nurses and management. These leaders represent staff and advocate for their concerns. One Canadian study showed that first-line nurse leaders can positively influence staff perceptions of the work environment and, in turn, improve nurse retention rates and job satisfaction (Laschinger et al., 2009). First-line nurse leaders are typically recruited directly from staff nurse positions, emphasizing the importance of systematically recruiting, educating, and supporting staff nurses to fulfill these critical leadership positions. In turn, first-line nurse leaders are often a source for management positions. The following Research Perspective indicates that empowerment-based leadership can be taught and is important to strengths-based leadership development.

RESEARCH PERSPECTIVE

Resource: MacPhee M, Dahinten V, Hejazi S, et al. Testing the effects of an empowerment-based leadership development programme: part 1—leader outcomes. *Journal of Nursing Management*, 2014; 22(1): 4–15.

A nursing leadership development program for front-line nurse leaders was developed and tested over a 4-year period (2006–2010) in British Columbia (MacPhee & Bouthillette, 2008). An empowerment framework was used to teach self-empowerment and staff empowerment behaviours to novice leaders with less than 3 years' experience (MacPhee et al., 2011). Leaders who participated in the programme were asked to complete a survey at the start of the programme and 1 year later; their

Continued

responses were compared with those of a similar group of novice leaders who filled out surveys but did not attend the programme. Leaders who attended the programme reported the use of significantly more leader-empowering behaviours than those leaders who did not attend the programme. This study showed that empowerment strategies are teachable.

Implications for Practice

Other research has shown that leaders' use of empowering behaviours is associated with more engaged staff and healthier work environments (Wong & Laschinger, 2013). Because empowerment strategies are teachable, organizations should invest in leadership development programmes that use these successful, evidence-informed approaches. Empowerment is discussed in more detail in Chapter 12. One highly recognized and respected Canadian nurse researcher, Dr. Heather Laschinger, devoted her research career to studying workplace empowerment and the importance of empowerment to nurse leaders, staff, and patient outcomes. See the tribute to Dr. Laschinger's life work at http://www.longwoods.com/content/24987.

How can we prepare nursing students before graduation to consider the importance of leadership, management, and followership roles? One nursing programme in Alberta used simulations to teach senior nursing students about leadership/followership roles (Pollard & Wild, 2014). Because management competencies typically require additional education and experience beyond the first few years of nursing, faculty members focused on students' appreciation of lead-

ership and followership. Simulation provides students with opportunities to try out different strategies in a safe place, and time is allotted for practice, reflection, and debriefing. In the Alberta programme, simulation exercises were based on students' clinical experiences. After role playing leader and follower roles in the simulation, students were asked to identify and to evaluate the fundamental leadership and followership competencies within a team context. The purpose of these simulation exercises was to foreground how leadership and followership competencies are both necessary for effective, collaborative teamwork. Some leader/follower competencies recognized by the students were: communications, such as giving constructive feedback, succinct reporting of critical information, and use of appreciative inquiry; and teamwork, such as showing respect, being civil, and engaging in shared problem solving and decision making. Evaluation of student learning found that students could recognize the importance of leadership and followership competencies within clinical contexts, and they valued a strengths-based, positive approach to leadership and followership. Finally, students "reported that participating in the activities was realistic and they felt like the decisional complexities experienced in the class were likely to be the ones they would also need to deal with in their future practice" (2014, p. 624). What is unknown is whether or not these students went on to enact strengths-based leadership–followership roles in their clinical practice. Using simulations with deliberate self-reflection and group debriefing, however, are strategies for better preparing nursing students for the complexities ahead.

CONCLUSION

This chapter covered the key theories, styles, attributes, and competencies related to strengths-based leadership, management, and followership. This chapter began with a focus on the strengths and unique assets of our Canadian health care system. Deficits and inequalities exist in Canada's health care system, but we must build on our societal strengths, such as the *Canada Health Act*; the promotion of the social determinants of health; and the desire to eradicate social exclusion. Strengths-based leadership begins within each of us.

A SOLUTION

Terry realized that she was not getting the mentorship support she needed to effectively transition into a new graduate nurse role on the medical-surgical unit. She connected with some of her friends, former classmates, who were working in other units in her hospital or in other organizations. She asked her friends about their transition experiences and supports. One hospital, in particular, sounded ideal to her: a new graduate internship over 6 months with an assigned senior nurse mentor. Terry applied to this hospital, and when she received an interview for a medical-surgical unit position, she had a list of questions ready to ask the nurse manager of the unit.

❓ A SOLUTION—cont'd

She also asked whether she could visit the unit and shadow a nurse during a shift to get to know the unit better. During the interview process, the manager provided details about the transition-to-practice internship program, and she answered all of Terry's questions in a respectful and supportive fashion. She even said: "We know becoming a nurse is a challenging time for new graduates, and we want you to feel supported by our team and our organization."

The manager granted Terry's request for a shadow experience and she met Terry during her shadow day to introduce Terry to the clinical nurse leader and educator. Terry received introductions to the staff and other health care professionals, and she observed lots of positive nurse-leader dialogue throughout her experience.

She was most impressed by the leader's presence, especially during shift report. The leader checked out staff assignments to be sure staff were comfortable with their workloads. The leader and manager were both present for a safety huddle mid-shift to discuss nurses' safety concerns. Terry was excited to receive an offer from the manager of this unit, and six months post-orientation, she continues to believe that she made the right move. Reflecting on her initial decision to work on a unit where she did her last practicum, Terry realized that she was too anxious for a job; she failed to consider all the factors associated with a positive work experience, particularly the presence of a strengths-based leader and collaborative team dynamics.

▌ THE EVIDENCE

In a qualitative interview and focus group study with Canadian nurse leaders and new graduates from seven provinces, new nurses and leaders identified similar factors associated with effective transition to practice: supportive unit cultures with welcoming and helpful staff, formal orientation programmes or internships, and mentors who provided constructive feedback and advice (Regan et al., 2017). Other facilitators for successful transition included lower new graduate: patient ratios, opportunities to request orientation extensions, and managerial efforts to evaluate and ensure nurse–job fit. Some new graduates have ideals to work on specific units, but they may not have the capabilities to do so. During interviews, managers will often ask specific questions and review new graduates' curriculum vitae (i.e., a resume with nursing courses and practicums) to ensure a fit with the work environment and the patient population. Effective fit between new graduates and their first employment experience makes a difference with respect to successful transition to practice and to retention. New graduate attrition attributed to workplace stressors or poor job fit is a serious loss to the nursing profession (Phillips et al., 2014).

The qualitative study by Regan and colleagues (2017) also identified major barriers to successful transition including short or no orientations, heavy workloads and understaffing, and uncivil staff behaviour. Fortunately, there is some good news for new graduates. Because new graduates are a valuable investment in our nursing future, organizations and their nurse leadership are advocating for more investment in evidence-based strategies that are associated with effective transition and retention. In a related Canadian survey that followed new graduates over their first year of practice (Laschinger et al. 2016 cited in Regan et al. 2017), new graduates reported that their work life was "relatively positive." New graduates reported access to resources and high levels of support (Regan et al., 2017, p. 253). The researchers concluded that new graduate nurses are a valuable human resource, and nurse leaders and health care organizations must ensure their successful integration within the workplace. They also noted the implications of not advocating for new graduate transition supports. "Nurse leaders at all levels of the organization need to be attuned to the transition needs of new graduates in the promotion of quality outcomes for patients. Moreover, retention of new graduates has a direct impact on the cost of turnover and stability in the workforce" (Regan et al., 2017, p. 253).

✳ NEED TO KNOW NOW

- Grow your emotional intelligence (EI). Know your own values (EI self-awareness). Practice self-reflection and control (EI regulation) of your own emotions.
- Be positive. Strengths-based leadership begins with a positive attitude—of looking for ways to build on positives. Practice positive psychology strategies, such as appreciative inquiry.
- Develop your leadership competencies. In addition to leading within (#1 earlier), leading others depends on relational skills or knowing how to develop and maintain positive relationships with your peers, other health care professionals, patients, and their families.
- Develop your followership competencies. Practice speaking up and using effective communications in interactions with your team and leadership. Effective followership depends on your proactive efforts to support your leader and team whenever possible.
- Seek out strong leader role models and formal leadership development opportunities: they are important components to becoming a strengths-based leader.

▌CHAPTER CHECKLIST

This chapter presents the case that nurses require the competencies, knowledge, skill, and abilities to move in and out of leader, manager, and follower roles with ease, whether in clinical or administrative positions.

- Emotional intelligence (EI) is about knowing one's own and others' feelings and emotions. Emotional intelligence is as critical to professional practice as are cognitive and technical skills.
- Multiple theories are used to understand leadership, management and followership within in today's complex health care environments. We especially need strengths-based, authentic, transformational, and transactional leaders.
- Authentic leadership is a root construct in leadership theory, meaning that authenticity, being genuine and sincere, is the foundation for strengths-based leadership. Other styles that add to leader effectiveness include transactional leadership (similar to effective management) and transformational leadership.
- Transformational leaders influence nurses to go beyond the status quo, by inspiring and motivating them with ideals and values that resonate with nurses' professional values and goals.
- Transactional leaders ensure nurses have necessary resources and supports to provide safe, quality care. They are visible, present, and supportive. Transactional leaders are synonymous with effective managers.
- Complexity science does not refer to the complexity of the decision to be made or to the work environment in isolation, but rather to examining how systems adapt and function: many possible ideas and actions unfold in a nonprescriptive, nonlinear manner.
- Proactive followers make significant contributions to organizations by working collaboratively with their leaders, managers, and teams. Followers are not passive.
- Systematic succession planning and formal leadership development opportunities are critical to the future of nursing leadership.

▌TIPS FOR LEADING, MANAGING, AND FOLLOWING

- Competency frameworks, when available, can be useful tools for determining whether you have the knowledge, skills, and attitudes associated with certain roles and responsibilities.
- You can use the leader, manager, and follower competencies and attributes in this chapter to create your own checklist. Look for these behaviours in others and use these competencies to guide your own leader, manager, and follower self-development.

Visit the Evolve website for Suggested Readings, Internet Resources, and additional resources related to the content in this chapter: http://evolve.elsevier.com/Canada/Yoder-Wise/leading/.

REFERENCES

Agote, L., Aramburu, N., & Lines, R. (2016). Authentic leadership perception, trust in the leader, and followers' emotions in organizational change processes. *Journal of Applied Behavioural Science, 52*(1), 35–63.

Anderson, D., Sweeney, D., Williams, T., et al. (2012). *An introduction to management science, quantitative approaches to decision making.* London: Cengage Learning.

Antonakis, J., & House, R. (2013). The full-range leadership theory: The way forward. In Bruce J. Avolio, & Francis J. Yammarino (Eds.), *Transformational and charismatic leadership: the road ahead 10th anniversary edition (monographs in leadership and management Vol 5.* (pp. 3–33). Emerald Group Publishing Limited.

Avolio, B., & Bass, B. (1991). *The full range leadership development programs: Basic and advanced manuals.* Binghamton, NY: Bass, Avolio, & Associates.

Avolio, B., & Gardner, W. (2005). Authentic leadership: Getting to the root of positive forms of leadership. *The Leadership Quarterly, 16*(3), 315–338.

Baker, S. (2007). Followership: The theoretical foundation of a contemporary construct. *Journal of Leadership & Organizational Studies, 14*(1), 50–61.

Baxter, C., & Warshawsky, N. (2014). Exploring the acquisition of nurse manager competence. *Nurse Leader, 12*(1), 46–51 59.

Beauvais, A., Brady, N., O'Shea, E. R., & Quinn Griffin, M. (2011). Emotional intelligence and nursing performance among nursing students. *Nurse Education Today, 31*, 396–401.

Bennett, K., & Sawatzky, J. V. (2013). Building emotional intelligence: A strategy for emerging nurse leaders to reduce workplace bullying. *Nursing Administration Quarterly, 37*(2), 144–151.

Blake, R., Mouton, J., Barnes, L., et al. (1964). Breakthrough in organization development. *Harvard Business Review, 42*(6), 133–155.

Boyatzis, R., & McKee, A. (2005). *Resonant leadership: Renewing yourself and connecting with others through mindfulness, hope, and compassion.* Boston, MA: Harvard Business School Press.

Burns, J. (1978). *Leadership.* New York: Harper & Row.

Burns, J. M. (2000). Leadership and followership: Complicated relationships. In B. Kellerman, & L. R. Matusak (Eds.), *Cutting edge: Leadership 2000.* College Park, MD: The James MacGregor Burns Academy of Leadership.

Canadian Nurses Association. (2012). A nursing call to action. http://www.cna-aiic.ca/en/on-the-issues/national-expert-commission/report-and-recommendations.

Canadian Nurses' Association. (2017). Code of ethics for registered nurses. https://www.cna-aiic.ca/~/media/cna/page-content/pdf-en/code-of-ethics-2017-edition-secure-interactive.pdf?la=en.

Chinn, P., & Kramer, M. (2007). *Integrated knowledge development in nursing* (7th ed.). St. Louis, MO: Mosby.

Cummings, G., MacGregor, T., Davey, M., et al. (2010). Distinctive outcome patterns by leadership style for the nursing workforce and work environments: A systematic review. *International Journal of Nursing Studies, 47*(3), 363–385. https://doi.org/10.1016/j.ijnurstu.2009.08.006.

Donaldson, S., Dollwet, M., & Rao, M. (2015). Happiness, excellence and optimal human functioning revisited: Examining the perr-reviewed literature linked to positive psychology. *The Journal of Positive Psychology, 10*(3), 185–195.

Falk-Rafael, A., & Betker, C. (2012). Witnessing social injustice downstream and advocating for dealth equity upstream: "the trombone slide" of nursing. *Advances in Nursing Science, 35*(2), 98–112.

Farmanova, E., Kirvan, C., Verma, J., Mukerji, G., Akunov, N., & Samis, S. (2016). Triple Aim in Canada: developing capacity to lead to better health, care and cost. *International Journal for Quality in Health Care, 28*(6), 830–837.

Feo, R., Conroy, T., Marshall, R., Rasmussen, P., Wiechula, R., & Kitson, A. (2016). Using holistic interpretive synthesis to create practice-relevant guidance for person-centred fundamental care delivered by nurses. *Nursing Inquiry, 24*(2), e12152.

Fiedler, F. A. (1967). *A theory of leadership effectiveness.* New York: McGraw-Hill.

Fischer, S. (2016). Transformational leadership: a concept analysis. *Journal of Advanced Nursing, 72*(11), 2644–2653.

Gorgens-Ekermans, G., & Brand, T. (2012). Emotional intelligence as a moderator in the stress burnout relationship: A questionnaire study on nurses. *Journal of Clinical Nursing, 21*, 2275–2285.

Gottlieb, L., Gottlieb, B., & Shamian, J. (2012). Principles of strengths-based leadership for strengths-based nursing care: A new paradigm for nursing and healthcare for the 21st century. *Canadian Journal of Nursing Leadership, 25*(2), 38–50.

Government of Canada. (2017). *Canada's health care system.* https://www.canada.ca/en/health-canada/services/canada-health-care-system.html.

Government of Canada. (2017). *What Makes Canadians Healthy or Unhealthy?.* https://www.canada.ca/en/public-health/services/health-promotion/population-health/what-determines-health/what-makes-canadians-healthy-unhealthy.html#evidence.

Hart, P., Brannan, J., & De Chesnay, M. (2014). Resilience in nurses: an integrative review. *Journal of Nursing Management, 22*, 720–734.

Hast, A., DiGioia, A., & Thompson, D. (2013). Utilizing complexity science to drive practice change through patient- and family-centered care. *Journal of Nursing Administration, 43*(1), 44–49.

Hersey, P., & Blanchard, K. (1977). *The management of organizational behavior* (3rd ed.). Englewood Cliffs, NJ: Prentice Hall.

House, R. J., & Mitchell, T. R. (1974). Autumn). Path-goal theory of leadership. *Journal of Contemporary Business, 3*, 81–97.

Institute for Healthcare Improvement Open School. (2018). Mindfulness in clinical practice e-series. http://www.ihi.org/education/IHIOpenSchool/resources/Pages/PFC-103-Incorporating-Mindfulness-into-Clinical-Practice.aspx.

Jackson, D., Firtko, A., & Edenborough, M. (2007). Personal resilience as a strategy for surviving and thriving in the face of workplace adversity: a literature review. *Journal of Advanced Nursing, 60*, 1–9.

Jennings, B., Scalzi, C., Rodgers, J., et al. (2007). Differentiating nursing leadership and management competencies. *Nursing Outlook, 55*, 169–175. https://doi.org/10.1016/j.outlook.2006.10.002.

Kelley, R. (1988). In praise of followers. *Harvard Business Review, 66*, 142–148.

Kinsman, L., Rotter, T., Stevenson, K., Bath, B., Goodridge, D., & Westhorp, G. (2014). "The largest Lean transformation in the world": The implementation and evaluation of Lean in Saskatchewan healthcare. *Healthcare Quarterly, 17*(2), 29–32.

Kong, L.-N., Qin, B., Zhou, Y.-Q., Mou, S.-Y., & Gao, H.-M. (2014). The effectiveness of problem based learning on nurses' students critical thinking: A systematic review and meta-analysis. *International Journal of Nursing Studies, 51*, 458–469.

Kramer, M., Brewer, B., Halfer, D., et al. (2013). Changing our lens: Seeing the chaos of professional practice as complexity. *Journal of Nursing Management, 21*(4), 690–704.

Laschinger, H., Finegan, J., & Wilk, P. (2009). Context matters: The impact of unit leadership and empowerment on nurses' organizational commitment. *Journal of Nursing Administration, 39*(2), 228–235.

Laschinger, H., Wong, C., Cummings, G., & Grau, A. (2014). Resonant leadership and workplace empowerment: The value of positive organizational cultures in reducing workplace incivility. *Nursing Economic$, 32*(1), 5–15 44.

Laschinger, H., Wong, C., & Grau, A. (2012). The influence of authentic leadership on newly graduated nurses' experiences of workplace bullying, burnout and retention outcomes: A cross-sectional study. *International Journal of Nursing Studies, 29*(10), 1266–1276.

Laschinger, H., Wong, C., Regan, S., Young-Ritchie, C., & Bushell, P. (2013). Workplace incivility and new graduate nurses' mental health: The protective role of resiliency. *Journal of Nursing Administration, 43*(7/8), 415–421.

Lewis, S. (2011). *Positive psychology at work: How positive leadership and appreciative inquiry create inspiring organizations.* Sussex, UK: John Wiley & Sons, Ltd.

Lucas, V., Laschinger, H., & Wong, C. (2008). The impact of emotional intelligent leadership on staff nurse empowerment: The moderating effect of span of control. *Journal of Nursing Management, 16*, 964–973. https://doi.org/10.1111/j.1365-2834.2008.0856.x.

MacPhee, M., & Bouthillette, F. (2008). Developing leadership in nurse managers: The British Columbia Nursing Leadership Institute. *Canadian Journal of Nursing Leadership, 21*(3), 64–75.

MacPhee, M., Dahinten, V., Hejazi, S., et al. (2014). Testing the effects of an empowerment-based leadership development programme: Part 1—leader outcomes. *Journal of Nursing Management, 22*(1), 4–15.

MacPhee, M., Skelton-Green, J., Bouthillette, F., et al. (2011). An empowerment framework for nursing leadership development: Supporting evidence. *Journal of Advanced Nursing, 68*(1), 159–169. https://doi.org/10.1111/j.1365-2648.2011.05746.x.

Mortier, A., Vlerick, P., & Clays, E. (2016). Authentic leadership and thriving among nurses: the mediating role of empathy. *Journal of Nursing Management, 24*, 357–365.

Merrill, K., Pepper, G., & Blegen, M. (2013). Managerial span of control: A pilot study comparing departmental complexity and number of direct reports. *Canadian Journal of Nursing Leadership, 26*(3), 53–67.

Mintzberg, H. (1990). March). The manager's job: Folklore and fact. *Harvard Business Review*, 1–13.

OECD. (2017). Health at a Glance 2017: OECD Indicators for Canada. http://www.oecd.org/canada/Health-at-a-Glance-2017-Key-Findings-CANADA.pdf.

Orak, R., Farahani, M., Kelishami, F., Seyedfatemi, N., Banihashemi, S., & Havaei, F. (2016). Investigating the effect of emotional intelligence education on baccalaureate nursing students' emotional intelligence score. *Nurse Education in Practice, 20*, 64–69.

Phillips, C., Kenny, A., Esterman, A., & Smith, C. (2014). A secondary data analysis examining the needs of graduate nurses in their transition to a new role. *Nurse Education in Practice, 14*(2), 106–111.

Pollard, C., & Wild, C. (2014). Nursing leadership competencies: Low-fidelity simulation as a teaching strategy. *Nurse Education in Practice, 14*(6), 620–626.

Por, J., Barriball, L., Fitzpatrick, J., & Roberts, J. (2011). Emotional intelligence: Its relationship to stress, coping, well-being and professional performance in nursing students. *Nurse Education Today, 31*, 855–860.

Porter-O'Grady, T., Clark, S., & Wiggins, M. (2010). The case for clinical nurse leaders: Guiding nursing practice into the 21st century. *Nurse Leader, 8*(1), 37–41.

Porter-O'Grady, T., & Malloch, K. (2007). *Quantum leadership: A resource for health care innovation* (2nd ed.). Sudbury, MA: Jones and Bartlett Publishers.

Regan, S., Wong, C., Laschinger, H., Cummings, G., Leiter, M., & Read, E. (2017). Starting out: Qualitative perspectives of new graduate nurses and nurse leaders on transition to practice. *Journal of Nursing Management, 25*(4), 246–255.

Registered Nurses Association of Ontario (RNAO). (2013). *Best practice guidelines for developing and sustaining nursing leadership*. Toronto, ON: RNAO.

Roberts, L., Dutton, J., Spreitzer, G., Heaphy, E., & Quinn, R. (2005). Composing the reflected best self portrait: Building pathways for becoming extraordinary in work organizations. *Academy of Management Review, 30*(4), 712–736.

Roche, M., Luthans, F., & Haar, J. (2014). The role of mindfulness and psychological capital on the well-being of leaders. *Journal of Occupational Health Psychology, 19*(4), 476–489.

Shendell-Falik, N., Fienson, M., & Mohr, B. (2007). Enhancing patient safety: Improving the patient handoff process through appreciative inquiry. *Journal of Nursing Administration, 37*(2), 95–104.

Spano-Szekely, L., Quinn Griffin, M., Clavelle, J., & Fitzpatrick, J. (2016). Emotional intelligence and transformational leadership in nurse managers. *Journal of Nursing Administration, 46*(2), 101–108.

Spreitzer, G., Sutcliffe, K., Dutton, J., Sonenshein, S., & Grant, A. (2005). A socially embedded model of thriving at work. *Organization Science, 16*(5), 537–549.

Steger, J., Manners, G., & Zimmerer, T. (1982). Following the leader: How to link management style to subordinate personalities. *Management Review, 71*, 49–51 (22–28).

Stogdill, R. M. (1948). Personal factors associated with leadership: A survey of the literature. *Journal of Psychology, 25*, 35–71.

Storch, J., Makaroff, K., Pauly, B., & Newton, L. (2013). Take me to my leader: The importance of ethical leadership among formal nurse leaders. *Nursing Ethics, 20*(2), 150–157.

Sturmberg, J., & Martin, C. (Eds.). (2013). *Handbook of systems and complexity in health*. New York: Springer Publishing.

Taylor, F. (1947). *Management science*. New York: Harper and Row.

Trajkovski, S., Schmied, V., Vickers, M., & Jackson, D. (2013). Using appreciative inquiry to bring neonatal nurses and parents together to enhance family-centred care: A collaborative workshop. *Journal of Child Health Care, 19*(2), 239–253.

Turner, S. (2014). The resilient nurse: An emerging concept. *Nurse Leader*, 71–73, 90.

Tyczkowski, B., Vandenhouten, C., Reilly, J., Bansal, G., Kubsch, S., & Jakkola, R. (2015). Emotional intelligence and nursing leadership styles among nurse managers. *Nursing Administration Quarterly, 39*(2), 172–180.

Uhl-Bien, M., Marion, R., & Mckelvey, M. (2008). Complexity leadership theory: Shifting leadership from the industrial age to the knowledge era. In M. Uhl-Bien, & R. Marion (Eds.), *Complexity leadership part 1: Conceptual foundations* (pp. 185–224). Charlotte, NC: Information Age Publishing.

Uhl-Bien, M., Riggio, R., Lowe, K., & Carsten, M. (2014). Followership theory: A review and research agenda. *Leadership Quarterly, 25*(1), 83–104.

Ulrich, B., Lavandero, R., & Early, S. (2014). Leadership competence: perceptions of direct care nurses. Nurse Leader. *Nurse Leader, 12*(3), 47–50.

Vroom, V., & Yetton, P. (1973). *Leadership and decision-making*. Pittsburgh, PA: University of Pittsburgh Press.

Walton, D. (2012). *Introducing emotional intelligence: A practical guide*. London: Icon Books Ltd.

Watkins, S., Dewar, B., & Kennedy, C. (2016). Appreciative Inquiry as an intervention to change nursing practice in in-patient settings: An integrative review. *International Journal of Nursing Studies, 60*, 179–190.

Weberg, D. (2012). Complexity leadership: A healthcare imperative. *Nursing Forum, 47*(4), 268–277.

Wong, C., Cummings, G., & Ducharme, L. (2013). The relationship between nursing leadership and patient outcomes: A systematic review update. *Journal of Nursing Management, 21*, 709–724.

Wong, C., & Laschinger, H. (2013). Authentic leadership, performance, and job satisfaction: The mediating role of empowerment. *Journal of Advanced Nursing, 69*(4), 947–959.

Yukl, G. (2006). *Leadership in organizations* (6th ed.). Upper Saddle River, NJ: Pearson Education.

2

Developing the Role of Leader

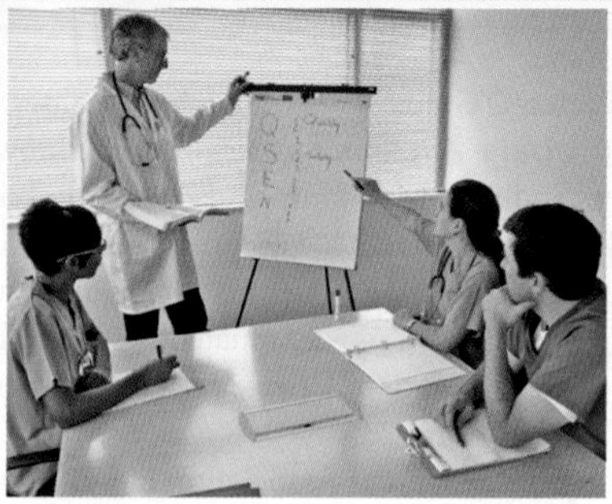

Maureen Cava, Sara Lankshear

This chapter focuses on the role of leadership to the nursing profession. How nursing leadership is critical at the system level to ensure outcomes and drive innovation will be highlighted. A description of the current state of leadership theories and frameworks that students can employ to build their leadership competencies are discussed. How to build your role as a leader will be addressed by using exercises and reflections.

OBJECTIVES

- Describe the importance and value of leadership in nursing.
- Explain some of the key competencies needed for nursing leadership in the twenty-first century.
- Analyze the current leadership theories and frameworks.
- Describe the impact of leadership on nurses, clients, organizations, and the health system.
- Determine opportunities to develop your leadership style and competencies.

TERMS TO KNOW

leadership
leadership framework
leadership styles
outcomes

A CHALLENGE

Lauren is team leader on her unit and has been in this role for less than 2 years. Her manager has been tasked to lead the implementation of nursing huddles as a way of improving nursing team communication. The nursing team is quite diverse in terms of age, years of experience, and areas of expertise. When the nursing huddles were initially introduced, there was a mixed reaction from the staff, with some quite opposed to the idea. Lauren is now faced with the challenge of introducing this change to her colleagues. As the team leader, how should Lauren deal with this situation?

INTRODUCTION

The Importance of Leadership in Nursing

The time has come for nurses to think about nursing in the context of the larger health care system, towards broader and bolder approaches to clients, populations and the system at large. Cummings's (2012, p. 3325) definition of **leadership** in this context is, "being able to see the present for what it is, see the future for what it could be and then take action to close the gap between today's reality and the preferred future of tomorrow." As Villeneuve and MacDonald (2006, p. 84) point out, nurses will be expected to be strong advocates for patients, families, communities, and social issues.

Moving the talk about activism to action will demand strong, visible, and charismatic nurse leaders. The recent opioid crisis, gun violence, and increased awareness of the health disparities of indigenous and new immigrant populations are examples of areas where nurses have and need to continue to raise their voices to advocate for change. They also indicate that these nurses must be "more representative of the Canadian population—both from a gender and ethnic perspective." Villeneuve and MacDonald (2006) further suggest that nurses across the country represent the diversity of Canadians.

For this to occur those nurses in key nursing leadership positions within the national, provincial, and territorial organizations, professional associations and unions, and other health stakeholders, must come together to advance and realize this new vision for nursing leadership.

Health care globally is changing enormously and will require nurses to become agents of change to provide leadership and direction at the micro (e.g., point of care), meso (e.g., professional and organizational) and macro (e.g., policy) levels. Some of the changes include: climate change and environmental issues; technological and scientific advances; labour market expectations; migration; differing disease trends and changes to the burden of disease; demographic shifts; and the commodification and prioritization of health (All-Party Parliamentary Group on Global Health, 2016).

As Daly et al. (2015) indicate, leadership is a highly prized commodity in health care where nurses play a central role to ensure the health system is effective and functional. As Garling (2008; cited in Daly, 2015) highlights, the demands affecting the health care system, and the increasing politicization and scrutiny of health care dollars, underscore the importance of having leaders that are confident, competent, and courageous. As health care organizations deal with fiscal constraints, community scrutiny, and socio-political pressures nursing leadership is of critical importance. Nurses can navigate the complex milieu of health, develop creative and innovative new models of care, and provide courageous and brave voices to ensure that health services are equitable and accessible (Daly, 2015).

Nursing leadership must occur at all levels in the system, from clinical practice, education and administration to research and policy development. The Canadian Nurses Association (2009) identified the importance of effective leadership in affecting nurses' quality of work life, but also its impact on the entire health system. As the International Council of Nurses (ICN, 2013) outlines

in its scope of nursing practice, national nursing associations must support and advocate for nurses to have the necessary competencies, evidence, and peer support to function in all levels of the health system. This will enable the profession to provide competent leadership and innovation in practice.

THE NEW COMPETENCIES FOR NURSE LEADERS

Nurses must develop new competencies and leadership skills both within areas nursing of practice and in collaboration with the other health partners and consumers. Essential skills include emotional intelligence, judgement and decision making, negotiation, critical thinking, people management, complex problem-solving, data management, competence in technology, and political acuity. New leaders will need to be adaptive and creative and bring stakeholders from many fields together to solve the "wicked problems" facing health care today. Identifying and testing new approaches will begin to address the complex challenges that will continue to arise in health care (Solman, 2017). Please refer to Chapter 1 for further discussion on competencies required of nurse leaders.

Nurses at every level must develop these competencies to achieve excellent health outcomes. Chunharas and Davies (2016) propose that a new agenda on leadership in health should encompass the following:
- Interactive leadership, which includes different actors within the health system
- Empowerment of operational leaders to look at new mechanisms and build a learning health system
- Involvement of communities, patients, and families in the heath dialogue
- Increasing evidence and research to understand leadership in different health systems.

Leadership must happen at every level so that nurses can provide quality care and positive outcomes in every practice area where they work. They must lead to improve work processes at the point of care, create new practice models, collaborate with stakeholders to develop policy and legislation that allow nurses to work to full capacity, lead nursing curricula to prepare nurses, translate and apply research and best practice, develop new and innovative models of care, and, finally, have a role on institutional and policy boards where critical health decisions are made (Institute of Medicine, 2011). This report further elaborates that nurse leaders of the future must have skills and knowledge related to population trends and have competencies that may expand what has traditionally been included in nursing curricula. For example, skills and knowledge related to finance, communication, social media, system design, philanthropy, law, and design are now considered important for student and new graduate nurses, as well as experienced nurses who may be engaged in graduate studies or other forms of professional development. Rosser, et al. (2017) report that the growth of effective leadership at all levels of nursing can be achieved through successful collaboration and support for robust connections between education and practice to promote quality care.

Ekstom and Idvall (2015) describe how new registered nurses experience their leadership role within the care team. Being a team leader is challenging for the novice leaders who described feeling inadequate and lacking the necessary experience to lead and not having access to the necessary supports or mentors to assist in their development as leaders. Yet, they also identified the importance of being self-aware, learning from personal experience and the value of team work and effective collaboration in their leadership roles supporting patient care.

Novice leaders may also experience the "imposter phenomenon," self-doubt in one's ability to function adequately in one's role. This may prevent nurses from taking advantage of leadership opportunities because of feelings of inadequacy. Christensen et al. (2016) found that nursing students experienced mild to moderate feelings of imposter phenomenon despite the number of clinical practice hours and amount of preparation. Aubeeluck et al. (2016) suggest that all nurses may experience imposter phenomenon at various stages of their career and this may be a typical reaction in transitioning from student to registered nurse or from one role to another.

To support leadership at all levels of the organization, it is important that student and early-career nurses determine their unique leadership goals and that they also be afforded the support and opportunities to develop leadership competencies.

LEADERSHIP, HEALTH INFORMATICS, AND SOCIAL MEDIA

Health Informatics and social media are two areas in which nurses must take a leadership role to build knowledge and skills. Hussey et al. (2015) suggest that nursing

informatics competencies is one method to support nurses globally an addressing the new health challenges of the future. At a basic level this means having the ability to retrieve the best available evidence, use communication and other technology effectively, and understand information management. The health agenda for nurses can potentially transform health care by addressing population health solutions and care delivery models. The American Organization of Nurse Executives (2015) also reinforces that technology and information management competencies are key to shaping expert nursing leadership and bringing about innovation in health care. With the increased use of social media by nurses, nurse regulators have developed various resources, guidelines and position statements to assist nurses in their practice. The International Nurse Regulator Collaborative (INRC, 2014) identifies common expectations for nurses when using social media and provides six "P"s of social media use:

1. Keep it **positive.**
2. Maintain the **privacy** of others.
3. Keep it **professional.**
4. Keep is **person free**—no specific reference to others.
5. Protect your **professionalism.**
6. Always **pause** before **posting.**

Social media has the potential to become a useful tool for contemporary nurse leaders. The rise of digital literacy, including social media literacy, has exploded with most people using computer platforms and smart mobile devices to connect to Twitter, Facebook, Instagram, YouTube, LinkedIn, and the like. It is a space where you can participate at the individual micro level, or on a much larger macro scale through monitoring tools, data exploration and crowd sourcing (Moorley & Chin, 2016). Social media is allowing more engagement between nurses, patients and other health care providers, as it facilitates engagement of ideas and allows evidence, opinions, expertise, and resources to be shared globally. It is important that student and registered nurses alike focus on developing their digital and interpersonal skills to become social media leaders. Through the use of data and social media listening tools, nurses can begin to understand and gain insight into a variety of issues. By using social media, nurses become visible and accessible role models (Moorley & Chin, 2016). More research is needed to understand how nurses lead in this new digital world, and what the impact is on the health care environment and patient care.

LEADERSHIP STYLES FOR TODAY

Leadership styles will evolve as you develop from a novice to expert nurse and may change based on your area of practice and practice setting (e.g., research, education, policy, administration). Therefore, it is important to be aware of the various leadership styles that you can draw upon.

The nursing literature identifies many leadership styles, which have been categorized by Cummings (2012) as either task-focused or relational. The task-focused style includes autocratic, transactional, instrumental, and laissez-faire leadership, while relational leadership centres more on people and relationships and includes transformational, emotionally intelligent, resonant and participatory leadership. Refer to Chapter 1 for a description of task-focused leadership styles, such as transactional leadership.

TASK-FOCUSED LEADERSHIP STYLES

Autocratic Leadership

An autocratic leader is often described as being close-minded, controlling and seeking power. Typically, these leaders do not consider input from others, and negative reinforcement, blame, and punishment are common (Pullen, 2016). Although sometimes viewed as being a negative leadership style, this approach can be vital in times of crisis when clear direction is required (Bish, 2015; Scully, 2015).

Laissez-faire and Instrumental Leadership

Laissez-faire leadership uses a hands-off approach, allowing others do the leading. Often decisions are left for others and responses are reactive and not proactive (Cope & Murray, 2017). Laissez-fair leaders usually do not make things happen, rather letting things happen and do not usually address problems or assist others to make improvements (Pullen, 2016). Instrumental leadership tends to focus on choosing a strategy and resources to solve a problem. Leaders with this style aim to maintain productivity and complete tasks that are in line with the organization's strategic direction (Hooijberg, 2014).

RELATIONAL LEADERSHIP STYLES

In addition to the transformation leadership style described in Chapter 1, relational leadership styles also include emotional intelligence, resonant and participatory leadership.

Emotional Intelligence Leadership

This type of leader can manage and reflect on their emotions and engage in rational decision making to effect co-operation and change in the work environment by building collaboration and teamwork. Emotionally intelligent leaders are very good at dealing with conflict, can manage the emotional aspects of patient care and staffing, and display confidence when challenging situations arise (Karimi & Rada, 2015). Evidence shows that emotionally intelligent nursing leaders can assist with retaining top talent, promote intraprofessional teamwork, ensure effective use of resources and time, increase team motivation and innovation, and develop trust among nurses (Coladonato, & Manning, 2017).

Resonant Leadership

Brendel and Bennett (2016) describe resonant leadership as being based on mindfulness and emotional intelligence, present in the moment, and open and responsive without judgement. These leaders also use coaching and development of trust, utilizing the attributes of emotional self-awareness, relationship management, socio-political awareness, and self-management (Squires et al. 2010, Laschinger et al. 2014, Boyatzis & McKee, 2006).

Participatory Leadership

This type of leadership considers the opinions of individuals and communities and their skills, experience and knowledge. It is based on respect and aims to optimize the collective strengths of people. The World Health Organization (WHO) has encouraged health care organizations to embrace participatory leadership as a means to strengthen health care systems (WHO, 2016). See Table 2.1 for exemplars of the various leadership styles.

APPROACHES TO LEADERSHIP

Agile Leadership

As organizations deal with changes at an alarming rate, leaders need to develop new skills to succeed. This development results in a new reality of leadership, one that Orski (2017) describes as the "agile leader." The agile leader "has the ability to anticipate the need for change and take effective action in conditions never witnessed" (Orski, 2017, p. 44). The development of agile leaders is based on four principles:

1. Visionary thinking and having the ability to state the reason why.

TABLE 2.1	**Leadership Styles Exemplars**
Leadership Style	**Exemplars/Behaviours**
Task oriented	• Provides clear direction • Little to no consultation with others • Autocratic
Laissez-faire	• Hands over decision making to others • Reactive not proactive • Does little to address the problem
Emotional intelligence	• Builds collaborative teams • Is very self-aware • Employs rational decision making
Resonant	• Open and accessible • Responsive without being judge-mental • Self-aware
Participatory	• Considers the opinions of others • Respectful • Optimizes the collective strengths of others

TABLE 2.2	**Diplomatic Leader: Essential Attributes**
Attributes	**Essential Competencies**
Culture development	• Ensuring diversity within the team, including diversity of opinions and perspectives • Creating a safe environment that values sharing of ideas
Collaboration	• Helping keep the team on track • Active involvement to resolve competing interests or priorities
Connection	• Development of a sense of "we" • Leader viewed as active and committed member of the team
Centredness	• Keeping focused on the objectives • Allowing time for self and team reflection • Celebrating successes
Communication, candour and clarity	• Clear communication that inspires desired behaviour • Providing clear sense of purpose • Honest, open communication to create a sense of camaraderie
Consistency	• Consistency in communication and actions • Demonstration of the importance of the work of the team
Curiosity	• Fostering curiosity through team discussions • Enabling the ability to make choices and adapting as required

Modified from Prestia, A.S. (2017). The art of leadership diplomacy. *Nursing management*, 48(4), 52-55.

2. Having a clear and strategic focus on what is required to achieve the desired goal.
3. Following through by creating the specific steps that need to be taken.
4. Following up through the use of clear metrics to monitor results.

Diplomatic Leadership

Leadership involves the ability to effectively manage teams to achieve desired outcomes. Diversity in teams requires leaders who can identify the synergies within the teams and build upon them to achieve success. Prestia (2017) describes nine essential attributes of a truly diplomatic leader. These are: culture development, collaboration, connection, centredness, clarity, communication, candour, consistency, and curiosity. Team effectiveness, innovation, and success depend on the ability of leaders to diplomatically harness the abilities of each team member towards achieving a common desired goal. See Table 2.2 for examples of the essential attributes of a diplomatic leader

Embodied Leadership

This is an evolving new approach to leadership described by Brendel and Bennett (2016) where individuals learn ways to deepen awareness of the mind and body as an

interdependent system to remain grounded, engaged, and open. This can then build resilience and resourcefulness and potentially improve relationships in complex environments. They further elaborate that if leaders are operating from habit and *not* listening to their mind and body, their actions may be inauthentic and disconnected from their intentions. This model of leadership may provide a deeper human connection with teams and address some of the challenges in the health care environment.

Shared Leadership

James (2011) suggests that rather being centralized at the top, there is a need for leaders to be distributed within and across all levels of the organization. This requires people to see themselves as leaders despite their lack of formal positional power. Informal leaders are those individuals that can see the work that needs to be done, work effectively with others, and influence those with formal positional power to achieve the desired outcomes. Nurses at all levels of the organization have the distinct ability to provide leadership that focuses on enabling best practice that supports optimal patient outcomes and good quality practice settings. This can be achieved by identifying the issues of importance, engaging others, sharing knowledge and expertise, and using shared problem-solving to arrive at solutions. Nurses embody leadership any time they advocate for their patients, their practice setting, and/or their profession. Lusardi (2012) identified the importance of strong clinical leadership at the unit level to apply evidence-based practices to support nursing practice.

EXERCISE 2.1

1. What is your definition of leadership? What do you think are important competencies needed to be a leader in nursing today?
2. Begin to reflect on the leadership style that best resembles you.
   a. What qualities or competencies do you have?
   b. What qualities or competencies do you need to further develop?

THE IMPACT OF LEADERSHIP

Nursing leadership is essential for improving and sustaining outcomes at the patient, professional, and organizational levels. Nurse researchers have provided a wealth of evidence that supports the impact of leadership.

Patient Outcomes

Wong et al. (2013) conducted a systematic review to examine the relationship between nursing leadership practices and patient outcomes. In this study, a leader was defined a nurse in a formal leadership role at any level of the organization who is involved in the direct supervision of other nurses. Twenty studies were included in the review, which identified a variety of patient satisfaction and patient safety outcomes associated with various leadership styles.

Patient Satisfaction

Leadership was positively associated with patient satisfaction in seven studies, with both relational and transactional leadership styles showed to have a positive association with patient, resident, and/or family satisfaction. Transactional leadership in nursing homes was positively associated with family satisfaction with resident care, in that transactional leaders may provide more direction and clear work expectations regarding care.

Patient Safety Outcomes

Four studies identified the link between transformation and resonant leadership styles and decreased patient mortality. Decreased medication errors, patient falls, incidence of pressure ulcers, and infection rates were associated with positive leadership styles, with a transformational leadership style being the most frequently described.

These findings support the idea that relational leadership styles are associated with positive patient outcomes. The positive relationship between both relational and transactional styles may indicates the benefits of a leadership practices that include elements of different styles in achieving desired outcomes.

Nurse Outcomes

A systematic review conducted by Cummings et al. (2010) included 53 studies that demonstrated the relationship between leadership and nurse-related outcomes within five distinct categories of satisfaction, such as work, role, relationships, health and wellbeing, work environment and effectiveness. Relational focused leadership styles, such as resonant and transformational, were associated with higher nurse satisfaction and higher satisfaction with their leader. Transformational leader styles were associated with higher degrees of organizational commitment and intent to stay, higher overall staff health, and lower reported levels of anxiety, emotional exhaustion, job tension, and stress. Transformation and resonant leadership styles were also associated with higher levels of role clarity, team functioning, and nurse–physician collaboration.

Practice Setting Related Outcomes

Nursing leadership is critical to the ability to deliver high quality patient outcomes, overall unit effectiveness and organizational sustainability (Australian College of Nursing, 2015). Leadership at all levels of the organization plays a key role in the creation and sustainability of healthy work environments. Shirey (2017) described that the leadership practices for creating and sustaining healthy work environments included four themes: quality leadership (e.g., people-focused rather than task-focused styles), relational exchanges (e.g., quality of the relationship between managers and staff), environmental elements (e.g., supportive structures and access to resources), and contextual factors (e.g., organizational culture and climate).

RESEARCH PERSPECTIVE

Resource: Wong, et al. The relationship between nursing leadership and patient outcomes: a systematic review update. *Journal of Nursing Management,* 2013; 21(5); 709–724.

This systematic review included 20 studies that examined the relationship between nursing leadership practices and patient outcomes. The results of the systematic review documented the evidence of a relationship between relational leadership and a variety of positive patient outcomes, although future testing of leadership models that examine the mechanisms of influence on outcomes is warranted.

Implications for Practice
Efforts by organizations and individuals to develop transformational and relational leadership reinforces organizational strategies to improve patient outcomes.

DEVELOPING FUTURE LEADERS

The knowledge, skills and attributes required for effective leadership are multi-faceted and complex. As such, leadership is a skill that does not simply involve formal education, but is developed over time. Nursing students have the opportunity within and outside their nursing education to articulate and identify those skills that will enable them to become nursing leaders of the future. Organizations also have a role to play in identifying and developing potential future leaders.

Role of the Emerging Leader

Individuals who aspire to become nursing leaders need to assume responsibility for their own learning and development through identifying those competencies they require to embark on this leadership journey. Simpson et al., (2011) encourage individuals to engage in reflective learning practices, including journaling, coaching conversations, use of assessment tools (e.g., 360-degree feedback), and building an individualized leadership plan.

Emerging leaders can seek out mentors who are themselves established leaders, and who can be extremely valuable in assisting the future leader to develop their values and learn how to integrate their own personal style into the culture of the workplace or, more broadly, the whole profession. They can also help the future leader begin to develop a stronger sense of self (Simpson et al., 2011).

There are other ways for individuals to enhance their leadership journey. A tangible way is for nurses to develop an action plan for career advancement. This may mean engaging more intentionally in their nursing education through career planning and development, or, if already a registered nurse, looking at higher education courses, such as a masters or doctoral degree program. Leaders may also consider earning certificates in a nursing specialty area. Attending courses, workshops and conferences (e.g., CNSA or other professional conferences) is another way of enhancing your leadership abilities (Pullen, 2016).

Leaders of the future may also seek opportunities to engage new partners in fields such as business, philanthropy, consumer groups, national health associations, and government, as well as capitalize on personal connections and relationships. This involvement will allow nurses' voices across the career continuum to be heard in areas of quality improvement, health promotion, and care coordination See Fig. 2.1.

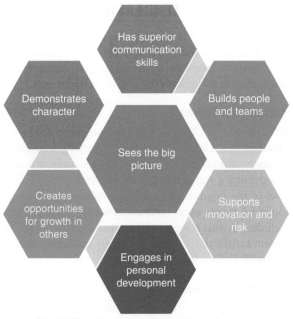

Fig. 2.1 Transformational leadership behaviours.

Role of the Organization

Organizations must also recognize and nurture the development of future nurse leaders. By doing so, they will be rewarded with leaders who can motivate, inspire change, and work with interprofessional colleagues in a shared vision of an environment of empowerment (Scully, 2015). Scully further articulates that "clinical leaders are crucial to the success of patient care initiatives: good leaders produce good care" (p. 443). If organizations identity and nurture future leaders, excellence in patient and family-centred care can be achieved. Some organizations specifically incorporate leadership expectations in every job description, from front-line practitioner to senior management, and use the performance management cycle to reinforce and strengthen leadership behaviours.

Health care organizations can be also successfully recruit and retain leaders to achieve their strategic priorities. Ongoing support in the area of leadership development is vital to organizational effectiveness (Cummings et al., 2010). Organizations that celebrate and communicate leadership accomplishments recognize leadership as a core function of the organization. Projects and accountability for results demonstrates commitment to building internal leadership capacity (Simpson, 2011).

Organizations can also provide education focused on how to foster innovation, creativity and change by developing new leader competencies, including building coalitions, developing intra- and inter-organizational partnerships and networks, and measuring system outcomes. Introducing new leaders to novel techniques to engage patients and families and incorporating feedback and information is increasingly important in changing the health care landscape (Health Workforce Australia, 2012).

Failure to effectively develop and use nursing leaders within and across the health care system will have a negative impact on the system's ability to meet the future demands on health care (Australian College of Nursing, 2015).

EXERCISE 2.2 Reflecting upon the leadership qualities and competencies you identified in Exercise 2.1:
1. Examine the website of one of your practice placements to see what professional development resources and opportunities are available to help nurses build up their leadership competencies.
2. Examine the website of a provincial or national nursing professional association to see what resources they offer for leadership development of their members.

EXAMPLES OF LEADERSHIP DEVELOPMENT FRAMEWORKS

LEADS

LEADS in a Caring Environment framework (LEADS) was developed in 2006 to address the need for a Canadian approach to leadership that would support leaders functioning within an increasingly complex environment with increasingly complex health system challenges. The LEADS framework is built around capabilities, as opposed to competencies, because competency implies the minimum standard required, whereas capacity includes competence but also implies the capacity for more (Dickson, 2008). The LEADS framework consists of the following five capacities:

1. Leads self: Effective leadership is associated with capabilities that can be learned by conscious and intentional effort.
2. Engages others: Without willing, energized, and engaged followers, a leader is unable to accomplish results on any significant scale.
3. Achieves results: Leaders are accountable for managing the resources of the organization to achieve results.
4. Develops coalitions.
5. Systems transformation: Leaders generate the strategic ability to create the changes required to address fiscal, technological, and professional challenges experienced by health care organizations.

Table 2.3 provides a brief description of the LEADS domains and sub capacities.

EXERCISE 2.3 Review the LEADS capacities outlined in Table 2.3 and consider which of the capacities you can begin to develop further and consider how you would work on this in your current program year.

THE IMPACT OF LEADS

The 2014–2016 LEADS Impact Study conducted by Vilches et al. (2016) involved five organizations and aimed to determine how the LEADS framework was being implemented and its associated impacts. Participants described the various effects and impacts for each of the LEADS domains (see Table 2.4). Although the impacts cited here were experienced at an organizational level, these effects are also pertinent to students as they work within interprofessional, collaborative teams.

TABLE 2.3   LEADS Capacities

LEADS	Capabilities within each component
Leads self	1. Self-awareness 2. Manages self 3. Develops self 4. Demonstrates character
Engages others	1. Fosters the development of others 2. Contributes to the creation of a healthy organization 3. Communicates effectively 4. Builds teams
Achieves results	1. Sets direction 2. Strategically aligns decisions with vision, values, and evidence 3. Acts to implement decisions 4. Assesses and evaluates
Develops coalitions	1. Purposefully builds partnerships and networks to create results 2. Mobilizes knowledge 3. Demonstrates a commitment to customers and service 4. Navigates socio-political environments
Systems transformation	1. Demonstrate systems/critical thinking 2. Encourage and support innovation 3. Orient themselves strategically to the future 4. Champion and orchestrate change

From Canadian College of Health Leaders. (2010). Lead self. The root of the matter: What every health leader should know. Retrieved from https://leadersforlife.ca/uploaded/web/Resources/summaries/EN/LEADS_LeadSelf_ExecutiveSummary_EN_2.pdf

THE LEADERSHIP CHALLENGE

Kouzes and Posner (2012) developed The Leadership Challenge as a framework of easily applied, measurable and teachable leadership behaviours. Known worldwide as the most practical model of leadership development, the five leadership practices enable the development of leadership potential in all formal or informal leaders, at any level of an organization (http://www.leadership-challenge.com/about.aspx). The five practices included in the framework are:
1. Model the way.
2. Inspire a shared vision.

TABLE 2.4   LEADS: Effects and Impacts

LEADS Domain	Effects and Impacts
Leads self Engages others Achieves results Develops coalitions Systems transformation	• Provided insights into own characteristics, strengths, and styles. • Increased insights about self and therefore able to communicate more effectively with others. • Having the increased awareness of how to balance personal style with that of others. • Better able to get tasks done by knowing how to identify and call upon resources. • Increased willingness to reach out to and collaborate with others (people and departments). • Increased opportunities to work together to solve a joint challenge or achieve a goal. • Helped reach beyond roles to engage with others.

Modified from Vilches, S., Fenwick, S., Harris, B., Lammi, B. & Racette, R. (2016). Changing health organizations with the LEADS leadership framework: Report of the 2014–2016 LEADS impact study. Ottawa, Canada. Retrieved from https://leadscanada.net/document/1789/Mitacs_LEADS_Summary_Report_EN_2017_FINAL.pdf

3. Challenge the process.
4. Enable others to act.
5. Encourage the heart.

Pullen (2016) applied these leadership practices when describing leadership in nursing practice. Table 2.5 provides exemplars of each of the leadership practices in action that can be used by students and novice nurses as they further develop their leadership practices.

EXERCISE 2.4 Kouze and Posner (2010) state that one of the fundamental truths about leadership is that you must believe that you can have a positive impact on others, and you must believe in yourself. Therefore, for leadership to begin, you must believe you can make a difference. Please reflect about your personal best leadership experience and determine which of the leadership practices and actions you applied and how?

TABLE 2.5 Leadership Practices	
Leadership Practices	**Practices in Action**
Model the way	• Set the example by aligning your actions with your values • Value and respect each person • Demonstrate a commitment to excellence • Inspire your colleagues through your actions
Inspire a shared vision	• Envision an exciting future that will improve nursing practice • Enlist others by tapping into shared passions and aspirations • Celebrate all contributions • Cultivate team spirit by discussing the ideal future with colleagues
Challenge the process	• Take risks • Look for opportunities to reflect upon and improve nursing practice using evidence • Respectfully question "why" things are done in a certain way
Enable others to act	• Foster collaboration within the nursing intraprofessional team and broader interprofessional team • Invest in the development of self and others • Encourage colleagues to participate in decision making
Encourage the heart	• Celebrate contributions and successes • Regularly express your appreciation and respect for the contributions of your colleagues • Inspire others to accept the invitation to leadership

Modified from: Pullen, R.L. Jr. (2016). Leadership in nursing practice. *Nursing Made Incredibly Easy*, 14(3), 26–31; Kouzes, J.M., & Posner, B.Z. (2012). *The leadership challenge: How to make extraordinary things happen in organizations*. 5th ed. San Francisco, CA: Jossey-Bass; Fischer, S.A. (2017). Developing nurses' transformational leadership skills. *Nursing Standard*, 31(51), 54–63.

DOROTHY WYLIE HEALTH LEADERS INSTITUTE (DWHLI)

The Dorothy Wylie Health Leaders Institute (DWHLI) was established in 2001 by nurse leaders Julia Scott, Bev Simpson and Judith Skelton-Green, in response to the pressing need to strengthen leadership competencies for emerging nurses at the point of care. The DWHLI is a four-day residential event with structured virtual follow-up over several months and includes a capstone project. Content areas include The Leadership Challenge, emotional intelligence, project leadership, and leading change.

The emphasis on the capstone project allows for the application of leadership principles to a current challenge or opportunity within the practice setting. This supports the importance of leadership development that is deeply embedded and driven out of the context and the real time challenges experienced by leaders (James, 2011).

In response to the importance of interprofessional collaboration and leadership, the DWHLI expanded in 2005 to include individuals from all health care disciplines, and 2018, the DWHLI partnered with the Canadian Nurses Association (CNA) to provide this unique Canadian leadership program to health care leaders from all disciplines across the country (https://health-leadersinstitute.ca/).

DWHLI has an impact on participants in areas such as increased confidence, seeing themselves as leaders, understanding the language of leadership, increased listening and communication skills, and the development of networking skills (Snell, 2010). Additionally, the importance of an invitation to leadership along with the necessary supports gives confidence to the emerging leader and allows them to see themselves in a different light (Simpson, 2011).

The DWHLI is just one example of the many extracurricular opportunities available for leadership development. Student and novice nurses need to continually keep an eye out for support and resources for ongoing leadership development that may be provided by their organization, professional associations, and/or unions.

? A SOLUTION

To address this scenario, consider the following questions:

1. How can Lauren identify her own leadership style and determine what style or approach would work best to help her achieve success?
2. What **leadership framework** might assist Lauren in accomplishing her goal?
3. How will Lauren know what the impact this will have on staff and patient outcomes?

   For Lauren to be successful, it is vital for her be aware of and reflect upon her own feelings about the nursing huddles as this could impact her ability to effectively lead the project and support her peers. She needs to consider both the advantages and challenges of introducing the nursing huddles, focusing on the impacts for patients and nurses. Lauren would benefit from reviewing the literature on nursing huddles/team communication strategies to have the necessary evidence as a resource when communicating with her colleagues. This will also help in determining the indicators of success that can be used for quality monitoring.

Lauren then needs to determine her own leadership style—does she tend to sit back and let others take the lead, for instance, or does she take charge without consideration of others? As a peer leader, it is important for Lauren to determine what degree of consultation and input she needs to obtain from her peers. An autocratic approach, for example, might not garner the support from them that she needs. Her manager has made it clear that the nursing huddles must be implemented, but the "how" is open for discussion. Do determine the "how" Lauren can draw from the LEADs framework and The Leadership Challenge to guide her actions and approach. Both the frameworks and the principles within them can help Lauren navigate the complexities of leading from within.

To promote teamwork, Lauren may consider asking her manager to support her attending the Dorothy Wylie Health Leadership Institute with another staff member where they can both further the development their leadership skills and the action plan for the implementation of the nursing huddles.

THE EVIDENCE

- Health care globally is changing rapidly, and nurses must be agents of change to provide leadership and direction.
- Nursing leadership must occur at all levels in the system from clinical and educational to administration and policy.
- Health informatics and social media are two areas where nurses need to assume leadership roles to build knowledge and skills.

- Many leadership styles are described in the literature, and nurses need to incorporate multiple styles into their own practice depending on the arena in which they are working.
- Nursing leadership is critical in order for good quality patient outcomes to be realized and for healthy work environments to be sustained.
- Collaboration and intersectional partnerships across all sectors will enable a functional health care system for the future.

✳ NEED TO KNOW NOW

- Leadership styles vary; a combination of leadership styles is required to navigate complex environments.
- There is a need for leaders at all levels.
- Leadership styles have significant impact on patient, nurse, and organizational outcomes.
- Leadership frameworks assist in the identification and development of leadership competencies.

- Nurses need to develop leadership competencies using a great variety of strategies and resources.
- New leadership competencies will be required for nurse to lead in the twenty-first century.
- Students can begin their leadership development the first day of their nursing education.

CHAPTER CHECKLIST

Nursing leadership is essential for improving and sustaining outcomes at the patient, professional, and organizational level.

- There are many leadership styles that can be learned and practised.

- There are many leadership approaches, yet no one style fits all leaders or all scenarios.
- Leadership development is a life-long process.

TIPS FOR BECOMING A LEADER

- Take advantage of all leadership opportunities.
- Take risks and learn from your experience—positive and negative.

- Seek out a mentor and learn from them.

Visit the Evolve website for Suggested Readings, Internet Resources, and additional resources related to the content in this chapter: http://evolve.elsevier.com/Canada/Yoder-Wise/leading/.

REFERENCES

All-Party Parliamentary Group on Global Health. (2016). *Triple Impact: How Developing Nursing will Improve health, Promote Gender Equality and Support Economic Growth.* Retrieved from: http://www.who.int/hrh/com-heeg/digital-APPG_triple-impact.pdf?ua=1.

American Organization of Nurse Executives (AONE). (2015). *AONE Nurse Executive Competencies.* Chicago, IL Retrieved from: http://www.aone.org/resources/nec.pdf.

Aubeeluck, A., Stacey, G., & Stupple, E. J. (2016). Do graduate entry nursing student's experience 'Imposter Phenomenon'? An issue for debate. *Nurse Education in Practice, 19*, 104–106.

Australian College of Nursing. (2015). *Nurse leadership.* Canberra: ACN.

Bish, M. (2015). Leadership and management frameworks and theories. In *Leading and managing health services: An australian perspective* (pp. 16–26). Port Melbourne: Cambridge University Press.

Boyatzis, R., & McKee, A. (2006). Inspiring others through resonant leadership. *Business Strategy Review, 17*(2), 15–19.

Brendel, W., & Bennett, C. (2016). Learning to embody leadership through mindfulness and somatics practice. *Advances in Developing Human Resources, 18*(3), 409–425.

Canadian Nurses Association. (2009). *Nursing Leadership Position Statement.* Retrieved from: https://www.cna-aiic.ca/~/media/cna/page-content/pdf-en/nursing-leadership_position-statement.pdf.

Christensen, M., Aubeeluck, A., Fergusson, D., Craft, J., Knight, J., Wirihana, L., et al. (2016). Do student nurses experience imposter phenomenon? An international comparison of final year undergraduate nursing students readiness for registration. *Journal of Advanced Nursing, 72*(11), 2784–2793.

Chunharas, S., & Davies, D. S. C. (2016). Leadership in health systems: a new agenda for interactive leadership. *Health Systems & Reform, 2*(3), 176–178.

Coladonato, A. R., & Manning, M. L. (2017). Nurse leader emotional intelligence: How does it affect clinical nurse job satisfaction? *Nursing Management, 48*(9), 26–32.

Cope, V., & Murray, M. (2017). Leadership styles in nursing. *Nursing Standard, 31*(43), 61–70. https://doi.org/10.7748/ns.2017.e10836.

Cummings, G. (2012). Editorial: Your leadership style--how are you working to achieve a preferred future? *Journal of Clinical Nursing, 21*(23-24), 3325–3327. https://doi.org/10.1111/j.1365-2702.2012.04290.x.

Cummings, G. G., MacGregor, T., Davey, M., Lee, H., Wong, C. A., Lo, E., et al. (2010). Leadership styles and outcome patterns for the nursing workforce and work environment: a systematic review. *International Journal of Nursing Studies, 47*(3), 363–385.

Daly, J., Jackson, D., Rumsey, M., Patterson, K., & Davidson, P. M. (2015). Building nursing leadership capacity: An Australian snapshot. *Nurse Leader, 13*(5), 36–39.

Dickson, G. (2008). *Genesis of the Leaders for Life Framework.* Vancouver, BC: Health Care Leaders Association of BC. Retrieved from: http://chlnet.ca/wp-content/uploads/leads_genesis.pdf.

Ekström, L., & Idvall, E. (2015). Being a team leader: newly registered nurses relate their experiences. *Journal of Nursing Management, 23*(1), 75–86.

Health Workforce Australia. (2012). *Leadership for the Sustainability of the Healthcare System: Part 1 – A Literature Review*. Adelaide, Australia Retrieved from: http://www.springboard.health.nsw.gov.au/content/uploads/2014/07/leadership-for-sustainability-of-health-sector-literature-review-012012.pdf.

Hooijberg, R. (2014). *Instrumental Leadership: the Nuts and Bolts of Leadership*. Lausanne, Switzerland: International Institute for Management Development. Retrieved from: https://www.imd.org/research/publications/upload/38-Instrumental-leadership.pdf.

Hussey, P., Adams, E., & Shaffer, F. A. (2015). Nursing informatics and leadership, an essential competency for a global priority: eHealth. *Nurse Leader, 13*(5), 52–57.

Institute of Medicine. (2011). *The future of nursing: Leading change, advancing health*. Washington, DC: National Academies Press.

International Council of Nurses (ICN). (2013). *Position Statement: Scope of Nursing Practice*. Retrieved from: http://www.icn.ch/images/stories/documents/publications/position_statements/B07_Scope_Nsg_Practice.pdf.

International Nurse Regulator Collaborative. (2014). *Position Statement: Social Media Use: Common Expectations for Nurses*. Retrieved from: https://www.inrc.com/INCR_Socia_Media_Use.pdf.

James, K. T. (2011). Leadership in context lessons from new leadership theory and current leadership development practice. *Commission on Leadership and Management in the NHS. The King's Fund*. Retrieved from: https://pdfs.semanticscholar.org/3767/091aa22b9020c7a-328534f69719ae6adcab3.pdf.

Karimi, L., & Rada, J. (2015). Emotional intelligence and self-awareness. *Leading and Managing in Health Services, 55*.

Kouzes, J. M., & Posner, B. Z. (2012). *The leadership challenge: How to make extraordinary things happen in organizations* (5th ed.). San Francisco, CA: Jossey-Bass.

Laschinger, H. K. S., Wong, C. A., Cummings, G. G., & Grau, A. L. (2014). Resonant leadership and workplace empowerment: The value of positive organizational cultures in reducing workplace incivility. *Nursing Economics, 32*(1), 5.

Lusardi, P. (2012). So you want to change practice: Recognizing practice issues and channeling those ideas. *Critical Care Nurse, 32*(2), 55–64.

Moorley, C., & Chinn, T. (2016). Developing nursing leadership in social media. *Journal of Advanced Nursing, 72*(3), 514–520. https://doi.org/10.1111/jan.12870.

Orski, K. (2017). What's your agility ability? *Nursing Management, 48*(4), 44–51. https://doi.org/10.1097/01.NUMA.0000511922.75269.6a.

Prestia, A. S. (2017). The art of leadership diplomacy. *Nursing Management, 48*(4), 52–55.

Pullen, R. L. (2016). Leadership in nursing practice. *Nursing Made Incredibly Easy, 14*(3), 26–31. https://doi.org/10.1097/01.NME.0000481442.05288.05.

Rosser, E. A., Scammell, J., Bevan, A., & Hundley, V. A. (2017). Strong leadership: The case for global connections. *Journal of Clinical Nursing, 26*(7/8), 946–955. https://doi.org/10.1111/jocn.13562.

Scully, N. J. (2015). Leadership in nursing: The importance of recognising inherent values and attributes to secure a positive future for the profession. *Collegian, 22*(4), 439–444. https://doi.org/10.1016/j.colegn.2014.09.004.

Shirey, M. R. (2017). Leadership practices for healthy work environments. *Nursing Management, 48*(5), 42–50.

Simpson, B., Green, J. S., & Scott, J. (2011). Promising practices in leadership development. *Nursing Leadership (Toronto, Ont.), 24*(3), 26–38.

Solman, A. (2017). Nursing leadership challenges and opportunities. *Journal of Nursing Management, 25*(6), 405–406. https://doi.org/10.1111/jonm.12507.

Snell, A. (2010). *Synopsis of the Downstream Evaluation Research Study for the Dorothy M. Wylie Nursing and Health Leaders Institutes*. Retrieved from: https://healthleadersinstitute.ca/pdf/DownstreamEvaluationResearchProjectSynopsis.pdf.

Squires, M., Tourangeau, A., Spence Laschinger, H. K., & Doran, D. (2010). The link between leadership and safety outcomes in hospitals. *Journal of Nursing Management, 18*(8), 914–925. https://doi.org/10.1111/j.1365-2834.2010.01181.x.

Vilches, S., Fenwick, S., Harris, B., Lammi, B., & Racette, R. (2016). *Changing health organizations with the LEADS leadership framework: Report of the 2014-2016 LEADS impact study*. Ottawa, Canada Retrieved from: https://leadscanada.net/document/1789/Mitacs_LEADS_Summary_Report_EN_2017_FINAL.pdf.

Villeneuve, M., & MacDonald, J. (2006). Toward 2020: visions for nursing setting the stage for the future. *Canadian Nurse, 102*(5), 22–23.

Wong, C. A., Cummings, G. G., & Ducharme, L. (2013). The relationship between nursing leadership and patient outcomes: a systematic review update. *Journal of Nursing Management, 21*(5), 709–724.

World Health Organization (WHO). (2016). *Open Mindsets: Participatory Leadership for Health*. Retrieved from: http://www.who.int/alliance-hpsr/resources/publications/participatory-leadership/en/.

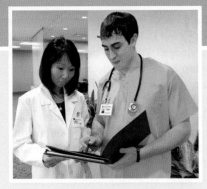

3

Developing the Role of Manager

Lisa Ashley, Wendy A. Gifford, Nancy Lefebre

This chapter identifies key concepts related to the roles of the nurse manager. It describes the different types of nurse manager roles within the Canadian health care environment. It also presents the basic manager functions, illustrates management principles inherent in professional practice, and identifies competencies for the nurse manager. Role development is crucial to forming the right questions to ask in a management or clinical situation to help identify problems and anticipate needs. This chapter provides an overview of practical skills for nurse managers, including the ability to make evidence-informed decisions, manage change, create positive work environments, and manage resources.

OBJECTIVES

- Analyze the roles and functions of a nurse manager within the Canadian health care context.
- Describe the relationship of nurse managers with others.
- Analyze management of health care settings.
- Understand management resource allocation and distribution.
- Identify the behaviours associated with professionalism in the nurse manager's role.

TERMS TO KNOW

healthy work environment
informatics
interactional justice
leader

manager
organizational culture
quality indicators
quality practice environment

role theory
situational leadership

❓ A CHALLENGE

In home health care, staffing presents a unique challenge to point-of-care nurse managers. Flexibility and creativity are needed to develop optimal staffing that ensures client safety while meeting budget expectations. Within the organization where Robert is a senior nurse manager, staff are recruited to work in defined geographical areas and are assigned clients in those specified areas. However, the challenge is that the number of clients to be seen each day varies, depending on the number of clients that are discharged from hospital or referred from community agencies. Unlike hospitals that have a fixed capacity, home health care has "no guaranteed number" of clients.

Therefore all referred clients are admitted and cared for regardless of the pre-existing workload or the number of staff working. Therefore it is particularly hard for Robert to determine the number of staff required each day to ensure safe and effective nursing care with an acceptable workload. Any changes made to staffing must align with the budget while maintaining or improving client and staff satisfaction. The challenges for Robert are *not* to cut positions at the point of care while avoiding unsafe increases in the number of clients assigned to each nurse.

What would you do if you were the nurse manager in this situation?

INTRODUCTION

Chapter 1 provided a general overview of leading and managing. This chapter looks at management from different perspectives. Management theory has undergone numerous changes in the past century. In the early 1900s, the theory of scientific management—a theory based on the idea that there is one best way to accomplish a task—was embraced. Role theory began with management theory, and although changes in health care delivery are no doubt affecting the roles of nurse managers, role theory remains relevant. Conway's (1978) historic definition, "role theory represents a collection of concepts and a variety of hypothetical formulations that predict how actors will perform in a given role, or under what circumstances certain types of behaviours can be expected" (p. 17), is still appropriate.

Early management theories discounted concern for workers' psychological needs and focused mainly on productivity and efficiency. Between 1930 and 1950, management and leadership research centred on physical and psychological "traits" such as gender, height, appearance, and intelligence, and authoritarianism differentiated leaders from non-leaders (House & Aditya, 1997). Much of the current leadership literature in health care focuses on behaviours rather than traits, emphasizing the need for managers to integrate and support clinical staff to use research evidence in their decision-making (Gifford et al., 2007; Gifford et al., 2018; Yuki, 2006).

Participative and humanistic management and leadership theories were the dominant perspectives into the 1970s. These perspectives emphasized human relationships, workers' needs, and staff motivation. Situational leadership theories emerged in the late 1970s and early 1980s and continue to be drawn on today. The premise is that no single "best" leadership style exists, but rather, effective leaders and managers adapt their behaviours based on the situation (i.e., the individual, group, and work context) (Hersey et al., 2008). An example of a situational theory is path-goal theory, which contends that the manager will engage in different types of behaviours, depending on the goals of staff and the organization. Effective managers adapt their behaviours based on the individual and group, in addition to the task, job, or goals that need to be accomplished (Hersey et al., 2008).

What is involved in managing? A self-appraisal might lead a potential nurse manager to ask the following questions: Do I have career goals that include gaining experience and education to become a nurse manager? What specific knowledge, skills, and personal qualities do I need to develop to be most effective in practice? Do I have a mentor who can guide me in this direction? Does the organization I work for have succession planning? Consider also, what is the role of the nurse manager? Some nurse managers would cite decision making and problem solving as major duties, for which maintaining objectivity is sometimes a challenge. Others would cite collaboration, especially with other professional groups and departments, to enhance good quality patient care and outcomes. Truly effective care is the result of efforts by the total health care team. Good collaboration includes honesty, directness, and listening to others' points of view. However, management in nursing is more complex than this.

THE MANAGEMENT ROLE

Management is a generic function that includes similar basic tasks in every discipline and in every society. However, a defining characteristic of all nurse managers is that they must be well grounded in nursing practice. In Canadian health care organizations, nurse managers work primarily in point of care or executive positions. Point-of-care nurse managers, often referred to as *managers*, *supervisors*, or *head nurses*, are individuals in a first-level administrative position who manage staff providing direct client care (Jeans & Rowat, 2005, p. 9). Point-of-care nurse managers are responsible for ensuring nursing standards are met, managing one or more nursing units or areas; the number of people they supervise directly, or their span of control, sometimes exceeds 100 nursing staff. Doran et al. (2004) found that the mean span of control for point-of-care nurse managers in seven Canadian hospitals was 81 staff (ranging from 36 to 258 staff). In contrast, senior nurse managers hold executive positions and are often referred to as *directors*, *administrators*, *vice-presidents*, or *chief nursing officers* (Meyer et al., 2014; O'Brien-Pallas et al., 2004). Senior nurse managers are typically in charge of nursing and/or client care and control a large proportion of an organization's operational budget. Because of the large numbers of nurses employed in health care organizations (nurses frequently exceed 50% of all employees), senior nurse managers often have the largest span of control of all health care administrators.

In 1974, Canadian management consultant Peter Drucker identified the following five basic manager functions:

1. Establishes objectives and goals for each area and communicates them to the persons who are responsible for attaining them.
2. Organizes and analyzes activities, decisions, and relations needed and divides them into manageable tasks.
3. Motivates and communicates with the people responsible for various jobs through teamwork.
4. Analyzes, appraises, and interprets performance and communicates the meaning of measurement tools and their results to staff and superiors.
5. Develops people, including self.

Table 3.1 shows how these basic management functions apply to the nurse manager.

Managers develop initiatives that focus on the individual. Their aim is to enable the person to develop their abilities and strengths to the fullest and to achieve excellence. Thus a manager has a role in helping people develop realistic goals. Goals should be set sufficiently high, yet also be attainable. Active participation, encouragement, and guidance from the manager and the organization are necessary for the person's developmental efforts to be fully productive. Often, nurse managers who are successful in motivating staff provide a work environment that facilitates goal accomplishment and personal satisfaction.

Leadership is an integral part of a manager's role. The nurse manager must possess the qualities of a good leader: knowledge, integrity, ambition, good judgement, courage, stamina, enthusiasm, communication skills, planning skills, and administrative abilities. Although differences between management and leadership roles have long been debated, some overlap exists between management and leadership competencies (see Chapter 1). Moreover, it is widely accepted that managers are in positions of leadership and that leadership is part of the manager's role.

The International Council of Nurses defines leadership as "having a vision, or a clear view of what future state to aim for, and then being able to inspire confidence and motivate others so they share the vision and goals and work together to try to accomplish them" (Shaw, 2007, p. 35). Managers exemplify leadership by holding themselves accountable to set a direction, develop a vision, and communicate the new direction to staff

| TABLE 3.1   Basic Manager Functions and Nurse Manager Functions ||
Basic Manager Functions	Nurse Manager Functions
Establishes and communicates goals and objectives	Delineates objectives and goals for assigned area
	Communicates objectives and goals effectively to staff members whose work will help attain goals
Organizes, analyzes, and divides work into tasks	Assesses and evaluates activities on assigned area
	Makes sound decisions about dividing up daily work activities for staff
Motivates and communicates	Role-models and emphasizes the importance of being a good team player
	Provides positive reinforcement and recognition
Analyzes, appraises, and interprets performance and measurements	Completes performance appraisals of individual staff members
	Communicates results to staff and management
Develops people, including self	Addresses staff development continuously through mentoring and preceptorships
	Integrates evidence-informed decision making into their role, role-models the use of research and clinical best practices, and is involved in research
	Furthers self-development by engaging in reflective practice, attending educational programs, and seeking specialty credentialing

From Drucker, P. F. (1974). *Management tasks, responsibilities and practices*. New York: Harper & Row.oi.

(Canadian Nurses Association, 2009). Managers are uniquely positioned to be leaders in health care delivery and address complexity and change. Complex issues are addressed by planning, budgeting, and setting target goals that promote healthy practice environments to ensure the provision of safe, competent, and ethical care (Canadian Nurses Association, 2017). Managers plan and organize, secure staffing, monitor outcomes, solve problems, and build coalitions with interprofessional colleagues to meet goals. A more detailed comparison of leadership and management roles appears in Chapter 1.

EXERCISE 3.1 In a small group, discuss the services required in a hospice to provide safe, compassionate, and ethical nursing care. As a nurse manager, you have a fixed budget. What factors would you consider in determining appropriate staffing? Consider the acuity of the clients, their needs, and the type of health care providers required, such as nurses, personal support workers, and other allied health care providers. Identify how a manager could contribute to the cost-effectiveness of these services.

The literature abounds with the complexities nurse managers face when leading staff. One example is creating a positive work environment that includes multiple generations of nurses: Baby Boomers, Generation Xers, and Generation Yers (Nexters, Millennials, or the Millennium Generation) (refer to Chapter 2 for further information on these generations). Carver and Candela (2008) discuss the importance of nurse managers having a strategy to increase job satisfaction, decrease nurse turnover, and increase organizational commitment by considering generational differences.

Managers who know how to relate to the different generations can improve the work environment for nurses and the interprofessional team. This idea was confirmed in a Canadian study of acute care nurses conducted by Widger et al. (2007) where data were collected from 8207 registered Ontario nurses and registered practical nurses made up of Baby Boomers, Generations Xers, and Generation Yers. Although Baby Boomer nurses showed a high degree of job satisfaction, Generation X and Y nurses did not. The study suggested that if nurse managers want to be more successful in establishing job satisfaction in younger generations, they must consider the following:

1. Creating a shared governance structure in which nurses are encouraged to make decisions
2. Providing opportunities for self-scheduling.
3. Providing opportunities for career development as well as supporting education.

The nurse manager is the "environmentalist" of the unit. In other words, the nurse manager is always assessing the context and work environment in which practice occurs and is responsible for creating and sustaining a healthy work environment for the delivery of safe patient care (a function that requires innovation and adaptability). Quality practice environments are practice settings that promote healthy work environments, maximize the health and well-being of nurses and clients, focus on client centred care, and organizational and system performance (Canadian Nurses Association & Canadian Federation of Nurses Unions, 2014a; 2014b; 2014c). Evidence-informed transformational leadership practices help nurse managers create healthy work environments (MacPhee & Bouthilette, 2008). These practices include:

1. Building relationships and trust.
2. Creating an empowering work environment.
3. Creating an environment that supports knowledge development and integration.
4. Leading and sustaining change.
5. Balancing competing values and priorities.

In today's health care environments—which are often riddled with high ambiguity, uncertainty, and complexity—a manager must be concerned with relationships to be successful in day-to-day operations. Building relationships and trust is foundational to a healthy work environment and quality patient care. A visible and credible point-of-care nurse manager who builds trust and positive relationships with staff can improve morale and staff motivation while increasing the quality of patient care (Jeans & Rowat, 2005). Respect for the worth of others and fairness are key components of trust (Mishra & Spreitzer, 1998). Canadian researchers have shown that when nurses feel respected, they have higher trust in management, higher job satisfaction, lower emotional exhaustion, and higher ratings of quality of care (Laschinger, 2004). Transformational leadership practices of managers have been shown to improve patient care and retention of new nurses, whereas abusive leadership leads to poorer quality of care and strong intention to leave for early career nurses (Lavoie-Tremblay et al., 2015).

Through their role, nurse managers help staff develop their abilities and strengths fully to achieve excellence in client care. Nurse managers who build relationships and trust through their interactions with staff foster work environments that empower staff, increase motivation to succeed, and improve work effectiveness and performance (Regan et al., 2015; Gifford et al., 2018).

Management Competencies

What constitutes good management in nursing? What competencies are required for nurse managers? These questions continue to challenge the profession. They are also particularly salient today, as nurse leaders increasingly contribute to the development of the health care system through their influence on practice, policies, and quality work environments. Although the nurse manager's role is important to the integrity of Canadian health care, a number of factors affect the nurse manager's ability to acquire and maintain the necessary skills and competencies. For example, a nurse manager cannot fulfill their role without a supportive work environment, clear and reasonable expectations, a reasonable workload, and access to ongoing education programs and mentorship. Udod et al. (2017) found that working with limited resources, responding to continuous change, and senior management's disconnection from practice were role stressors, whereas planful problem solving, reframing situations, and having social supports were coping strategies.

According to the literature, the following competencies are important to nurse managers: interpersonal skills, collaboration expertise, analytical thinking, seeing the big picture, resource management, information technology, awareness of the political arena and knowledge and skills in the areas of clinical practice and overall leadership (Jeans & Rowat, 2005; Gifford et al., 2018). To understand the competencies required for nurse managers, the Canadian Nurses Association (CNA) commissioned a nationwide study that included interviews and surveys with 629 senior nurse managers, point-of-care nurse managers, and staff nurses (Jeans & Rowat, 2005). The top six competencies for nurse managers were as follows:

1. Accountability for professional practice.
2. Verbal communication.
3. Team-building skills.
4. Leadership skills.
5. Conflict resolution.
6. Knowledge of ethical and legal issues (Jeans & Rowat, 2005).

EVIDENCE-INFORMED DECISION MAKING

The responsibility of nurse managers also includes active participation in research and facilitating the use of research in their own administrative practices and in staff's clinical practice. National policies clearly articulate that nurses must use research evidence in their decision making to ensure high-quality care and positive outcomes for clients (Canadian Nurses Association, 2010). As part of ongoing quality improvement, nurse managers have a fundamental role in helping staff use research evidence in their clinical practice. When managers are involved in quality and safety improvement initiatives, the success of those initiatives is higher than when managers are not involved (Fleiszer et al, 2016; Ovretveit, 2005). Nurse managers can help staff use research evidence in their practice decision making by valuing research, role modelling, providing encouragement, ensuring policies are based on research and are up to date, and monitoring practice and client outcomes (Gifford et al., 2018; Gifford et al., 2017).

Through collaboration with nurse researchers and academic institutes, nurse managers are in a strategic position to participate in research and identify priority gaps in care that could be examined through nursing research. When nurses participate in research, they are more likely to value and subsequently use research findings in their own practice (Black et al., 2015; Tranmer et al., 2002).

Nurse managers also have a responsibility to use research in their own management decision making. Evidence-informed management reflects the application of empirical research evidence and other forms of evidence in everyday management decision making. Interdisciplinary work is being done in Canada to develop strategies to support evidence-informed management (Canadian Health Services Research Foundation, 2007; Lavis et al., 2015; Marquez et al., 2018). For evidence-informed management to occur, nurse managers require access to research findings as well as to process and outcome data from their own organization. Health care informatics—the use of technology and information systems to support improvements in client care and health care administration—is a powerful tool that nurse managers can use to access research related to their own management practice (see "Informatics" later in the chapter).

EXERCISE 3.2 In your current area of work, speak to a nurse manager and staff nurse and identify the type of health care informatics being used. How is the data being collected? How is the data being used within the clinical area? Brainstorm how data might be used more effectively to improve person-centred care.

MENTORING

A manager is also concerned about preparing successors. Cherry and Jacob (2008) include the role of mentoring as another that nurses in leadership and management positions must embrace. Mentoring has been defined as "an intense interpersonal exchange between a senior experienced colleague (mentor) and a less experienced junior colleague (protégé) in which the mentor provides support, direction, and feedback regarding career plans and personal development" (Russell & Adams, 1997, p. 2). Mentoring is a voluntary, interactive, mutually beneficial, and multi-faceted relationship that assists staff with setting realistic, attainable goals (McNamara et al. 2014; Cherry & Jacob, 2008; CNA, 2004). A meta-analysis of 43 studies on mentoring in diverse settings, including health care, found that individuals who had been mentored had higher career and job satisfaction, had stronger intentions to stay with an organization, and were more likely to be committed to their career, compared with individuals who had not been mentored (Allen et al., 2004).

Mentorship is critical for preparing new leaders and is a key component of career planning and professional development that has a positive impact on job satisfaction and the retention of staff (Cooper & Wheeler, 2010; Cummings et al., 2008). Through mentoring, nurse managers can boost staff self-confidence, helping staff gain professional satisfaction when they reach their goals. Nurse managers give clinical guidance to their staff, and they can be instrumental in assisting them with their present work and their career development.

ORGANIZATIONAL CULTURE

Managers play a key role in shaping and nurturing organizational climate and culture (Aarons & Sawitzky, 2006; Aarons et al., 2014). They do this by providing clarity for staff about the organization's vision and mission, its values, and desired culture. The role of the nurse manager models behaviours that are consistent and aligned with the culture. Engaging nurses in decision making and designing changes that impact their work and working environments are additional ways nurse managers shape culture and support nurses' involvement.

In the ever-changing environment of health care, nurse managers need to understand the organizational culture of their work environment and how it supports their workplace's mission and goals. Organizational culture can be described as the implicit knowledge or values and beliefs within the organization that reflect the norms and traditions of the organization. Organizational culture is discussed in more detail in Chapter 10. Respect is a moral principle that implies valuing another person's dignity and worth, and in organizational theory it is a core value of organizational culture. In a random sample of 500 staff nurses working in Ontario teaching hospitals, Laschinger (2004) examined nurses' perceptions of respect. The instruments used addressed interactional justice (the perceived fairness of the quality of interactions by people who are affected by decisions and subsequent outcomes) and included structural empowerment, respect, work pressures, emotional exhaustion, and work effectiveness. In a 52% response rate, 280 questionnaires were returned. The results revealed that the nurses did not consider that their managers shared information about imminent changes in their work environment or showed compassion for the nurses' responses to the changes. The study highlighted the importance of a positive organizational culture and good interpersonal relationships between managers and staff for nurses to feel respected and supported in their work environment.

DAY-TO-DAY MANAGEMENT CHALLENGES

Nurse managers who meet day-to-day management challenges must be able to balance three sources of demand: client needs, staff needs, and upper management requests. They have to both ensure that staff members have opportunities to provide upper management with input regarding changes that affect them, and make unit and staff needs known to upper management (CNA, 2017). Consumers of health care services today are much better educated and accustomed to providing input into decisions that affect them. Nurse managers must respect the persons' and families' requests yet maintain care in the broad context of safety and efficiency. Staff members need recognition and independence when carrying out their roles and responsibilities. Nurse managers need to have a sense of when to relinquish control, thus allowing decision making at the point of care.

Nurse managers must be perceived as credible in the areas they manage. A critical factor in being an excellent nurse manager is understanding how to make decisions that ensure optimal client outcomes, involve persons and families in the plan of care, and allocate resources in a fair and ethical manner. Sometimes, decisions are made to meet one important client-care need at the expense of another. That is an important message to convey to staff.

> **EXERCISE 3.3** Select a nurse manager and a staff nurse follower in one of your clinical areas. Observe them over a certain time (e.g., 2 to 4 hours). Compare the management styles and behaviours they exhibit. Is power shared or centralized? Are interactions positive or negative? What is the nature of their conversations? Is there a link between your observations and the characteristics of managers, leaders, and followers? Review the observed characteristics and behaviours of each nurse: Where were they similar? Where were they different? Describe any times where each nurse demonstrated or used more than one type of characteristic or behaviour.

Workplace violence

Nurse managers continue to be responsible for ensuring the safety of their staff and clients. Workers in high-risk areas, such as the emergency department, require special attention. For nurse managers, "special attention" translates to their staff receiving adequate on-the-job training to recognize, prevent, and effectively intervene in workplace violence. Such training may include effective techniques relating to crisis intervention and handling highly agitated people who may be carrying a weapon. Four types of violence encountered by nurses in the workplace:

1. Worker to worker.
2. Person and family.
3. Personal relationship.
4. Criminal intent (Registered Nurses' Association of Ontario, 2009).

From the point of hiring through to a potential disciplinary process, nurse managers have a responsibility to assess employees and the workplace to help avert violence and the conditions that lead to it. Senior nurse managers are ultimately responsible for promoting and supporting a workplace free of violence; however, point-of-care managers must have the knowledge and competencies to prevent, identify, and respond to potential and actual workplace violence (Canadian Nurses Association & Canadian Federation of Nurses Unions, 2014). Refer to Chapter 26 for further information on this topic.

MANAGING HEALTH CARE SETTINGS

Managing health care settings is always challenging for nurse managers, and the current nursing shortage has made the challenge paramount. Nurse managers are key in creating and maintaining a healthy work environment that keeps stress to a minimum, so that the staff can achieve optimal work satisfaction. However, to be effective, nurse managers must also be able to reduce their own stress in the work environment. (See Research Perspective box.)

In Canada and the United States, professional organizations are speaking out about the need to create work environments that are more conducive to nurses providing safer client care (Canadian Nurses Association & Canadian Federation of Nurses Unions, 2014; Registered Nurses' Association of Ontario, 2013). For this to happen, change is required from those in leadership roles, beginning with top-level senior managers and filtering through the hierarchy to point-of-care unit managers. Five management practices have been found to be effective when instituting change in complex organizations:

1. Managing the change process actively.
2. Balancing the tension between efficiency and reliability.
3. Creating a learning environment.
4. Creating and sustaining trust.
5. Involving the workers in the work redesign and the workflow decision making.

Staff members often look to the nurse manager to lead them in addressing workplace issues with higher levels of senior management. To do this, the nurse manager must address power sources and define power-based strategies in the work environment, such as organizing other nurse managers with similar concerns. They must also effectively influence the power holders so that needed change can occur. It is essential for nurse managers to ensure that staff members have an opportunity to provide feedback to senior management and simultaneously advocate for staff needs. In their interviews of 24 nurse leaders, Antrobus and Kitson (1999) found that effective nurse leaders act as interpreters and translators for the macro issues of senior organizational decision makers and the micro issues of practice. For example, point-of-care managers translate staff issues (such as workload) into language and priorities that are understood by senior management (such as costs and client safety). They also interpret senior management decisions and then translate them into language and actions that are meaningful to staff (such as staffing and scheduling). Through this process, effective nurse managers position issues and concerns in ways that are meaningful to the audience they are targeting, be it point-of-care staff, senior managers, or organizational decision makers. Refer to Chapter 19 for an in-depth discussion on leading change.

Staff members also look to the nurse manager to lead them in ethical, value-based management. The nurse manager's commitment to the mission and vision of the organization must be demonstrated in everyday behaviour, not merely recited on special occasions. This ongoing commitment lends stability in a time of constant change. In other words, although the strategies and approaches to address an issue may change, the core values remain the same, and the actions and decisions of the nurse manager must reflect the mission and vision of the organization. Therefore the nurse manager must understand how the work of the unit supports the mission, values, and goals of the organization. Without this understanding, which is almost palpable, staff nurses may be sceptical about the nurse manager's commitment to the organization and to them. Nurse managers must translate their commitment so that staff know they are valued in accomplishing the work of the unit that furthers the mission of the organization. One way of demonstrating that employees are valued is through recognition. Recognizing staff's efforts is part of effective management practice (Yuki, 2006). Employees who have exceeded expectations in meeting the needs of the client, department, or institution deserve recognition. Recognition may occur in many forms, for example, personal memos or "Bravo Cards" that acknowledge communication, performance, personal leadership, respect, teamwork, or staff's efforts to implement best practices.

RESEARCH PERSPECTIVE

Resource: Shirey, M.R., Ebright, P.R., & McDaniel, A.M. (2013). Nurse manager cognitive decision-making amidst stress and work. *Journal of Nursing Management, 21*(1), 17–30.

Through a qualitative, descriptive study, Shirey et al. (2013) looked at the decision-making processes that nurse managers use to address stressful situations amidst complexity in the workplace. Twenty-one nurse managers from three US acute care hospitals were interviewed using a "Critical Decision Method" where managers were asked to recollect one difficult situation that provided the focus for the interview and analysis to capture factors that influenced their decision making. Three sub-themes highlighting expert-novice differences guided nurse managers' decision making amidst stress and work complexity:

1. Self-reflective questions guide nurse manager cognitive decision making: Only the two most experienced nurse managers were found to challenge assumptions and expectations and seek clarification on "Why are we doing this?"
2. Salient factors influence cognitive decision making: Although all nurse managers "were alert to environmental cues," only the more experienced ones were able to assess those cues and look at synergies to understand the situation they were immersed in.
3. Effects of stress on nurse manager cognitive decision making: The negative effects of stress on work-related

decision making was reported by all nurse managers and included inattention to detail, worry about making errors, and command/control leadership "do as I say" leadership tactics.

Although all of the managers loved their jobs, they did feel a work–life imbalance, and although more studies are needed pertaining to stress in nurse managers, this study supports the need that other studies have found—that is, to re-examine and redesign the nurse manager position, which is crucial to their contributions to the overall organization.

Implications for Practice

The findings of the study, as in earlier work by Shirey et al. (2008) suggests that nurse managers' experience in the role, the organizational context, and situation factors impact decision-making processes. Nurse managers use a series of self-reflective questions to guide their decision-making processes in stressful situations. The stress that nurse managers feel may not only affect their physical well-being, but also their family life. Several other studies (i.e., Cummings, 2013) have shown similar results, and the nursing profession needs to address the study findings and develop concrete plans that reduce nurse manager stress. Nurse managers are not expendable, and nursing needs to re-examine and develop mechanisms that reduce the stress in these essential management leaders.

> **EXERCISE 3.4** In your organization you have been charged with establishing a recognition program for the staff members who gave endless hours to their community during a crisis situation. Speak to managers within your organization to see how they would approach establishing this recognition program. What resources would you need, and where would you go to seek the needed resources? How would you want to be recognized in a similar situation?

MANAGING RESOURCES

Many of the concepts inherent in managing resources are addressed in depth elsewhere in this book, but the key point is that the nurse manager must manage resources and integrate these efforts with others. The practice settings of tomorrow will no doubt continue to include in-hospital care; however, numerous innovative practice models operating from a community-based framework are emerging. Predictors of positive outcomes for quality patient care include:

1. All-care settings where clients receive comprehensive interprofessional care.
2. Precise outcome-oriented quality assurance processes, such as critical pathways.
3. Concerted efforts to control spiralling health care costs by ensuring the provision of effective evidence-informed health care.

Other practice models, differentiated practice, shared governance, and restructured work environments make use of all levels of health care personnel.

The nurse manager is responsible for managing all resources designated to the unit of care. This includes all personnel, health care providers, and others, under the nurse manager's span of control (see also Chapter 10). Delegation and interdisciplinary collaboration are essential to the nurse manager's role and are covered in Chapter 27. The wise nurse manager quickly determines that a unit must function economically and, in so doing, realizes that many opportunities exist to reshape how nursing is delivered. Sare and Ogilvie (2010) have envisioned nursing in the twenty-first century based on a business paradigm with the goal of empowering the profession. Nurse managers also act as EntrepreNurses and innovation agents of health care. The EntrepreNurse is someone who trailblazes innovation and leadership by embracing new ideas, models

of care, and technology, both within the health system and adjacent businesses. Nurse managers, together with nurses, represent the largest segment of health care workers and are uniquely qualified to be innovation activators, influencers, disrupters, designers, collaborators, and scalers. They can lead the way as new solutions are identified and introduced into health systems. Sare and Ogilvie suggested combining existing nursing theories with business theories to depict the nurse as a change agent in health care. For Sare and Ogilvie, nurses must know and be able to apply fundamental business practices to take a stronger position within their organizations. Why are business theories important to the role of the nurse manager? The answer is simple yet germane: because many tenets of business theories, such as management, leadership, personnel, and systems, are inherent in the role of the nurse manager.

Budget and personnel have always been considered critical resources. However, as technology improves, informatics must be integrated with budget and personnel as a critical resource element. Basing practice on research findings (evidence-informed care), networking with other nurse managers, sharing concerns and difficulties, and being willing to step outside of tradition, can assist future nurse managers in decisions about resource use.

INFORMATICS

Informatics in health care is constantly changing and growing. Much technology and many systems are available to health care organizations to assist in improvements. Electronic medical records give quick and ready access to current and retrospective clinical patient data. Electronic patient classification systems allow managers to better measure the acuity of nursing areas, as well as assist in budget planning and the need for resources. New technologies, such as Smart Beds, are being used in some hospital settings; they have computers that do things such as weigh patients, help prevent pneumonia and bed sores, and replace the manual process of documenting patients' vital statistics. Smart Beds have the capacity to collect information for nurses, thus creating real time for nurses to think critically about what to do regarding the data.

The accessibility and use of the Internet facilitate the education of staff, clients, and their families. Nurse managers must stay abreast of, and in touch with, changing technologies in health care, such as Artificial Intelligence, mechanical learning, robotics and chat bots, and be ready to advocate and defend the need for them to make improvements. In addition, managers must role model early adoption of new technology to demonstrate its value to staff. Older generations of nurses (e.g., Baby Boomers) may not have had the same exposure to electronic informatics systems as Generation X and Generation Y nurses, and therefore may have more difficulty adapting to new electronic technologies (for more on technology in nursing, see Chapter 13). Nurse managers have a key role to play in introducing these technologies along with new models of care.

BUDGETS

Budgetary allocations, whether they are related to the number of dollars available to manage a unit or related to full-time equivalent employee formulas, may be the direct responsibility of nurse managers. For highly centralized organizations, only senior managers at the executive level decide on budgetary allocations. Within less hierarchical organizations with "flat" organizational structures and decentralized management decision-making responsibilities, point-of-care nurse managers with responsibilities for client care manage fiscal resources for their designated unit. Nurse managers require business and

---

EXERCISE 3.5 While in your clinical placement, examine the information system used by that health care setting. What type of information system is used? Are paper (hard copy) and computer sources used? What can you assume about the budget, based on the physical appearance of the setting? Does any equipment appear dated? How do the employees (and perhaps volunteers) function? Do they seem motivated? Ask two or three to tell you, in a sentence or two, the purpose (vision and mission) of the organization. Can you readily identify the nurse manager? What does the nurse manager do to manage the three critical resources of personnel, finances, and technological access?

---

financial skills to prepare and justify detailed budgets that reflect the short-term and long-term needs of their unit.

Perhaps the most important aspect of a budget is the provision for a mechanism that allows nurse managers to have some budgetary control, such as decision making at the point of service, which does not require previous hierarchical approval.

QUALITY INDICATORS

The nurse manager is constantly concerned with the quality of care that is being delivered on their unit. Using data to identify nursing's contribution to quality care is an important part of the nurse manager's role and requires reliable and valid nursing-sensitive indicators and outcomes. In the late 1970s, data sets, such as the Universal Minimum Health Data Set and the Discharge Abstract Database (DAD), were developed, but they did not include information specific to nursing care, thereby rendering nurses' contribution to client care and outcomes invisible (Doran et al., 2011). To address this information gap, initiatives have been undertaken in Canada and around the world to develop nursing minimum data sets (NMDSs). For example, the American Nurses Association (ANA) developed the National Database of Nursing Quality Indicators (NDNQI) (www.nursingquality.org). The NDNQI measures are specifically concerned with client safety and aspects of quality of care that may be affected by changes in the delivery of care. The quality indicators (measurable elements of quality that specify the focus of evaluation and documentation) address staff mix and nursing hours for acute care settings, as well as other care components. The NDNQI project is designed to assist health care organizations identify links between nursing care and client outcomes. Participating organizations collect and adhere to certain core measures concerned with quality and outcomes of care. Hospitals are compared with other hospitals across the United States in these measurements. Examples of the core measures are practices associated with acute myocardial infarctions, care for clients with congestive heart failure, and care associated with the treatment of pneumonia.

Work is underway to advance NMDSs and develop core measures of nursing-sensitive indicators for a national nursing report card (for more information, visit http://nhsru.com/publications/toward-a-national-report-card-in-nursing-a-knowledge-synthesis). Nursing-sensitive indicators are a set of generic outcomes relevant for adult populations in acute care, home care, long-term care, and complex continuing care settings, and include, for example, pain, nausea, dyspnea, fatigue, pressure ulcers, and falls (Doran et al., 2011). Databases of nursing-sensitive indicators in Canada include the Health Outcomes for Better Information and Care project in Ontario (HOBIC) and Canada-HOBIC (C-HOBIC), which involves Saskatchewan and Manitoba (http://c-hobic.cna-aiic.ca/about/default_e.aspx).

Nurse managers are constantly concerned with the quality of care that is being delivered on their unit.

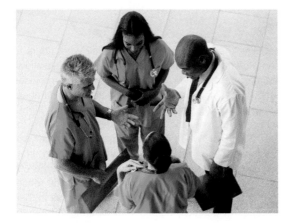

Nurse managers are constantly concerned with the quality of care that is being delivered on their unit.

PROFESSIONALISM

Nurse managers must set examples of professionalism, which include academic preparation, roles and related competencies, and increasing autonomy. Nursing is a self-regulating profession in Canada, which means that provincial and territorial governments delegate to the nursing profession the power to regulate itself in the interest of the public. To this end, the CNA developed the *Code of Ethics for Registered Nurses* (CNA, 2017), which articulates the specific values and ethical responsibilities expected of registered nurses in Canada. The code of ethics serves as a framework through which nurse managers can understand nursing's accountability to those who receive care and advocate for quality work environments

that enable the provision of safe, compassionate, and ethical care (CNA, 2008). Professional nursing within an ethical framework also involves endeavouring to address broad aspects of social justice that are associated with health and well-being. For example, a nurse manager's professional philosophy should include patient rights. The primary values within the code of ethics that support patient rights include preserving dignity, promoting and respecting informed decision making, and maintaining privacy and confidentiality (CNA, 2008).

> **EXERCISE 3.6** Consider this work situation: Mr. Jafri, a client who had foot surgery 3 days ago, has asked Daniel, a novice nurse on a surgical orthopedic unit, several times during his 12-hour day shift for some medication for pain. Daniel's assessment of Mr. Jafri leads him to believe that he is not experiencing that much pain. Although the client does have an oral medication order for pain, Daniel independently decides to administer a placebo by subcutaneous injection and documents his medication intervention. Mr. Jafri does not receive any pain relief from this subcutaneous medication. When Daniel is relieved by the 12-hour night nurse, Daniel, gives them a report of his intervention concerning Mr. Jafri's pain. The following morning, the night nurse reports Daniel's medication intervention to you, the nurse manager. If you were the nurse manager how would you address Daniel's behaviour? What would you do? What resources would you use to handle Daniel's behaviour? How would you demonstrate professionalism?

Professionalism is all-encompassing; the way a manager interacts with personnel, other disciplines, clients, and families reflects a professional philosophy. Professional nurses are ethically and legally accountable for the standards of practice and nursing actions delegated to others. Conveying high standards, holding others accountable, and shaping the future of nursing for a group of health care providers are inherent behaviours in the role of a nurse manager.

Nurse managers are the closest link to direct care staff. They set the tone, create the work environment, and manage, while providing professional role-modelling to develop future managers and leaders (see Theory Box for two approaches to motivating employees). They influence staff members' decisions to stay or leave. Nurse managers are critical to the success of any health care setting.

THEORY BOX

Theory X/Theory Y

Theory/Contributor	Key Idea	Application to Practice
Skelton-Green, J., Simpson, B., Scott, J.	Leading self	Be knowledgeable about the care delivery models in your work setting, best practices, policies and procedures, and scopes of practice for your team. Consider your values and ethics and how they relate to your work environment.
	Leading teams	To effect change it is important to exemplify passion, conviction and confidence in your teams.
	Leading change	Provide as much information as you can, and if you are not able to, explain why. Provide the support and resources to empower others to lead and accept change. Build relationships and cultivate stakeholders.

From Skelton-Green, J., Simpson, B., Scott, J. (2007). An integrated approach to change leadership. *Canadian Journal of Nursing Leadership, 20*(3), 1–15.

A SOLUTION

As senior nurse manager, Robert looked at the current processes and developed a plan to allow for maximum flexibility of nursing staff, maintenance of patient quality care and continuity, and promotion of staff satisfaction. His solution was to create a staffing model that allowed flexibility in the staffing of geographical areas and self-scheduling, while maintaining an adequate mix of full-time and part-time staff.

The geographically based approach allowed nurse managers to assign nurses to specific areas and use a "group practice" or team model approach to care of the client. Through group practice, nurses became familiar with a distinct physical area and built their knowledge of locations and resources that reduced travel time between clients. Having flexibility in the staffing of geographical areas meant that the nurse managers could assign nurses outside their prescribed geographical areas or receive staff into prescribed geographical areas as the demand for services increased or decreased in different areas. However, this approach was only possible because nurses and nurse managers from different regions worked together as a team, collaborating and accepting accountability to meet the care needs of the population.

The foundation of this model is nurse self-scheduling and using all nurses to their full scopes of practice. Self-scheduling means nurses can select their work hours to accommodate their and their family's needs, while allowing a balance between work and home. This provides greater job satisfaction while ensuring adequate numbers of licensed nursing staff each day. The use of the "right" number of full-time and part-time staff also allows for greater flexibility; when client numbers go up, staff can be increased, and when client numbers go down, staff can work outside their geographical area, take time off, or share a reduced workload with other staff. The model is further complemented by using a mix of nurses to their full scopes of practice; nurses with differing competencies are able to manage their own caseload or share appropriate clients with other nurses as needed.

The changes Robert made allowed for the full use of all nursing staff and improved job satisfaction and an appreciation of staff for the skills and knowledge each group brings to the care team. Since implementing the new staffing model, staff nurses and nurse managers have reported increased job satisfaction, greater stability and continuity in their workload, and a better work–life balance.

Would this be a suitable approach for you? Why or why not? What might you do differently?

THE EVIDENCE

Hall et al. (2008) conducted a quasi-experimental study in Ontario to understand how interventions designed to improve nursing work environments impact client and nurse outcomes. The study involved 16 nurse managers, 1137 patients, and 296 observations by registered nurses. Data were collected pre-intervention and 3 and 6 months postintervention. Interventions included enhancing documentation, improving linen supply, increasing availability of stock medications, and improving communication related to patient transfers and basic equipment needs for staff. The most significant finding was an increase in how nursing staff felt about the quality of their work life. After participation in the intervention, nurses reported higher perceptions of their work and work environment. Patients' perceptions of the quality of care also increased significantly as a result of the change interventions. Study results made it apparent that nurse managers can positively influence nursing staff's perceptions of nurses' work environments. In addition, positively impacting nursing staff increases patients' perceptions of quality of care.

✳ NEED TO KNOW NOW

1. Understand and respect the individual needs of the different generations of nurses working together in health care settings.
2. Engage in a unit-based, shared-governance council inclusive of staff, allowing for empowerment.
3. Provide professional development opportunities and support for furthering education.
4. Encourage, support, and model the use of evidence-informed practice.
5. Participate in the rewarding and recognition of nursing staff.

CHAPTER CHECKLIST

The role of the nurse manager is multi-faceted and complex. Integrating clinical concerns with management functions, synthesizing leadership abilities with management requirements, and addressing human concerns while maintaining efficiency are the challenges facing the nurse manager. Thus, the nurse manager's role is to ensure effective operation of a defined area, contribute to the overall mission of the organization, and create an environment that supports quality of care for persons and their families.

The basic functions of a manager are as follows:

- Establishes and communicates goals and objectives.
- Organizes, analyzes, and divides work into tasks.
- Motivates and communicates.
- Analyzes, appraises, and interprets performance and measurements.
- Develops people, including self.
  A nurse manager is responsible for the following:
- Relationships with those above themselves, peers, and staff for whom they are accountable.
- Professionalism.
- Management of resources.
- Application of evidence-informed decision making.
- Role-modelling.

TIPS FOR IMPLEMENTING THE ROLE OF NURSE MANAGER

Aspects of the role of the nurse manager include being a leader as well as a follower. To be effective in the role, the nurse manager must be dedicated to the following:

- A management philosophy that values people.
- A commitment to person-focused quality of care outcomes that include evidence-informed processes and health outcomes of the client.
- The desire for ongoing learning about health care change and its effect on the nurse manager's role and functions.

Visit the Evolve website for Suggested Readings, Internet Resources, and additional resources related to the content in this chapter: http://evolve.elsevier.com/Canada/Yoder-Wise/leading/.

REFERENCES

Aarons, G. A., Ehrhart, M. G., Farahnak, L. R., & Sklar, M. (2014). Aligning leadership across systems and organizations to develop a strategic climate for evidence-based practice implementation. *Annual Review of Public Health, 35*, 19.

Aarons, G. A., & Sawitzky, A. C. (2006). Organizational culture and climate and mental health provider attitudes toward evidence-based practice. *Psychological Services, 3*(1), 61.

Allen, T. D., Eby, L. T., Poteet, M. L., et al. (2004). Career benefits associated with mentoring for protégés: A metaanalysis. *Journal of Applied Psychology, 89*, 127–136. https://doi.org/10.1037/0021-9010.89.1.127.

Antrobus, S., & Kitson, A. (1999). Nursing leadership: Influencing and shaping health policy and nursing practice. *Journal of Advanced Nursing, 29*, 746–753. https://doi.org/10.1046/j.1365-2648.1999.00945.x.

Black, A. T., Balneaves, L. G., Garossino, C., Puyat, J. H., & Qian, H. (2015). Promoting evidence-based practice through a research training program for point-of-care clinicians. *Journal of Nursing Administration, 45*(1), 14–20. https://doi.org/10.1097/nna.0000000000000151.

Canadian Health Services Research Foundation. (2007). *Is research working for you? A self-assessment tool and discussion guide for health services management and policy organizations*. Ottawa, ON: Author.

Canadian Nurses Association. (2004). *Achieving excellence in professional practice. A guide to preceptorship and mentorship*. Ottawa. ON.

Canadian Nurses Association. (2009). *Position statement. Nursing leadership*. Ottawa, ON. Available from: https://www.cna-aiic.ca/-/media/cna/page-content/pdf-en/nursing-leadership_position-statement.pdf?la=en&hash=F8CECC6A2D52D8C94EAF939EB3F9D56198EC93C3.

Canadian Nurses Association. (2010). *Evidence-informed decision making and nursing practice: CNA position statement*. http://www.cna-aiic.ca/CNA/documents/pdf/publications/PS113_Evidence_informed_2010_e.pdf.

Canadian Nurses Association. (2017). *2017 Edition code of ethics for registered nurses*. Ottawa. ON Retrieved from: https://cna-aiic.ca/~/media/cna/page-content/pdf-en/code-of-ethics-2017-edition-secure-interactive.pdf?la=en.

Canadian Nurses Association & Canadian Federation of Nurses Unions. (2014a). *Joint position statement—practice environments: maximizing outcomes for clients, nurses and organizations*. Ottawa, ON.

Canadian Nurses Association & Canadian Federation of Nurses Unions. (2014b). *Joint position statement—workplace violence and bullying*. Ottawa, ON.

Canadian Nurses Association & Canadian Federation of Nurses Unions. (2014c). *Joint position statement. Practice environments: maximizing outcomes for clients, nurses and organizations*. Ottawa, ON. Available from: http://cna-aiic.ca/~/media/cna/page-content/pdf-en/practice-environments-maximizing-outcomes-for-clients-nurses-and-organizations_joint-position-statement.pdf.

Carver, L., & Candela, L. (2008). Attaining organizational commitment across different generations of nurses. *Journal of Nursing Management, 16*(8), 984–991.

Cherry, B., & Jacob, S. R. (2008). *Contemporary nursing, issues, trends and management*. St. Louis, MO: Mosby.

Conway, M. E. (1978). Theoretical approaches to the study of roles. In M. E. Hardy, & M. E. Conway (Eds.), *Role theory: Perspectives for health professionals* (pp. 17–28). New York, NY: Appleton-Century-Crofts.

Cooper, M., & Wheeler, M. M. (2010). Building successful mentoring relationships. *Canadian Nurse, 106*(7), 34–35.

Cummings, G. (2013). Nursing leadership and patient outcomes. *Journal of Nursing Management, 21*(5), 707–708.

Cummings, G. G., Olson, K., Hayduk, L., et al. (2008). The relationship between nursing leadership and nurses' job satisfaction in Canadian oncology work environments. *Journal of Nursing Management, 16*(5), 508–518.

Doran, D., McCutcheon, A. S., Evans, M. G., et al. (2004). *Impact of the manager's span of control on leadership and performance*. Ottawa, ON: Canadian Health Services Research Foundation.

Doran, D., Mildon, B., & Clarke, S. (2011). Towards a national report card in nursing: A knowledge synthesis. *Nursing Leadership, 24*, 38–57.

Drucker, P. F. (1974). *Management tasks, responsibilities and practices*. New York, NY: Harper & Row.

Fleiszer, A. R., Semenic, S. E., Ritchie, J. A., Richer, M. C., & Denis, J. L. (2016). A unit-level perspective on the long-term sustainability of a nursing best practice guidelines program: An embedded multiple case study. *International journal of nursing studies, 53*, 204–218.

Gifford, W., Graham, I. D., Ehrhart, M. G., Davies, B. L., & Aarons, G. A. (2017). Ottawa Model of Implementation Leadership and Implementation Leadership Scale: mapping concepts for developing and evaluating theory-based leadership interventions. *Journal of Healthcare Leadership, 9*, 15–23.

Gifford, W. A., Squires, J. E., Angus, D. E., et al. (2018 Accepted). *Managerial Leadership for Research use in Nursing and Allied Health Care Professions: a Systematic Review Implementation Science*.

Gifford, W. A., Davies, B. L., Edwards, N., et al. (2007). Managerial leadership for nurses' use of research evidence: An integrative review of the literature. *Worldviews on Evidence-Based Nursing, 4*, 126–145.

Hall, L. M., Doran, D., & Pink, L. (2008). Outcomes of interventions to improve hospital nursing work environments. *Journal of Nursing Administration, 38*(1), 40–46.

Hersey, P., Blanchard, K. H., & Johnson, D. E. (2008). *Management of organizational behavior: Leading human resources* (9th ed.). Upper Saddle River, NJ: Pearson Prentice Hall.

House, R. J., & Aditya, R. N. (1997). The social scientific study of leadership: Quo vadis? *Journal of Management, 23*, 409–473.

Jeans, M. E., & Rowat, K. M. (2005). *Competencies required of nurse managers.* Ottawa, ON: Canadian Nurses Association.

Laschinger, H. K. (2004). Hospital nurses' perception of respect and organizational justice. *Journal of Nursing Administration, 34*(7–8), 354–363.

Lavis, J. N., Wilson, M. G., Moat, K. A., et al. (2015). Developing and refining the methods for a 'one-stop shop' for research evidence about health systems. *Health Research Policy and Systems, 13*(10). https://doi.org/10.1186/1478-4505-13-10.

Lavoie-Tremblay, M., Fernet, C., Lavigne, G., & Austin, S. (2015). Transformational and abusive leadership practices: impacts on novice nurses, quality of care and intention to leave. *Journal of Advanced Nursing, 72*(3).

MacPhee, M., & Bouthilette, F. (2008). Developing leadership in nurse managers: The British Columbia Nursing Leadership Institute. *Nursing Leadership, 21*, 64–75.

Marquez, C., Johnson, A., Jassemi, S., et al. (2018). Enhancing the uptake of systematic reviews of effects: What is the best format for health care managers and policy-makers? A mixed-methods study. *Implementation Science, 13*(84), 14.

McNamara, Fealy, Casey, et al. (2014). Mentoring, coaching and action learning: Interventions in a national clinical leadership development program. *Journal of clinical nursing, 23.* https://doi.org/10.1111/jocn.12461.

Meyer, R. M., O'Brien-Pallas, L., Doran, D., Streiner, D., Ferguson-Paré, M., & Duffield, C. (2014). Boundary spanning by nurse managers: Effects of managers' characteristics and scope of responsibility on teamwork. *Nursing Leadership, 27*(2), 42–55.

Mishra, A., & Spreitzer, G. (1998). Explaining how survivors respond to downsizing: The roles of trust, empowerment, justice and work redesign. *Academy of Management Review, 23*, 567–588.

O'Brien-Pallas, L., Murphy, G. T., Laschinger, H., et al. (2004). *Survey of employers: Health care organizations' senior nurse managers.* Ottawa, ON: The Nursing Sector Study Corporation.

Ovretveit, J. (2005). Leading improvement. *Journal of Health Organization and Management, 19*, 413–430.

Regan, S., Laschinger, H. K. S., & Wong, C. (2015). The influence of empowerment, authentic leadership, and professional practice environments on nurses' perceived interprofessional collaboration. *Journal of Nursing Management.* https://doi.org/10.1111/jonm.12288. Advance online publication.

Registered Nurses' Association of Ontario. (2009). *Preventing and managing violence in the workplace.* Toronto, ON: Author.

Registered Nurses' Association of Ontario. (2013). *Developing and sustaining nursing leadership.* Toronto, ON: Author.

Russell, J. E. A., & Adams, D. M. (1997). The changing nature of mentoring in organizations: An introduction to the special issue on mentoring in organizations. *Journal of Vocational Behaviour, 51*, 1–14.

Sare, M. V., & Ogilvie, L. A. (2010). *Strategic planning for nurses: change management in health care.* Boston, MA: Jones and Bartlett Publishers.

Shaw, S. (2007). *International council of nurses: nursing leadership.* Oxford: Blackwell.

Shirey, M. R., Ebright, P. R., & McDaniel, A. M. (2008). Sleepless in America: Nurse manager cognitive decision-making amidst s cope with stress and work complexity. *Journal of Nursing Administration Management, 38*(3), 125–131.

Tranmer, J. E., Lochhaus-Gerlach, J., & Lam, M. (2002). The effect of staff nurse participation in a clinical nursing research project on attitude towards, access to, support of and use of research in the acute care setting. *Canadian Journal of Nursing Leadership, 15*, 18–26.

Udod, S. A., Cummings, G., Care, W. D., & Jenkins, M. (2017). Impact of role stressors on the health of nurse managers a Western Canadian context. *Journal of Nursing Administration, 47*(3), 5.

Widger, K., Pye, C., Wilson, B., et al. (2007). Generational differences in acute care nurses. *Nursing Leadership, 20*(1), 49–61.

Yuki, G. A. (2006). *Leadership in organizations* (6th ed.). Upper Saddle River, NJ: Pearson Prentice Hall.

4

Nursing Leadership in Indigenous Health

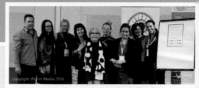

International Alliance of Indigenous Nurses

*R. Lisa Bourque Bearskin, Andrea Kennedy,
Danielle Bourque, Domonique Bourque*

This chapter focuses on nursing leadership when working with Indigenous populations in Canada. It stems from oral teachings of many Indigenous nurses and traditional knowledge holders who speak to the importance of authenticity in life-giving forces from their own experiences, language, and culture as touchstones to uncovering truth and developing leadership when working in diverse First Nations, Inuit, and Métis communities. This chapter provides an overview of Indigenous peoples in Canada, health care service delivery decolonization, Indigenization, and Truth and Reconciliation to prepare nursing leaders for the future.

OBJECTIVES

- Recognize the unique diversity of Indigenous populations in Canada.
- Understand how health care services are delivered to Indigenous populations.
- Describe how cultural safety and humility cultivate authentic nursing leadership relationships with Indigenous individuals, families, communities, and nations.
- Relate nursing leadership to Indigenous health priorities and worldviews.
- Create meaning through an Indigenous Nursing Knowledge perspective.

- Describe how all nurses may engage in leadership through reconciliation.
- Identify Indigenous rights in relation to health as outlined in the United Declaration on the Rights of Indigenous Peoples.
- Understand Indigenous relations in establishing traditional wellness practices.
- Relate the importance of decolonization to nursing practice, leadership, and health care.
- Consider how nurse leaders support Indigenous populations in designing services and programs to meet the diverse needs of Indigenous populations in Canada.

TERMS TO KNOW

colonization	equity	Inuit
cultural humility	First Nations	leadership
cultural safety	Indian Act	Métis
decolonization	Indigenous	reconciliation
deficit-based approach	Indigenous Nursing Leadership	social justice

？ A CHALLENGE

Community health nurses provide and offer a wide variety of programs and services to support, manage, and prevent the prevalence of type II diabetes. In preparation for a community workshop on diabetes, Spencer, the community health nurse working in a Métis settlement, prepares a presentation on best practices in diabetes education. Spencer begins by addressing the high prevalence of type II diabetes in Indigenous communities and focuses on statistics, genetics, and personal lifestyle risk factors. As Spencer continues the presentation, people start to leave. One participant asks Spencer, "How can I eat right if I don't have access to the proper foods?" Spencer is unsure how to respond but suggests eating 5–7 servings of fresh fruit and vegetables is the recommended guideline. Spencer further suggests that healthy grocery shopping tips, such as planning and using coupons, will help.

Knowing that community health nurses play a pivotal role in supporting, managing, and providing culturally relevant diabetes information, what could Spencer do differently to ensure the provision of culturally appropriate health care services where individuals and families feel safe?

If you were the nurse, how might you avoid this medical model approach to mitigate furthering stereotyping of Indigenous peoples?

How can nurses address health indicators specific to Métis settlements?

What other information would have helped Spencer prepare for the presentation on diabetes education to Indigenous communities?

How would cultural humility and cultural safety influence the nursing approach?

INTRODUCTION

This chapter describes how nursing and leadership intertwine with the knowledge and experiences of Indigenous nurses, scholars, and advocates. Such connections reveal a holistic way of being, respecting the central importance of Indigenous populations' health to Indigenous nations and nursing. Contributions by Indigenous nursing embody a spirit of knowledge: a pattern of knowing, being, and doing that is symbiotically and spiritually united. Indigenous nurses' understanding represents the 'sinew' that binds collective knowledge of Indigenous peoples that connect our ancestral past, present, and future (Bourque Bearskin et al., 2016). Indigenous populations in Canada are taking on revitalized leadership roles that build resilient communities, establish relational practice, and liberate women as moral authorities (Kenny & Fraser, 2012). Specific to nursing are the words of the eminent Indigenous nursing leader Jean Goodwill (1975) who stated, "Speaking together is a collective expression of the concerns, thoughts, and aspiration that you hold for further generations of Indigenous peoples in Canada. Our contributions live in the manifestation of alternate approaches to life that come from the original inhabitants of this land" (p. 10) as a means to legitimizing the contribution of Indigenous nurses in Canada and their influence on nursing practice. Over four decades ago, Goodwill initiated a call for action with nursing and government to collectively reduce health disparities and promote

equity for Indigenous populations. Today, this work still resonates in efforts by Indigenous peoples and non-Indigenous allies and is reflected in the United Nations Declaration of Rights of Indigenous Peoples (UNDRIP) (2008) and the Truth and Reconciliation Commission of Canada (TRC) (2015a).

The Canadian Nurses Association (CNA) (2009) defines nursing leadership as an ongoing commitment to positive change within the discipline and for those we serve. All nurses have the capacity for leadership. During this critical time in Canadian history, positive change may be realized by moving forward together in reconciliation with Indigenous populations. CNA and the Canadian Indigenous Nurses Association (CINA) (2016) signed a partnership accord "to advance Indigenous nursing" and promote health equity with Indigenous populations. Nurses are called upon to understand the impact of colonization for all people, and critically appraise entrenched systems that interfere with equity, including marginalization of Indigenous nursing knowledge. A nursing leadership response is rooted in upholding social justice at micro/interpersonal, meso/community, and macro/system levels. This includes skill development related to cultural safety, conflict mediation, human rights and anti-racism, advocacy for cross-jurisdictional health care rights, and sustainable holistic health care services (Truth and Reconciliation Commission of Canada, 2015a). With Indigenous nursing knowledge central, positive change is cultivated through dynamic interplay of education, standards, research, and politics: nursing leadership in Indigenous health is a political act. This chapter will explore three main concepts and principles:

1. Indigenous populations and health
2. Indigenous nursing knowledge and leadership
3. Reconciliation

INDIGENOUS POPULATIONS AND HEALTH

Diverse Indigenous Populations in Canada

In Canada, over 1.6 million people self-identify as Indigenous. As outlined in Section 35 of the 1982 Constitution Act of Canada, First Nations, Inuit, and Métis are terms that reflect current Canadian legislation. However, it is important to recognize each of these distinct groups as unique. Among the Indigenous population in Canada, 58.4% are First Nations peoples (Registered and/or Treaty), 35.1% are Métis peoples, 3.9% are Inuit peoples, and the remaining 2.7% are of other Indigenous identities (Statistics Canada, 2017). The First Nations population who do not hold Treaty status (or are not Registered or non-status) are not accounted for in these statistics due to the definition outlined in the Indian Act and further discussed later in the chapter. In today's context, it is very important for Canadians to know the distinct names of the Nations instead of lumping these distinct groups into one definition.

From a decolonizing perspective, it is important to consider a broader understanding of the term *Indigenous* as follows:

- "Self-identification as Indigenous peoples at the individual level and accepted by the community as their member.
- Historical continuity with pre-colonial and/or pre-settler societies
- Strong link to territories and surrounding natural resources
- Distinct social, economic or political systems
- Distinct language, culture and beliefs
- Form non-dominant groups of society
- Resolve to maintain and reproduce their ancestral environments and systems as distinctive peoples and communities" (United Nations Permanent Forum on Indigenous Issues, n.d. p. 1).

According to the World Health Organization (2007), Indigenous peoples globally have retained social, cultural, economic, and political characteristics distinct from the dominant societies in which they live, representing a rich diversity of spirituality, traditions, and languages. Over 370 million Indigenous peoples are acknowledged as the inheritors, practitioners, and holders of unique cultural ways of relating to other people and their environment, yet they remain among the poorest and most marginalized populations.

Despite experiencing such hardships, Indigenous peoples in Canada remain steadfast in their resurgence and desire to reclaim traditional lands and resources. Specific attention is put on developing meaningful social, economic, and political policies and practice using Indigenous language, methodologies, and traditional knowledge to support the restoration of communities' wellness through Indigenous sovereignty (Manuel & Dierrickson, 2017). Even traditional healing practices have been sustained in their survival since time immemorial. Traditional wellness and healing practices rooted in ancestral knowledge are handed down from generation to generation and improve Indigenous peoples' sense of well-being (Fiedeldey-Van Dijk et al., 2016; Marsh et al., 2018). Specifically, traditional women's teachings and birthing practices (George et al., 2018), water and health revitalization (Bradford et al., 2017), and land-based pedagogies (Redvers, 2016) are considered promising practices that support cultural revitalization and carry a transformative energy and momentum, shifting focus from biomedical to holistic wellness in health care. Strengths of Indigenous peoples' knowledge counters the deficit-based approach that dominates health care assumptions and statistical landscape of numbers and figures.

According to the 2016 Census of Population (Statistics Canada, 2018), several trends point to the revitalization of Indigenous peoples and the corresponding need for nursing to be prepared to work with such diverse populations. Almost 5% of the overall population is Indigenous, with increased self-identification, life expectancy, and relatively higher fertility rates (para 4). Indigenous populations are relatively younger, with rapid growth at four times the rate compared with the non-Indigenous population. Since 2006, there has been a 42.5% increase in Indigenous peoples, with the expected population to exceed 2.5 million within the next 20 years.

Indigenous populations live in urban, rural, and remote settings, with over 600 First Nation communities, 8 Métis settlements, and the Inuit territory of Nunavut; urbanization of this population has been on the rise for decades. Indigenous families live in a variety of settings including multi-generational, homes, with 17.9% of children living with grandparents, almost twice as often as non-Indigenous children; and 34% of children live with a lone parent, compared with 17% of non-Indigenous children. Language is central to Indigenous knowledge and culture, and over the past 10 years there has been a 3.1% resurgence in over 70 Indigenous languages among 260000 speakers. Ongoing barriers include overrepresentation of almost half the children placed in foster care and 20% of Indigenous population living in homes needing major repairs. While educational attainment is on the rise for high school and post-secondary, the Indigenous population still lags behind the non-Indigenous population. Strengths of the Indigenous population must be considered alongside systemic discrimination related to policies and practices of colonization, including the Indian Act.

Historical and Structural Markers of Indigenous Health

Nursing leadership questions surrounding Indigenous knowledge need to be connected to the experiences of colonization, intergenerational historical trauma, identity, displacement, decolonization, equity, and power. First Nations, Inuit, and Métis peoples in Canada continue to be the most legislated, over-researched, and marginalized population in Canada (Logan McCallum, 2017). No other cultural group has seen this level of interference. Such interference continues today in Canada, with neglect of Indigenous knowledge and human rights through deeply entrenched Eurocentric systems. Nurses are called to reflect on their colonial worldview, and how this shapes their interpretation of the nature of being, knowing, and doing. If nurses deny the legitimacy of the Indigenous worldview and the reality of Indigenous history in Canada, they subsequently deny our capacity for human rights and ethical practice with Indigenous peoples.

Over the past 500 years, Indigenous peoples, as the original inhabitants of Canada, have undergone extensive racism through the process of colonization (Paradies, 2016; Reading, 2018). In the pre-contact era prior to the 1500s, Indigenous peoples lived in highly structured societies. In the post-contact era after arrival of European settlers, Indigenous peoples set out to develop strong economic trade deals and respectful relationships with the newcomers. Tension was held in respecting self-determination amidst growing interdependence. The Royal Proclamation (1763) recognized Treaty Rights and land title for Indigenous peoples, with a foundation for self-determination and respectful relations. However, the British monarchy put the settler government in control of Indigenous peoples. In the 1800s, European cultural domination overshadowed negotiated Treaty Rights and relationships. The first residential school opened in 1849. Further to this, the Gradual Civilization Act (1857), the British North American Act (1867), and the Indian Act (1876) were enforced to regulate every aspect of Indigenous peoples' lives. By the mid-1900s, attendance at residential school was compulsory, traditional activities were outlawed and punished by jail, and ceremonial items were destroyed. Amendments to the Indian Act were regularly made in support of deeper assimilation and dispossession of Indigenous peoples.

In the 1950s, amendments to the Indian Act granting limited rights for Indigenous peoples were initiated, but assimilation practices continued. Thousands of Indigenous children were apprehended and adopted without their parents' consent into primarily non-Indigenous families and communities: this resulted in the 'Sixties Scoop' (Sinclair, 2007). After years of political advocacy by Indigenous leaders, the Constitution Act of Canada (1982) was revised to recognize existing Treaty Rights and that First Nations, Inuit, and Métis people were recognized as original inhabitants. After a long struggle by Indigenous women, Bill C-31 (1985) was introduced as an amendment of the Indian Act, which advanced gender equality and shifted control to support Indigenous peoples to identify their own membership (Dickason & McNab, 2009). Further to this, the question of inherent constitutional rights resurfaced during the Meech Lake Charlottetown Accord (1990). Finally, in 2016, the Government of Canada endorsed its adoption of the United Declaration on the Rights of Indigenous Peoples (UNDRIP) (United Nations, 2008). Signaling a turn in Canada's collective social consciousness and commitments to social justice, in 2018, private members Bill C-262 adopting UNDRIP passed in the Canadian parliament. The government's renewed commitment to reconciliation is about respecting the original relationships with Indigenous peoples that set the foundation of Canadian society. This brief historical context is not the intent of this chapter but important for nurses to understand the longevity and historical impact this legacy of legislation has on the health of First Nations, Inuit, and Métis peoples. For further information refer to the Canadian government website Department of Justice—Principles respecting the Government of Canada's relationship with Indigenous peoples. From the start of residential schools, an abundance of concerns and inquiries led to The Bryce Report on Health Conditions in Residential Schools (1907), documenting the deplorable conditions faced by Indigenous children who were living in residential schools (First Nations Child and Family Services of Canada, 2016). Until recently, such reports have gone largely unnoticed and without commensurate action. Since this first report there has been a significant number of recommendations outlining many diverse solutions, for example: the assimilation policy known as the White Paper (1969); the "Royal Commission on Aboriginal Peoples" (1999), a five volume report including over 400 recommendations on improving relationships, health, and sovereignty; the Kelowna Accord (Government of Canada 2006) outlining economic, housing, and health solutions to reducing health disparities and improving the quality of life; and the more recent Truth and Reconciliation Commission of Canada Calls to Action (2015a). These policy reports highlight the structural determinants of health and emphasize systemic factors and policy issues that continue to be detrimental to the health of First Nations, Inuit and Métis peoples.

Reading (2018) and Reading and Wien (2009) suggest that the strongest predictors of Indigenous health inequities are historical connections to social determinants of health, which includes the past, present, and future. Authors characterized the social determinants of health for Indigenous people as distal, intermediate, and proximal. Proximal determinants of health are those with a direct impact on any aspect of health—such as access to adequate food, water, and soil; proper housing; education; income; social support networks; culture; and gender. Intermediate determinants, such as the inability to access health care and education, result in the decreased likeliness of individuals' developing healthy behaviours or having the necessary opportunities to secure employment. This impact extends to a lack of cultural continuity in traditional and intergenerational connectedness that is often cited as a primary cause of many of the social problems that Indigenous populations face. However, it is the distal determinants of health, which include political, economic, social, and historical contexts, that

influence both the intermediate and proximal determinants of health. Historically, many of these distal determinants of health, such as colonialism and racial and social exclusion, have created social inequalities that are detrimental to the self-determination of Indigenous peoples in Canada. The next section provides a glimpse into how the Indian Act policy shaped the delivery of health services both past and present.

> **EXERCISE 4.1** Complete an online search using the following key terms: Indigenous, colonization, systemic racism, intergenerational trauma, and access to health care, to determine what you might consider to be important determinants of health. Reflect back on historical and structural factors that impact the health of Indigenous peoples.
>
> What social determinants of health appear to be having the greatest impact upon the health of Indigenous peoples?

The Indian Act

The Indian Act (1876) is Canadian federal legislation that governs all matters pertaining to Indigenous peoples. This legal document dictates how Indigenous peoples are governed and identified and determines what services will be provided to Indigenous peoples under Canadian law. The Indian Act is grounded in Eurocentric assimilation, dispossession, and domination, and is the root of systemic racism for Indigenous peoples in Canada.

"Our Indian legislation generally rests on the principle that the aborigines are to be kept in a condition of tutelage and treated as wards or children of the State . . . the true interests of the aborigines and of the State alike require that every effort should be made to aid the Red man in lifting himself out of his condition of tutelage and dependence, and that is clearly our wisdom and our duty, through education and every other means, to prepare him for higher civilization by encouraging him to assume the privileges and responsibilities of full citizenship" (Department of the Interior, Annual Report for the year ended 30th June, 1876 (Parliament, Sessional Papers, No. 11, 1877), p. xiv).

In 1879, the government commissioned Nicholas Flood Davin to conduct the *Report on Industrial Schools for Indians and Half-Breeds* (Truth and Reconciliation Commission of Canada, 2015b). This report generated recommendations to extend government-funded and church-run day-school programs for "Indian and half-breed" children. This residential school system policy further inspired government assimilation efforts by forcibly removing children from their families, homes, and communities. The goal was to create boarding schools that were self-sufficient through "farming, raising cattle and mechanical trades . . . (and) directed towards the destruction of Aboriginal spirituality" (p. 27). In 1883, Minister Hector Langevin echoed support of this assimilation policy by stating:

"If you wish to educate these children you must separate them from their parents during the time that they are being educated. If you leave them in the family they may know how to read and write, but they still remain savages, whereas by separating them in the way proposed, they acquire the habits and tastes—it is to be hoped only the good tastes— of civilized people" (TRU, 2015b, p. 29).

Deplorable conditions in residential schools were seldom reported by inspectors and principals, with a long-standing refusal from the government and churches to assume responsibility to address harms, including widespread abuse, malnutrition, disease, injury, and death. In 1938, ongoing assimilation and cultural genocide is illustrated in a letter written by residential school administrator Reverend A.E. Caldwell to a local Indian agent:

"The problem with the Indians is one of mortality and religion. They lack the basic fundamentals of civilized thought and spirit, which explains their child-like nature and behavior. At our school we strive to turn them into mature Christians who will learn how to behave in the world and surrender their barbaric way of life and their treaty rights which keep them trapped on their land and in a primitive existence. Only then will the Indian problem in our country be solved" (Rev. A. E. Caldwell to Indian Agent P.D. Ashbridge, 1938, cited in Annett, 2001, p. 26).

It was not until the 1960s that residential schools were re-evaluated, and apologies from the government and churches began in the 1980s. The Davin Report was maintained until 1969, and the last residential school closed in 1996. It wasn't until 2005 that the Indian Residential School Settlement (IRSSA) was reached. Five key outcomes of the IRSSA included a financial compensation for students who attended and suffered abuse, a national inquiry established through the Truth and Reconciliation Commission of Canada, Health and Healing Foundation, and a commemoration fund. The Indian Act and residential schools' policies created a tragic legacy of rampant disparities, human rights violations, and intergenerational trauma leading to significant barriers for the health of Indigenous populations (Lovoie et al., 2010). These patterns of politics continue to shape Indigenous health care services, and nursing has the power to create positive change and promote health and social justice at micro, meso, and macro levels. However, nursing leadership will not be able to establish cultural safe care if it is not fully aware of the continued legacy of oppression of Indigenous peoples in Canada. Nursing leaders' obligation and opportunity will be further discussed in the section on Reconciliation.

Health Care System with Indigenous Populations
Health Care Delivery

Indigenous health care delivery in Canada is "made up of a complicated 'patchwork' of policies, legislation and agreements that delegate responsibility between federal, provincial, municipal and (Indigenous) governments in different ways in different parts of the country" (National Collaborating Centre for Aboriginal Health (NCCAH), 2013, p. 6). Health care service delivery was a key feature of Treaty agreements made with Treaty 6 in 1876, known as the "Medicine Chest Clause". It is under this clause that the federal government promised to provide health care services to First Nations peoples. And it is under this clause that interpretation remains debatable, as Indigenous peoples believe health care is a Treaty right whereas the federal government believes it is a fiduciary responsibility. Within this context, nursing services were first provided to First Nations community in the early 1920s, which led to the development of the Department of Health and Welfare in late 1940 to oversee the delivery of health care services (Lovoie et al., 2010; Richmond and Cook, 2016).

The federal government Health Act (1984) is in place to ensure the universality, accessibility, portability, comprehensiveness, and public administration of health care. The Canada Health Transfer provides federal funding for 13 provincial and territorial governments to provide insured services for medically necessary hospital, physician, and health care (Government of Canada, 2016).

However, jurisdiction over health policy, funding, and service delivery for First Nations and Inuit populations flows from the federal government as per the Indian Health Policy (1979) and Non-Insured Health Benefits Renewed Mandate (1997) (Government of Canada 2014; 2018a). While provinces and territories are mainly responsible for hospital and physician services, Health Canada – First Nations and Inuit Health Branch (FNIHB) funds federal health services for First Nations and Inuit peoples and communities, including about 200 remote areas (NCCAH, 2013); the federal government is currently transitioning "FNIHB programs and direct resources to DISC" (Department of Indigenous Services Canada) (Government of Canada, 2018c). Since the government determines who qualifies as status/registered/treaty Indian under the Indian Act (1876), Indigenous and Northern Affairs Canada registers eligible First Nations and Inuit peoples; Métis and non-status First Nations peoples are excluded from federal health benefits. Health Canada: FNIHB (now DISC) provides health services, including community-based health promotion and disease prevention programs, with limited primary, urgent, and hospital care; non-insured health benefits include vision and dental care, prescription medications, medical equipment, and transport (Government of Canada, 2018b). Federally funded Indigenous health service provision has been in constant change since implementing the Health Transfer Policy (1989). The transfer of health services aligns with UNDRIP articles on Indigenous sovereignty but varies significantly from Nation to Nation. For instance, one community can be completely transferred, another integrated (meaning they only control the delivery of certain programs), and then another community is fully controlled by DISC.

One example of an integrated approach to health care service delivery is the All Nations Healing Hospital. This interagency organization in Treaty 4 is owned and operated by 15 First Nations. File Hills Qu'Appelle Tribal Council, Touchwood Agency Tribal Council in

affiliation with Saskatchewan Health authority provides services to 11 First Nations communities. Leadership values and governance structures are built on partnerships and relationships with numerous agencies. The model of health care is responsive, innovative, collaborative, and inclusive to facilitate a culturally safe and inviting environment. Services include a holistic bundle of primary, secondary, and tertiary health care services. Unique to this hospital is its cultural program, including access to traditional wellness knowledge holders. Programs include acute care, palliative care, mental health counselling, podiatry, emergency amenities, dental, and diagnostic and telehealth services. All Nations' Healing Hospital is owned and operated by the File Hills Qu'Appelle Tribal Council and Touchwood Agency Tribal Council and is funded through an operating agreement with the Regina Qu'Appelle Health Region. Fort Qu'Appelle Health Services has an interagency service relationship with File Hills Community Health Services, Lakeview Lodge, and the community health services of local First Nations. Unfortunately, without a clear national plan or policy to effectively coordinate transfers, First Nations and Inuit populations have inconsistent funding and service gaps leading to challenges in accessing equitable health care (Allan & Smylie, 2015; NCCAH, 2013).

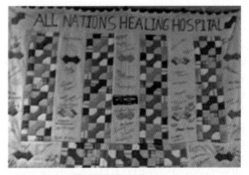

All Nations Healing Hospital

RESEARCH PERSPECTIVE

Resource: Camargo Plazas, Cameron, B. L., Milford, K., Hunt, L. R. Bourque Bearskin, R. L., & Santo Salas, A. (2018). Engaging Indigenous youth through popular theatre: Knowledge mobilization of Indigenous peoples' perspectives on access to health care services. *Action Research.* Retrieved from http://journals.sagepub.com/doi/10.1177/1476750318789468; Cameron, B. L., Camargo Plazas, M. d. P., Santos Salas, A., Bourque-Bearskin,

L., & Hungler, K. (2014). Understanding inequalities in access to healthcare services for aboriginal people: a call for nursing action. *Advances in Nursing Science* special issue on Health Equities. 37:3.

A group of community leaders, researchers, and students led by Dr. Brenda Cameron (Principle Investigator) at the University of Alberta initiated a series of research

RESEARCH PERSPECTIVE—cont'd

enquiries aimed at improving access to health care services and reducing disparities for Indigenous peoples. Known as the Access Research team, this diverse group of members used a combination of Indigenous, interpretive, community-based participatory, and action research methodologies to examine the experiences of Indigenous peoples' access to health care services in urban, rural, and inner-city settings. A program advisory committee that included eminent scholar Elder Rose Martial (Cold Lake First Nations), researchers, service providers, program planners, service managers, community members, and trainees collaborated for this research program. Meetings with the advisory members were conducted through teleconference and face-to-face on a regular basis.

Four qualitative studies were completed during this project. The research process was informed by relational ethics, principles Ownership, Control, Access, and Possession (OCAP), Alberta Aboriginal Capacity and Developmental Research Environments (ACADRE), Network Ethical standards, and the Canadian Institute of Health Research (CIHR) Guidelines for Health Research with Indigenous populations.

1. In the first study on Indigenous peoples' health care experiences, a rigorous data analysis process was established. This required non-Indigenous researchers to identify patterns of key concepts, then return to Indigenous researchers to check for accuracy of themes and concepts from initial interpretation of results. Findings from initial exploratory studies of Indigenous peoples' experience in urban, inner city, and rural areas revealed a critical need to develop culturally safe comprehensive care strategies.

2. The second qualitative intervention study involved placement of two Indigenous Community Health Representatives (CHRs), one in a rural and one an urban emergency department, to support the effectiveness of improving Indigenous people's experiences accessing health care services. With further validation of the first study, findings highlight how Indigenous CHRs were able to improve the access experience for both the Indigenous client and the health care professionals, which resulted in reduced stigmatized and racialized care. Recognizing the CHR intervention as a promising practice, the rural hospital implemented an Indigenous Liaison position, and used study findings to lobby for additional CHR positions.

3. The third project based on the rural CHR study findings study focused on using popular theatre as an action research approach to disseminate research findings. A community symposium was organized, and local high school students were actively involved in the creation of a play to make meaning of the data collected

4. The fourth research activity was a secondary analysis of data sets using a social determinants of health framework specific to Indigenous populations. Based on the overall research program, key findings include the following:
   - Communication barriers
   - Enduring hardship associated with being Indigenous and speaking an Indigenous language
   - Dissatisfaction with emergency care due to lack of attention to complex needs
   - Frustration with waiting time compared to non-Indigenous patients
   - Racialization of care
   - Lack of understanding of Indigenous culture and traditional practices
   - Lack of understanding of how Indigenous social determinants of health impinge on the experience of access to emergency care.

Overall, a lack of respect within the interaction with emergency staff and not being treated as a person or equal human being because of their Indigenous status were prevailing themes that permeated many stories and prevented clients from disclosing their concerns, fears, and health history.

Implications for Practice

Indigenous health research in Canada is making an important contribution to improving nursing practice and supporting culturally safe delivery of health care services that are more culturally congruent with Indigenous ways of knowing, being, and doing. By addressing the historical structural barriers through nursing research, the production and mobilization of knowledge from an Indigenous perspective creates meaningful opportunities for Indigenous peoples to be involved in the design, delivery, and dissemination of research. Nursing leaders working with Indigenous communities need to invest in rebuilding trusting relationships, creating relational accountability, and ensuring that reciprocity in the research process is mutually beneficial to all involved.

Policy gaps rooted in systemic racism lead to jurisdictional disputes within and between federal and provincial/territorial government payments for First Nations and Inuit health. A tragic illustration was Jordan River Anderson from Norway House Cree Nation, a young boy with a complex medical condition who needlessly spent the last two years of his life in hospital until he died at age five: provincial and federal governments were locked in disagreement over who should pay for Jordan's home care (Blackstock, 2012). In 2007, Jordan's Principle was unanimously passed in the House of Commons as a "child-first principle . . . to resolve jurisdictional disputes involving the care of First Nations children" (Blackstock, 2012, p. 368). In 2016, the Canadian Human Rights Tribunal ruled that the Government of Canada discriminated against First Nation children and did not fully implement Jordan's Principle; the federal government continued to delay essential health care services to First Nations children, and non-compliance orders continued until 2017. The federal government established a short-term fund and staff for timely coordination of expenses related to Jordan's Principle until 2019 (Government of Canada, 2018b). While this may sound promising, a long-term, coherent plan is needed to ensure that all Indigenous peoples have access to medically necessary health care.

There is a common misconception that Indigenous peoples do not pay taxes and get free health care and education: this is not true. However, Indigenous peoples do pay a high price in poor health outcomes that are related to inequitable health service delivery. Amidst health disparities, Allan and Smylie (2015) in *First Peoples, Second Class Treatment* outline several innovative approaches that are reforming Indigenous health care. These are:

- Health services, programs and systems directed by Indigenous peoples (e.g. British Columbia First Nations Health Authority)
- Community-directed Indigenous services related to health (e.g. housing supports)
- Community-based and health-impacting services and programs (e.g. Indigenous program within mainstream health centre)
- Interventions at the level of mainstream institutions (e.g. Indigenous patient navigators)
- Promising interventions and training responses (e.g. cultural safety) (pp. 10–11).

Indigenous health reform respects self-determination and shifts service delivery to Indigenous peoples-centred community-driven approaches. Such reform is needed to positively impact the determinants of health and address systemic racism in health care.

Systemic Barriers to Health Care

The legacy of colonialism, systemic racism, and all other forms of discrimination present, apparent or silent, within our current health care system contributes and sustains proliferation of health and social inequities faced by Indigenous populations in Canada. Literature confirms that despite efforts by the health care sector to integrate cultural competence, Indigenous populations continue to experience both individual and systemic discrimination when seeking care (Allan & Smylie 2015; Browne et al., 2011; Browne et al., 2016). For example, in a study looking at inequalities in access to health care services for Indigenous peoples in urban hospitals, it found numerous reports of racism, stigmatization, intimidation, harassment, and deep fear with health care providers (Cameron et al., 2014; McGibbon & Etowa, 2009). As a result, Indigenous populations experience difficult and limited access to health care. These experiences reinforce that trusting health care relationships are critical to addressing ongoing inequities in access to health care and have a role in mitigating future harm for Indigenous populations seeking health care (Jacklin et al., 2017).

Access to appropriate and responsive health care services is clearly chartered in the Canada Health Act (1984) and is essential to achieving overall improvements in the health status amongst Indigenous populations (Browne et al., 2011). Yet, as the Indigenous population continues to grow, so do inequities, which rate as one of our nation's most serious shortcomings (Institute on Governance, 2013). Indigenous populations living in Canada are more likely to be unemployed, living in housing in need of major repairs, have experienced physical, emotional, or sexual abuse, and been a victim of a violent crime (Canadian Human Rights Commission, 2010). Further, Indigenous populations have an increased chance of obesity, cancer, hepatitis, HIV, and an altered level of mental health (Canadian Human Rights Commission, 2010).

The most recent First Nations Regional Health Survey (First Nations Information Governance Centre, 2018) represents responses from 250 communities with over

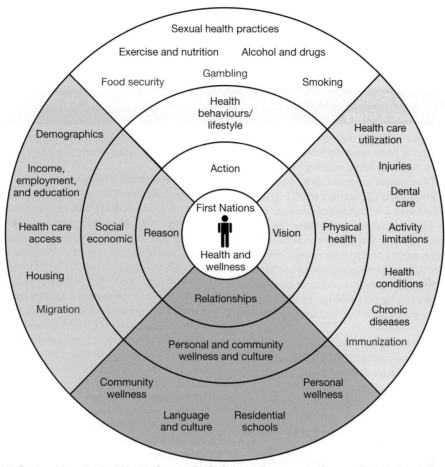

Fig. 4.1 Regional Longitudinal Health Survey (RHS) Cultural Framework. (Source: First Nations Information Governance Centre (FNIGC) (2012). First Nations Regional Health Survey (RHS) 2008/10: National report on adults, youth, and children living in First Nations communities. p. 9. Retrieved from https://fnigc.ca/sites/default/files/docs/first_nations_regional_health_survey_rhs_2008-10_-_national_report.pdf)

20 000 First Nations children (0–11 years), youth (12–17 years), and adults (18 years and older). Fig. 4.1 illustrates the health and wellness of First Nations peoples. Data collection is represented through a holistic framework that represents "total health of the total person within the total environment" (p. 8). Findings confirm ongoing disparities related to "education, employment and housing" (p. 15), access to safe drinking water, chronic disease, and oral health. The "intergenerational negative effects of Residential Schools . . . were found in relation to self-rated general and mental health, suicidal thoughts and substance abuse" (p. 140). Positive trends include increased educational attainment, personal income, and self-reported mental health. Resiliency is noted through sharing traditional Indigenous culture and language

and participating in community-related events. Nurses need to consider this culturally attuned health survey methodology and findings on Indigenous population strengths held in tension with persistent gaps in health outcomes.

The combination of health and social disparities and rapidly growing population is positioned to create a spike in incidence of Indigenous health-related challenges. Nurses share an ethical obligation to support reconciliation and restorative justice by truthfully recognizing harm and being accountable to repair such harm; this will lead to improved health and right to self-governance of Indigenous peoples, which is congruent with the nursing *Code of Ethics* (Canadian Nurses Association, 2017; Mahara et al., 2011).

Canadian nurses need to be aware of the unique history and context of Indigenous populations in order to provide equitable, effective, and culturally safe care to promote health with Indigenous peoples. Recognizing the effects of structural oppression and systemic violence will assist nursing leaders to advocate for social change so that improving health care services become a collective action. See Box 4.1.

BOX 4.1   Practice Scenario: Nursing Leadership and Enacting Culturally Safe Health Care – Brian Sinclair's Story

It has been ten years since the unlawful death of Brian Sinclair, an Indigenous man, resulting from the discrimination and racism he faced while seeking medical care. Brian Sinclair did not receive adequate care at the Health Science Centre Emergency Department (HSC-ED) in September 2008. Brian was a wheelchair-bound man with a long-term Foley catheter in place, necessitated by a complication relating to a treatable bladder infection. Brian first went to a community health centre seeking medical support. The health care professionals believed Mr. Sinclair required more urgent care that could not be provided at the health centre, so he was referred to the HSC-ED, provided with transportation (a taxi) and a letter outlining his condition.

According to video footage, Brian Sinclair arrived at the HSC-ED at 2:53 p.m. on September 19, 2008, where he was triaged. Unfortunately, there was no appropriate documentation or record of Brian being triaged, which led to his 34-hour wait, not being seen by an ER physician or nurses. Once Mr. Sinclair was finally acknowledged after concerns being voiced by several other patients, it was too late, and rigor mortis had already set in. The cause of death was from acute peritonitis relating to severe cystitis or inflammation of the bladder. It was confirmed that no drugs or alcohol were in his system, as security and staff's main reason for not addressing his condition was based on the assumption that he was drunk and just sleeping it off, as he had nowhere else to go. There was little documentation of the events leading up to Mr. Sinclair's death other than the video footage, which gives rise to how he was treated while trying to access medical care.

The Brian Sinclair Working Group

According to the "Out of Sight" Interim Report, the Brian Sinclair Working Group was created to examine the role of racism in the death of Brian Sinclair and the inquest that followed. The Brian Sinclair Working Group developed recommendations focused on racism within the health care system and improving care for Indigenous patients. An important focus of this comprehensive group is on the ongoing structural and systemic anti-Indigenous racism within the health and legal systems using various presentations, public forums, and op-eds.

The Legal System's Response

According to the "Out of Sight" document, the legal system's focus needed to be on the ongoing systemic anti-Indigenous racism in health and legal systems. The investigation started in 2010 and concluded in 2012, but unfortunately no one was held accountable for Brian Sinclair's death; rather it was to be used as an education case to "learn" from. Police did not investigate Sinclair's death until his family pressured authorities. When the Sinclair's family requested a retrial or for the crown's decision to be publicly made, their requests were denied. The health care system and legal system failed Mr. Sinclair and his family: both were supposed to instill a sense of security and safety, but the opposite was experienced.

The Inquest Proceedings

The purpose of the inquest was to determine facts relating to Brian Sinclair's death and to identify changes in how his death could have been prevented. Initially, a public inquiry was called to address how Indigenous people are treated within the health care system; however, the government of Manitoba refused, putting forward a need for an inquiry. There were two phases in Mr. Sinclair's inquest. This first phase focused on answering questions about circumstances of Brian Sinclair's death. This phase took place over 34 days and included 74 witnesses, most of whom attested to staff at HSC-ED making assumptions and holding biases about Mr. Sinclair. However, when staff testified, they mentioned never seeing Mr. Sinclair and stated that racism was not a factor as they treat everyone the same. The second phase focused on the health care system and its response to Mr. Sinclair's death. This phase was completed in 13 days and included 9 or 10 witnesses. This phase's focus was shifted from the original mandate, solely concentrating on the HSC-ED triage process and the delays in care as well as staffing levels, even though these posed no problem to the other 150 patients who received treatment that same weekend.

BOX 4.1   Practice Scenario: Nursing Leadership and Enacting Culturally Safe Health Care – Brian Sinclair's Story—cont'd

Next Steps and Recommendations

There is a clear objective for future work to focus on addressing racism and discrimination in the health care system. The inquest developed recommendations, some more significant than others: the family and organizations are disputing some recommendations, as they are not inclusive for Indigenous patients. Recommendations outlined in the report are as follows:

Interim Recommendation

"Recommendation #1: We urge the federal government to implement a national, overarching, explicit anti-racist policy to be adopted at all levels of all healthcare systems operating in Canada, including provincial and territorial systems and those under federal purview (the First Nations and Inuit Health Branch of Health Canada and Veterans Affairs)." (p. 10)

Overall Recommendation

"Recommendation #2: Manitoba Health and other provincial/territorial Health Departments across Canada adopt an explicit anti-racism policy in which the Health Departments and Regional Health Authorities (RHAS), develop anti-racism implementation plans and report on progress in their annual reports. These policies shall include specific actions, remediation and supports to assist systems and healthcare workers and administrators. Further, the authorities will advance these requirements to all contract service provider systems, consultants, contractors and others involved in the capital development of health service in Canada." (p. 10)

Union and Professional Organization Recommendation

"Recommendation #3: That unions and nursing and medical professional organizations issue clear and unequivocal position statements of zero tolerance for racism in the workplace. Further, mechanisms to receive complaints and concerns by Indigenous patients need to be adequately developed to eliminate and reduce the harms of racism at multiple levels, including in organizational policies and practices and at the point of care. The nursing and medical colleges in Manitoba must develop process-

es to support positive behaviour changes by healthcare providers to foster equitable healthcare for Indigenous people. Professional accountability and performance management strategies are needed to ensure that repeat actions of racism warrant severe disciplinary actions accordingly." (p. 11)

"Recommendation #4: All health professional schools must adopt an anti-racism curriculum and share best practices in relation to curriculum development with an emphasis on cultural safety for First Nations, Métis and Inuit communities. Further, schools must increase the number of visible First Nations, Métis and Inuit healthcare students, faculty and administrators and commit to anti-racist policies to improve the experience of all learners. Learners, administrative staff and faculty members who are member of communities historically affected by oppressions will all benefit by adoption and implementation of the recommendations. Collaboration with continuing health education offices in the institutions offer excellent ways to address the ongoing behaviour and attitudinal changes that foster excellent in-care for Indigenous patients in healthcare practices." (p. 11)

Significance to Practice

Write a letter to the Minister of Indigenous Health Services in Canada answering the following questions to explain why addressing systemic racism in health care requires our immediate attention.

1. What nursing practice of standards were addressed in this situation? Why is this important to nurses and how they deliver care to an Indigenous patient?
2. Is there significance in using an inquest versus a public inquiry? What are the advantages and disadvantages for Brian Sinclair's case?
3. How could training in anti-racism, cultural safety, and cultural humility have helped prevent the death of Brian Sinclair?
4. Do you think the recommendations are adequate to address relevant Indigenous population needs?
5. What are some examples of how these recommendations can be implemented, or are they already implemented elsewhere?

Resource: Brian Sinclair—Ignored to Death in Winnipeg Manitoba (2017). *Out of sight: Interim report of the Sinclair Working Group.* Retrieved from http://ignoredtodeathmanitoba.ca/

History of Indigenous Women in Nursing

According to the Aboriginal Nurses Association of Canada (2016), from time immemorial, customs and practices of Indigenous women hold a distinct and prominent role within Indigenous societies, both as life givers and through traditional knowledge of medicines establishing a sound knowledge base for traditional healing practices of First Nations, Inuit, and Métis peoples (Anderson, 2001; Anderson et al., 2003; Burnett, 2010; Drees, 2013; Robbins & Dewar, 2011). Since the origins of nursing are influenced by the nature of our social context, Indigenous ways of knowing heavily influenced how health care services were originally delivered in Canada (Donahue, 2011; McCallum 2014). Early evidence shows how discoveries in westernized medicine originated from Indigenous peoples' care for the sick, which generated early ideas on nursing care and medical treatment (Donahue, 2011). The documented relationship between missionaries and Indigenous healers was not clearly understood, and by the early 1900s the rapid influx of settlers coupled with advances in westernized medicine fundamentally transformed the relationship between Indigenous peoples and early nursing leaders.

The story of Indigenous nurses in Canada is a remarkable one. Through a historical analysis of Indigenous nurses, McCallum (2007, 2008, 2014) explains how disparities were created and sustained in knowledge development of nursing. During the first half of the twentieth century, many hospitals, nursing stations, outposts, and health centres serving First Nations, Inuit, and Métis communities came to rely on the labour of Indigenous nurses, despite restricted nursing education for Indigenous peoples until the late 1950s. However, at the discretion of residential school principals and Department of Indian Affairs, some women were supported to attain a nursing education. During this time, most Indigenous nurses found jobs in hospitals. Indigenous nurses also enlisted to serve in the Canadian and United States militaries in both World War I and World War II. Charlotte Edith Anderson Monture from Six Nations is a well-known First Nations nurse who, after being denied education in Canada, went to New York to complete nurse training in 1914; she then served in World War I, and is recognized as Canada's first Indigenous registered nurse.

The second generation (1950–1970) of Indigenous nurses was marked by the nursing profession opening doors to men and married women, with a notable expansion in the number of licensed practical nurse and registered nurse aid programs and community health representatives, which many Indigenous nurses used as stepping stones to higher education. For example, the opening quote by nurse leader Jean Goodwill from Poundmaker First Nation is of importance, given her place in history as one of the first Indigenous registered nurses to complete training in Canada, in 1954. However, for the most part, Indigenous women felt isolated and discriminated against because of their identity (Etowa et al., 2011). This exposed Indigenous nurses to seemingly subtle yet harmful forms of racism reinforced through the Indian Act. For example, First Nations peoples were disenfranchised as Canadians against their will if they were educated or married to non-status men. This meant that an educated First Nations woman was no longer considered to be a member of her community or could identify as First Nation person because a First Nations woman's status was defined by her husband. As a result, many racialized policies penalized Indigenous people who publicly self-identified. Because of this societal and legal punishment, there were likely far more Indigenous nurses during this period than we can ever know about. Those who went into nursing during this time serve as important role models and inspirations to Indigenous nurses later in the century. During the next two decades of political activism, the search for true "equality" began with growing calls for recognition of Treaty Rights. This led to development of many organizations and advocacy groups reclaiming their Indigenous lands and approaches to education, health, and rights as sovereign nations.

The third generation (1971–1991) of Indigenous nurses found their collective voice by coming together for their first nursing conference to share ideas about Indigenous identity, laws, and language and their influence on nurse's approaches to primary health care, health promotion, prevention, treatment, and education. During the 1980s, a significant development in the field of Indigenous nursing practice was cross-cultural nursing. Cross-cultural approaches permitted discussion of the impact of cultural difference from the patients' perspective and the health care provider. Cross-cultural care required an understanding of illness not only within the patient's cultural context but also within that patient's experience of colonialism. Indigenous nurses bore more than their fair share of the weight of the work of defining, teaching, and practising cross-cultural care, because of what Jean Goodwill called their "unique expertise". During this period, Indigenous nurses found for themselves a space in the nursing profession as respected critics and providers of health care services to First Nations, Inuit, and Métis peoples. They also developed an Indian nurse identity, which combined a strong belief in social and cultural responsibility with a professionalizing nursing ethic.

The fourth generation (1991–2011) of Indigenous nurses made significant commitments and achievements despite chronic underfunding in all sectors delivered to First Nations, Inuit, and Métis communities. For example, federal transfer of health care services to First Nations communities had symbolic consequences for nurses who transferred their positions from federal to local; these nurses suffered serious pay cuts, lost extended employment benefits, and were isolated geographically. The most significant change in Indigenous nursing and education during this period is the concerted effort to change health professions' attitudes, knowledge, and ability to deliver culturally appropriate and safe health services to Indigenous populations. This work continues with the next generation of Indigenous nurses, by increasing efforts towards cultural safety, equity, self-determination, decolonization, reconciliation, and integration of Indigenous knowledge.

Canadian Indigenous Nurses Association

Nurses are the backbone of the health care system and are central to First Nations, Métis, and Inuit communities. Based on 2016 National Household Survey data, a joint project undertaken by the Canadian Indigenous Nurses Association (CINA) and the University of Saskatchewan College of Nursing (2018) identified statistics and trends related to Indigenous nurses in Canada. In 2016, there were 9695 Indigenous nurses in Canada, representing 3% of the registered nursing workforce, from approximately 4.3% of the total Canadian population. A higher proportion of Indigenous health care professionals are registered nurses (74.5%) compared to the non-Indigenous health professionals (59%). An interesting trend is that overall, Indigenous nurses are younger than the average non-Indigenous nurses, noting the opportunity for this newest generation to influence change.

CINA is the longest-standing Indigenous Health Professional Organization in Canada that is governed by a Board of Directors whose vision mission is to improve the health of First Nation, Inuit, and Métis peoples, by supporting First Nation, Inuit and Métis nurses and by promoting development and practice of Indigenous Health Nursing

(ANAC, 2016). In advancing this mission, CINA engages in activities related to recruitment and retention, member support, consultation, research, education, and policy directives. Through its members, CINA brings 40 years of experience and wisdom regarding both Indigenous ways of knowing regarding health and well-being and culturally safe nursing practice. As such, CINA has collaborated successfully with many partners at international, national, and regional levels over the years. CINA, believes in "authentic Indigenous partnerships" with Indigenous rights holders and non-Indigenous stakeholders that are inclusive of values grounded in diverse Indigenous philosophies that place relationality, respect, and reciprocity at the core of self-determination (2016). This approach is in keeping with the United Nations' Declaration on the Rights of Indigenous Peoples (2008) in recognition of "the urgent need to respect and promote the inherent rights of Indigenous peoples which derive from their political, economic and social structures and from their cultures, spiritual traditions, histories and philosophies." CINA processes are inclusive of an Indigenous worldview and endeavour to collectively work together to promote the principle of "for and by" Indigenous peoples and situates partners as Indigenous allies. Centred on building relationship values of respect, reciprocity, and self-determination, collaborative processes include identification of common goals and objectives and mutual benefit to each organization and the nurses they represent.

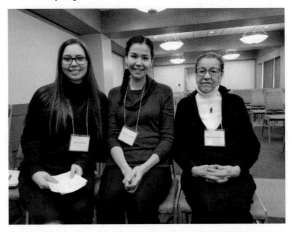

Past, Present and Future Indigenous Nursing Leaders

Cultural Humility and Cultural Safety

Nurses need an approach that uses the process of cultural humility to achieve cultural safety outcomes. The First

Nations Health Authority (2018) defines cultural humility as "a process of self-reflection to understand personal and systemic biases and to develop and maintain respectful processes and relationships based on mutual trust." Nurses are reflective lifelong learners who share a commitment to social justice. These qualities make nurses well positioned to integrate the process of cultural humility in practice: reflecting on self-worldview, while taking a learner's perspective of openness, respect, and curiosity when holding stories and experiences with Indigenous peoples. Building mutual trust through the process of cultural humility is a required foundation for the outcome of cultural safety at all levels: patients, health care professionals, and health organizations and systems. Cultural humility requires nurses to be egoless, aware of power imbalances, understand diversity, and be willing to change when confronted with difference (Foronda et al., 2015). It is important for nurses to engage with humility and consider that our two national official languages do not represent the 60 distinct languages of Canada's Indigenous peoples. For example, the "double work" (Møller, 2016, p. 92) of Inuk nurses in Nunavut who speak Inuktitut needs to be acknowledged, as their communication supports culturally safe care: "language carries culture and culture carries . . . the entire body of values by which we come to perceive ourselves and our place in the world" (Ngũgĩ, 1986, cited in Møller, 2016).

Stemming from seminal work on cultural safety by Indigenous Māori nurse scholar Ramsden (2002), three national sister organizations, Canadian Indigenous Nurses Association (CINA) (former Aboriginal Nurses Association of Canada), Canadian Nurses Association (CNA), and the Canadian Schools of Nursing Association (CASN), are strengthening collaboration for Indigenous nursing and education. Together, they developed a framework to guide nursing education and practice based on Indigenous knowledge, cultural humility, and relational ethics to support cultural safety (see Fig. 4.2). The First Nations Health Authority (2018) defines cultural safety as "an outcome based on respectful engagement that recognizes and strives to address power imbalances inherent in the health care system. It results in an environment free of racism and discrimination, where people feel safe when receiving health care" (p. 5).

Cultural safety was originally coined by Māori nurses in New Zealand and arose because of poor health outcomes of Indigenous peoples who were subjected to unsuitable and unsafe health care services (Nursing Council of New Zealand 2005; Ramsden, 2002; Woods 2010). Health experiences and inequities amongst Indigenous peoples in Canada are no different. The cultural competency/safety curriculum framework is a tool to help nurses address health disparities and power imbalances between students/patients and health care professionals by examining social-historical and political factors influencing the health care system. It is critical for all nurses to understand culturally safe care because it goes beyond benefiting one group. Cultural safety is the foundation to address health inequities and the gap in Indigenous knowledge throughout nursing practice. Six core competencies and indicators outlined in the CINA, CNA, and CASN framework (ANAC, 2009) are:

1. **Postcolonial understanding:** requires an in-depth understanding of how colonization impacts the lives of Indigenous peoples and the relationship between residential schools and intergenerational trauma.

2. **Communication:** applies to nursing interactions with First Nation, Inuit, and Métis peoples where listening and responding to the needs of Indigenous peoples is central to building trust.

3. **Inclusivity:** attention to who might be excluded or marginalized as part of the engagement process and relationship building with First Nations, Inuit, and Métis peoples.

4. **Respect:** consideration for First Nation, Inuit, and Métis students, their families, and communities for who they are, their uniqueness, diversity, and use of traditional approaches to health.

5. **Indigenous knowledge:** recognition of traditional knowledge and oral histories as having a place in education. This includes an understanding of First Nations, Inuit, and Métis ontology, epistemology, and cosmologies.

6. **Mentoring and supporting students for success:** central to teaching and learning process where opportunities to learn from traditional knowledge holders or elders alongside western education fosters their success.

Each of the core competencies is supported by four guiding principles of *respect, relevance, reciprocity*, and *responsibility* (Kirkness & Barnhardt, 2001) to maintain First Nations, Inuit, and Métis cultural integrity, experiences, relationships, and participation in education and practice. Furthermore, cultural safety is action oriented and supports nursing leadership and advocacy in promoting social justice of colonized and marginalized populations.

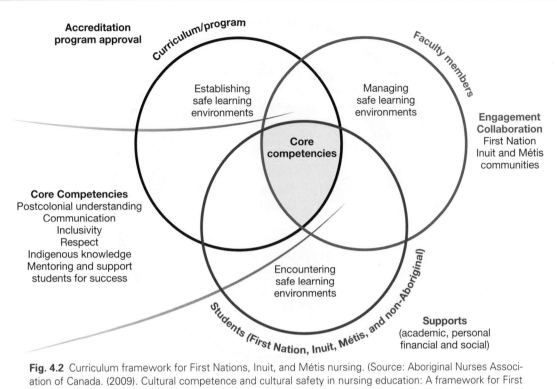

Fig. 4.2 Curriculum framework for First Nations, Inuit, and Métis nursing. (Source: Aboriginal Nurses Association of Canada. (2009). Cultural competence and cultural safety in nursing education: A framework for First Nations, Inuit, and Métis nursing. p. 6. Retrieved from https://www.cna-aiic.ca/~/media/cna/page-content/pdf-en/first_nations_framework_e.pdf)

It is important to critique and raise caution on common approaches to culture. For example, "cultural awareness or cultural sensitivity" is limited, as this leads to a potentially fixed and narrow understanding of cultural traits. This way of focusing on difference creates *othering* and does not invite nurses to reflect on how their worldview and sociopolitical-historical context impacts health care (ANAC, 2009). Nurses need to move beyond this approach and engage in active learning and practice. *Cultural competence* may also be limited, as reducing culture care to skill development risks oversimplifying cultures and lacks action to address related inequities. Moreover, there may be a risk of perpetuating colonization if westernized nursing and health care continues to be merely adapted for Indigenous peoples, rather than deeply examining and reforming systems. With this in mind, cultural humility and cultural safety are necessary approaches to promote health by authentically addressing the historic legacy of colonization that has resulted in widespread health inequity amongst Indigenous populations.

A growing concern about achieving culturally safe nursing practice in Indigenous populations has led to increasing research on trauma informed care. Evans-Campbell (2008) explains how a "Colonial Trauma Response" strategy supports Indigenous communities' resurgence of healing and developing resilience in the face of colonial oppression. Wesley-Esquimaux and Smolewski (2004) describe historical trauma as an accumulation of violence experienced over generations, which leads to a sense of learned helplessness and an array of social and cultural disruptions. Not only has it caused the separation of families, but it has also prevented the transmission of knowledge and language. In terms of policy change at the organizational level, Bowen and Murshid (2016) argue that "trauma-informed social policy should move beyond broad notions of trauma as a universal experience and address its specific sociopolitical and economic roots as well as its disproportionate impacts among marginalized populations" (p. 224). Key principles in implementing trauma informed social policy include: safety, transparency, collaboration and

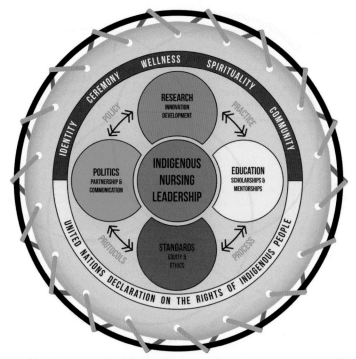

Fig. 4.3 Indigenous Nursing Leadership Model. (Source: L. Bourque Bearskin, 2017 (Beaver Lake, Cree Nation) adapted with art gifted by J. Bear Chief, 2018 (Blackfoot, Siksika Nation))

support, empowerment, choice, and intersectionality. Incorporating these principles into a broader approach can assist nurses in advocating for change that disrupts the trauma-informed health disparities as seen in Indigenous populations in Canada.

INDIGENOUS NURSING KNOWLEDGE AND LEADERSHIP

Indigenous Nursing Ways of Being and Knowing

Indigenous nurses in Canada have been combining Western education with a firm grounding in their own territory, land-based teachings, languages, cultures, community life, and healing traditions that shape Indigenous nursing knowledge to advance the current context of nursing practices (Bourque Bearskin, et al., 2016; CINA, n.d.). Indigenous ways of knowing and being have survived extensive attempts at extermination, continued colonization, and assimilation (Battiste, 2013; Monchalin, 2016). Indigenous societies throughout the world have sustained their unique worldviews and knowledge

systems and are being recognized and validated by mainstream societies (Barnhardt and Kawagley, 2005). Indigenous ways of knowing and being are inextricably linked through language, traditional laws, and spirituality of the intellectual, mental, and physical relationship Indigenous peoples have individually and collectively with the land. These ways of knowing are informed by the stories of knowledge holders and elders who carry the history of ancestors from one generation to the next (Weber-Pillwax, 1999).

Indigenous ways of knowing and being, found in ceremonies, songs, and dreams in unique ways of understanding our relationship to the spiritual world, are essential to Indigenous peoples' identity (Cardinal 2001; Steinhauer, 2008; Weber-Pillwax, 2003). Indigenous ways of knowing and being are self-generating and are tied to a place and those who live in that space (Basso, 1996; Donald, 2012; Ermine, 1995; Sinclair, 2013). Battiste & Youngblood Henderson (2000) explain that as Indigenous peoples, "we carry the mysteries of our ecologies and their diversity in our oral traditions, in our ceremonies, and in our art; we unite these mysteries in the structure of our languages and our ways of knowing" (p. 9). Indigenous peoples who live in accordance with natural laws learn through language, demonstration, observation, self-reflexive thinking, and experiences embedded in stories about compassion, humility, and intelligence that are deeply rooted (Archibald, 2008; Baskin, 2016; Battiste, 2002; Castellano, 2000; Hart, 2002; Lighting, 1992; Tuhiwai Smith, 1999/2012; Weber-Pillwax, 1999, 2001, 2003; Wilson, 2008). Indigenous ways of knowing and being are "inherently, political, reformative, relational and deeply personal approaches that must be located in the chaos of colonial interfaces to create spaces for Indigenous knowledge within existing and new curricula" (Phillips et al., 2005, p. 7). The activities and actions of Indigenous peoples in communities throughout the world show that a significant shift is underway in which Indigenous ways of knowing are being recognized as consisting of complex knowledge systems with an integrity of their own and one that lies no further than the self (Ermine, 1995).

Rooted in nursing, an Indigenous worldview must begin with a common vision guided by collective values and priorities of the community: "Aboriginal People must maintain the integrity of their traditional knowledge" (Dion Stout et al., 2001, p. 2; Dion Stout, 2012). Indigenous nurses must create and stand by their own Indigenous perspective stemming from experiences situated in traditions and customs shaped by their ancestors, land, and mental, emotional, physical, and spiritual relationships with each other (Bill, 2012; Dion Stout & Downey, 2006; Struthers, 1999, 2003). This includes all generations—*past present and future*—and cycles in time and space for the manifestation of compassion and respect in the development of self-understanding associated with identity formation. Indigenous knowledge is the manifestation of human knowledge, heritage, and consciousness and is a means

---

EXERCISE 4.2 Review and reflect on this passage by Elder John Crier: a Cree knowledge holder and Elder from Samson Cree Nation in Maskwacis Alberta Canada:

We do not come to be by random design, but rather by a greater design, that flows from the rhythm of life, from the stories of the people, the collective whole. We need to be emotionally, intellectually, physically, and spiritually connected to the world of speech and language because speaking through the spirit will enable us to bring back new forms of life that add to the great mystery of life. Language sets the foundation of our existence as nehiyawak (four souls) or iyiniw (first people). The Cree term wahkohtowin refers to the acts of being in relationships (kinship). It enfolds everything around us and can be symbolized as a circle or container (boundaries) in which we live, and dwell. It becomes a way of living in ceremony. The first step is to find meaning in the structure of ideas that are embedded in the words. You take that in so that you feel it and own it so that you give yourself permission to speak the language. A Cree life is about preparation to be in good standing to the Great Lawmakers. The land determines part of our identity. The songs are the expressions of the spirit, which comes through in our vocal cords. Vocalization become the means of expression body language then comes through the eyes. The Cree word "maskihkiwiskwewiw" for nurse is generally interpreted to mean "medicine woman" in English. In Cree, this is a narrow translation, as it does not capture the original intention or significance of traditional healers. For example, the word "maskihki" means "medicine", and if you further break it down again to "askiy", which means "land or Earth". The second part of the word, "skwew" which means women come from the word "iskotew" meaning fire or spirit. These teachings help us to understand how Indigenous knowledge is rooted in language and highlight the unique contributions of Indigenous health providers, including Elders, traditional wellness holders, and healers. (personal communication March 27, 2010 as cited in Bourque Bearskin, 2014).

1. Write a journal reflection using these guiding questions to critically examine your own personal knowledge, skills and attributes and how they influence your nursing leadership capabilities.
2. How do Indigenous knowledge systems compare and contrast with your understanding of knowledge?
3. What strategies can you implement, as a nursing leader, in your everyday practice?
4. Think about some of the biases and assumptions you have about Indigenous peoples, Indigenous knowledge or Indigenous rights. What are some ways to "check" your biases and the assumptions that you have adopted?
5. What are some potential barriers and/or tensions you anticipate in implementing nursing leadership when working in Indigenous communities?

of ecological order (Battiste & Youngblood Henderson, 2000). Indigenous knowledge is not the same as having knowledge of Indigenous peoples. A teaching from a renowned Indigenous scholar reminds us that "Indigenous Knowledge is in our being as lived. It is at the intersection of ontology (state of being) and epistemology (state of knowledge) where we need to be to explore deeply our thoughts, because it is here where the people hold the knowledge" (personal communication, Network Environments of Indigenous Health Research Graduate Conference, June 2010). Recognizing that we share the impact of colonization and hold the lineage of our ancestors, this teaching is applicable to all people. If nurses understand the original Latin term Indigenous to mean "originating in the region or country where found" (Bahr, 2005, p. 154), all nurses can situate themselves out of respect and as a method of gaining trust.

Indigenous Nursing Leadership

Indigenous nurses working in Indigenous communities become the connection and link to the health care system as stewards of Indigenous nursing knowledge and recognize the four priorities to improving Indigenous health in Canada: *practice, education, research* and *policy* (Bourque Bearskin, 2014; Bourque Bearskin et al., 2016; CINA 2016). This *Indigenous Nursing Leadership Model* (see Fig. 4.3) was developed from research with Indigenous nurse scholars who helped inform key features of Indigenous nursing knowledge (Bourque Bearskin, 2014; Bourque Bearskin et al., 2016). Although this is not a new concept, originally discussed by CINA board of directors in the early 1980s, this model illustrates important aspects of nursing that are unique to Indigenous communities. Indigenous nurses have a very holistic (spiritual, intellectual, emotional, and physical) way of addressing health, which not only involves the individual but also requires nurses to include the family, specific nation's values, and society assumptions as a whole. Indigenous nurses recognize being Indigenous as a political act which supports self-understanding, community healing, and self-determination within the context of health in advancing culturally secure health care services.

Indigenous nursing scholarship is a crucial and critical role in implementing an effective and efficient comprehensive health care system. Foundational to Indigenous nursing knowledge is the implementation of the UNDRIP (2008) so nursing is inclusive of Indigenous peoples' language and knowledge, and the protocols of local nations merged in a holistic and meaningful way. Supporting the transformation of nursing practice, education, administration, and research to shift emphasis from *individualized care in hospital* to *family care in communities* requires a broad systemic approach. Systems of health care require nurses to be attentive to Indigenous protocols, practice, process, and policy in nursing practice (see Fig. 4.3).

- *Protocols:* important and necessary for respecting and honouring peoples of the land and recognition of territory in printed materials, public meetings, and engagements; respecting protocol ensures the voice of local knowledge holders, prevents pan-Indigenous thinking, recognizes self within settler colonialism, and honours Indigenous peoples.
- *Practice:* clinical experiences, self-awareness, language used, and colonial terms that position local people; addressing colonial influences and learning about health through Indigenous ways of knowing.
- *Process:* sincere and deep respect for ways of being, knowing and doing with Indigenous peoples and communities; equity that rejects tokenism; *nothing about us without us.*
- *Policies:* formalizing systems-level opportunities for success by creating advocacy statements on cultural safety, equity, recruiting, and retaining Indigenous student nurses and faculty, and TRC Calls to Action.

Nursing leadership in clinical practice, education, research, management, and policy must be grounded in an appreciation of culture and an understanding of the historical and political context and diversity amongst Indigenous peoples. Self-determination, tradition, culture, language, and the relationship to the land are distinct determinants of health and wellness (Adelson, 2005; Reading & Wien, 2009). Self-determination is considered the cornerstone of progress towards improving health and economic and social conditions. The importance of historically ground visions, autonomy of community members, and community voice in decision making are essential for effective health leadership and governance.

Future nursing leaders in health care will continue to benefit from developing their capabilities in leadership. There is a significant amount of literature about nursing leadership that outlines the specific use of competencies in clinical practice and management.

While much literature is about achieving excellence in nursing leadership, little evidence exists on **Indigenous nursing leadership**. Best practices in excellence in nursing leadership need to be identified, mastered, and incorporated into new ways of doing things as nurses of the future. While there are many lists about the components of leadership, they generally include the following:

- Engaging in authentic self-awareness to become a critical reflexive leader (Alexander & Lopez, 2018).
- Creating a shared vision and managing organizational change.
- Improving results through teamwork and collaborative relationships (Orchard et al., 2017).
- Influencing others through advocacy and effective communication (Galuska, 2016).
- Developing leadership skills in others through succession planning and mentoring (Waxman & Delucas, 2014).

Indigenous nursing leadership integrates these components, while founded on several key elements including the following:

- Collectivist worldview based on relationships, holism, and interconnection.
- Fluid lifelong commitment to learning, community, service, and caretaking.
- Collaborative strengths-based, and non-hierarchical approach.
- Knowledge of Indigenous land, stories, community, values, and history as continuous.
- Indigenous knowledge woven with discernment alongside Westernized ways.
- Spiritual leadership through families, elders, and community.
- Liberation from oppression and promotion of equity (Kenny, 2012).

It is important to distinguish leadership theories that are aligned with Indigenous health and Indigenous nursing knowledge such as *strength-based*, *relational*, *collective*, and *transformative* leadership theories (Brookes, 2015; Gottleib et al., 2012; Opsina & Foldy, 2015; Orchard et al., 2017). These theories reflect the nature of Indigenous nursing (Doyle & Hungerford 2015; Henry & Wolfgramm, 2018; Kenny & Fraser, 2012). Shared principles include *interconnected relationships*, *common purpose*, *shared knowledge*, *capacity development*, *mutual responsibility*, *community service*, and *collective action*. Findings by Bourque Bearskin (2014; 2016) extends understanding of Indigenous nursing knowledge and leadership to

include *Indigeneity, relationality, self-understanding, collaboration* and the *pedagogy of service* as essential features to working with Indigenous communities.

EXERCISE 4.3 You are a nurse hired by the Government of Nunavut to work in an isolated Inuit community. You have many clients that require home care visits. One of the clients is a young mother who has just arrived back home with her one-week-old baby, after giving birth down south in an urban hospital. Upon further review of her records, you realize that none of her children have been immunized and the mother is requesting the nurse to immunize her children at home. You are aware of the immunization policy, which states nurses are unable to immunize in the home. You are aware that this single mom has struggled with depression. You are concerned about this health risk to the other children, especially since you heard of a recent measles outbreak in the city where this mother just gave birth. You call the senior public health official to request special permission, but they reiterate that you are unable to give immunization at home and the mother must bring the children in to the clinic. As a nursing leader in this Inuit community working with vulnerable families, what leadership skills would you draw on to ensure the safety of the family unit? Use the following questions to reflect on your approach.

1. How do you create open, trusting, and inclusive spaces where families are welcomed?
2. When was the last time you took a risk?
3. Do you consider yourself courageous?
4. When was the last time you inspired others to be courageous and take risks to serve others with care, compassion, and love?
5. When was the last time you were vulnerable and shared this vulnerability with your team?
6. How have you grown together, learned, and improved health care services?
7. How have you led, served, and supported others to do the same?

Relational Practice as Nurse Leaders

Indigenous nursing leadership honours relationships within our whole nursing discipline and cultivates genuine collaborative, strength-based holistic health promotion with communities. Being an effective leader in Indigenous health requires nurses to have a high level of emotional intelligence to understand the historical impact of intergenerational trauma to help manage relationships, emotions, and feelings of individuals, families, and communities. These skills must be coupled

TABLE 4.1   Respectful Practice

R Reflect deeply on your own cultural values and beliefs.

E Examine and question assumptions and biases in practice.

S Share and recognize ethical space of nurse–patient relationship.

P Participate and celebrate cultural uniqueness.

E Engage in relationship building.

C Create open and trusting environments.

T Treat people with dignity and compassion.

Source: Bourque Bearskin, R.L. (2011). A critical lens on culture in nursing practice. *Nurse Ethics, 18*(4), p. 557. https://doi.org/10.1177/0969733011408048.

with critical self-awareness skills to remain confident, courageous, and willing to take risks to challenge the hegemony and bureaucracy of Indigenous health politics. Nurses are encouraged to be authentic and willing to courageously show their vulnerabilities and whole self to help establish trusting therapeutic relationships (Bourque Bearskin, 2011). See Table 4.1.

Relational practice as described Henry and Wolfgramm (2018) explains how the experience of Indigenous leaders offers new ways of understanding broader complex leadership dynamics. Relational leadership includes the embodiment of identity and culture, enacting of organizational (industry) goals and cultural dimension to support Indigenous leaders' ways of being, knowing, and doing. Furthermore, identity includes an understand the importance of genealogical recital, which portrays one's identification of who they are and where they come from in relation to family, territory, language, ancestors, and spiritual and social spheres. Identifying as an Indigenous person or ally is imperative to developing strong relational leadership when working with Indigenous communities; this helps locate and position oneself so that respect is enacted and power dynamics are neutralized. With reference to industry dimensions, enacting relational leadership requires training and mentorship, and open dialogue on the politics and presence of Indigenous peoples in organizations to support knowledge sharing locally and internationally. The macro or larger contextual concerns focus on the consequences of colonialism, institutional racism, and sovereignty as key factors encountered through the individual and collective experience. This contribution offers nursing leaders a way in which Indigenous

worldviews and holistic understanding are affirmed. Relational leadership is a process of social construction that emerges from Indigenous ways of being and doing that examines cultural identity, organizational structural, and contextual dimensions of leadership.

Colleagues Stewart and Warn (2017) explore the influence of indigeneity on Indigenous leaders and found that distinct emerging Indigenous leadership attributes are relationally based. Indigenous leaders are innovative when it comes to working with communities while functioning in non-indigenous systems of governance. Conceptualizations of enacting leadership stemming from this study included demonstrating patience, being a role model, helping people, listening, humility, appropriate communication, and self and territorial acknowledgement. Specific leadership tasks include being the "bridge" or liaison between two worldviews while remaining true to one's own identity and cultural context. Tasks also include embracing change, gaining trust, and supporting individual communities to take ownership and responsibility for their own programming. Key findings are that culture is a leadership resource, and Indigenous leadership must be part of the collective, as opposed to one individual leader, when engaged with Indigenous populations.

In accordance with Indigenous nursing leadership (Bourque Bearskin, et al., 2016; Desjarlais, 2011; Lowe & Struthers, 2001; Struthers, 1999; Kurtz, 2013, Parent, 2010) the Canadian Interprofessional Health Collaborative (2010), overall goal of interprofessional collaboration is to provide improved health outcomes through developing and maintaining interprofessional working relations. It is a process of supporting health care users to be active participants in health care decision making. Collaborative leadership requires both the health care provider and the health care recipient to interact in the following ways:

- Work together to improved patient/client/family/community-centred care.
- Strengthen interdependent working relationships through responsive communication.
- Clarify roles and responsibilities of individual, family, community, and health care providers.
- Facilitate effective, high-functioning teams through role modelling healthy group processes.
- Establish a climate of mutual respect for collaborative leadership practice amongst all participants.

- Creating a climate of trust, self-awareness, and personal responsibility that supports effective conflict resolution.

Similarly, a strength-based approach shared by Gottlieb et al. (2012) recognizes the values of shared responsibility and commitment to family- and community-centred care, which arise out of respect for individual, family, and community decision making and reciprocity in terms of benefiting from the delivery of health care services that promotes family wellness and holistic care.

Developing nursing leadership skills is a continuous process of assessment, planning, implementing, and evaluating an individual's attributes to enhance self-understanding. Levey et al. (2002) outline four key aspects of self-discovery, which include growing awareness of one's intellectual, emotional, spiritual, and physical capabilities. This process helps leaders determine which behaviours are inconsistent with their values and which behaviours embody their values. Self-awareness helps leaders determine their strengths and areas needing improvement and become highly effective leaders for their organization.

RECONCILIATION

Indigenous Human Rights in Relation to Health

Grandmother Doreen Spence is from Saddle Lake, Cree Nation. She is a traditional healer and a retired nurse. When denied admission to nursing school, she applied as a landed immigrant by documenting her birthday as the date she landed in Canada. Doreen graduated from nursing in 1959, and spent over 40 years practising in urban, rural, and remote areas. Since 1994, Doreen has served as a presiding Elder for the United Nations Working Group on Indigenous Populations. She is part of the original group who travelled to Geneva and demanded the concerns of Indigenous peoples be heard by the United Nations. Doreen worked with global Indigenous brothers and sisters to draft the United Nations Declaration of Rights for Indigenous Peoples (2007). She has dedicated her life to service with local-to-global communities as a human rights and peace activist, to build understanding, collaboration, and reconciliation between all peoples. Doreen continues to work closely with nursing students and faculty to integrate Indigenous knowledge and reconciliation within academia and health systems, and was recognized with an honorary Bachelor of Nursing degree

from Mount Royal University. She encourages all nurses to embrace their leadership potential with a loving intention as a central guiding force.

According to the United Nations Permanent Forum on Indigenous issues, "*Cultural rights are of particular relevance for indigenous peoples given that indigenous peoples are culturally distinct from the majority societies in which they live. Cultural rights involve protection for traditional and religious practices, languages, sacred sites, cultural heritage, intellectual property, oral and traditional history, etc. And, economic, social, and cultural rights are deeply rooted in the lands, territories and resources as well as the life ways of Indigenous peoples*" (United Nations Permanent Forum on Indigenous Issues, 2015). The United Nations Declaration on the Rights of Indigenous Peoples (UNDRIP) (2008) emphasizes these rights as indispensable to the survival, dignity, and well-being of Indigenous people. This provides a framework for standards to ensure Indigenous peoples remain distinct to pursue economic, social, education, and health priorities as sovereign nations.

In keeping with UNDRIP (2008), Indigenous health includes the active participation in the design, delivery, and implementation of primary health care services. Under this approach nursing leaders and the populations they serve need to be intimately involved in determining what services and programs improve access to health care and strengthen effectiveness and efficiency of service delivery. This includes services such as traditional wellness, health promotion across the life span, and home care services that protect against illness and alleviate suffering. Partnerships and relationships between and amongst communities, health care systems, federal and provincial governments, institutions, health care professionals, and community rights holders are initiated, developed, and maintained. Principles of Indigenous engagement where the nurse acts as a "bridge" and "brings together" many health care professionals and disciplines required to support innovative and effective research initiatives then lead to increased understanding of critical Indigenous health issues. Nurses who build community capacity by creating culturally appropriate health practice standards and policy to foster local, regional, and national partnerships in Indigenous health service delivery through the implementation of UNDRIP contribute to reducing disparities and inequities in Indigenous health. Addressing equity in Indigenous health requires a deepened knowledge base of why leadership is needed to address Indigenous health disparities. We need to be asking questions such as: What do these health disparity pathways and indicators look like? What is the most effective way to mobilize Indigenous nursing leadership? Does this culturally diverse leadership improve health care services?

EXERCISE 4.4 Nurses are often the first contact someone has with the health care system and are bound by practice standards to protect and promote the health of populations. Knowing that UNDRIP emphasizes the importance of health professionals appreciating the link between Indigenous rights and the strength and resiliency of Indigenous peoples, nursing leaders will be required to ensure this is acted upon in the health care setting. Nurses who familiarize themselves with UNDRIP will recognize it enhances care and is more likely to bring about positive health outcomes and increased adherence to care plans for continued health. Under this approach, clients are driving access to health care services and programs that strengthen the efficiency of service delivery models that include these elements: promote wellness, protect against illness, and develop appropriate interventions that meet the needs of individuals, families, and communities as distinct populations.

Interview a senior nursing leader using the following guiding questions:

1. In which areas is Canada falling short and in which areas are nurses making progress in upholding standards set out in the United Nations Declaration of Rights for Indigenous Peoples (UNDRIP, 2008)?
2. How can we work to encourage all Canadian governments to use UNDRIP as the standard of practice by which to work with Indigenous communities?
3. What challenges do you foresee in using UNDRIP in your work?
4. How can we overcome obstacles to implementing the standards set out in UNDRIP?
5. What future support/connections do you think you will need in using UNDRIP in your work?

Social justice is the cornerstone of health equity and intended for nurses in all domains of administration, education, acute care, home care, community, public health, research, and policy. The CNA Code of Ethics (2017) states, "nurses uphold principles of justice by safeguarding human rights, equity and fairness and by promoting the public good" (p. 15). However, in the case of Indigenous peoples, health and wellness continues to be the poorest across all groups of people in Canada

(Health Council of Canada 2012; King, 2010; Royal College of Physician and Surgeons of Canada, 2012). According to the United Nations Human Rights Office of the High Commissioner (2014), Indigenous populations experience wide array of "devastating human rights violations" (p. 4) exacerbated by unresolved historical issues, overcrowded housing, high population growth rates, high poverty rates, and the geographic remoteness of many communities. There is growing evidence to show the link of poor health status is related to the historical context and ongoing racism and oppression of Canada's colonial health care system (Allan & Smylie, 2015; Greenwood et al. 2018; Health Council of Canada, 2013).

Reutter and Kushner (2010) encourage nurses to advocate for a social justice population health approach because the emphasis on the nurse–patient relationship over the years has not addressed the root causes of these health inequities. Understanding inequities in the health care system creates a contextual understanding of structures, process and policy issues, and analysis of how the current system influences diverse populations. Duncan and Reutter (2006) found that the move from a social model of care to a business model created more disparities for all in access to health care services. Nursing leaders need to advocate for action that requires a shift of thinking from the individual to the collective community within the socio-political economy to decrease health disparities. This collective approach challenges and requires nurses to attend to power and politics and make a difference in the health of communities or populations.

Reconciliation Process

All Canadians are responsible for taking up the global focus as expressed in the United Nations Declaration on the Rights of Indigenous Peoples (UNDRIP) (2008) out of respect for the inherent rights of Indigenous peoples. This mandate is clearly outlined in the Truth and Reconciliation of Canada Commission (8) (2015a) report that calls all levels of government to take up the 94 Calls to Action. In specific regard to health, the TRC explains how the residential school system denied people of their rights to education and health care. This "double denial" has originated in government policy and continues today. From 1831 to 1996, denial of such rights led to cultural genocide of Indigenous peoples in the legacy of government-funded/church-run residential schools: over 150 000 children were taken from their families, up to 6000 died, with 80 000 survivors remaining today.

Numerous cases of the holistic long-standing harm to residential school survivors was brought forward to the courts. Refusal of the federal government to address these cases forced the Supreme Court of Canada to resolve the growing issue. In 2007, residential school survivors and Indigenous organizations, including the Assembly of First Nations, lobbied to create the Indian Residential Schools Settlement Agreement, including establishing the Truth and Reconciliation Commission. In 2008, a formal apology was issued by the Prime Minister, and the residential school survivors' claim for restorative justice began through a process of truth and reconciliation to document the historical legacy of residential schools. For six years, TRC commissioners held private, community, regional, and national events across Canada to gather statements about experiences of residential school (TRC, 2015c). With overwhelming turnout at each event, thousands of people gathered for the opportunity to share their truth. The commissioners spent over 300 days at local health centres across 77 communities and received over 6750 statements from survivors, family members, communities, former residential school staff, government workers, and other Canadians. What was learned from peoples' experience in residential schools was that there was a legacy of intergenerational trauma that significantly contributed to disparities in education, language, health, income, social relationships, racism, and systemic discrimination. Still today there is a disproportionate apprehension of Aboriginal children into the child welfare system, imprisonment of Indigenous peoples, and victimization of survivors and their families (Sinclair, 2007; Blackstock, 2011).

Nurses have a collective responsibility to learn the *Truth* from TRC statement gatherings and engage in a restorative justice process of *Reconciliation* by upholding the Calls to Action (TRC, 2015a). Nurses need to understand and enact the 10 founding principles of TRC to guide the ongoing reconciliation process between Indigenous and non-Indigenous peoples.

1. Enact the United Nations Declaration on the Rights of Indigenous Peoples.
2. Support self-determination through the recognition of human rights.
3. Foster healing relationships by redressing past harms.
4. Advance constructive action that addresses legacies of colonialism.
5. Promote equity and inclusivity between Indigenous and non-Indigenous Canadians.
6. Share responsibilities in maintaining respectful relationships.
7. Acknowledge Indigenous knowledge systems and Indigenous knowledge holders.
8. Revitalize culture to support Indigenous oral histories, laws, and protocols.
9. Create partnerships that are accountable and transparent, with shared resources.
10. Engage in public education to advance collaboration with Indigenous peoples.

While all Calls to Action relate to the social determinants of health, the section explicitly dedicated to health includes the following items:

1. Recognize that the state of health is directly related to Canadian policy of assimilation and colonization.
2. Identify measurable goals in consultation with Indigenous peoples.
3. Acknowledge distinct needs and diversity of First Nations, Inuit, and Métis peoples.
4. Sustainable funding for existing and new programs that are working.
5. Enhance access to traditional healing practices.
6. Recruit and retain more Aboriginal health care providers.
7. Mandatory human rights and anti-racism training in health education.

Nursing leaders who are committed to taking up these "Calls to Action" in nursing focus on the strengths of individual and community attributes by recognizing that personal agency and power dynamics influence health care delivery. Engagement strategies that inspire the human spirit by uplifting the whole community require truth telling, decolonization, and social justice expressions of nursing care

Research done on barriers and facilitators to implementing the TRC Calls to Action within a university health faculty (Kennedy et al, 2018) revealed how colonized dominionization (ownership of expertise) is a barrier to our responsibility in shared caretaking of knowledge to promote health with families, communities, and populations. This research led to an Indigenous knowledge mobilization strategy for reconciliation, guided by retired nurses and Elders Grandmother Doreen Spence (Saddle Lake, Cree Nation) and Roy Bear Chief (Blackfoot,

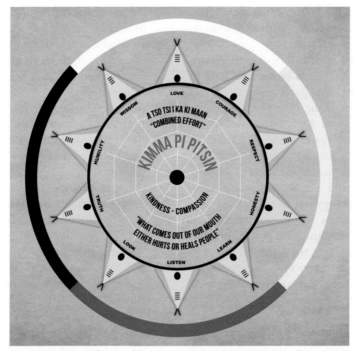

Fig. 4.4 Kimma pi pistin teachings. (Source: Kimma pi pitsin teachings (2018) by Elder Roy Bear Chief (Siksika Nation) with artwork gifted by Jillian Bear Chief (Siksika Nation))

Siksika Nation). Roy is a residential school survivor, and his teachings of central kindness/compassion—*kimma pi pitsin*—situates us in a combined effort working collectively in reconciliation to uphold seven sacred teachings of *truth, humility, wisdom, love, courage, respect, and honesty* (Anishinaabe Elder Dave Courchene) through *looking, listening, and learning* (see Fig. 4.4). When we work together in reconciliation, we build interconnected ways of being and knowing; when we work in silos, we move away from relational building. Roy illustrates this with a teaching he received at a conference presentation by Wilton Littlechild: "Reconciliation is like walking down the railroad tracks. If we walk alone, we lose balance and fall. But if we hold hands, we will go a long way together" (person communication by Elder Roy Bear Chief with Wilton Littlechild).

Nursing Leadership and Reconciliation

As our health care system continues to grow and change, so does the role of nursing. Nurses are continuously adapting with the evolving health care system and are paramount in becoming leaders in an interprofessional and interdisciplinary team (Curtis et al., 2011; Parse, 2015). Leading and organizing care represent a large portion of the nurse's role (Ekström & Idvall, 2015). Therefore it is imperative that nurses entering the workforce

take necessary steps to develop strong leadership skills. Authentic relational, collective, and strength-based leadership skills are needed to facilitate reconciliation between Indigenous and non-Indigenous people living in Canada. Nursing leadership roles in reconciliation are social justice–centred and include a relational ethic, respecting and upholding the need for self-determination with all peoples, including Indigenous populations.

After decades of intergenerational trauma stemming from colonization, every Canadian needs to understand the widespread legacy trauma has had on individuals, families, communities, and systems of health, education, and justice. Nurses may commemorate residential school survivors by upholding the concept that "Every Child Matters" and honouring a child whose orange shirt was taken away on their first day of residential school at St. Joseph Mission in William Lake, B.C. Nurses need to be vigilant and to act, so this vision becomes reality in health care, with our mantra "Every Patient, Family and Community Matters."

There are four key actions nurses can take that stem from an intentional integration of the personal, professional, and political where we engage in authentic, reciprocal, and meaningful relationships.

1. **Full Presence:** Listening, knowing, being, and doing. Listen to the people, hear the suffering, and be aware

of your own bias. Know how these biases unfold in your day-to-day practice and how they influence your current perceptions and approaches. Be present, help people exercise their personhood, and inspire them by giving them space to speak their language, tell their stories, and direct their own care.

2. **Lifelong Learning and Action**: Do everything you can to ensure reconciliation remains endless. As Justice Murray Sinclair stated, "Education got us into this mess, education will get us out." Familiarize yourself with the United Nations Declaration on the Rights of Indigenous Peoples so that when you are developing policy you are informed about what is working and what is not, and always remember that policy is not made to be static. Listen to what is not working in the system and be prepared to enact social justice by grounding your decisions in the UNDRIP (2008).

3. **Reflexivity**: Be prepared to engage in self-reflexive thinking asking yourself why this policy is important, and does it work to improve access to health care or create more barriers. As nurses, take a stand on Indigenous rights to health and support the redesigning and improvement of quality of nursing care delivered to Indigenous populations.

4. **Advocacy for Equity:** Every nurse must enact their leadership by taking up the call for mandatory Indigenous nursing education as nurses who advocate for health equity recognize and understand the impact that legislated identities and the influence of colonization has had on the overall wellness of First Nations, Inuit, and Métis peoples.

Decolonization of Nursing Practice, Leadership and Health Care

It is important to recognize that Canadian nursing education and practice are deeply colonized and to understand how entrenched Eurocentric systems lead to domination rather than social justice and equity. Decolonization is considered with respect to the "ethical space of engagement" (Ermine, 2007), noting the opportunity for Western and Indigenous peoples to collaborate through truthful reflection, deepened awareness, and mutual respect. Scholar Michael Yellow Bird from Sahnish and Hidatsa Nations conceptualizes decolonization as both an event and process:

> "**Event** – As an event, decolonization concerns reaching a level of critical consciousness, an active understanding that you are (or have been) colonized and are thus responding to life circumstances in ways that are limited, destructive, and externally controlled.
>
> **Process** – As a process, decolonization means engaging in the activities of creating, restoring, and birthing. It means creating and consciously using various strategies to liberate oneself, adapt to or survive oppressive conditions; it means restoring cultural practices, thinking, beliefs, and values that were taken away or abandoned but are still relevant and necessary to survival; and it means the birthing of new ideas, thinking, technologies, and lifestyles that contribute to the advancement and empowerment of Indigenous Peoples." (Waziyatawin & Yellow Bird, 2012, p. 3)

To engage in reconciliation and decolonization, we must understand how settler colonialism (Barker, 2012) has pervasive roots in the displacement of Indigenous ways of being and knowing at micro, meso, and macro levels. Within nursing, questions around Indigenous knowledge are centred on the experience of colonization and intertwined with questions of identity, displacement, decolonization, equity, and power. This critical reflection and awareness is the first step in the ongoing process of decolonization for Indigenous and non-Indigenous people alike (Regan, 2010).

McKillop at al. (2012) describe how the domination of a Eurocentric perspective intentionally and unintentionally undermined their own Indigenous knowledge. European domination marginalized and disclaimed Indigenous knowledge and legitimized Eurocentric knowledge through "cognitive imperialism" (Battiste, 2005; 2013).

Even in accessing nursing post-secondary studies, preparing students for university, barriers continue to be rooted in their ongoing experiences of colonization and marginalization (Smith et al., 2011). Sherwood and Edwards (2006) emphasize how nurses need to integrate decolonization in health care as a critical reflective thinking skill-set used to critique Western cultural paradigms that inform our perceptions of and assumptions about Indigenous peoples. Study findings by Bourque Bearskin (2014) illustrate how Indigenous nursing scholars collectively acknowledge decolonization as a process to address social issues. Decolonization within the wider framework of self-determination is needed to articulate questions to explore the ethical space of Indigenous ways of being, knowing, and dwelling in nursing.

McGibbon et al. (2014) articulate the importance of critical analysis of "nursing's participation in colonial processes and practices . . . based on the examination of politics and power of the structural determinants of health" (p. 179). The authors urge nurses to consider decolonization as an immediate imperative for positive change and advancement within our discipline and practice, so that nurses may authentically cultivate social justice and equity. Nursing decolonization emphasizes integration of postcolonial theories by doing the following:

- *Focusing on colonized subjectivities and imperialism* to challenge oppressive Eurocentric systems, with action that reclaims Indigenous identity and knowledge in nursing.
- *Applying a critical social science perspective* to question power structures that adversely impact health outcomes, with action that is re-centred on equity to re-pattern complex health determinants.
- *Committing working toward decolonization* to address the colonial nature of Canadian nursing, with action that "involves affirming and activating paradigms of Indigenous knowledge" (McGibbon et al., 2014, pp. 180–182).

Working toward decolonization requires honest reflection of beliefs and assumptions, including how racism and white privilege are personal-to-systemic barriers in promoting health and upholding nursing ethics. Honest reflection challenges the ideology that nurses treat everyone equally and reframes this mindset more accurately as an aspirational goal. Nurses need to address how colonized nursing knowledge and practice perpetuates inequity, equipped with knowledge and skills to move forward in a relational (Bourque Bearskin, 2011) and ethical space of engagement (Ermine, 2007). Such decolonizing practices are consistent with a social innovation approach (Mason et al., 2015; Murray et al., 2010) to create positive change at all levels:

1. Micro: individual practice.
2. Meso: teams, departments, and facilities.
3. Macro: health, education, social, and political systems.

In nursing education, CINA, CNA and the Canadian Association of Schools of Nursing (2013) developed a framework for nurses addressing and integrating Indigenous knowledge that is respectful and responsive to the needs of Indigenous populations. Strategies are aimed at social justice, anti-racist education, and cultural safety through the building of respectful relationships in the context of the historical, social, political, and economic determinants of health. According to Waite and Nardi (2017), nursing colonialism in North America results in racism and continues to shape the knowledge, attitude, and skills of nurses' leadership. The authors outline specific strategies to decolonize the nursing profession, which include moving beyond the ally role and becoming an *accomplice* to deconstructing white privilege and mobilizing anti-racist practice and policy. An accomplice is described as someone who optimizes inclusion, critiques organizations' public persona, maintains a process of knowledge development, and not only recognizes white silence but takes action to identify and change ethnocentric education and practice. These strategies are direct actions confronting and revealing marginalizing nursing practices and health inequities that have been generated and sustained by colonialism, and destroying structural racism.

The Federation of Post-Secondary Educators of BC (McFarlane & Schabus, 2017) published a decolonization resource manual titled *Whose Land Is It Anyways.* This resource was inspired by the late Arthur Manuel, a prominent and humble Indigenous activist who spent his entire life advocating for Indigenous rights. He is well known for his leadership from the local to the international arenas, serving with his Neskonlith Indian band, Shuswap Nation Tribal Council, and UN Permanent Forum on Indigenous Peoples. This resource explains how the grassroots defenders of decolonization are the undoing of colonization, and that what is needed to achieve decolonization is land reclamation and returning to the teachings of Indigenous knowledge holders and Elders (Manuel, 2017). Decolonization is about safety and protection of those who suffer from violence, and celebrating the resilience, strength, and authentic belonging that makes partners of and honours Indigenous women and two-spirited people (Jacobs 2017; McNeil-Seymour, 2017). Decolonization is "heart-centered and does not look like Indigenized heteropatriarchy . . . it is a call-in to ensure our ways forward in nation and community revision are decolonized, equitable and sovereign" (McNeil-Seymour, 2017, p. 56). Decolonization is about land-based pedagogy, international advocacy for human rights, and reclaiming Indigenous knowledge (Coulthard, 2017; Schabus, 2017; Palmater, 2017).

Bill Mussell (2008), a residential school survivor, student of Paulo Freire, and national leader in mental health, describes decolonization as a building block for reconciliation. It begins with a process of self-discovery, truth-telling, and relationship mending between Indigenous and non-Indigenous Peoples. His story, like so many, is difficult to hear, but this recognition of the historical trauma and injustice needs to happen at every level—personal, community, and systemic. He states, "If reconciliation is to work, restoration of Indigenous languages, cultures social structures and traditional institution for governance must occur" (p. 324).

Nurses can make the difference: we must choose to be vigilant and not continue the victimization of Indigenous peoples. We can do this by engaging in decolonization and reconciliation as nurse leaders. Together we may rewrite and re-right the Canadian narrative in support of equity with Indigenous peoples to move beyond the ascriptions that have been embedded into our flesh to working toward "achieved wellness" (Dion Stout, 2012). Nurses can nurture this transformation so that peoples and systems can begin doing the work that is responsive to the needs of Indigenous populations.

CONCLUSION

In the collective effort of nursing leaders, it is crucial to engage in decolonization and reconciliation to advance health equity. The first step is engaging in learning about diverse Indigenous populations and health and truthfully reflecting on connections to practice. Nurses

💡 A SOLUTION

The struggles faced by many First Nations, Inuit, and Métis communities to sustain and deliver comprehensive, effective, and culturally safe health care services that are rights- and strengths-based is an issue of global concern. Nursing leaders committed to taking up the challenge of decolonization and Indigenization in nursing practice begin with addressing inequitable access to health care by disrupting the impacts of stereotyping, biases, and discrimination in nursing.

From a position of cultural humility, Spencer begins with self-reflection of assumptions and biases in preparation for engaging with the Métis community. Spencer considers how western-dominated systems shape societal views and health care services. Spencer recognizes the importance of challenging stereotypes and providing respectful nursing care, noting that generalizing Indigenous health inequities may lead to inaccurate and disrespectful assumptions. Learning from the community is key for empowerment and health promotion. To address specific health indicators unique to Métis settlements, Spencer seeks out community members with knowledge about local determinants of health, including social, economic, and political factors. Together they explore how such factors contribute to health equity and disparities experienced by Métis peoples. Following this assessment Spencer gains a more fulsome understanding of key factors influencing diabetes with this Métis settlement. In follow-up, Spencer fosters partnerships between the local, provincial, and national diabetes organizations that enhance local participation in the design and delivery of diabetes education. Going beyond the typical format for diabetes education, Spencer uses a client-centred nursing approach and recognizes that relational and collaborative leadership skills help in engaging in meaningful ways as a means of creating culturally safe working relationships. In addition, Spencer applies a strengths-based approach to guide the assessment in order to begin with positive community health indicators and resilience. From this stance, health challenges may be explored with a collaborative solution-oriented approach in partnership with the community. Furthermore, explicit respect of cultural identity will empower community members to consider their own health practices while learning about westernized diabetes care. Essentially Spencer's enactment of cultural humility is a process that helps nurses provide safe and effective care founded on trust and respect of cultural identity. This is established through ongoing reflection and learning with Indigenous clients and communities, noting the impact of personal and systemic discrimination. Nurses become skilled in recognizing how their own privilege, biases, and approach unfolds in practice and influences health promotion with Indigenous populations. Cultural safety is the outcome of trust and respecting cultural identity, resulting in services and workplaces that are safe, respectful, and free of discrimination.

What is your next step— what is your personal, professional, or political Call to Action to advance decolonization and indigenization in nursing practice?

need to stop problematizing Indigenous culture and peoples and demand equitable health service delivery. Rooted in cultural safety, nurses need to focus on the strengths and personal/community attributes of personal agency, power dynamics in health care systems, and authentic engagement strategies that uplift the whole community. The history and contribution of Indigenous nursing knowledge must be recognized and integrated within nurse education and practice, noting how this advances the nursing discipline. We must remain grounded and strong in our support of ongoing decolonization and reconciliation efforts by upholding the UNDRIP (2008) and TRC (2015a) Calls to Action. Vigilance in nursing is the astute attention to detail and its surroundings. As nurse leaders, it is important to ask: What is the contribution of vigilance in nursing and how do we communicate this vigilance? If we are taking a social justice stance in nursing leadership, we need to ignite a conversation with the goal of developing ownership for our actions with Indigenous populations, including relations with Indigenous nurses.

THE EVIDENCE

The growing evidence revealing Canada's dark history of abuse and attempted genocide of Indigenous peoples has lasting impacts on Indigenous health equity. Health inequities and disparities cut across a wide range of major health outcomes and health determinants and have been exacerbated by Indigenous health policy. The influence between colonialism, racism, and nursing leadership is relatively new concept that disrupts older ideas about nursing leadership and the delivery of effective and culturally relevant health care for Indigenous peoples. Enhancing nurses' understanding of colonialism, using a critical lens to undertake self-exploration and an analysis of Indigenous and mainstream knowledge and practices within complex health systems is imperative. Historically, Indigenous and Western knowledge is perceived as existing on opposite ends of a spectrum. But instead of being viewed as opposites, they can be perceived as complementary elements that support holistic nursing practice. Zeran (2016) describes achieving such a balance through involving a council of elders to assist in understanding Indigenous ways of knowing, establishing a culture of inclusivity, and greater exposure to alternative perspectives and ways of being as an essential aspect of understanding Indigenous nursing knowledge. Furthermore, understanding the experiences, values, traditions, and history of Indigenous nurses highlights how predetermined attitudes and actions put others at risk for cultural harm, and how Indigenous identity is essential to enhancing professional practice (Bourque Bearskin et al., 2016). In a critical review by Rozendo et al. (2017) on social and health inequalities in the nursing curriculum, social justice, cultural competence, advocacy, cultural safety, and social responsibility were the main elements identified that contribute to reducing social and health inequalities. The authors highlighted the need for nurses to understand how health inequalities are produced and sustained, especially in nurses' approach to taking action. Nurses need to continue to equip themselves with critical knowledge of how to confront the root causes of inequalities so that they can take part in the political change. This review reinforces the idea that nurses lack an understanding of culturally informed care, especially when it comes to marginalized and vulnerable populations, as nurses do not know how to properly care and provide resource for this patient population. It is evident there is an absence of Indigenous content within the nursing standards for professional practice and that minimal research has been done from an Indigenous perspective. While the ideal of the "Calls to Action" outlined in the TRC is to ensure health education specifically addresses Indigenous history and health disparities exists, this has not yet been met and is an area where nursing leadership in Indigenous health can flourish. In advancing the discourse on Indigenous health, we are in the midst of change and a shift in mainstream society is acknowledging that Indigenous ways of knowing, reconnecting, and rebuilding relationships is necessary to support the social justice movement of Indigenous peoples.

✳ NEED TO KNOW NOW

- Understand the diversity of Indigenous populations in Canada.
- Promote culturally safe care, respecting traditional health practices.
- Engage in lifelong learning and relationship-building with Indigenous populations.

- Be responsive to Indigenous nursing knowledge and how this guides nursing leadership and promotes health for all.
- Understand Indigenous human rights and how to engage effectively in reconciliation.
- Promote equity in nursing and health.

CHAPTER CHECKLIST

Nursing leadership in Indigenous health is a relatively new area of study. This chapter provides an overview of key concepts important in understanding the complexities of Indigenous health, Indigenous nurses' knowledge, and reconciliation. Nursing leaders must challenge the status quo and never be complacent in delivering health care services that are harmful to Indigenous populations. In the spirit of reconciliation, all nurses have the capacity for leadership and must acknowledge and address Indigenous human rights. The nurse must be able to do the following:

- Understand the diversity of Indigenous populations beyond the legislative definitions.
- Transform the current deficit-based approach in nursing to a strengths- and rights-based practice.
- Recognize that health inequities and disparities are rooted in colonization.

- Articulate the negative consequences of Indigenous health policies on Indigenous populations.
- Create supportive environments where innovation and possibilities to change health care systems are enhanced.
- Incorporate the history and socialization of Indigenous nurses in Canada.
- Lead with a clear understanding of principles that embraces cultural humility as a means to achieving cultural safety.
- Appraise key elements of Indigenous Nursing Knowledge and relational nursing leadership skills.
- Engage in decolonization and reconciliation as an ongoing process in maintaining human rights in relations to Indigenous health.
- Advocate for the adoption of the United Nations Declaration on the Rights of Indigenous Peoples in health care.

TIPS FOR LEADING WITH EQUITY

Since Canadian nurses lead practice in various settings with Indigenous populations, nurses need to do the following:

- Implement a rights- and strengths-based approach based on the United Nations Declaration of Rights for Indigenous Peoples (2007).
- Recognize and acknowledge Indigenous traditional territories.
- Uphold inclusivity and respectful collaboration "not for us without us."
- Describe effective techniques for leading with cultural safety.

- Help address the cultural needs and rights of patients and colleagues.
- Embrace principles relating to cultural safety and humility to promote human rights and equity.
- Commit to lifelong learning with Indigenous populations.
- Advocate for capacity development and the sharing of human and financial resources.
- Promote knowledge sharing of both traditional Indigenous and Western based health care services.

Visit the Evolve website for Suggested Readings, Internet Resources, and additional resources related to the content in this chapter: http://evolve.elsevier.com/Canada/Yoder-Wise/leading/.

REFERENCES

Aboriginal Nurses Association of Canada (ANAC). (2016). *Ninanâskomânânak kâkinîkânohtêcik we are grateful for the first leaders*. Ottawa: Author.

Aboriginal Nurses Association of Canada. (2009). *Cultural competence and cultural safety in nursing education*. Ottawa, ON: Aboriginal Nurses Association of Canada. http://www.anac.on.ca/Documents/Making%20It%20Happen%20Curriculum%20Project/FINALFRAMEWORK.pdf.

Adelson, N. (2005). The embodiment of inequity: Health disparities in Aboriginal Canada. *Canadian Journal of Public Health, 96*, S45–S61.

Alexander, C., & Lopez, R. P. (2018). A thematic analysis of self-described authentic leadership behaviors among experienced nurse executives. *Journal of Nursing Administration, 48*(1), 38–43.

Allan, B., & Smylie, J. (2015). *First Peoples, second class treatment: The role of racism in the health and well-being of Indigenous peoples in Canada*. Toronto: The Wellesley Institute.

Anderson, K. (2001). *A recognition of being: Reconstructing Native womanhood*. Toronto, ON: Sumach Press (Original work published 2000).

Anderson, J., Perry, J., Blue, C., Browne, A., Henderson, A., Khan, K. B., et al. (2003). Rewriting cultural safety within the postcolonial and postnational feminist project. Toward new epistemologies of healing. *Advances in Nursing Science, 26*(3), 196–214.

Annett, R. K. D. (2001). *Hidden from history: The Canadian holocaust. The untold story of the genocide of Aboriginal Peoples by the Church and State in Canada. A summary of ongoing, independent inquiry into Canadian Native 'Residential Schools' and their legacy*Port Alberni, BC: The Truth Commission into Genocide in Canada. http://canadiangenocide.nativeweb.org/genocide.pdf.

Archibald, J. (2008). *Indigenous storywork: Educating the heart, mind, body and spirit*. Vancouver, BC: UBC Press.

Bahr, A. M. B. B. (2005). *Religions of the world. Indigenous religions*. Philadelphia: Chelsea House Publishers.

Barker, A. (2012). Locating settler colonialism. *Journal of Colonialism & Colonial History, 13*(3), 1–11.

Barnhardt, R., & Kawagley, A. O. (2005). Indigenous knowledge systems and Alaska Native ways of knowing. *Anthropology and Education Quarterly, 36*(1), 8–23.

Baskin, C. (2016). *Strong helpers' teachings: The value of Indigenous Knowledges in the helping professions* (2nd ed.). Toronto: Canadian Scholars' Press.

Basso, K. H. (1996). *Wisdom sits in places: Landscape and language among the Western Apache*. Albuquerque, NM: UNM Press.

Battiste, M. (2013). *Decolonizing education: Nourishing the learning spirit*. Saskatoon, SK: Purich.

Battiste, M. (2005). *Indigenous knowledge: Foundations for First Nations*. Saskatoon: University of Saskatchewan. https://www2.viu.ca/integratedplanning/documents/IndegenousKnowledgePaperbyMarieBattistecopy.pdf.

Battiste, M., & Youngblood Henderson, J. (2000). *Protecting Indigenous knowledge and heritage: A global challenge*. Saskatoon, SK: Purich.

Battiste, M. (2002). *Indigenous knowledge and pedagogy in First Nations education: A literature review with recommendations. National Working Group on Education, Our Children: Keepers of the Sacred Knowledge*. Ottawa, ON: Indian and Northern Affairs Canada.

Bill, L. (2012). Ceremony and the Indigenous field. In F. Mason Boring (Ed.), *Connection to our ancestral past. Healing through family constellations, ceremony and ritual* (pp. 49–59). Berkeley, CA: North Atlantic Books.

Blackstock, C. (2011). The Canadian Human Rights Tribunal on First Nations child welfare: Why if Canada wins, equality and justice lose. *Children and Youth Series Review, 33*(1), 187–194.

Blackstock, C. (2012). Jordan's principle: Canada's broken promise to First Nations children? *Paediatrics & Child Health, 17*(7), 368–370.

Bourque Bearskin, R. L. (2011). A critical lens on culture in nursing practice. *Nurse Ethics, 18*(4), 548–559. https://doi.org/10.1177/0969733011408048.

Bourque Bearskin, L. R. (2014). *Mâmawoh Kamâtowin, "Coming together to help each other in wellness". Doctoral thesis*. Edmonton: University of Alberta.

Bourque Bearskin, R. L., & Downey, B. (2016, May). *Indigenous nursing Knowledge: A Call to Action for Nursing Educators*. Toronto Ontario: CASN Biennial Canadian Nursing Education Conference. https://www.casn.ca/wp-content/uploads/2016/02/Program-2016-SB-FINAL-revised-p-142.pdf.

Bourque Bearskin, R. L., Cameron, B., King, M., Weber-Pillwax, C., Dion Stout, M., Voyageur, E., et al. (2016). Mâmawoh Kamâtowin, "Coming together to help each other in wellness": Honouring Indigenous Nursing Knowledge. *International Journal of Indigenous Health, 11*(1), 18–33. https://doi.org/10.18357/ijih111201615024.

Bowen, E., & Murshid, N. S. (2016). Trauma informed social policy: A conceptual framework for policy analysis and advocacy. *American Journal of Public Health, 106*(2), 223–229.

Bradford, L. E. A., Zagozewski, R., & Bharadwaj, L. (2017). Perspectives of water and health using photovoice with youths living on reserve. *The Canadian Geographer, 61*(2), 178–195. https://doi.org/10.1111/cag.12331.

Brookes, S. (2015). *The selfless leader: A compass for collective leadership*. New York: Palgrave Macmillan.

Browne, A. J., Smye, V. L., Rodney, P., Tang, S. Y., Mussell, B., & O'Neill, J. (2011). Access to primary care from the perspective of Aboriginal patients at an urban emergency department. *Qualitative Health Research, 21*(3), 333–348.

Browne, A. J., Varcoe, C., Lavoie, J., Smye, V., Wong, S. T., Krause, M., et al. (2016). Enhancing health care equity with indigenous populations: Evidence–based strategies from an ethnographic study. *BMC Health Services Research, 16*(1), 544.

Burnett, K. (2010). *Taking medicine: Women's healing work and colonial contact in Southern Alberta, 1880-1930*. Vancouver: UBC Press.

Cameron, B. L., Martial, R., King, M., Santos Salas, A., Bourque Bearskin, R. L., Camargo Plazas, P. M., et al. (2014). *Access Research Community Report: Reducing health disparities and promoting equitable access to health care service for Indigenous peoples. Communitsy Report*. Edmonton, AB: University of Alberta, Faculty of Nursing.

Cameron, B. L., Camargo Plazas, M. D. P., Santos Salas, A., Bourque Bearskin, R. L., & Hungler, K. (2014). Understanding inequalities in access to health care services for Aboriginal people: A call for nursing action. *Advances in Nursing Science, 37*(3), E1–E16.

Canadian Association of Schools of Nursing. (2013). *Educating nurses to address socio-cultural, historical, and contextual determinants of health among Aboriginal Peoples*. Ottawa: Author. https://casn.ca/wp-content/uploads/2014/12/ENAHHRIKnowledgeProductFINAL.pdf.

Canadian Human Rights Commission. (2010). *Report on equality rights of Aboriginal people*. Ottawa: Author.

Canadian Indigenous Nurses Association (C.I.N.A.). (2016). *Nothing for us-without us. Indigenous Nurse Newsletter (Spring)*. Ottawa: Author.

Canadian Indigenous Nurses Association. (n.d.). Canadian Indigenous Nurses Association (CINA). http://indigenousnurses.ca/.

Canadian Indigenous Nurses Association & University of Saskatchewan College of Nursing. (2018). *Aboriginal nursing in Canada*. http://indigenousnurses.ca/sites/default/files/inline-files/Nursing_AborigNursing_sheet_2018_3.pdf.

Canadian Interprofessional Health Collaborative. (2010). *A national interprofessional competency framework*. Vancouver: Author.

Canadian Nurses Association. (2009). *Position statement: Nursing leadership*. https://www.cna-aiic.ca/~/media/cna/page-content/pdf-en/nursing-leadership_position-statement.pdf?la=en.

Canadian Nurses Association. (2017). *Code of ethics for registered nurses*. Ottawa: Author.

Canadian Nurses Association and Canadian Indigenous Nurses Association. (2016). *National nursing associations sign partnership accord in spirit of authentic Indigenous collaboration*. https://www.cna-aiic.ca/en/news-room/news-releases/2016/national-nursing-associations-sign-partnership-accord-to-improve-indigenous-health.

Cardinal, L. (2001). What is an Indigenous perspective? *Canadian Journal of Native Education, 25*, 180–182.

Castellano, M. B. (2000). Updating Aboriginal traditions of knowledge. In B. L. Hall, G. J. S. Dei, & D. G. Rosenberg (Eds.), *Indigenous knowledges in global contexts: Multiple readings of our world* (pp. 21–36). Toronto: University of Toronto Press.

Coulthard, G. (2017). Dechinta-Bush University: Land-based education and Indigenous resurgence. In R. McFarlane & N. Schabus (Eds.), *Decolonization handbook. Whose land is it anyway?* (pp. 57–61). Vancouver: Federation of Post-Secondary Education.

Curtis, E. A., de Vries, J., & Sheerin, F. K. (2011). Developing leadership in nursing: Exploring core factors. *British Journal of Nursing, 20*(5), 306–309.

Desjarlais, J. (2011). *Walking in multiple worlds: Stories of Aboriginal nurses*. Edmonton, AB: Doctoral Dissertation.

Dickason, O., & McNab, D. (2009). *Canada's First Nations: A history of founding peoples from earliest times*. Don Mills, ON: Oxford University Press.

Dion Stout, M. (2012). Discourse: Ascribed health and wellness, "Atikowisi miýw-ayawin," to achieved health and wellness, "Kaskitamasowin miýwaayawin": Shifting the paradigm. *Canadian Journal of Nursing Research, 44*(2), 11–14.

Dion Stout, M., & Downey, B. (2006). Nursing, Indigenous peoples and cultural safety: So what? Now what? *Contemporary Nurse, 22*, 327–332.

Dion Stout, M., Stout, R., & Rojas, A. (2001). *Thinking outside the box: Health policy options for NAHO to consider: Roundtable report*. Ottawa, ON: National Aboriginal Health Organization.

Donahue, P. (2011). *Nursing, the finest art: An illustrated history* (3rd ed.). Iowa City, IA: Mosby Elsevier.

Donald, D. (2012). Indigenous Métissage: A decolonizing research sensibility. *International Journal of Qualitative Studies in Education, 25*(5), 533–555.

Doyle, K., & Hungerford, C. (2015). Leadership as a personal journey. An Indigenous perspective. *Issues in Mental Health Nursing, 36*(5), 336–345.

Drees, L. M. (2013). *Healing histories: Stories from Canada's Indian hospitals*. Edmonton, AB: The University of Alberta Press.

Duncan, S., & Reutter, L. (2006). A critical policy analysis of an emerging agenda for home care in one Canadian province. *Health and Social Care in Community, 14*(3), 242–253.

Ekström, L., & Idvall, E. (2015). Becoming a team leader: Newly registered nurses relate their experiences. *Journal of Nursing Management, 23*(1), 75–86.

Ermine, W. (1995). Aboriginal epistemology. In M. Battiste, & J. Barman (Eds.), *First Nations education in Canada: The circle unfolds* (pp. 101–112). Vancouver: University of British Columbia Press.

Ermine, W. (2007). Ethical space of engagement. *Indigenous Law Journal, 6*(1), 193–203.

Etowa, J., Jesty, C., & Vukic, A. (2011). Indigenous nurses' stories: Perspectives on the cultural context of Aboriginal health care work. *The Canadian Journal of Native Studies, 31*(2), 29–46.

Evans-Campbell, T. (2008). Historical trauma in American Indian/Native Alaska communities: A multilevel framework for exploring impacts on individuals, families, and communities. *Journal of Interpersonal Violence, 23*(93), 316–338.

Fiedeldey-Van Dijk, C., Hall, L., Mykota, D., Farag, M., & Shea, B. (2016). Honoring Indigenous culture-as-intervention: Development and validity of the Native Wellness Assessment. *Journal of Ethnicity in Substance Abuse.*

First Nations Health Authority. (2018). *Cultural humility.* http://www.fnha.ca/wellness/cultural-humility#learn.

First Nations Child and Family Caring Society of Canada. (2016). *Dr. Peter Henderson Bryce: A story of courage. Information Sheet. Ottawa: Author.* https://fncaringsociety.com/sites/default/files/Dr.%20Peter%20Henderson%20Bryce%20Information%20Sheet.pdf.

First Nations Information Governance Centre (2018). *National report of the First Nations regional health survey. Phase 3: Volume 1.* Ottawa: Author. Retrieved from: http://fnigc.ca/sites/default/files/docs/fnigc_rhs_phase_3_national_report_vol_1_en_final_web.pdf

Foronda, C., Baptiste, D. L., & Reinholdt, M. (2015). Cultural humility: A concept analysis. *Journal of Transcultural Nursing, 27*(3), 210–217.

Department of the Interior, Annual Report for the year ended 30th June, 1876 (Parliament, Sessional Papers, No. 11, 1877), p. xiv.

Galuska, L. (2016). Advocating for patients: Honoring professional trust. *AORN – Association of perioperative Registered Nurses, 104*(5), 410–416.

George, J., Macleod, M., Graham, K., Plain, S., Bernards, S., & Wells, S. (2018). Traditional healing practices in two Ontario first nations. *Journal of Community Health, 43*(2), 227–237.

Goodwill, J. (1975). *Speaking together: Canada's native women.* Ottawa: Department of the Secretary of State.

Gottlieb, L. N., Gottleib, B., & Shamian, J. (2012). Principles of strengths-based nursing leadership for strengths-based nursing care: A new paradigm for nursing and healthcare for the 21st century. *Nursing Leadership, 25*(2), 38–50.

Government of Canada. (2006). *Aboriginal Roundtable to Kelowna Accord: Aboriginal Policy negotiations 2004-2006.* https://lop.parl.ca/content/lop/ResearchPublications/prb0604-e.pdf.

Government of Canada. (2014). *Indian health policy.* https://www.canada.ca/en/indigenous-services-canada/corporate/first-nations-inuit-health-branch/indian-health-policy-1979.html.

Government of Canada. (2014). *Canada's health care system.* Ottawa, ON: Author. http://www.hc-sc.gc.ca/hcs-sss/pubs/system-regime/2011-hcs-sss/index-eng.php.

Government of Canada. (2016). *Canada's health care system.* https://www.canada.ca/en/health-canada/services/canada-health-care-system.html.

Government of Canada. (2018a). *Indigenous services Canada.* https://www.canada.ca/content/canadasite/en/indigenous-services-canada.html.

Government of Canada. (2018b). *Indigenous health.* https://www.canada.ca/en/services/health/aboriginal-health.html.

Government of Canada. (2018c). *2018-2019 Departmental plan: Health Canada.* https://www.canada.ca/en/health-canada/corporate/transparency/corporate-management-reporting/report-plans-priorities/2018-2019-report-plans-priorities.html.

Greenwood, M., de Leeuw, S., & Lindsay, N. (2018). Challenges in health equity for Indigenous peoples in Canada. *The Lancet, 391*(10131), 1645–1648.

Hart, M. A. (2002). *Seeking mino-pimatisiwin: An Aboriginal approach to helping.* Halifax, NS: Fernwood.

Health Council of Canada. (2012). *Empathy, dignity, and respect: Creating cultural safety for Aboriginal people in urban health care.* Toronto: Author.

Health Council of Canada. (2013). *Canada's most vulnerable: Improving health care for First Nations, Inuit, and Métis Seniors.* Toronto: Author.

Henry, E., & Wolfgramm, R. (2018). Relational leadership – an Indigenous Māori Perspective. *Leadership, 14*(2), 203–219.

Institute on Governance. (2013). *Beyond Section 35 BC symposium summary.* Ottawa: Author.

Jacklin, K. M., Henderson, R. I., Green, M. E., Walker, L. M., Calam, B., & Crowshoe, L. J. (2017). Health care experiences of Indigenous people living with type 2 diabetes in Canada. *Canadian Medical Association Journal, 189*(3), E106–E112.

Jacobs, B. (2017). Decolonizing the violence against Indigenous women. In R. McFarlane & N. Schabus (Eds.), *Decolonization handbook. Whose land is it anyway?* (pp. 47–51). Vancouver: Federation of Post-Secondary Education.

Kennedy, A., McGowan, K., & El Hussein, M. (2018). *Grounded theory of barriers and facilitators to implementing Truth and Reconciliation (2015) Calls to Action with Health Faculty: Moving forward with together with Kimma Pi Pitsin.* Unpublished manuscript: Mount Royal University.

Kenny, C. B. (2012). Liberating leadership theory. In C. B. Kenny, & T. N. Fraser (Eds.), *Living indigenous leadership: native narratives on building strong communities* (pp. 1–14). Vancouver: UBC Press.

Kenny, C. B., & Fraser, T. N. (2012). *Living indigenous leadership: Native narratives on building strong communities.* Vancouver: UBC Press.

King, M. (2010). Chronic diseases and mortality in Canadian Aboriginal peoples: Learning from the knowledge. *Chronic Diseases in Canada, 31*(1), 2–3.

Kirkness, V. J., & Barnhardt, R. (2001). The Four Rs – Respect, Relevance, Reciprocity, Responsibility. In R. Hayoe, & J. Pan (Eds.), *Knowledge across cultures: A contribution to dialogue among civilizations* (pp. 1–18). Hong Kong: Comparative Education Research Centre, The University of Hong Kong. https://www.afn.ca/uploads/files/education2/the4rs.pdf.

Kurtz, D. L. (2013). Indigenous methodologies: Traversing Indigenous and Western worldviews in research. *AlterNative: An International Journal of Indigenous Peoples, 9*(3), 217–230.

Levey, S., Hill, J., & Green, B. (2002). Leadership in healthcare and the leadership literature. *Journal of Ambulatory Care Management, 25*(2), 68–75.

Lightning, W. C. (1992). Compassionate mind: Implications of a text written by elder Louis Sunchild. *Canadian Journal of Native Education, 19*(2), 215–253.

Logan McCallum, M. J. (2017). Starvation, experimentation, segregation, and trauma: Words for reading Indigenous health history. *Canadian Historical Review, 98*(1), 96–113.

Lovie, J., Forget, E., & Browne, A. (2010). Caught at the crossroads: First nations health care, and the legacy of the indian act. *Pimatisiwin: A Journal of Aboriginal and Indigenous Community Health, 8*(1), 83–94.

Lowe, J., & Struthers, R. (2001). A conceptual framework of nursing in Native American culture. *Journal of Nursing Scholarship, 33*(3), 279–283.

Mahara, M. S., Duncan, S. M., Whyte, N., & Brown, J. (2011). It takes a community to raise a nurse: Educating for culturally safe practice with Aboriginal peoples. *International Journal of Nursing Education Scholarship, 8*(17), 1–13.

Manuel, W. (2017). From dispossession to dependency. In R. McFarlane & N. Schabus (Eds.), *Decolonization handbook. Whose land is it anyway?* (pp. 18–21). Vancouver: Federation of Post-Secondary Education.

Manuel, R., & Derrickson, R. (2017). *The reconciliation manifesto recovering the land and rebuilding the economy.* Toronto: James Lorimer and Company Ltd.

Marsh, T. N., Marsh, D. C., Ozawagosh, J., & Ozawagosh, F. (2018). The sweat lodge ceremony: A healing intervention for intergenerational trauma and substance use. *The International Indigenous Policy Journal, 9*(2). https://ir.lib.uwo.ca/ iipj/vol9/iss2/2.

Mason, C., Barraket, J., Friel, S., O'Rourke, K., & Stenta, C.-P. (2015). Social innovation for the promotion of health equity. *Health Promotion International, 30*(S2), ii116–ii124.

McCallum, M. J. L. (2007). *Twice as good: A history of Aboriginal nurses.* Ottawa: Aboriginal Nurses Association of Canada.

McCallum, M. J. L. (2008). *Labour, modernity and the Canadian state: A history of Aboriginal women and work in the mid-twentieth century.* PhD thesis, The University of Manitoba.

McCallum, M. J. L. (2014). *Indigenous Women, Work, and History.* Winnipeg. MB: University of Manitoba Press.

McGibbon, E. A., & Etowa, J. B. (2009). *Anti-racist health care practice.* Toronto: Canadian Scholars' Press.

McGibbon, E., Mulaudzi, F. M., Didham, P., Barton, S., & Sochan, A. (2014). Toward decolonizing nursing: The colonization of nursing and strategies for increasing the counter-narrative. *Nursing Inquiry, 21*(3), 179–191.

McFarlane, R., & Schabus, N. ((Eds.). (2017). *Decolonization handbook. Whose land is it anyway?* Vancouver: Federation of Post Secondary Education. http://www.fpse.ca/sites/default/files/news_files/Decolonization%20Handbook.pdf.

McKillop, A., Sheridan, N., & Rowe, D. (2012). New light through old windows: Nurses, colonist, and indigenous survival. *Nursing Inquiry, 20*(30), 265–276.

McNeil-Seymour, J. (2017). Two-spirit resistance. In R. McFarlane & N. Schabus (Eds.), *Decolonization handbook. Whose land is it anyway?* (pp. 52–56). Vancouver: Federation of Post Secondary Education.

Monchalin, L. (2016). *The Colonial Problem: An Indigenous Perspective on Crime and Injustice in Canada.* Toronto: The University of Toronto Press.

Møller, H. (2016). Culturally safe communication and the power of language in Arctic nursing. *Études/Inuit/Studies, 40*(1), 85–104.

Murray, R., Caulier-Grice, J., & Mulgan, G. (2010). *The open book of social innovation.* Social Innovation Series: Ways to Design, Develop and Grow Social Innovation. London, UK: The Young Foundation.

Mussell, W. J. (2008). Decolonizing education: A building block for reconciliation. In M. B. Castellano, L. Archibald, & M. DeGagne (Eds.), *From truth to reconciliation. Transforming the legacy of residential schools* (pp. 323–338). Ottawa: Aboriginal Healing Foundation.

National Collaborating Centre for Aboriginal Health (NCCAH). (2013). *An overview of Aboriginal health in Canada*. Prince George, BC: Author. https://www.ccnsa-nccah.ca/docs/context/FS-OverviewAboroiginal-Health-EN.pdf.

Nursing Council of New Zealand. (2005). *Guidelines for cultural safety, the Treaty of Waitangi, and Maori health in nursing education and practice*. http://www.nursingcouncil.org.nz/Cultural%20Safety.pdf.

Orchard, C., Sonibare, O., Morse, A., Collin, J., & Al-Hamad, A. (2017). Collaborative leadership, part 1: The nursing leaders role within interprofessional teams. *Nursing Leadership*, *30*(2), 14–25.

Ospina, S., & Foldy, E. G. (2015). Enacting collective leadership in a shared-power world. In J. Perry, & R. Christensen (Eds.), *Handbook of public administration* (3rd ed., pp. 489–507). San Francisco: Jossey-Bass.

Palmater, P. (2017). Decolonization is taking back our power. In R. McFarlane & N. Schabus (Eds.), *Decolonization handbook. Whose land is it anyway?* (pp. 73–78). Vancouver: Federation of Post-Secondary Education.

Paradies, Y. (2016). Colonization, racism and Indigenous health. *Journal of Population Research*, *33*(1), 83–96.

Parent, M. L. (2010). *A study on nursing education: A consensus on ideal programs for Aboriginal students*. Doctoral dissertation, Capella University.

Parse, R. R. (2015). Interdisciplinary and interprofessional: What are the differences? *Nursing Science Quarterly*, *28*(1), 5–6.

Philips, J., Whatman, S., Hart, V., & Winslett, G. (2005). *Decolonising university curricula – reforming the colonized spaced in which we operate. Indigenous Knowledge Conference, Reconciling academic priorities with Indigenous realities*. Wellington, NZ: University of Wellington.

Plazas, C., Cameron, B. L., Milford, K., Hunt, L. R., Bourque Bearskin, R. L., & Santo Salas, A. (2018). *Engaging Indigenous youth through popular theatre: Knowledge mobilization of Indigenous peoples' perspectives on access to health care services*. Action Research. http://journals.sagepub.com/doi/10.1177/1476750318789468.

Ramsden, I. (2002). *Cultural safety and nursing education in Aoetearoa and Te Waipounamu. Doctoral* thesis, Victoria University of Wellington.

Reading, C. L. (2018). Structural determinants of Aboriginal Peoples' Health. In M. Greenwood, S. de Leeuw & N.

Lindsay (Eds.), *Determinants of indigenous peoples health beyond the social* (2nd ed., pp. 3–17). Vancouver: Canadian Scholars.

Reading, C. L., & Wien, F. (2009). *Health inequalities and the social determinants of Aboriginal peoples' health*. Prince George: National Collaborating Centre for Aboriginal Health.

Redvers, J. (2016). *Study: Land-based practice for Indigenous health and wellness in the Northwest Territories, Yukon, and Nunavut*. Yellowknife, YT: Institute for Circumpolar Health Research (ICHR). http://www.ichr.ca/research/land-based-practice-forindigenous-health-and-wellness-in-the-northwest-territories-yukon-and-nunavut.

Regan, P. (2010). *Unsettling the settler within: Indian residential schools, truth telling and reconciliation in Canada*. Vancouver: UBC Press.

Reutter, L., & Kushner, K. F. (2010). 'Health equity through action on the social determinants of health': Taking up the challenge in nursing. *Nursing Inquiry*, *17*(3), 269–280.

Richmond, C., & Cook, C. (2016). Creating conditions for Canadian aboriginal health equity: The promise of healthy public policy. *Public Health Reviews*, *37*(2), 1–16.

Robbins, J. A., & Dewar, J. (2011). Traditional indigenous approaches to healing and the modern welfare of traditional knowledge, spirituality and lands: A critical reflection on practices and policies taken from the Canadian Indigenous example. *The International Indigenous Policy Journal*, *2*(4), 1–17.

Royal College of Physicians and Surgeons of Canada. (2012). *Disparities in health outcomes and inequities in the quality of health care services for Aboriginal Peoples (Discussion paper)*. http://www.royalcollege.ca/portal/page/portal/rc/common/documents/policy/ih_discussion_paper_e.pdf.

Royal Commission on Aboriginal Peoples. (1996). *Looking forward looking back* (Vol. 1). Ottawa: Author. http://data2.archives.ca/e/e448/e011188230-01.pdf.

Rozendo, C. A., Santos Salas, A., & Cameron, B. (2017). Review: A critical review of social and health inequalities in the nursing curriculum. *Nurse Education Today*, *50*, 62–71.

Schabus, N. (2017). Going international to decolonize. In R. McFarlane & N. Schabus (Eds.), *Decolonization handbook. Whose land is it anyway?* (pp. 62–67). Vancouver: Federation of Post Secondary Education.

Sherwood, J., & Edwards, T. (2006). Decolonisation: A critical step for improving Aboriginal health. *Contemporary Nurse: A Journal for the Australian Nursing Profession*, *22*(2), 178–190.

Sinclair, R. (2007). Identity lost and found: Lessons from the sixties scoop. *First Peoples Child & Family Review*, *3*(1), 65–82.

Sinclair, J. R. (2013). *The footprints of our ancestors: Exploring the reconnection to My Cree ancestors (âniskôtapânak) and ancestral land in the Lesser Slave Lake Area.* Doctoral dissertation, ProQuest, UMI Dissertations Publishing (NS27694).

Sinclair, R. (2007). *Identity lost and found: lessons from the sixties scoop. First Peoples Child & Family Review, 3*(1), 65–82.

Smith, D., McAlister, S., Gold, S. T., & Sullivan-Bentz, M. (2011). Aboriginal recruitment and retention in nursing education: A review of the literature. *International Journal of Nursing Education Scholarship, 8*(1), 1–22.

Statistics Canada. (2018). *First Nations People, Métis and Inuit in Canada: Diverse and growing populations.* http://www.statcan.gc.ca/pub/89-659-x/89-659-x2018001-eng.htm.

Statistics Canada (2017). *Table 1. Aboriginal identity population, Canada, 2016.* Retrieved from: https://www150.statcan.gc.ca/n1/daily-quotidien/171025/t001a-eng.htm

Steinhauer, N. R. (2008). *Natwahtaw: Looking for a Cree model of formal education. (Doctoral Dissertation).* Library & Archives Canada (NR45610).

Stewart, J., & Warn, J. (2017). Between two worlds: Indigenous leaders exercising influence and working across boundaries. *Australian Journal of Public Administration, 76*(1), 3–17.

Struthers, R. (1999). *The Lived Experience of Ojibwa and Cree Women Healers.* Doctoral Dissertation, University of Minnesota. UMI No. 9929523-331.

Struthers, R. (2003). The artistry and ability of traditional women healers. *Health Care for Women International, 24,* 340–354.

Truth and Reconciliation Commission of Canada. (2015a). *Truth and Reconciliation Commission of Canada: Calls to Action.* Winnipeg: Author. http://www.trc.ca/websites/trcinstitution/File/2015/Findings/Calls_to_Action_English2.pdf.

Truth and Reconciliation Commission of Canada. (2015b). *What we have learned. Principles of Truth and Reconciliation.* Winnipeg: Author. http://www.trc.ca/websites/trcinstitution/File/2015/Findings/Principles_2015_05_31_web_o.pdf.

Truth and Reconciliation Commission of Canada. (2015c). *The survivors speak.* http://nctr.ca/assets/reports/Final%20Reports/Survivors_Speak_English_Web.pdf.

Tuhiwai Smith, L. (1999/2012). *Decolonizing methodologies: research and Indigenous peoples* (2nd ed.). London, UK: University of Otago Press.

United Nations. (2008). *United Nations Declaration on the Rights of Indigenous Peoples.* https://www.un.org/esa/socdev/unpfii/documents/DRIPS_en.pdf.

Who are indigenous peoples? *Indigenous Peoples, Indigenous Voices. FACTSHEET.* Retrieved from: http://www.un.org/esa/socdev/unpfii/documents/5session_factsheet1.pdf

United Nations Human Rights, Office of the High Commissioner for Human Rights. (2014). *Special Rapporteur on the rights of Indigenous peoples.* http://www.ohchr.org/en/issues/ipeoples/srindigenouspeoples/pages/sripeoplesindex.aspx.

United Nations Permanent Forum on Indigenous Issues. (2015). *Economic, social and cultural rights.* http://www.un.org/esa/socdev/unpfii/documents/2015/media/escr.pdf.

Waite, R., & Nardi, D. (2017). Nursing colonialism in America: Implications for nursing leadership. *Journal of Professional Nursing* (22 December 2017), doi.org/10.1016/j.profnurs.2017.12.013.

Waxman, K. T., & Delucas, C. (2014). Succession planning: Using simulation to develop nurse leaders for the future. *Nurse Leader, 12*(5), 24–28.

Waziyatawin, & Yellow Bird, M. (2012). Introduction. Decolonizing our minds and actions. In Waziyatawin & M. Yellow Bird (Eds.), *For Indigenous minds only: A decolonization handbook* (pp. 1–14). Santa Fe, NM: School for Advanced Research.

Weber-Pillwax, C. (1999). Indigenous research methodology: Exploratory discussion of an elusive subject. *Journal of Educational Thought, 33*(1), 31–45.

Weber-Pillwax, C. (2001). Coming to an understanding: A panel presentation: what is Indigenous research? *Canadian Journal of Native Education, 25*(2), 166–174.

Weber-Pillwax, C. (2003). *Identity formation and consciousness with reference to Northern Alberta Cree and Métis Indigenous people.* Doctoral Dissertation, Library & Archives Canada (NQ82179).

Wesley-Esquimaux, C. C., & Smolewski, M. (2004). *Historic trauma and Aboriginal healing.* Ottawa, ON: Aboriginal Healing Foundation. http://www.ahf.ca/downloads/historic-trauma.pdf.

Wilson, S. (2008). *Research is ceremony: Indigenous research methods.* Winnipeg: Fernwood.

Woods, M. (2010). Cultural safety and the socioethical nurse. *Nursing Ethics, 17*(6), 715–725.

World Health Organization. (2007). *Fact sheet. Health of Indigenous peoples.* http://www.who.int/mediacentre/factsheets/fs326/en/.

Zeran, V. (2016). Cultural competency and safety in nursing education: A case study. *Northern Review* (43), 105–115.

5

Patient Focus

Sandra Regan

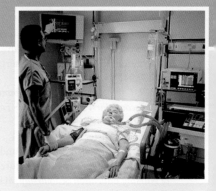

Patient focus is a broad concept. In this chapter, patient is broadly defined to include any and all of those who are interacting with nurses to receive nursing care. Patients include individuals, families, non-professional caregivers, communities, and populations. To meet the public mandate of nursing, nurses in all roles must maintain a focus on patients and patient care. In its simplest form, nursing must work to the benefit of patients. In its more complex form, nursing must focus on patients by applying professional standards to patient-centred care, patient safety, and patient outcomes. Patient focus is also central to effective nursing leadership and management initiatives.

OBJECTIVES

- Understand how nursing professional standards and codes of ethics guide nurses' practice.
- Identify key values of patient-centred care.
- Understand how nurse leadership and management can implement initiatives that promote patient-centred care.
- Describe nursing's role in patient safety and a culture of safety.
- Identify the key organizations and resources that support a patient focus.
- Understand how nursing-sensitive outcomes are used to enhance a patient focus.
- Apply various resources to analyze a patient-safety situation.

TERMS TO KNOW

adverse event	culture of safety	patient- or client-centred care
code of ethics	harmful event	patient safety
collaborative practice	nursing-sensitive outcomes	professional standard

❓ A CHALLENGE

Jack is a new nurse manager of a medical unit in a regional hospital. The unit has recently undergone staff mixture changes to increase the use of care aides and practical nurses (PNs) and reduce the number of registered nurses (RNs) working at any one time. Although teamwork is encouraged, it is not the reality. PNs have also been asked to assume an expanded scope of practice because of the decrease in RNs and are feeling overwhelmed. RNs are regularly seen admonishing PNs and care aides for decision making about care. Care aides and PNs have responded to the negative attitudes of selected RNs by avoiding working closely with them.

What might Jack do to help build a stronger patient focus in this medical unit?

SAFE, COMPETENT, AND ETHICAL PRACTICE

As members of a regulated profession, nurses are accountable to the public. Provincial and territorial governments have delegated to their respective nursing regulatory bodies the responsibility to regulate the profession in the public interest. One means for the nursing profession to achieve accountability is through the provision of safe, competent, and ethical nursing care. Details of the regulatory frameworks affecting nursing practices are further outlined in Chapters 7 and 21 Nursing regulatory bodies, among their various duties, are responsible for establishing, monitoring, and enforcing the professional standards that govern the practice of nursing. A professional standard is an "authoritative statement that sets out the legal and professional basis of nursing practice" (College of Nurses of Ontario, 2009, p. 3). "The primary purpose of standards is to identify for nurses, the public, government, and other stakeholders the desired and achievable level of performance expected of nurses in their practice, against which actual performance can be measured" (Association of Registered Nurses of Newfoundland and Labrador, 2007, p. 2).

While each provincial and territorial nursing regulatory body has developed its own professional standards, standards between jurisdictions share many similarities. For example, standards commonly include statements regarding accountability and responsibility, the competent application of knowledge, continuing competence, ethics, nurse–patient relationships, and interdisciplinary collaboration. In addition to defining standards, nursing regulatory bodies set out indicators that describe how nurses demonstrate they have met each standard. In some cases, indicators have been developed that are relevant to nurses working in particular domains of practice, such as administration and education. See Box 5.1 for an example of a professional standard and its associated indicators for nurses working in administration.

Patient focus is also integrated in the entry-level competencies for nurses that guide curriculum development and implementation in nursing education programs. These entry-level competencies are developed through collaboration among nursing regulatory bodies in Canada. The competencies are grounded in a standards-based conceptual framework—professional responsibility and accountability, knowledge-based practice, ethical practice, service to the

BOX 5.1 Example of a Professional Standard and Indicators for Nurses in an Administrative Role

The British Columbia College of Nursing Professionals provides indicators to demonstrate how each of its professional standards is applied in four areas of practice. Standard 3 and its indicators for administration appear here.

Standard 3: Client-Focused Provision of Service
Provides nursing services and works with others to provide health care services in the best interest of clients.

Indicators for Administration
1. Communicates, collaborates, and consults with nurses and other members of the health care team about the provision of health care services.
2. Educates others about the nurse's role in the coordination of client care.
3. Develops policies that outline the responsibility and accountability for all involved in the appropriate assignment of clients and client care activities.
4. Develops policies that provide direction for nurses on appropriate delegation of nursing activities to other members of the health care team.
5. Develops supporting policies for appropriate regulatory supervision.
6. Guides, directs, and seeks feedback from staff and others involved in the planning, delivery, and evaluation of health care services as appropriate.
7. Directs and participates in changes to improve client care and administrative practice.
8. Takes appropriate action in situations of incompetent or impaired practice or unethical conduct up to and including reporting to the regulatory body; guides others in reporting such practices.
9. Understands and communicates the role of nursing in the health of clients.
10. Assists clients, colleagues, students and others to learn about nursing practice and health care services.

British Columbia College of Nursing Professionals. (2018). *Professional standards for registered nurses and nurse practitioners*. Vancouver, BC: Author.

public, and self-regulation—with the patient central to the framework (Black et al., 2008). If you are not already familiar with the entry-level competencies for registered, practical, or psychiatric nurses in your province or territory, you can access them on your nursing regulatory body's website (see Table 5.1 for a list of nursing regulatory bodies).

In addition to professional standards, nurses have codes of ethics that guide their practice. A code of ethics is a statement of a set of values that help guide nurses in ethical practice. The Canadian Nurses Association (CNA) has developed and periodically revises its *Code of Ethics for Registered Nurses*. Practical nurses and psychiatric nurses can find codes of ethics at their provincial association websites. The most universally adopted nursing code in Canada, the CNA's *Code of Ethics for Registered Nurses*, is divided into two parts: Part One sets out the nursing values and core ethical responsibilities, and Part Two describes ethical endeavours that are meant to guide nurses in addressing societal issues, such as inequity (CNA, 2017). Provincial and territorial registered nursing regulatory bodies have incorporated the CNA's code of ethics in one form or another, and Part One is usually found in their professional standards. A summary of Part One appears in Box 5.2.

EXERCISE 5.1 Familiarize yourself with the professional standards and code of ethics set out by the relevant nursing regulatory body in your province and territory. You can also review the entry-level competencies for registered nurses, practical nurses, or psychiatric nurses. A list of the provincial and territorial nursing regulatory bodies can be found at the end of this chapter. How do these standards, entry-level competencies, and codes of ethics inform your role as a nurse? As a future leader? As a follower? How do they guide how you view the patient?

PATIENT-CENTRED CARE

The focus of nursing practice has always been the patient, which includes striving for excellence in patient care. However, historically the needs of the organization or even those of health care providers, including nurses, have at times been placed above those of the patient in decision making about care. Workplace examples include interdisciplinary non-cooperation or competition, communication breakdown, adversarial staff, fear of reprisal for taking opposing views, inflexibility, job dissatisfaction, and emphasis on workplace issues that are not associated with improving patient care and patient participation. Often attitudes affecting patient care are entrenched in organizational cultures and become part of the unstated organizational philosophy of care. Nurses play an important role in influencing these philosophies for the benefit of patients and

---

BOX 5.2   Canadian Nurses Association's Code of Ethics for Registered Nurses

The Canadian Nurses Association's Code of Ethics for Registered Nurses sets out the following nursing values and ethical responsibilities:

1. *"Providing safe, compassionate, competent, and ethical care.* Nurses provide safe, compassionate, competent, and ethical care.
2. *Promoting health and well-being.* Nurses work with persons who have health care needs or are receiving care to enable them to attain their highest possible level of health and well-being.
3. *Promoting and respecting informed decision making.* Nurses recognize, respect, and promote a person's right to be informed and make decisions.
4. *Honouring dignity.* Nurses recognize and respect the intrinsic worth of each person.
5. *Maintaining privacy and confidentiality.* Nurses recognize the importance of privacy and confidentiality and safeguard personal, family, and community information obtained in the context of a professional relationship.
6. *Promoting justice.* Nurses uphold principles of justice by safeguarding human rights, equity, and fairness and by promoting the public good."* (Canadian Nurses Association, 2017).
7. *Being accountable.* Nurses are accountable for their actions and answerable for their practice.

Nurses in all domains of practice bear the ethical responsibilities identified under each of the seven primary nursing values.

Note: This represents only one part of the code of ethics for registered nurses, the nursing values and ethical responsibilities part, which are articulated through seven primary values and accompanying responsibility statements in the Code of ethics for registered nurses (2017). The core values make up the code and the responsibility statements are intended to help nurses apply the code.
Canadian Nurses Association. (2017). Code of Ethics for Registered Nurses (2017 Edition). Toronto, ON: Author. © Canadian Nurses Association. Reprinted with permission. Further reproduction prohibited.

---

positive patient outcomes. They also maintain responsibility for identifying and changing systemic factors that hinder patient-centred care. Collaborating with patients and their families in respectful and meaningful ways may require shifting how organizations and health care providers view the patient. Finding effective ways within an organization to promote a philosophy of patient-centred care is an important strategy for maintaining focus or refocusing on the patient and their family.

BOX 5.3 Governance and Management Activities That Support Patient-Centred Care

For managers and governors to support patient-centred care, they must focus on the following:

1. Indicators that capture patient-centredness accurately and comprehensively.
2. Health science education programs that build patient-centred care into the core of their curricula and the formative apprenticeship experiences.
3. Explicit goals and targets for achieving various elements of patient-centred care.
4. Regular patient surveys to monitor the evolution of patient-centred care and identify strengths and weaknesses.
5. Regular provider surveys to monitor their attitudes, expectations, and behaviours.
6. Organizational changes that promote systems thinking, collective accountability, and team-based care.
7. E-health and other technologies that facilitate communication, efficiency, and convenience.
8. Investments in system re-engineering that advance patient-centred care.
9. Progressively more robust policies to spread patient-centred care successes, e.g., mandatory open access scheduling, patient-driven e-health initiatives, transparent reporting of patient-centred care performance, etc.
10. A culture of patient-centred care that refuses to tolerate behaviours that do not put patients first.
11. Incorporating important patient-centred care criteria and measures into accreditation and regulatory employer standards and processes.

Adapted from Lewis, S. (2009). Patient-centred care: An introduction to what it is and how to achieve it: A discussion paper for the Saskatchewan Ministry of Health. Saskatoon: The Change Foundation. Retrieved from http://www.southeastlhin.on.ca/uploadedFiles/Public_Community/Board_of_Directors/Board_Committee/Collaborative_Governance_and_Community_Engagement/Ppatient-Centred-Care%20Steven%20Lewis%202009.pdf.

Patient- or client-centred care is "an approach in which the patient is viewed as a whole person; it is not just about delivering services and involves advocacy, empowerment, and respecting the patient's autonomy, voice, self-determination, and participation in decision making" (Registered Nurses' Association of Ontario, 2015, p. 75). The Registered Nurses' Association of Ontario (RNAO) identified four themes that form the foundation of patient- or client-centred care, these being:

1. Establishing a therapeutic relationship for true partnership, continuity of care, and shared decision making.
2. Care is organized around, and respectful of, the person.
3. Knowing the whole person (holistic care).
4. Communication, collaboration, and engagement (RNAO, 2015, pp. 21–22).

Client-centred care is the foundation of nursing education and practice. For example, the competencies required for entry-level registered nurse practice are based on the principle of client-centred care to prepare nurses to provide safe, competent, and ethical care (College and Association of Registered Nurses of Alberta, 2013).

Managers and senior health care leaders must make patient-centred care a priority in their roles of making policies, ensuring system accountability, and quality improvement (Baker et al., 2016; Lewis, 2009). A number of activities can be implemented to enact these roles,

and nurses can support or implement many of them. For example, nurses can lead changes that promote team-based and collaborative care, create a culture that discourages behaviours that do not put patients first, and identify and change policies to align with themes, such as those identified by RNAO (2015) and other identified provincial professional bodies. Other areas that leaders must focus on to enable patient-centred care appear in Box 5.3.

COLLABORATIVE PRACTICE

Nurses have always worked alongside other health care professionals. However, working alongside others and working as team are different. According to the World Health Organization (2010), collaborative practice "happens when multiple health workers from different professional backgrounds work together with patients, families, careers, and communities to deliver the highest quality of care" (p. 7). Interprofessional collaboration or collaborative practice has been identified as important for both patient-centred care and patient safety (Weller et al., 2014). Being able to effectively work in a collaborative practice means that nurses need to be able to understand their role and that of others, communicate effectively with other team members, and know how to resolve conflicts (Canadian Interprofessional Health Collaborative,

2010). You will learn more about collaborative practice and interprofessional teams in Chapters 20 and 27.

PATIENT SAFETY

When patients come into contact with the health care system, they place a great deal of trust in those providing care to them. They expect the provision of safe care and have a reasonable expectation that they will not be harmed in the process. In 2000, the Institute of Medicine (IOM), a US-based organization, released *To Err Is Human: Building a Safer Health System*. The IOM report stated that in the United States, nearly 100 000 hospital deaths annually were attributed to adverse events. According to the Canadian Patient Safety Institute (n.d.) online glossary of terms, an **adverse event** is "an event that results in unintended harm to the patient and is related to the care and services provided to the patient rather than to the patient's underlying condition." The outcome of an adverse event might be disability, extended length of stay, or even death.

Baker et al. (2004) conducted the first Canadian study of adverse events (The Canadian Adverse Events Study). They conducted a chart review in 20 randomly selected Canadian hospitals in British Columbia, Alberta, Ontario, Quebec, and Nova Scotia in 2000 to provide a national estimate of the incidence of adverse events. They found that the adverse events rate was 7.5 per 100 hospital admissions. This means that an adverse event was experienced in 7.5% of hospital admissions. They further estimated that 36% of the adverse events were preventable and approximately 9250 to 23 750 of the adverse events that ended in death were preventable. It's essential to keep in mind that nursing's mandate to provide safe, competent, and ethical care carries with it an expectation that nurses will contribute to patient safety. Building on this important research, the Canadian Institute for Health Information (CIHI) and Canadian Patient Safety Institute recently reported on **harmful events**, "an unintended outcome of care that may be prevented with evidence-informed practices and this is identified and treated in the same hospital stay" (2016, p. 7). According to reports in 2014–2015, Canadian patients experience harm in 1 of every 18 hospitalizations. Harmful events were grouped into four categories: health care/medication–associated conditions (37%), health care–associated infections (37%), procedure-associated conditions (23%), and patient accidents (3%) (CIHI, 2016).

The World Health Organization (n.d.) defines **patient safety** as "the absence of preventable harm to a patient during the process of health care." Research on adverse events has highlighted the importance of safety in health care organizations and led health care leaders in the United States and Canada to have a more progressive approach to quality and patient safety. Health care organizations typically monitor adverse events through incident-reporting systems. These reporting systems permit the identification of trends and patterns in adverse events, which can in turn lead to activities that foster improvements in the health care facility. Quality improvement is discussed further in Chapter 22. The CIHI tracks medication and intravenous fluid incidents through the National System for Incident Reporting (NSIR). The NSIR is a secure and anonymous tracking system that supports local regional, provincial, and national efforts to understand how to improve the health care system. You can visit CIHI's website (http://www.CIHI.ca) for more information (the site includes a video on the NSIR). In addition to incident reporting, many health care facilities have created specific roles and departments charged with leading initiatives on patient safety and creating a culture of safety. Creating a culture of safety is essential to reducing adverse events in the Canadian health care system. Wiseman and Kaprielian (2005) suggest that "in a **culture of safety** the focus is on effective systems and teamwork to accomplish the mutual goal of safe, high-quality performance. When something goes wrong, the focus is on what (or how), rather than who, is the problem. The intent is to bring process failures and system issues to light, and to solve them in a non-biased non-threatening way" (para. 1).

What does a culture of safety look like? In their review of the literature on safety culture, Halligan and Zecevic (2011) list the following attributes as common features of a culture of safety:

- Leadership commitment to safety.
- Open communication founded on trust.
- Organizational learning.
- A non-punitive approach to adverse event reporting and analysis.
- Teamwork.
- Shared belief in the importance of safety (p. 340).

Studies have found that when health care facilities create a culture of safety, their staff are more willing to report adverse events (Vogus et al., 2010). This

LITERATURE PERSPECTIVE

Resource: Bishop, A., & Macdonald, M. (2017). Patient involvement in patient safety: A qualitative study of nursing staff and patient perceptions. *Journal of Patient Safety, 13*(2), 82–87.

How can health care organizations improve their culture of patient safety? The authors conducted focus groups with nursing staff and patients in two hospitals in Eastern Canada to understand perceptions of safety. Their analysis identified four themes:

1. Wanting control: Both patients and nurses described patients as knowing enough about their health care.
2. Feeling connected: Both patients and nurses need to connect with one another. This occurs through respect and sharing information.
3. Encountering roadblock: Patients perceived that nursing staff were too busy to answer questions or spend time with them while nurses reported that their workload prevented them from interacting with patients in a meaningful way.
4. Sharing responsibility for safety: Both patients and nurses identified their roles in improving safety. For patients, these roles included asking questions and advocating for their well-being. Nurses considered their role in improving safety as engaging in teamwork and improving communication.

Implications for Practice

Nurses can contribute to patient safety by sharing information, showing respect, and involving patients in their care.

EXERCISE 5.2 Reflect on a recent clinical experience you have had in your nursing education program. Based on what you have read about attributes of a culture of safety, how do these attributes align with your clinical experience? Were you aware of how to report an adverse event? Did you encounter any activities that promote the ideal of a culture of safety? How is patient safety discussed in the mission, vision, or mandate of the organization? Is there a specific role or department in the organization responsible for patient safety?

---

willingness is because they understand that the focus is on addressing issues in the system and not blaming individuals. The CNA (2009) position statement on patient safety is as follows: "Although individual competency may be a contributing factor, and individuals remain accountable for their own actions, it is increasingly evident that system competency plays a major role in patient safety. Only when adverse events and near misses are disclosed can they be analyzed in a collaborative manner by the health-care team and other stakeholders to identify and address problems in the system" (p. 2). The position statement goes on to suggest that "strong leadership across the nursing profession is essential to moving forward cultural reform required to ensure the delivery of safe, quality care in professional environments" (p. 2). Whether nurses are front-line staff (followers and leaders) or hold formal leadership positions, all have a role in achieving a culture of safety. Some examples of activities health care organizations can implement to support a culture of safety include establishing Quality Improvement (QI) teams, having regular team "huddles" on the unit, debriefing adverse events when they occur, and requiring completion of a surgical safety checklist. See the Literature Perspective for more on how health care organizations can create a culture of safety.

Nurses are in a unique position to lead and manage patient safety; they are with the patient 24 hours a day, seven days a week. Few health care providers are positioned with such a patient focus. Nurses in follower and leadership roles can identify safety issues originating at the unit or patient level and give voice to these issues at the organizational level (Jones et al., 2016; Tregunno et al., 2009). Creating a culture attuned to patient safety requires a number of leadership skills, such as understanding change processes, being able to manage conflict, and having an understanding of quality and patient safety practices. However, nurse leaders need support and resources to take up this important role.

Canadian Patient Safety Institute

The Canadian Patient Safety Institute (CPSI) was established in 2003 by Health Canada to support improvements in patient safety and quality. CPSI's vision, "safe healthcare for all Canadians," is supported by the following strategic priorities:

- Improve the safety of patient care in Canada through learning, sharing, and implementing interventions that are known to reduce avoidable harm.

- Build governance capability.
- Support networks.
- Increase capacity through evidence-informed resources and tools (Canadian Patient Safety Institute, n.d.a.).

The CPSI website is a rich resource for health care organizations as well as practitioners. CPSI's flagship program Safer Healthcare Now! supports front-line health care providers and the delivery system to improve the safety of patient care throughout Canada by implementing interventions known to reduce avoidable harm. The Safer Healthcare Now! program has resources for front-line health care providers and others who want to improve patient safety. The tools and resources at the CPSI website (http://www.patientsafetyinstitute.ca) are free and can be customized to an organization's needs. By incorporating safety competencies in their educational programs and professional development activities, health care leaders can ensure their staff have the knowledge, skills, and attitude to create a culture consistent with quality and patient safety. The CPSI's safety competencies appear in Box 5.4.

The CPSI's Effective Governance for Quality and Patient Safety: A Toolkit for Healthcare Board Members and Senior Leaders provides information on the drivers of quality and patient safety, references (including Canadian studies), and stories from health care organizations. Important drivers of quality and patient safety include access to information, evidence and research, and relevant measures. The drivers for effective governance for quality and patient safety appear in Fig. 5.1. Nurses can use this toolkit in their own workplace to ensure patient safety.

EXERCISE 5.3 Visit the CPSI website (http://www.patientsafetyinstitute.ca) and explore the Tools & Resources section. Using information found on the CPSI website, answer the following questions.

1. What percentage of home care clients experience an adverse event annually?
2. What are the five questions every patient should ask about their medications?
3. What do 220 000 Canadians develop each year and about 8000 die from annually?
4. What practice by health care workers can reduce the number of health care associated infections by 50%?
5. According to the Canadian Hand Hygiene Audit, what percentage of health care workers clean their hands?

BOX 5.4 Canadian Patient Safety Institute's Safety Competencies

The Canadian Patient Safety Institute (CPSI) created safety competencies that include six core competency domains:

Domain 1: Contribute to a Culture of Patient Safety— A commitment to applying core patient safety knowledge, skills, and attitudes to everyday work.

Domain 2: Work in Teams for Patient Safety—Working within interprofessional teams to optimize patient safety and quality of care.

Domain 3: Communicate Effectively for Patient Safety—Promoting patient safety through effective health care communication.

Domain 4: Manage Safety Risks—Anticipating, recognizing, and managing situations that place patients at risk.

Domain 5: Optimize Human and Environmental Factors—Managing the relationship between individual and environmental characteristics in order to optimize patient safety.

Domain 6: Recognize, Respond to, and Disclose Adverse Events—Recognizing the occurrence of an adverse event or close call and responding effectively to mitigate harm to the patient, ensure disclosure, and prevent recurrence.

Canadian Patient Safety Institute. (2011). The safety competencies. Retrieved from http://www.patientsafetyinstitute.ca/English/toolsResources/safetyCompetencies/Pages/default.aspx.

NURSING-SENSITIVE OUTCOMES

How do you know if what you are doing is making a difference for the patients you provide care for? How do health care organizations measure nursing's contribution to quality care? While nurses have long been interested in understanding how nursing practice influences patient outcomes, it is in the last decade that a growing body of research in Canada and elsewhere has begun to answer this question. Nursing-sensitive outcomes is the phrase used to describe patient outcomes that are sensitive to nursing practice or interventions. They are measured by indicators that reflect information on patient outcomes. Specifically, information is collected from patient charts or other sources, such as nurse staffing complements and discharge data. This information is entered into a database and is then categorized to

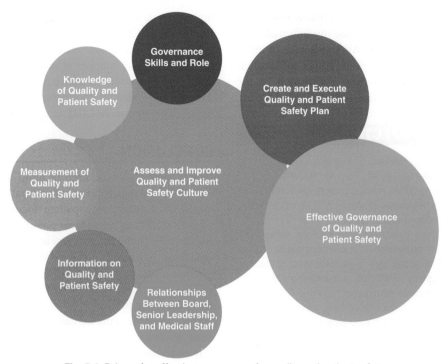

Fig. 5.1 Drivers for effective governance for quality and patient safety.

provide data on patient outcomes. Several broad categories of patient outcomes were identified by Doran (2011):

- *Functional status:* patients' perceptions of their day-to-day functioning. Examples: activities of daily living.
- *Self-care:* patients' perceptions and abilities to manage their care. Examples: medication administration, healthy eating.
- *Symptom management:* how well symptoms are managed. Examples: pain, fatigue.
- *Adverse patient outcomes:* occurrence and types of adverse events. Examples: hospital-acquired infections, patient falls, readmission to hospital, medication errors.
- *Patient satisfaction:* patient satisfaction with nursing care.
- *Mortality rates:* rates of death for specific, often preventable, causes. Examples: 30-day mortality rates, hospital standardized mortality ratio (pp. 1–18).

When information on patient outcomes is available, nurses can use it in a variety of ways at the individual, unit, and organization level. Patient outcome information is important for patient safety. Doran et al. (2004)

suggested the following uses for nurse-sensitive outcomes:

- Develop treatment plans for individual patients.
- Evaluate different approaches to patient care.
- Inform best practices.
- Improve the quality of nursing care.
- Improve patient outcomes.
- Inform staffing policies and decisions.
- Assist organizations to balance the competing demands of access, cost, and quality (p. 3).

Nurse managers might use information about patient outcomes on a particular unit to design specific strategies or change policies to decrease an occurrence of an event, such as hospital-acquired infections. Or they might advocate for resources that support patient satisfaction or staffing to optimize patient functional status. Front-line nurses can use information about patient outcomes to design care plans for patients or evaluate interventions. Information about patient outcomes becomes an invaluable tool for nurses to support a patient focus and advocate for nursing resources to improve care delivery. See the Research Perspective for a study on patient-centred care and patient outcomes.

Various sources of information on patient outcomes exist, including the health care organization itself. Health care organizations collect a great deal of information about the patients admitted for care and use this information to assess how well they are doing. Another source of information is the Canadian Institute of Health Information (CIHI). CIHI collects and analyzes information on the health care system, including data collected by health care organizations, to support decisions that will improve the health system. CIHI is able to identify trends and patterns that provide information on how well the health system is performing in a number of respects, including patient safety and some nurse-sensitive outcomes. You can have a look at the variety of information available on Canada's health care system at the CIHI website (http://www.cihi.ca).

RESEARCH PERSPECTIVE

Resource: Sidani, S., Reeves, S., Hurlock-Chorostecki, C., van Soren, M., Fox, M., & Collins, L. (2017). Exploring differences in patient-centered practices among healthcare professionals in acute care settings. *Health Communication*, 33(6): 715–723.

In this study, the researchers examined the extent to which health care professionals implement patient-centred care (PCC) in acute care organizations in Canada. They were particularly interested in examining different health care professionals with respect to three PCC components: holistic care, collaborative care, and responsive care. The researchers used survey data from 328 health professionals in four groups: physicians, nurses, social workers, and other health care professionals working in 18 Ontario hospitals. The study findings showed differences in how health care professionals implemented the three PCC components. For example, physicians reported higher scores for enacting holistic care than the other three groups while nurses, physicians, and other health care professionals had higher scores for providing responsive care. The study showed that health care providers vary in their provision of patient-centred care components.

Implications for Practice
The researchers suggest that supports such as interprofessional education sessions and clinical guidelines may enhance the ability of health care professionals to provide patient-centred care.

CONCLUSION

As you read this book, keep in mind that student and registered nurses need to maintain a patient focus. Some means of maintaining a patient focus include asking yourself questions about how power and responsibility are shared with the patient; how input is actively encouraged from the patient and how communication is shared; whether a patient's individuality, cultural needs, values, and life issues have been taken into account; what efforts are being made to include patients who are not presenting for care at the expected care points; and what is being done to enhance prevention and health promotion. Nurses across the career continuum, including those in leadership and administrative roles, need to stay patient focused. They also need to actively engage with patients across the continuum of care in care planning, coordination, and implementation—respecting patient values and preferences—to enhance the impact and quality of care while acting ethically. Nurse managers and other leaders need to facilitate a change in practice whereby nurses are accountable to patients. Health care delivery systems in Canada must emphasize patient centredness and create a culture of safety. Nurses must respond positively and adapt to these changes. Even organizationally focused goals must ultimately address patient needs (the raison d'être of all health care organizations).

❓ A SOLUTION

In Canada, the US, and many other countries, having a mix of different staff is a reality. Care and due process in introducing these changes can help make the transition easier. Supporting nursing care that is patient focused and patient centred helps ensure that staffing conflicts and tensions do not adversely affect the care the public receives. Patient-centred care helps direct staff energy in productive ways, and patient-centred care, combined with appreciative inquiry, helps shift the focus on abilities and away from deficits. This situation clearly requires manager involvement. Team building is required. Asking staff to express their concerns using reference to *the patient* rather than *I* is one means of shifting the focus. Asking individuals to "walk in another's shoes" and consider what it is like to be the other health care provider and to identify what skills and abilities the other person brings to the unit is another technique. Jack and his staff should look for ways to modify the culture of care in the medical unit to foster patient centredness, collaborative practice, and a culture of safety.

What other techniques might you suggest for improving patient focus and a culture of care in this work environment? What is the role and responsibility of student nurses in contributing to improving patient-focused care?

TABLE 5.1	**Provincial and Territorial Nursing Regulatory Bodies**		
Province/ Territory	Registered Nurses	Licensed/Registered Practice Nurses	Registered Psychiatric Nurses (British Columbia, Alberta, Saskatchewan, and Manitoba)
British Columbia	British Columbia College of Nursing Professionals www.bccnp.ca	British Columbia College of Nursing Professionals www.bccnp.ca	British Columbia College of Nursing Professionals www.bccnp.ca
Alberta	College and Association of Registered Nurses of Alberta http://www.nurses.ab.ca	College of Licensed Practical Nurses of Alberta http://www.clpna.com	College of Registered Psychiatric Nurses of Alberta http://www.crpna.ab.ca
Saskatchewan	Saskatchewan Registered Nurses' Association http://www.srna.org	Saskatchewan Association of Licensed Practical Nurses http://www.salpn.com	Registered Psychiatric Nurses Association of Saskatchewan http://www.rpnas.com
Manitoba	College of Registered Nurses of Manitoba http://www.crnm.mb.ca	College of Licensed Practical Nurses of Manitoba http://www.clpnm.ca	College of Registered Psychiatric Nurses of Manitoba http://www.crpnm.mb.ca
Ontario	College of Nurses of Ontario http://www.cno.org	College of Nurses of Ontario http://www.cno.org	
Quebec	Ordre des infirmières et infirmiers du Québec http://www.oiiq.org	Ordre des infirmières et infirm- iers auxiliares du Québec http://www.oiiaq.org	
New Brunswick	Nurses Association of New Brunswick http://www.nanb.nb.ca	Association of New Brunswick Licensed Practical Nurses http://www.anblpn.ca	
Nova Scotia	College of Registered Nurses of Nova Scotia http://www.crnns.ca	College of Licensed Practical Nurses of Nova Scotia http://www.clpnns.ca	
Prince Edward Island	Association of Registered Nurses of Prince Edward Island http://www.arnpei.ca	Licensed Practical Nurses Asso- ciation of Prince Edward Island http://www.lpna.ca	
Newfoundland and Labrador	Association of Registered Nurses of Newfoundland and Labrador http://www.arnnl.ca	College of Licensed Practical Nurses of Newfoundland & Labrador http://www.clpnnl.ca	
Northwest Terri- tories	Registered Nurses Association of Northwest Territories and Nunavut http://www.rnantnu.ca		
Yukon	Yukon Registered Nurses Association http://www.yrna.ca		

▌ THE EVIDENCE

Nurses have an integral role in promoting patient safety. In 2007, the symposium 'Advancing Nursing Leadership for a Safer Healthcare System' was held in Toronto. Jeffs et al. (2009) summarized the themes emerging from the research presented at this symposium. They identified four future directions for nursing, including focusing on the patient in patient safety, broadening the knowledge base on patient safety beyond acute care, linking healthy work environments and a culture of patient safety, and bridging evidence-informed research and practice. Nurses continue to lead the way for patient safety in direct care, education, research, and leadership.

※ **NEED TO KNOW NOW**

- Know how and where to access resources related to patient- or client-centred care, patient safety, and patient outcomes.
- Contribute to an organization that is accountable to patients and their families.
- Understand how evidence regarding nursing-sensitive outcomes can be used to advocate for patient-centred care and patient safety.

- Know and apply the eight values forming the foundation of patient-centred care in nursing.
- Know and apply the six safety competencies in your nursing practice.

CHAPTER CHECKLIST

Through a philosophy of patient centredness, creating a culture of patient safety, and attending to patient outcomes, nurse leadership and management can advocate for a patient focus and support all nurses to practise in a safe, competent, and ethical manner.

- Nurses in all roles must maintain a patient focus. Foundational to the patient focus, nurse leaders and followers must practise according to the professional standards and code of ethics.
- Nurse leaders and followers play an important role in influencing organizational culture for the benefit of patients and positive patient outcomes. They also maintain responsibility for identifying and changing systemic factors that hinder patient-centred care.

- Nurse leaders and followers play an important role in identifying potential safety issues and raising awareness of these issues to ensure early intervention and avoid significant and negative outcomes.
- Nurse leaders can use the safety competencies set out by the Canadian Patient Safety Institute to develop educational activities for staff; followers can use the safety competencies to identify gaps in their practice that need to be addressed.
- Organizations that offer support for the creation of a culture of patient safety include the following:
  - Canadian Patient Safety Institute
  - Canadian Nurses Association.

TIPS FOR PATIENT-FOCUSED LEADERSHIP

- Review the RNAO Best Practice Guidelines: *Person- and Family-Centred Care* and identify areas where your unit aligns with the themes of patient-centred care and areas for improvement.

- Be aware of the strategies your organization is focusing on to address patient safety.
- Know what patient outcomes are collected and reported for your unit.

Visit the Evolve website for Suggested Readings, Internet Resources, and additional resources related to the content in this chapter: http://evolve.elsevier.com/Canada/Yoder-Wise/leading/.

REFERENCES

Association of Registered Nurses of Newfoundland and Labrador. (2007). *Standards for nursing practice*. St. John's, NL: Author. http://www.arnnl.ca.

Baker, G. R., Norton, P., Flintoft, et al. (2004). The Canadian Adverse Events Study: The incidence of adverse events among hospital patients in Canada. *Canadian Medical Association Journal, 170,* 1678–1686. https://doi.org/10.1503/cmaj.1040498.

Baker, G. R., Fancott, C., Judd, M., & O'Connor, P. (2016). Expanding patient engagement in quality improvement and health system redesign: Three Canadian case studies. *Healthcare Management Forum, 29*(5), 175–182. https://doi.org/10.1177/0840470416645601.

Black, J., Allen, D., Redfern, L., et al. (2008). Competencies in the context of entry-level registered nurses' practice: A collaborative project in Canada. *International Nursing Review, 55,* 171–178.

Canadian Institute for Health Information, Canadian Patient Safety Institute. (2016). *Measuring patient harm in Canadian hospitals.* Ottawa, ON: Author. https://www.cihi.ca/sites/default/files/document/cihi_cpsi_hospital_harm_en.pdf.

Canadian Interprofessional Health Collaborative. (2010). *A national interprofessional competency framework.* Vancouver, BC: Author. http://www.cihc.ca/files/CIHC_IPCompetencies_Feb1210.pdf.

Canadian Nurses Association. (2017). *Code of ethics for registered nurses (2017 edition).* Toronto, ON: Author. https://www.cna-aiic.ca/html/en/Code-of-Ethics-2017-Edition/files/assets/basic-html/page-3.html.

Canadian Nurses Association. (2009). *Position statement: Patient safety.* http://www.cnaaiic.ca/~/media/cna/page%20content/pdf%20fr/2013/07/26/10/48/ps102_patient_safety_e.pdf.

Canadian Patient Safety Institute. (n.d.a). About CPSI. Retrieved from: http://www.patientsafetyinstitute.ca/english/about/pages/default.aspx.

Canadian Patient Safety Institute. (n.d.b). Adverse event. Retrieved from: http://www.patientsafetyinstitute.ca/english/toolsresources/governancepatientsafety/pages/glossaryofterms.aspx.

College and Association of Registered Nurses of Alberta. (2013). *Entry-to-practice competencies for the registered nurse's profession.* Edmonton, AB: Author.

College of Nurses of Ontario. (2009). *Professional standards, revised 2009.* Toronto, ON: Author.

Doran, D. (2011). *Nursing outcomes: The state of the science* (2nd ed.). Sudbury, MA: Jones and Bartlett Learning.

Doran, D., Harrison, M. B., Laschinger, H., et al. (2004). *Collecting data on nursing-sensitive outcomes in different care settings: Can it be done? What are the benefits? Report of the nursing and health outcomes feasibility study.* Toronto, ON: University of Toronto.

Halligan, M., & Zecevic, A. (2011). Safety culture in healthcare: A review of concepts, dimensions, measures and progress. *BMJ Quality and Safety, 20*(4), 338–343. https://doi.org/10.1136/bmjqs.2010.040964.

Institute of Medicine. (2000). *To err is human: Building a safer health system.* Washington, DC: National Academy Press.

Jeffs, L., MacMillan, K., McKey, C., et al. (2009). Nursing leaders' accountability to narrow the safety chasm: Insights and implications from the collective evidence based on healthcare safety. *Canadian Journal of Nursing Leadership, 22*(1), 86–98.

Jones, A., Lankshear, A., & Kelly, D. (2016). Giving voice to quality and safety matters at board level: A qualitative study of the experiences of executive nurses working England and Wales. *International Journal of Nursing Studies, 59,* 169–176. https://doi.org/10.1016/j.ijnurstu.2016.04.007.

Lewis, S. (2009). *Patient-centered care: An introduction to what it is and how to achieve it: A discussion paper for the Saskatchewan Ministry of Health.* Saskatoon, SK: The Change Foundation. http://www.changefoundation.ca/docs/patient-centred-care-intro.pdf.

Registered Nurses' Association of Ontario. (2015). *Person- and family-centred care.* Toronto, ON: Author. http://rnao.ca/bpg/guidelines/person-and-family-centred-care.

Tregunno, D., Jeffs, L., McGillis Hall, L., et al. (2009). On the ball: Leadership for patient safety and learning in critical care. *Journal of Nursing Administration, 39* (7–8), 334–339. https://doi.org/10.1097/NNA.0b013e-3181ae9653.

Vogus, T. J., Sutcliffe, K. M., & Weick, K. E. (2010). Doing no harm: Enabling, enacting, and elaborating a culture of safety in health care. *Academy of Management Perspectives, 24*(4), 60–76. https://doi.org/10.5465/AMP.2010.55206385.

Weller, J., Boyd, M., & Cumin, D. (2014). Teams, tribes, and patient safety: Overcoming barriers to effective teamwork in healthcare. *Postgrad Medical Journal, 90,* 149–154. https://doi.org/10.1136/postgradmedj-2012-131168.

Wiseman, B., & Kaprielian, V. S. (2005). *What do we mean by a culture of safety?.* http://patientsafetyed.duhs.duke.edu/module_c/what_do_we_mean.html.

World Health Organization. (n.d.). Patient safety. Retrieved from: http://www.who.int/patientsafety/about/en/.

World Health Organization. (2010). *Framework for action interprofessional education and collaborative practice.* Geneva: Author. http://apps.who.int/iris/bitstream/handle/10665/70185/WHO_HRH_HPN_10.3_eng.pdf.

6

Ethical Issues

Nancy A. Walton

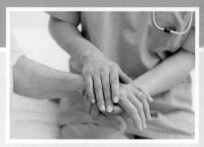

© Can Stock Photo Inc. / 4774344sean

This chapter highlights ethical concerns as they relate to the practice of nurses, student nurses, and leaders in nursing. Relational ethics, principles of bioethics, and codes of ethics are discussed. Nursing has been described as a "moral activity, a moral act, and even an ethical force in society" (Raya, 1990, p. 506), which means that nurses are expected to act ethically. This chapter also examines how ethical decision making can be applied to everyday clinical practice.

OBJECTIVES

- Define *ethics*.
- Discuss the principles of relational ethics.
- Analyze the bioethical principles of autonomy, justice, beneficence, and nonmaleficence.
- Apply nursing codes of ethics from a nurse manager's perspective.
- Explore ethical violations, dilemmas, and distress.
- Discuss how law, morality, and professional accountabilities can influence nurses' managerial and clinical decision making.

- Apply a framework to prevent and resolve ethical conflicts.
- Understand the ethical obligations of nurse managers and leaders.
- Analyze the role of clinical ethics committees.
- Understand the nurse manager's responsibility to develop policy using an ethical decision-making framework.

TERMS TO KNOW

autonomy
beneficence
bioethics
confidentiality
ethical dilemma
ethical violations

ethics
informed consent
justice
moral distress
moral residue
moral resilience

moral uncertainty
nonmaleficence
relational ethics
social justice

❓ A CHALLENGE

Medhat is a nursing manager of a busy postoperative cardiac surgery unit at a downtown hospital. The unit has initiated new care plans for surgical patients across the hospital to try to improve recovery time and reduce time to discharge. Today the unit needs to discharge a number of patients in order to accommodate the transfers from the Cardiovascular Intensive Care Unit (CVICU). Overnight, there were two emergency surgeries and the CVICU needs bed space. The resident on call did rounds this morning and discharged Carl, a 68-year-old man, who underwent coronary bypass and valve replacement seven days ago, with postoperative complications, including hypertension and abnormal cardiac rhythms. Carl is precariously housed, having lived between shelters, temporary housing, and the street for decades. Medhat is discharging Carl to a shelter, and while it is a better option than other possibilities, Medhat knows that Carl will have to vacate his bed and leave the shelter for a few hours each day and that he will not be monitored as closely as he has been in hospital. Carl continues to struggle with insomnia, fatigue, and oedema.

Medhat notes that Carl finds it difficult to get used to taking his new medications and seems forgetful and distracted, and at times sad and teary. Carl requires reminding, multiple times a day, about the new medications and other practices to support his recovery. From a medical perspective, Carl is relatively stable and ready for discharge, but from a nursing perspective, Carl requires additional help, education, and support. When Medhat talks to Carl about discharge, Carl reassures them, saying, "It's okay, I know you have to get me out of here. I've survived in shelters and on the street since before you were born! Don't worry about me." But Medhat is very worried, preferring to either keep Carl in hospital a few extra days or transfer Carl to a rehabilitation bed for further recovery, but neither of those options are a possibility today. The resident has now authorized the transfer of patients out of the ICU to the unit and the bed must be made available, quickly.

How would you deal with this situation if you were Medhat? What ethical principles could help guide your actions?

INTRODUCTION

Nurses and nurse managers are held to a high level of ethical accountability and are expected to act in a way that reflects ethical and compassionate practice, especially when making decisions regarding patient care. To be viewed as ethical, nursing decisions and actions are typically guided by three elements (Fig. 6.1):

1. Ethical principles and values.
2. Professional accountabilities.
3. The law.

These elements interconnect to influence the development of the nurse's ethical practice, which is demonstrated by the nurse's decisions and actions. It is also a reality that ethical decisions are based on the nurses' values, principles, and past experiences. Ethical decision making and ethical practice is challenging for nurses in today's complex health care environment. Rising patient acuity, complexity of care, resource allocation challenges, heavy workloads, recruitment and retention issues, ever-expanding treatment options, and evolving scope of practice can place extraordinary ethical demands on nurses (Bjarnason, 2011; Pavlish et al., 2011). Nurse managers and leaders should always view managerial decisions through not only a lens of professional obligations but also through an ethical lens in order to ensure that patients and nursing staff are both *cared for* and *cared about* in a manner that reflects high levels of mutual respect as well as valuing (Woods, 2012). This chapter provides an introduction to the ethical theories and principles that nurses and nurse leaders must consider when making decisions in a clinical setting. Relational ethics and the principles of bioethics are also explored, especially as they relate to the roles of nurse leader and manager.

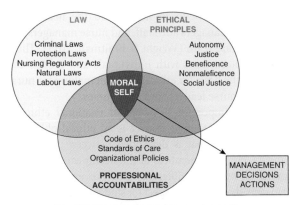

Fig. 6.1 The interface of law and morality.

THE RELATIONAL CONTEXT OF ETHICS

Ethics is a division of moral philosophy that involves the moral practices, beliefs, and standards of individuals or groups (Toren & Wagner, 2010). It includes consideration and evaluation of whether actions and intentions can be deemed as 'right' or 'wrong.' *Ethics* and *morality* are often considered to have the same meaning. However, *ethics* is a branch of philosophy that deals with what is right and wrong, whereas *morality* is the code of conduct advanced and accepted by a society, a group, or an individual (*Merriam Webster*, n.d.; *Stanford Encyclopedia of Philosophy*, 2011). Morality can be reflected in personal, cultural, and professional values, and it is based on ideas about right and wrong. Ethics can be divided into three branches:

1. Meta-ethics.
2. Normative ethics.
3. Applied ethics.

Meta-ethics explores the broader theory and meaning of morality and the foundation and scope of moral values, words, and practice (*Stanford Encyclopedia of Philosophy*, 2007). *Normative ethics* is concerned with the standards most people use to guide their behaviours (e.g., murder is wrong), and how they are determined (*Encyclopaedia Britannica*, n.d.). Finally, *applied ethics* relates to how we apply ethical principles to resolving real-life ethically challenging situations, such as how to provide ethically competent nursing care and how to engage in the responsible conduct of research that involves human participants. A division of philosophical thought within applied ethics is *bioethics*, which focuses on questions about science and human life, often in the context of health care with a focus on principles such as respect for autonomy, justice, beneficence, and nonmaleficence (Beauchamp & Childress, 2013; Risjord, 2014). Better understanding of ethics can help nurses and nurse leaders develop the strategies and enhance the skills and knowledge needed to engage in ethical decision making and ethically competent nursing practice.

In health care, the importance of human relationships in ethical decision making cannot be overemphasized. A key area of ethical nursing practice is the therapeutic relationship between the nurse and the patient (Beckett et al., 2007). Whether this relationship involves direct one-on-one care provided by a staff nurse or indirect care, as provided by a nurse manager or leader, relationships are central to nursing and nursing care. The relationships that develop between nurses and individuals, groups, and communities form the relational context of ethical practice. Although each relationship is unique and includes different individual experiences, thoughts, and actions, all can be grounded in the core elements of relational ethics.

BOX 6.1   Core Elements of Relational Ethics

- Engaged interactions.
- Mutual respect.
- Embodied knowledge.
- Uncertainty and vulnerability.
- Interdependent environment.

From Austin, W., Goble, E., & Kelecevic, J. (2009). The ethics of forensic psychiatry: Moving beyond principles to a relational ethics approach. *Journal of Forensic Psychiatry & Psychology, 20*(6), 835–850; Kunyk, D., & Austin, W. (2012). Nursing under the influence: A relational ethics perspective. *Nursing Ethics, 19*(3), 380–389; Shaw, E. (2011). Relational ethics and moral imagination in contemporary systemic practice. *Australian & New Zealand Journal of Family Therapy, 32*(1), 1–14.

RELATIONAL ETHICS

Relational ethics involves asking not only *What should I do?* but also *What should I do for others?* and *How do my actions affect those around me?* In an effort to answer these questions, relational ethics focuses on ethical actions within ethical dimensions of relationships. The core elements of relational ethics are engaged interactions, mutual respect, embodied knowledge, uncertainty and vulnerability, and interdependent environment (Austin et al., 2009; Kunyk & Austin, 2012; Shaw, 2011). According to a relational ethics approach, nurses must consider those who will be influenced or affected by their intentions, their words, and their actions (Falk-Rafael & Betker, 2012) (Box 6.1).

A relational ethics approach to nursing includes engaged interactions that promote the interpersonal aspects of relationships (Leung & Esplen, 2010; Olmstead et al., 2010). In nursing practice, engaged interactions are not confined to the nurse–patient relationship; they also occur between nurses and the health care team, nurse managers and staff, and nurse managers and the health care team (Wright & Brajtman, 2011). These engaged interactions with individuals and groups can help form the basis for ethical decision making for nurse managers, nurse leaders, and staff nurses.

Another important principle of relational ethics is mutual respect. Mutual respect is an ethical obligation in relationships that is developed between nurses and patients, families, members of the health care team, and among all nurses in different roles. For example, nurse managers show mutual respect for students, nurses, and the health care team by facilitating inclusive interprofessional team meetings to discuss and plan patient care. Team meetings provide an opportunity to demonstrate value for everyone's contributions and thereby demonstrate mutual respect—a critical aspect of effective teamwork. This is one example of how relationships that are based on mutual respect can help guide ethically sound actions.

Part of providing mutually respectful nursing care is the establishment and maintenance of the therapeutic relationship between patient and nurse. "Nurses build trustworthy relationships with persons receiving care as the foundation of meaningful communication, recognizing that building these relationships involves a *conscious* effort" (CNA, 2017, p. 8). Nurses should be aware of the challenges to the integrity of the nurse–patient relationship as well as the challenges of supporting ethically sound relationships in busy and complex health care environments. There are a number of both internal and external factors that can interfere or threaten the integrity of the nurse–patient relationship. External factors, such as high rates of turnover or casual nursing staff, staff shortages, consistently high workloads, unhealthy or hostile work environments, or poor staff morale might make it difficult to establish and sustain nurse–patient relationships. Internal factors might include fatigue, moral residue or moral distress, or a values conflict. While nurses have an obligation to demonstrate respect for the diverse values of the patients to whom they provide care, there may be situations in which nurses feel that mutually respectful or ethically sound care can not be provided. In these types of cases, nurses must be both reflective and self-aware, acknowledge the situation professionally, and work with the nurse manager to ensure that the patient is provided with appropriate nursing care. The CNA Code of Ethics refers to conscientious objection, a case in which a nurse may have personal objections to practising in certain types of situations or with certain procedures, such as medical assistance in dying, providing blood transfusions, or being involved in a situation in which accessible care is being refused. In cases where the nurse's personal values do not allow for moral acceptance of practices of the patient, a nurse is permitted to step back from a situation that involves a "conflict with their conscience" (CNA, 2017, p. 35) to work with the team to allow another nurse to take over care. A nurse in a situation of values conflict is obligated to provide safe, ethical, and competent care until other provisions can be made. Nurses should try to anticipate potential values conflicts ahead of time when and where possible (CNA, 2017). For example, a nurse who holds strong and deep personal feelings about the sanctity of life should reflect carefully about accepting a position on a unit in which medical assistance in dying is provided. But sometimes, nurses may find their personal values tested to the limit in situations with individuals or families, and must be able to be reflective, self-aware, realistic, and professional when faced with an ethically problematic or personally challenging situation.

EXERCISE 6.1 Lara is a new graduate nurse working nights in an emergency room in a downtown hospital. Tonight, is her fifth night in a row working and it is a very busy night. A patient is brought to the unit by ambulance accompanied by police officers and handcuffed to the stretcher rail. He is noticeably intoxicated and covered in blood. When Lara goes to help other team members move him to a bed, the patient swears and spits at them, yelling and laughing about "knifing" someone "who deserved it!" The police officers tell Lara and the team that the patient, who has previously been charged with domestic abuse and sentenced to prison time, was found in his home 10 days after getting out of prison, and after drinking heavily most of the day. The patients' 10-year-old daughter called emergency services after he reportedly stabbed his wife during a fight that became physical. His wife is in serious condition in another hospital and his daughter is in the care of children's services while other relatives are found. As they can't determine if all the blood on him is his wife's, the patient is here for an assessment before being taken to a holding cell by police. Lara knows that a nurse's role is to provide respectful, non-judgemental, and compassionate care to everyone (CNA, 2017). Lara also knows that, while some might be horrified by the patient's alleged actions and the gravity of the situation, domestic violence is a tragic and complex situation and that knee-jerk responses, assumptions, or judgements are not helpful. Lara grew up in a family situation that involved serious domestic violence, and when she was 14, Lara's mother was murdered by Lara's stepfather. Lara, realizing that this patient situation is already affecting her personally, steps into the clean utility room alone, takes some deep breaths, and then calmly and professionally approaches the nurse manager, Idil. Lara tells Idil that she knows she cannot provide good quality care to this patient, and briefly explains why, but will remain with the patient and the team and provide care until another nurse can be assigned.

In this case, do you think what Lara did was ethically sound? If you were Idil, how would you respond and what actions would you take? Reflect on and discuss some situations that might be potentially ethically problematic for you, as a nurse, in terms of providing care. What would you do if faced with a situation like Lara's?

BOX 6.2   The Core Elements of Relational Ethics Applied to Nursing Leadership

Core Elements	Nurse Leader's Role	Nurse Leader's Actions
Engaged interactions	Communicator	Attends and actively takes part in team meetings
	Counsellor	Fosters and facilitates nurse–patient therapeutic relationships
	Teacher	Provides ongoing professional development opportunities for patients and staff
	Decision maker	May be engaged in hospital ethics committees or other advisory or decision-making committees
Mutual respect	Negotiator	Participates actively in patient rounds
	Team builder	Facilitates interprofessional team meetings
	Patient advocate	Participates actively in discussions with patients and families about care
Embodied knowledge	Researcher	Participates in scholarship and engages in research
	Coordinator of care	Takes time to understand unique needs of patients and families
	Professional development supporter	Remains current by attending conferences and engaging in the literature
	Policy and procedure administrator	Engages with institutional policy and procedure committees
	Expert clinician	Engages in the literature and with multidisciplinary expert clinicians
Uncertainty and vulnerability	Advocate	Helps develop policy and procedures
	Consultant	Consults appropriately with allied health care team members, and local experts
	Risk manager	Advocates for quality care for all
Interdependent environment	Team leader	Applies code of ethics, values, and principles to practice
	Advocate for social justice	Actively participates in professional associations
		Actively participates in policy development

According to a relational ethics approach, the workplace is considered to be an interdependent environment that extends beyond the individual nurse and relationships to include more complex relationships that connect nurses to the health care system, communities, and the broader world—an idea described in the *International Council of Nurses Code of Ethics for Nurses* (2012). In an interdependent environment, all nurses, nurse managers, and leaders recognize individuals' and groups' social and political natures. This implies that nurse managers should involve different nurses and roles in matters of health policy and create an environment where nurses and the health care team are encouraged to apply their experience and professional values to the development of policy and standards of care. For example, since 2017, new policies and protocols have been required to be put in place at every publicly funded health care institution addressing medical assistance in dying. In many cases, nurse managers and leaders have been obligated to involve nurses who provide the direct care, and other members of the health care team, in the development of those policies and protocols to ensure they accurately reflect the needs of patients and that they are feasible and realistic within the context of the unit and institution. When developing or revising *any* type of

health policy, nurses should consider that within a relational ethics approach, each individual or stakeholder is social and brings both context and experience to the process of policy development.

Applying the principles of relational ethics to practice and managerial decisions related to patient care can help nurse managers think about the fundamental question: *What should I do for others?* In an effort to answer that this question, the relational ethics perspective focuses on the relationships that develop within the health care team as important in the development and maintenance of professional ethical practice. A relational ethics perspective can help nurse leaders and managers realize that relationships they have with others—nurses, other health care team members, patients, and families—are critical in the development and degree of effectiveness of the nurse managers' and leaders' roles and actions. A relational ethics approach helps nurse managers and leaders reflect on how they ought to act and think, and to consistently consider the relationships they have with their staff, patients, families, communities, and groups in an effort to provide ethically sound nursing care and make ethical decisions in the clinical setting. Box 6.2 shows how the core elements of relational ethics can be applied to nursing leadership.

THE PRINCIPLES OF BIOETHICS

Bioethics (also referred to as *biomedical ethics*) is a division of applied ethics rooted in biological research and medicine and increasingly concerned with questions related to health care. Four major principles of bioethics are: respect for autonomy, justice, beneficence, and nonmaleficence (Beauchamp & Childress, 2013). Bioethics applies to real-life situations for nurses, nurse leaders, and managers, such as ensuring patients have provided informed consent, supporting nursing staff in providing competent and safe patient care, and making resource allocation and priority-setting decisions.

Respect for Autonomy

Autonomy is derived from the Greek words *autos* ("self") and *nomos* ("rule"). Autonomy is the freedom and the right to choose what will happen to one's own person. Being autonomous means that we are allowed to be free to do as we wish in most situations, without influence, interference, or being forced to do something against our will. Ensuring respect for autonomy implies that each person is, in turn, afforded the ability and information about options to make decisions about their situations and meet their goals (Burkhardt et al., 2017; Yeo et al., 2010). Applying the principle of autonomy to nursing practice means that nurses have an ethical obligation to focus on a patient's unique needs, opinions, and preferences for care, while balancing the recommendations of the health care team and plan of care (Risjord, 2014). When nurses apply the principle of respect for autonomy to help guide their ethical practice, they recognize the right of patients to be actively involved in decisions about their own lives to the extent they are able. The role of nurses as advocates means that they must facilitate the inclusion of individuals and families in decision making about their care and lives. Helping people be actively involved in decision making and educated about their available options is a key nursing role in the process of obtaining informed consent. The term *informed consent* in health care refers to, typically, a formal process by which patients are actively engaged in making decisions about their care. By being informed of the proposed procedure or treatments, the expected outcomes, potential benefits, and risks of harm related to the proposed treatment or procedure, patients make an informed decision and thus exercise their autonomous wishes. The process of informed consent assures the legal protection of a patient's right to personal autonomy in regard to specific treatments and procedures. Obtaining consent formally, and usually in writing, is typical for invasive medical procedures (e.g., surgery, insertion of a temporary pacemaker, or a needle biopsy) and this is usually obtained by the medical practitioner who is doing the procedure or administering the treatment. The nurse's role is often to help ensure that the patient has provided informed consent and that any barriers to the integrity of the process have been addressed. For many types of routine nursing procedures, written informed consent is not necessary, but consent should still be obtained from the patient, in a less formal way. Each time a nurse approaches a patient to administer a medication, to check vital signs, or to change a dressing, the nurse should always first check in with the patient that they understand what is about to happen and that the immediate plan of care is acceptable to them at that point in time. Respecting patient autonomy means always ensuring that patients are not passive recipients of care, but rather that they are as involved as possible in all decisions that are part of their own health care experience. Informed consent and the nurse's role are discussed in more detail in Chapter 7.

EXERCISE 6.2 Gwen is a new graduate nurse working nights on an oncology unit. On rounds at 6 a.m., Gwen finds Zachary, a patient scheduled for surgery in a few hours, crying. Zachary admits to Gwen that the surgery is "terrifying" and says, "I'm afraid I won't live through it!" As Gwen sits and talks with Zachary, Gwen realizes that while Zachary signed the consent form, he doesn't have an understanding of the surgery, does not know why the surgery is necessary, and does not comprehend the potential risks and benefits. Zachary tells Gwen that "I don't want the surgery now" and goes on to say, "I'll just live with the cancer." Gwen knows that the surgeon visited Zachary last night briefly, that there was a very short conversation only about the surgery, and that Zachary reportedly had no questions at that time.

In this case, how can Gwen use the core elements of relational ethics and ensure Zachary's autonomy is respected, to help address this situation?

When nurse managers apply the principle of respect for autonomy to guide their ethical practice and managerial decision making, they recognize the importance of involving their staff in decisions that affect their work lives. Applying the principle of respect for autonomy suggests that nurse managers are aware of their responsibility to consider the needs of a diverse group of individuals who make up the staff of their unit or agency. For example, a nurse manager who is preparing the budget for the next two years should ask the unit staff to actively participate in developing a list of priority items to be purchased for their unit. By doing so, the nurse manager involves staff in decisions that affect them directly. In some cases, a decision must be made quickly and without extensive consultation, such as in the case of an emergency or crisis. An important part of building strong and sustainable teams in an ethically supportive environment is providing opportunities for staff to give meaningful input to help inform important decisions. Managers who respect the autonomy of their team members also respect their staff as individuals with personal goals and aspirations; for example, a manager respects and supports a staff nurse's right to request a leave of absence from work to return to school and complete her degree even though it means the unit will now be one staff member short.

One criticism of the principle of respect for autonomy is that it can lead to a focus on the rights or needs of one individual at the expense of the rights or needs of others. A relational approach to respect for autonomy recognizes that respecting the autonomy of one individual should not come at the expense of the autonomy of others and acknowledges that all individuals have different social, political, and economic backgrounds. Consider the example of the nurse who always insists on taking an early lunch break. Depending on the nursing workload assignment, the patient care situations, the staffing ratio, and the needs of others, it may not be convenient for that nurse to take an early lunch on every shift. While the nurse may also insist to the nurse manager that the nurse should be able to choose, the preference for an early lunch should not supersede other goals, or other members of the health care team's legitimate requests. The perceived rights of one can infringe on the rights of others. As such, respecting autonomy means respect not only for the individual but also for others. A relational approach to autonomy suggests that autonomy

can sometimes be best promoted through advocating for ongoing social change rather than through simply protecting an individual's freedom of choice (Kenny et al., 2010).

Justice

Justice refers to the principle that addresses how we treat others out of a sense of what we consider to be *fair*. There is no one way to think about justice or to decide what actions are more just than others, as justice can be subjective and highly dependent upon the lens through which you view a situation, a decision, or a process. Justice is a multi-faceted concept and may refer to how benefits and burdens are allocated (distributive justice); how laws, rules, and policies are created and applied (procedural justice); and how decisions are made about whether the rules themselves are fair (substantive justice). A sense of justice may guide the actions of nurses by promoting the principle that those who are poor, sick, and vulnerable should be given more help than those who have adequate resources, are healthy, and can defend their rights on their own. Patients are often vulnerable in the context of health care settings, and once they enter the health care system, nurses become their advocates, or their "voice," to help ensure they receive the best care for their individual situation. It is not enough that nurses support the principle of justice; they must actually engage in those good and right actions that show justice is being done. For example, if a nurse observes an unsafe practice, they must report it rather than ignore it. The principle of justice also suggests that benefits and burdens should be distributed in a just manner in society (distributive justice).

Nurse managers may refer to principles of distributive justice in their nursing practice and managerial decision making when they are working to ensure that staffing and workload are fairly distributed among the nursing staff. It is not enough to recognize that one nurse has a heavier workload than another; a nurse manager must look carefully at the workload of each nurse on every shift to ensure that the work is as evenly distributed as possible. It is important to consider that some nurses believe that equal distribution of work is unfair given that it does not take into account contextual factors such as patient acuity, complexity of care required for individual patients, or factors related to the individual nurse such as seniority or required accommodations.

Performance appraisals by nurse managers ought to be guided by principles of procedural justice and substantive justice. This means ensuring that, as much as possible, fair and transparent processes are in place regarding evaluations and performance appraisals. Objective information is used as an evaluative measure, and nurses are made aware of clear expectations upon which their performance will be appraised. In turn, those expectations and measures by which nurse will be evaluated should make sense given the professional context. There should be clear processes in place for a nurse to respond to a performance appraisal, set a plan for professional development, and be rewarded when performance is outstanding. By ensuring fair and transparent processes for evaluation, nurse managers follow principles of procedural and substantive justice.

The Canadian Nurses Association (CNA) considers social justice to be a key policy initiative and priority, noting clearly that the value of social justice is aligned with the professional values outlined in the CNA Code of Ethics newest revision (Canadian Nurses Association, 2010; 2017). Social justice refers to "the fair distribution of society's benefits, responsibilities, and their consequences. It is the relative position of one social group in relationship to others in society as well as on the root causes of disparities and what can be done to eliminate them" (CNA, 2006, p. 7 as cited in CNA, 2010, p. 10). In other words, nurses using a lens of social justice will have a keen awareness of inequity in terms of distribution of goods, burdens, and advantages as well as a recognition of the role of the nurse in exploring these differences and addressing contributing factors and social structures and systems that contribute to disparities and inequity (CNA, 2010; Myllykoski, 2011; Peter, 2011; Whitehead, 1991; Woods, 2012). Social justice principles are in keeping with a relational approach to ethics because the focus often extends beyond individuals to social groups and communities who may be affected by systems, social structures, practices, and policies that have the potential to create, sustain, or entrench social inequities and disparity. Nurse managers and leaders often have to make tough decisions about the allocation of scarce resources, and using the principles of social justice can help them make a case for allocating resources to certain patient populations.

EXERCISE 6.3 Clevance is a third-year nursing student doing a clinical placement in a policy unit of a local downtown public health agency, serving persons affected by poverty, food insecurity, addictions, and homelessness. The nurse manager tells Clevance that the agency has been allocated a small portion of additional funds for the next year and must use them to support a specific initiative. The staff have brought forth a number of ideas—starting a mother and baby drop-in program, expanding the clean needle exchange program, starting a literacy program, or hiring an additional temporary staff member so that they can increase their winter overnight shelter program for this year. The funds are one-time funds and will only support one initiative. As a project, the nurse manager asks Clevance to explore each initiative idea and make a recommendation on how the agency staff should spend this small allocation of funds.

What are some ways, from a social justice perspective, that Clevance could use to assess each project, given that only one can be funded?

Beneficence

Nurses are bound by a professional, legal, and ethical duty to provide high-quality, safe, and compassionate care. The principle of beneficence states that in all actions and intentions, we should aim to "do good." This principle is reflected in the provision of high-quality, holistic, and responsive nursing care based on competent and ethical practice that is sensitive to the needs of patients, families, and communities. Nurses working in all contexts must be educated in accredited nursing education programs and then maintain their competence through active practice and continuing professional education. Nurse managers have an obligation to support staff nurses in their pursuit of continuing competency as well as maintain their own competency in practice and management. In ensuring high-quality nursing care to all patients and patient groups as well as by maintaining a focus on the therapeutic relationship between individual nurses and patients, nursing as a profession is viewed by many as a highly beneficent profession.

The obligation to "do good" within the nurse–patient therapeutic relationship also means carefully assessing what patients may define as "good." Goodness is a subjective notion. It seems safe to assume that the intention of nurses in general is to do good, but it is also arguably true that each person's idea of what "good" may be, in a particular situation, will be quite different. The examination and assessment of what constitutes "good" in any particular case, for those involved, will help determine the most ethically sound action to be taken.

> **EXERCISE 6.4** Consider the case of a patient who is in the last stages of a lingering, painful, terminal illness and who is eligible for and considering medical assistance in dying. In discussion of the case with the health care team and family members at patient rounds, it is clear that some believe that life is sacred and should be preserved at all costs. Others believe that a peaceful death with family present is valued over continuing pain, dependence, and deterioration.
> Think about what you consider to be the "good" action in this hypothetical case. Would your idea of what constitutes "good" change if this were your family member, or yourself?

Nonmaleficence

The principle of nonmaleficence states that in all that we do and intend, we must "do no harm." This principle is reflected in all spheres of professional

> **EXERCISE 6.5** The side effects of many treatments, such as chemotherapy, may be experienced by some patients more severely than others, and each person may view any particular side effects as more harmful than others. For some patients, anemia is the most devastating side effect, while for others, painful swallowing and mouth sores may be difficult to tolerate. Still other patients may view the loss of hair as the most worrisome side effect of chemotherapy.
> Look up the most common side effects of chemotherapy and think about how you would discuss these with a patient who you are educating about treatment options. How would you explore the patient's values and their ideas of what constitutes harm related to the potential treatment, while facilitating them to make an autonomous decision about treatment?

practice and in administration, education, and research. Nurses in practice should be competent, be aware of any safety concerns for patients, and anticipate any potential risks of treatment. In addition, nurses in practice should always ensure that they explore the ideas of what constitutes "harm" from the patient's own perspective, acknowledging that this is an important part of respect for autonomy. Nurse managers are obligated to consider patient safety, but they must also consider staff safety and recognize their responsibility to establish safe, good-quality professional practice environments for all, including their staff. Nurse managers must help establish standards of practice and develop policies that promote a safe work environment with constructive systems for professional appraisal and professional development.

CODE OF ETHICS FOR NURSES

Nurses have access to several key documents that can guide their ethical conduct in practice, including codes of ethics for licensed practical nurses (LPNs) (called *registered practical nurses* in Ontario), registered psychiatric nurses (RPNs), and registered nurses (RNs). The Canadian Nurses Association (CNA), the International Council of Nurses (ICN), and provincial or territorial regulatory colleges have all developed or adopted codes of ethics, which guide the ethical conduct and ethical obligations of nurses, nurse managers, and nurse leaders. While each individual code of ethics may have different values, priorities, or obligations outlines, many of the principles are essentially the same as those identified in the CNA and the ICN code of ethics (CNA, 2017; ICN, 2012). An important part of exploring guidelines for practice for any nurse is seeking out and engaging in their specific provincial or territorial code of ethics.

The CNA *Code of Ethics for Registered Nurses* describes the ethical values that guide registered nurses' actions in all areas of nursing practice, including education, administration, research, policy, and clinical practice (CNA, 2015; 2017).

The CNA code states that nurses are ethically committed "to persons with health care needs and to those receiving nursing care" (CNA, 2017, p. 2). The code outlines seven primary values that serve as bases for

BOX 6.3 Elements of the ICN Code of Ethics Applied to the Nurse Manager's Role

Element	Nurse Manager's Role
People	Provide leadership that respects patient and staff rights and is sensitive to the values, customs, and beliefs of all people. Provide education for staff on ethical principles to guide practice. Ensure staff have adequate information to advocate for the patient's right to choose or refuse treatment. Maintain the confidentiality of staff information (e.g., professional appraisals)
Practice	Establish a working environment that promotes quality care. Establish a system for the professional appraisal of staff. Establish systems for the professional development of staff. Monitor and promote the personal health of staff.
Profession	Set standards and policies to guide ethical practice. Foster the use of research and evidence for practice. Promote participation in federal, provincial, territorial, and international nursing associations.
Co-workers	Create awareness of the benefits of interprofessional team collaboration. Support common professional ethical values and behaviours among staff. Prevent unsafe practices and work environments.

the relationships that nurses have with their patients, students, colleagues, and other members of the health care team, which are, for example, similar to those identified in the code of ethics for LPNs of British Columbia (College of Licensed Practical Nurses of BC, 2004) and the code of ethics for LPNs of Newfoundland and Labrador (College of Licensed Practical Nurses of Newfoundland and Labrador, 2011). Those values include a responsibility to provide safe, compassionate, competent, and ethical care and to intervene to address unsafe, noncompassionate, unethical, or incompetent practice or unsupportive working conditions (see Box

5.2). These seven values can clearly also be applied as guidelines for the conduct of nurse managers and leaders. For example, nurse managers are ethically obligated to ensure that nursing staff are providing safe, competent, and ethical nursing care—through the maintenance of "quality practice environments" (CNA, 2017, p. 5). To meet this obligation, nurse managers may need to provide support and resources for nurses dealing with ethical dilemmas, ensure professional development of all nursing staff in the area of ethics, and they may need to intervene if nursing staff are deemed to be engaging in unsafe, unethical, or incompetent nursing care.

The CNA Code of Ethics stresses the importance of nurses maintaining their competency while adhering to the values of the code. Nurses are expected to care for patients while collaborating with the team to plan that care. Nurses respect the wishes of their patients and share information to help patients make informed decisions. Nurses play key roles in advocating for patients, and in that role should intervene to preserve the dignity of patients by refraining from judgement and discrimination and from labelling, demeaning, or stigmatizing patients. Advocacy, according to CNA, goes beyond the individual nurse–patient relationship in that nurses are also expected to advocate for health care systems that are accessible and inclusive for those who may be vulnerable or marginalized and to eliminate social inequities (CNA, 2017). Nurses are expected to be accountable for their practice and to adhere to the values outlined in the CNA Code of Ethics, wherever they work.

The ICN Code of Ethics states that nurses have a moral obligation "to promote health, to prevent illness, to restore health, and to alleviate suffering" (ICN, 2012, p. 1). In the light of this moral obligation, the ICN has identified four principal elements that outline the standards of ethical conduct that guide nurses' actions, these being:

- Nurses and people
- Nurses and practice
- Nurses and the profession
- Nurses and co-workers.

Each of these principal elements can be applied by practising nurses, nurse managers, educators, and researchers. Box 6.3 demonstrates how the ICN code of ethics can be applied specifically to the nurse manager's role.

EXERCISE 6.6 Lionel is teaching a third-year leadership and nursing course for the first time. One of the key learning objectives is for students to understand and engage in a discussion of the Canadian Nurses Association Code of Ethics. Lionel remembers learning about codes of ethics as a student nurse and that the concepts therein didn't really resonate until Lionel was in full-time practice and grappling with difficult and ethically challenging situations. Lionel wants to help ensure that the key ideas and concepts of the CNA Code of Ethics "come alive" for the students, in discussions.

What are some strategies that helped you learn about codes of ethics? How can we better ensure that the ideas and concepts within the CNA Code of Ethics will resonate with students and remain with them as they begin their careers?

THE INTERDEPENDENT ENVIRONMENT OF NURSING: ETHICS AND THE LAW

Within a relational ethics approach to ethics, nurse managers and leaders must consider the interdependent environment that goes beyond the individual nurse to include connections to the community and globally. Recall that three factors, in addition to the individual patient context, can have an influence on nurses' managerial and clinical decision making: relevant laws, ethical principles, and professional accountabilities (see Fig. 6.1). A relational ethics approach promotes the idea that the workplace is an interdependent environment that fosters relationships that connect nurses to their patients, one another, members of the health care team, local and international professional organizations, the community, and globally.

Many laws affect nursing actions and decision making, including nursing regulation acts, common laws, natural laws, and labour laws. Some of these laws are discussed in more detail in Chapter 7. Laws are generally rooted in ethical and moral principles, but laws and morality can differ and even contradict one another. Many of today's laws have been influenced by ethical values that have been in existence for thousands of years, such as "thou shall not kill" and "do not steal." While there is a great deal of overlap between ethics and the law, there are some clear differences as well. There are lawful acts are considered arguably unethical, such as gossiping or lying. In turn, there are acts that are illegal, but arguably ethical, such as driving over the speed limit in order to transport an injured person to hospital or smashing a car window to rescue a dog left on a hot day.

As society's ethical values evolve, so can the relevant laws. It can be argued that the first laws of early society developed as a result of ethical inquiry into wrongful acts. Murder is one of the clearer examples of how society's ethical values have affected the development of laws that serve to punish wrongful acts. However, there is a continuing interface between law and ethics, whereby changing community standards, evolving dominant discourses, and a recognition of diverse ideas about ethics can effect a change in laws. A clear example is medical assistance in dying, once considered unethical and unlawful in Canada. Now, patients and their families can explore and request medical assistance in ending their lives (if certain criteria are met). The movement towards upholding the ethical principle of respect for autonomy that protects a patient's right to make decisions about his or her own care, and a movement towards recognizing the importance of quality of life, underpinned these changes in the law. In Quebec's Bill 52, we can see community standards and ethical principles reflected through ensuring that end-of-life patients are provided with care that is respectful of their dignity and autonomy (Quebec National Assembly, 2013).

The interface of law and ethics can also have an impact upon the professional accountabilities of nurses. Just as society's ethical values influence the law, so too laws and ethical values influence the professional accountabilities of nurses and nurse managers. For example, laws exist to ensure that patients provide informed consent, so those laws and the bioethical principle of respect for autonomy work together to influence the nurse–patient relationship.

Another example of how the law and ethical principles can have an impact upon professional accountabilities is confidentiality. Confidentiality can be viewed as both an ethical and a legal concept. It includes an ethical obligation for nurses to uphold the privacy and security of privately held personal information and a legal obligation under common law to protect personal information divulged to health care providers and not release that information without the patient's explicit permission (Cornock, 2011). Institutional or agency policies on privacy and confidentiality are based on laws such as the *Personal Health Information Protection Act, 2004* and the ethical principle of respect for autonomy. Given that both legal and ethical implications must be considered in policy development, such a policy would have to provide guidance on how to access, disclose, and handle patient information based on legal

BOX 6.4 Example of a Privacy and Confidentiality Policy

Values

Wellness Hospital is dedicated to protecting the privacy and confidentiality of personal health information. We are legally and ethically obligated to keep all information collected within our services confidential, including how we collect, use, access, maintain, and destroy personal information.

Principles

All personal health information collected at Wellness Hospital is to be held in the strictest confidence and only collected, used, or disclosed for reasons of patient care or education. Collecting, sharing, discussing, and disposing of information must be in accordance with relevant legislation, professional standards, and codes of ethics. Information to be kept confidential includes, but is not limited to, patients' personal health information or personal information and any financial information.

requirements found within the statutory law (Box 6.4). Confidentiality is discussed in further detail in Chapter 7.

While nurses should consider the interface between law and ethics when establishing professional standards and policies to guide actions in any practice setting, they also must be aware of changes in dominant discourses and the evolution of ethical norms in society that are often then reflected through changes in legislation and professional standards.

DEFINING ETHICAL PROBLEMS FOR NURSE MANAGERS

Nurse managers and leaders are faced with a variety of ethical issues and concerns that sometimes can be difficult to define, and staff nurses often turn to their managers for help with ethical concerns (Zuzelo, 2007). Being able to understand and express the ethical concern being experienced can help nurses discuss it further with colleagues. For example, is the situation one in which the autonomy of a patient is not being respected? Is the problem really an ethical problem or is it really a more practical problem? Is the situation one in which the nurse feels a sense of moral distress, knowing the right thing to do but being unable to do it (CNA, 2017; Jameton, 1984)? The CNA code of ethics suggests several terms that nurses can consider when they are expressing

ethical issues and concerns, including *ethical problem*, *ethical violations*, *ethical dilemmas*, and *ethical distress*.

At the simplest level, an ethical experience is a situation that creates a sense of moral uncertainty: "A situation where there are conflicts between one or more values and uncertainty about the correct course of action" (CNA, 2017, p. 7). An ethical problem may create feelings of discomfort and uneasiness for individual nurses. Situations that provoke moral uncertainty may be resolved by discussing the problem with the patient, colleagues, and health care team members.

LITERATURE PERSPECTIVE

Resource: Zuzelo, P. R. (2007). Exploring the moral distress of registered nurses. *Nursing Ethics, 14*(3), 344–359.

As the author notes, nurses are confronted every day with practice issues that can evoke moral distress. This research-based article describes the causes of nurses' moral distress and the frequency of morally distressing events in practice. The Moral Distress Scale was administered to 100 direct care nurses working in a variety of settings, including medical–surgical, maternal–child, and critical care units. The nurses in the study identified that the two most morally distressing events in their practice were related to working with "unsafe" levels of nursing staff and working with physicians who were not as competent as the complexity of patient care required. Comments from the nurses indicated that they resented it when physicians were reluctant to address death and dying concerns with patients and their families. Another very frequent distressing event for RNs was carrying out orders for unnecessary treatments and tests. RNs also identified that their nurse managers and supervisors were their most important supports when dealing with ethical issues.

Implications for Practice

Nurses practising in different settings and with different patient groups can all potentially experience moral distress. One example of a morally distressing event often reported by nurses in practice includes unsafe levels of staffing. Nurses rely on their nurse managers to provide advice and guidance on ethical concerns. Therefore making nurse managers aware of specific ethical issues may be an important first step in enhancing the ethical reasoning and moral assertiveness of nurses in practice. Nurse managers can also implement other strategies to address the moral distress of RNs, such as ethics rounds, improving access to ethics consultations, and increasing involvement of RNs on ethics committees.

Ethical violations "involve actions or failures to act that breach fundamental duties to the persons receiving care or to colleagues and other health care providers" (CNA, 2017, p. 7). Ethical violations reflect a nurse's neglect of moral obligations and a breach of duty (e.g., when a nurse discusses patient information publicly). **Ethical dilemmas** or questions "arise when there are equally compelling reasons for and against two or more possible courses of action, and where choosing one course of action means that something else is relinquished or let go" (CNA, 2017, p. 6). With ethical dilemmas, reasons exist for and against a particular course of action, but only one option can be selected (e.g., when deciding to continue treatment for a patient who is likely to die). Finally, **ethical (or moral) distress** "arises when nurses feel they know the right thing to do, but system structures or personal limitations make it nearly impossible to pursue the right course of action" (CNA, 2017, p. 6; Jameton, 1984; Webster & Baylis, 2000; Rodney, 2017).

Moral distress occurs when the nurse knows the right thing to do but cannot act on that insight. Experiencing moral distress that is unresolved can often provoke feelings of guilt, concern, or frustration; for example, a family wants their elderly and terminally ill mother resuscitated at all costs when the mother previously signed a "do not resuscitate order." Moral distress can result from unresolved or repeated ethical uncertainty or ethical violations. Repeated, unresolved ethical distress can ultimately result in professional dissatisfaction, poor staff morale affecting patient care, and sometimes in nurses leaving the workplace or the profession (Burston & Tuckett, 2013; Chiarella & McInnes, 2008; Rodney, 2017).

It is important for nurse managers and leaders to focus on the resources that are needed to help resolve the ethical concerns experienced by nursing staff. Managers must examine organizational barriers that may contribute to moral distress or prevent the resolution of ethical problems. Conflicts with health care team members, excessively heavy workloads, unsafe levels of staffing, inadequate resources, or a lack of clear and responsive policies can contribute to unresolved ethical dilemmas and ethical distress (Gaudine et al., 2011; Musto et al., 2015; Rodney, 2013; Rodney, 2017). Managers should ensure that nurses are supported in order to be safe, competent, and ethical practitioners who provide compassionate care. To that end, nurse managers must help ensure that nurses have a good understanding of the ethical principles and professional values that guide practice

and decision making in all nursing contexts. Nurse managers have an ethical obligation to support the continued professional development of nursing staff in understanding how ethical concepts and constructs apply to their practice. Providing informal and formal educational opportunities for nursing staff to discuss ethical situations in practice, or allowing time for exploration and discussion of ethically challenging situations, are two examples of initiatives that can help promote the awareness and resolution of ethical dilemmas and moral distress in practice. Finally, nurse managers should remember that part of their role is to be ethical role models for staff and to support staff in grappling with ethically challenging decisions in all aspects of professional practice.

LONG-TERM CONSEQUENCES OF EXPERIENCING MORAL DISTRESS

A great deal of focus in nursing is on moral distress, and two related concepts are important to acknowledge and understand. **Moral residue** and **moral resilience** are two consequences for nurses who experience moral distress. When situations of moral distress arise, feelings of frustration, guilt, anxiety, and anger can result. Over time, with unresolved situations of moral distress, feelings of powerlessness and compromise of self or personal values settle in and can become embedded into one's self-concept (Epstein & Delgado, 2010; Webster & Baylis, 2000). This is the "residue" that unresolved moral distress can leave behind—and when not addressed, is deeply concerning.

Moral resilience is a concept that has arisen out of the literature on moral distress and is still deemed to be a concept without a single or mutually agreed-upon definition (Young & Rushton, 2017). Rushton's continuing work on moral resilience asks key questions about the experience of moral distress and enquires why some who experience moral distress have resultant feelings of hopelessness, disempowerment, and despair while others can remain more positive, even resilient (Rushton, 2016). Recognizing that there are some people who experience situations that are morally distressing but are still able to find meaning, positive guidance, and hope, Rushton seeks to enquire how this happens and why it happens to some and not others. Better understanding the concept of moral resilience and how it is developed and nurtured may provide a path forward to examining and addressing moral distress in nursing.

EXERCISE 6.7 Consider an ethically challenging situation you have encountered in the context of your nursing practice – as a nursing student, new graduate nurse, staff nurse, or as a nurse leader or manager. Discuss the reasons you found the situation to be ethically challenging. Did you experience a sense of moral distress? If so, think about the cause of that feeling, while remembering the definition of moral distress. What are some ways you addressed the situation and what might you have done differently?

BOX 6.5 Steps in Ethical Decision Making

1. Clarify the need.
2. Identify all involved.
3. Arrange a meeting.
4. Select a facilitator or chair.
5. Identify areas of agreement.
6. Identify areas of disagreement.
7. Offer resources.
8. Seek outside advice if necessary.
9. Make a decision.
10. Implement the decision.

A MODEL FOR ETHICAL DECISION MAKING FOR NURSE MANAGERS AND LEADERS

Ethical decision making is not done in a vacuum. It is always carried out in the context of relationships, power and politics, particular settings, and social structures. Throughout the ethical decision-making process, values and often emotions can also have an effect upon those most involved and on the process of making decisions about ethically charged situations. Ethical decision-making models can help guide nurses through decision making and make sure that key steps are not missed. Additionally, ethical decision-making models can help nurses reflect on and apply relevant ethical values to the decision-making processes. In general, most ethical decision-making models follow similar steps and can be adapted to individual situations and contexts (Box 6.5). One example of a clear ethical decision-making model, grounded in nursing and nursing ethics, has been developed by Oberle and Raffin Bouchal and is described in the most recent version of the CNA *Code of Ethics* (CNA, 2017; Oberle & Raffin Bouchal, 2009). Effective nurse managers and nurse leaders should be familiar with these steps and be prepared to facilitate ethical reflection and the decision-making process.

One of the first steps in making ethical decisions is to *clarify the need* for the decision and its urgency; for example, the need to decide whether to provide experimental but high-risk treatment for a stable patient with a rare disease is different from the need to implement a do-not-resuscitate order of an acutely unstable terminally ill patient. Timelines for making the decision must be established and agreed upon by all who are involved, including the patient, family, and the health care team.

When clarifying the need for the decision, it is also important to collect all of the available information that will be used to make the decision (e.g., diagnostic test results, documentation of previous wishes regarding care). Once the need to make a decision has been clearly established, it is important to *identify all of those who are involved* and who are directly affected by the decision and *arrange a meeting* with them to discuss the decision-making process and options.

Discussing ethically difficult situations, such as removing a patient from a ventilator, can be a very difficult process for everyone involved. The health care team typically includes the patient and family, nurses, physicians, social workers, and other relevant health care providers, but when an ethical situation arises, the team may include a patient representative and a health care ethicist. Once the meeting has been arranged, it is appropriate for the group to *select a facilitator* who is not directly involved in the decision and can be impartial. The key to a productive meeting is to ensure that an open discussion and a safe environment exists in which all can comfortably express personal views.

The facilitator should establish key areas for discussion, including *areas of agreement* and *areas of disagreement* between members of the group. The roles and responsibilities of each member of the group should be established and clarified (e.g., patient representative, staff nurse, the unit's nurse manager). All members must be given the opportunity to express their views and be heard. If consensus cannot be reached, *outside advice may be necessary* (such as from a clinical ethics committee). Ideally, everyone should agree and understand the available options, and the implications of the decision that is being made. Consensus may be difficult to achieve, so the group must decide on how a final decision will be made, who will *make the final decision* (this is especially important if the patient is unable to express their own wishes), and how to *implement the* *decision*. The ethical decision-making process can help the group reflect on the ethical values that may have an impact upon the decision.

EXERCISE 6.8 You are a nursing student in your last semester of your degree program. In your clinical setting, you are providing care for a comatose patient, Josh, admitted to the neuro-trauma unit after a motor vehicle accident resulting in a severe brain injury. Along with your preceptor, you have become a source of information and comfort for the family at this difficult time. You have worked a few nights and have had "heart to heart" discussions with Josh's mom, who has identified with you after you told her during the first shift you met the family that you also have a son named Josh. At this time three successive electroencephalograms (EEGs) have revealed that Josh is now "brain dead," and the care team has begun discussions with his parents to remove all life support. After a number of difficult discussions, Josh's father has agreed to the removal of life support, but Josh's mother is adamant that such a decision can never be acceptable. Josh's father said at the last family meeting, "More than anything, Josh loved life. He has no quality of life here, like this. We have to let him go, to be at peace, even if it's the hardest thing we'll ever do." Josh's mother approaches you in the lobby coffee shop as you are on your break, appearing sad and reflective and admitting to you that they cannot live with this decision. "There is still so much life for Josh to live—how could we give up on that? Life is life, no matter what it might look like, even with machines. He's still warm, and he's still alive! You can't just give up on life. It's not right. You're a mother. You understand how precious life is—there must be a way to help them understand."

In a small group with your classmates, talk about what approaches you might use to help Josh's mother and family work towards a decision for Josh.

CONCLUSION

Ethical values and principles, moral thought, the law, and professional accountabilities all guide the decisions and actions of nurses, nurse leaders, and nurse managers. This chapter provides an introduction to the ethical principles that are important to consider when making decisions in clinical settings. Guidelines for ethical conduct have been presented and applied to the nurse manager's role, and a framework for ethical decision making has been outlined to help managers and decision makers engage in ethical reflection when decisions involving ethical concerns are required in practice.

❓ A SOLUTION

In this situation, Medhat is feeing "caught between" what is the right thing to do from Medhat's perspective and the demands and requirements of the institution. Medhat feels that the right thing to do would be to allow Carl a few more days in hospital or arrange for Carl to go to a rehabilitation centre in order to support the recovery process. Medhat is also aware of Carl's vulnerability and the fact that Carl faces consistent challenges and marginalization in everyday life. Finally, Medhat realizes that by sending Carl to a shelter today, Carl will face additional challenges that could be avoided. Medhat wants to provide compassionate and safe care to Carl—and to all patients on his unit—but Medhat feels that the new initiatives to move patients to discharge faster is not in the best interests of many of the patients that are on the cardiac surgical ward, in particular patients with complex medical or social support needs, like Carl. Medhat calls together the nurse manager in the CVICU and the resident and attending surgeon, and explains the concerns regarding Carl, while advocating for an additional two days in hospital to provide time to get social work involved with Carl and work towards getting him a bed in the rehabilitation hospital. Medhat reminds the resident and surgeon that if Carl has complications in the shelter, they will very likely simply send Carl to the emergency room and the patient will end up back in hospital. Medhat also reminds them that Carl has some particular needs and vulnerabilities and that the team has an ethical obligation to provide ethically sound and compassionate care in all cases. While the CVICU nurse manager is not happy that one of the ICU patients will not be able to transfer to the postoperative unit, they agree that calling in an extra staff member to cover the shifts in the CVICU is reasonable and necessary. They all agree that they feel considerable pressure to demonstrate improved unit statistics for time to discharge, and that in this case pressure made them overlook ethically sensitive and compassionate care to the individual patient. They reflect on the fact that this will no doubt happen again. Given this, they agree that, going forward, doing a better job in identifying patients with particularly complex medical or social support needs *pre-operatively* might help improve postoperative planning and ensure that patients' needs can be met more effectively in the recovery period, while also allowing them to meet their targets for time to discharge.

THE EVIDENCE

It is clear that nurse managers are often confronted with the need to make the most ethically sound decision for patients, for their staff, and for their nursing staff (Ganz et al., 2015; Toren & Wagner, 2010). They may ultimately experience a tension between meeting the needs of the institution, meeting the needs of their nursing staff, and meeting the needs of patients and families. This tension directly results from the role of manager, as managers are, of course, nurses in leadership positions who also have obligations to further the initiatives and values of the institution alongside the professional values of nursing. Nurses in all areas of practice, when confronted with ethical dilemmas, often find that the available options or alternatives are not completely satisfactory. While there may be clear justifications or reasons why each alternative might be acceptable, there may still be relevant ethical objections or problems associated with each option. Institutional values or priorities, which nurse managers are expected to support and promote, may not be aligned with, or may directly conflict with, nurses' professional—or even their personal—values. The role of nurse manager implies a number of often conflicting ethical obligations. Nurses in management roles, especially those in clinical areas, are obligated to ensure that patients, families, and communities are able to access safe, compassionate, and high-quality nursing care. To that end, nurse managers support their staff by creating opportunities to engage in ethical practice, and workplace environments that support optimal and responsive care. Those same nurse managers are also obligated to advocate for their own units and unit needs, often with some degree of "competition" with other managers, who are all advocating for finite resources and funds for their own areas. Additionally, nurse managers are involved in the administration of the institution and are expected to promote the values and priorities of the institution. Finally, at the level of the individual workplace, nurse managers are expected to not only ensure that patients, families, and communities have—overall—access to high quality care, but they are also obligated to be sensitive to unique or extenuating individual needs for particular patient-care situations. In many situations, nurse managers may experience conflicting obligations and duties, with little available guidance for how to resolve these ethical or values conflicts. Using an ethical decision-making model, being transparent about and encouraging discussions of potential conflicts in ethical obligations, and remaining aware of one's own professional and personal values, are some examples of ways to help work though these inevitable ethically challenging situations.

NEED TO KNOW NOW

- Know the ethical principles that can guide nursing practice, management, and leadership.
- Understand how the principles of relational ethics can be applied to nursing practice, leadership, and management.
- Use nursing codes of ethics to help guide your ethical practice and understand how the principles outlined in codes of ethics can be applied to the work of a staff nurse, nurse manager, or nurse leader.
- Understand that laws and professional accountabilities may have an impact upon your ethical nursing practice, leadership, and management.

- Develop a reflective process for working through ethical dilemmas in your own practice.
- Be aware of any institutional policies or procedures regarding ethical decision making in practice.
- Develop self-awareness of your own values and beliefs and identify good resources and professional mentors to whom to turn when you are involved in an ethically challenging situation or values conflict.

CHAPTER CHECKLIST

This chapter focused on ethical issues as they relate to the role of nurse managers and leaders. In particular, relational ethics was discussed with a focus on its core elements: engaged interactions, mutual respect, embodied knowledge, uncertainty and vulnerability, and interdependent environment. Nurses must consider the relationships they have with those who will be influenced by their thoughts and actions. The major principles of bioethics were also presented: autonomy, justice, beneficence, and nonmaleficence. An understanding of these ethical principles can help nurse managers and leaders develop the strategies they need to engage in ethical decision making and practice. Nurse managers experience a variety of ethical issues on a daily basis. Therefore it is important for managers and leaders to be aware of the strategies to deal with these issues, including the role of hospital ethics committees and how to establish a clear process for ethical decision making.

The following key concepts apply to ethical decision making in everyday clinical practice:

- Nurse managers' decisions and actions are guided by ethical principles, professional accountabilities, and, sometimes, the law.
- Ethics involves moral practices, beliefs, and standards of individuals or groups.
- Principles of relational ethics include engaged interactions, mutual respect, embodied knowledge, uncertainty and vulnerability, and interdependent environment.
- The major principles of bioethics are respect for autonomy, justice, beneficence, and nonmaleficence.
- Other related and important concepts to explore are ethical violations, ethical dilemmas, or ethical distress.
- Ethics committees can provide a framework to prevent and resolve ethical conflicts in practice.
- The steps in ethical decision making are: clarify the need, identify all involved, arrange a meeting, select a facilitator or chair, identify areas of agreement, identify areas of disagreement, offer resources, seek outside advice if necessary, make a decision, and implement the decision.

TIPS FOR DECISION MAKING AND PROBLEM SOLVING

- Reflect on the ethical principles and values that guide your practice and decisions.
- Seek guidance from professional nursing codes of ethics.
- Engage your colleagues and the health care team in open discussions about ethical concerns or challenges.
- Think about ensuring that ethical concerns are discussed, in addition to other types of concerns, at team rounds.

- Explore the nursing ethics literature to help understand more about ethically complex situations in nursing practice.
- Get to know your institution's bioethicist or clinical ethicist and consult the bioethics team or ethics committee when further guidance is needed.

Visit the Evolve website for Suggested Readings, Internet Resources, and additional resources related to the content in this chapter: http://evolve.elsevier.com/Canada/Yoder-Wise/leading/.

REFERENCES

Statutes

Personal Health. (Information Protection Act, 2004. SO 2004, c. 3, Sch. A. Retrieved from http://www.e-laws.gov .on.ca/html/statutes/english/elaws_statutes_04p03_ e.htm#BK65.

Texts

Austin, W., Goble, E., & Kelecevic, J. (2009). The ethics of forensic psychiatry: Moving beyond principles to a relational ethics approach. *Journal of Forensic Psychiatry & Psychology, 20*(6), 835–850.

Beauchamp, T. L., & Childress, J. (2013). *Principles of biomedical ethics* (7th ed.). New York: Oxford University Press.

Beckett, A., Gilbertson, S., & Greenwood, S. (2007). Doing the right thing: Nursing students, relational practice, and moral agency. *Journal of Nursing Education, 46*(1), 28–32.

Bjarnason, D. (2011). Moral leadership in nursing. *Journal of Radiology Nursing, 30*(1), 18–24.

Burkhardt, M. A., Nathaniel, A., & Walton, N. (2017). *Ethics and Issues in Contemporary Nursing.* Toronto, ON: Nelson.

Burston, A. S., & Tuckett, A. G. (2013). Moral distress in nursing: contributing factors, outcomes and interventions. *Nursing Ethics, 20*(3), 312–324.

Canadian Nurses Association. (2006). Social justice: A means to an end, an end in itself. *Canadian Nurse, 102*(6), 18–20.

Canadian Nurses Association. (2010). *Social justice: A means to an end...an end in itself* (2nd ed.). Retrieved from. https://www.cna-aiic.ca/~/media/cna/page-content/pdf-en/social_justice_2010_e.pdf.

Canadian Nurses Association. (2015). *Framework for the practice of registered nurses in Canada.* Retrieved from *https://www.cna-aiic.ca/~/media/cna/page-content/pdf-en/framework-for-the-pracice-of-registered-nurses-in-canada.pdf?la=en.*

Canadian Nurses Association. (2017). *Code of ethics for registered nurses: 2017 edition.* Toronto, ON: Author. Retrieved from https://www.cna-aiic.ca/~/media/cna/page-content/pdf-en/code-of-ethics-2017-edition-secure-interactive.

Chiarella, M., & McInnes, E. (2008). Legality, morality and reality: The role of the nurse in maintaining standards of care. *Australian Journal of Advanced Nursing, 26*(1), 77–83.

College of Licensed Practical Nurses of B.C. (2004). *CLPNBC code of ethics for LPNs: Companion guide.* Burnaby, BC: Author.

College of Licensed Practical Nurses of Newfoundland and Labrador. (2011). *Standards of practice and code of ethics for Licensed Practical Nurses of Newfoundland & Labrador.* St. John's, NL: Author.

Cornock, M. (2011). Confidentiality: The legal issues. *Nursing Children & Young People, 23*(7), 18–19.

Encyclopedia Britannica. (n.d.). *Normative ethics.* Retrieved from http://www.britannica.com/EBchecked/topic/418412/normative-ethics.

Epstein, E.G., Delgado, S., (Sept 30, 2010) "Understanding and Addressing Moral Distress" *OJIN: The Online Journal of Issues in Nursing* Vol. 15, No. 3, Manuscript 1.

Falk-Rafael, A., & Betker, C. (2012). Relational ethics in public health nursing practice. *International Journal for Human Caring, 16*(3), 63.

Ganz, F. D., Wagner, N., & Toren, O. (2015). Nurse middle manager ethical dilemmas and moral distress. *Nursing Ethics, 22*(1), 43–51.

Gaudine, A., LeFort, S., Lamb, M., et al. (2011). Ethical conflicts with hospitals: The perspective of nurses and physicians. *Nursing Ethics, 18*(6), 756–766.

International Council of Nurses. (2012). *The ICN code of ethics for nurses.* Geneva, Switzerland: Author.

Jameton, A. (1984). *Nursing practice: The ethical issues.* Englewood Cliffs, NJ: Prentice-Hall.

Kenny, N., Sherwin, S., & Baylis, F. (2010). Re-visioning public health ethics: A relational perspective. *Canadian Journal of Public Health, 101*(1), 9–11.

Kunyk, D., & Austin, W. (2012). Nursing under the influence: A relational ethics perspective. *Nursing Ethics, 19*(3), 380–389.

Leung, D., & Esplen, M. (2010). Alleviating existential distress of cancer patients: Can relational ethics guide clinicians? *European Journal of Cancer Care, 19*(1), 30–38.

Merriam-Webster. (n.d.). (Ethic. Retrieved from http://www.merriam-webster.com/dictionary/ethic/.

Musto, L. C., Rodney, P. A., & Vanderheide, R. (2015). Toward interventions to address moral distress: Navigating structure and agency. *Nursing Ethics, 22*(1), 91–102.

Myllykoski, H. (2011). Social justice: Who cares? *Alberta RN, 67*(4), 28–29.

Oberle, K., & Raffin Bouchal, S. (2009). *Ethics in Canadian nursing practice.* Toronto: Pearson.

Olmstead, D., Scott, S., & Austin, W. (2010). Unresolved pain in children: A relational ethics perspective. *Nursing Ethics, 17*(6), 695–704.

Pavlish, C., Brown-Saltzman, K., Hersh, M., et al. (2011). Nursing priorities, actions, and regrets for ethical situations in clinical practice. *Journal of Nursing Scholarship, 43*(4), 385–395.

Peter, E. (2011). Fostering social justice: The possibilities of a socially connected model of moral agency. *Canadian Journal of Nursing Research, 43*(2), 11–17.

Quebec National Assembly. (2013). *Bill 52: An act respecting end-of-life care.* Retrieved from http://www.assnat.qc.ca/en/travaux-parlementaires/projets-loi/projet-loi-52-40-1.html.

Raya, A. (1990). Can knowledge be promoted and values ignored? Implications for nursing education. *Journal of Advanced Nursing, 15*(5), 504–509.

Risjord, M. (2014). Nursing and human freedom. *Nursing Philosophy, 15*(1), 35–45.

Rodney, P. A. (2013). Seeing ourselves as moral agents in relation to our organizational and sociopolitical contexts: Commentary on "a reflection on moral distress in nursing together with a current application on the concept" by Andrew Jameton. *Journal of Bioethics Inquiry, 10*(3), 313–315.

Rodney, P. (2017). What we know about moral distress. *American Journal of Nursing, 117*((2) Supp.), S7–S10.

Rushton, C. H. (2016). Moral resilience: A capacity for navigating moral distress in critical care. *Ethics in Critical Care, 27*(1), 111–119.

Shaw, E. (2011). Relational ethics and moral imagination in contemporary systemic practice. *Australian & New Zealand Journal of Family Therapy, 32*(1), 1–14.

Stanford Encyclopedia of Philosophy. (2007). *Metaethics*. Retrieved from http://plato.stanford.edu/entries/metaethics/.

Stanford Encyclopedia of Philosophy. (2011). *The definition of morality*. Retrieved from http://plato.stanford.edu/entries/morality-definition/.

Toren, O., & Wagner, N. (2010). Applying an ethical decision-making tool to a nurse management dilemma. *Nursing Ethics, 17*(3), 393–402.

Webster, G., & Baylis, F. (2000). Moral residue. In S. B. Rubin, & Zoloth (Eds.), *Margin of error: The ethics of mistakes in the practice of medicine* (pp. 217–232). Hagerstown, MD: University Publishing Group.

Whitehead, M. (1991). The concepts and principles of equity in health. *Health Promotion International, 6*(3), 217–228.

Woods, M. (2012). Exploring the relevance of social justice within a relational nursing ethic. *Nursing Philosophy, 13*(1), 56–65.

Wright, D., & Brajtman, S. (2011). Relational and embodied knowing: Nursing ethics within the interprofessional team. *Nursing Ethics, 18*(1), 20–30.

Yeo, M., Moorhouse, A., Khan, P., & Rodney, P. (2010). *Concepts and cases in nursing ethics* (3rd ed.). Peterborough, ON: Broadview Press.

Young, P. D., & Rushton, C. H. (2017). A concept analysis of moral resilience. *Nursing Outlook, 65*(5), 579–587.

Zuzelo, P. R. (2007). Exploring the moral distress of registered nurses. *Nursing Ethics, 14*(3), 344–359.

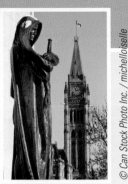

7

© Can Stock Photo Inc. / michelloiselle

Legal Issues

Nancy A. Walton with contributions by Lyle G. Grant

Legal issues have become a growing concern for nurses as nursing practice continues to expand in scope and involve higher degrees of expertise, autonomy, and accountability. Nursing practice is legally defined as distinct from and independent of other health care practices, and this distinction has also changed traditional views of nursing liability. Laws that are relevant to nursing practice cover areas such as the governance, rights of individuals, autonomy, privacy, informed consent, substitute decision making, records management, freedom of information, and labour relations. By viewing nursing practice through a legal lens, laws and the application of laws can add a perspective of not only certainty, but also, sometimes, complexity. A basic understanding of the laws that apply to nursing practice is an expectation of nurses in all contexts and practice areas. Nurse leaders need a strong working knowledge of the applicable areas of law to provide advice, guide decision making, and manage liability risk. This chapter provides an introduction to areas of law that are important for nurses in Canada. It is a given that the law and application of laws is a constantly changing landscape, and often laws must be viewed in the light of individual situations and contexts. It is impossible in one chapter, therefore, to describe and explain all relevant knowledge and information regarding legal aspects of nursing. Instead, the purpose here is to introduce relevant legal terms and concepts and increase your awareness of some highly relevant areas of law that may have an effect upon you as a student and a new graduate nurse.

OBJECTIVES

- Identify the sources of Canadian law.
- Identify key legal differences in nursing practice and nursing regulation.
- Identify key areas of liability of concern to nurses.
- Understand key areas where positive duties to act exist around reporting, risk management, and public protection.
- Understand how various legal matters—including negligence, malpractice, privacy, confidentiality, reporting statutes, employment law, and insurance—affect leading and managing roles in nursing.
- Describe the purposes and components of documentation and record keeping.

- Identify areas of law relevant to information and health record management, including responsibilities of leaders and managers.
- Describe how institutional policies, procedures, and protocols integrate patient care and legal responsibility.
- Understand legal obligations related to the nurse's role in medical assistance in dying.
- Understand the role of nurses and nurse leaders in developing institutional policies, procedures, and protocols that address legal issues.

TERMS TO KNOW

battery
circle of care
collective agreements
common law
confidentiality
duty of care
fiduciary
foreseeability
informed consent

legislation
liability
licensure
malpractice
medical assistance in dying
(MAID)
natural law
negligence
nursing practice act

personal liability
privacy
regulatory body
risk management
scope of practice
statute
statutory law
tort

? A CHALLENGE

Charlotte is a nurse practitioner who has relocated from Vancouver to a small Northern BC town, where she works in the only family health clinic. Over the past year she has been working and living in this new setting and has become a familiar face in town—and on her days off, when she heads to the grocery store or the local diner, she is often greeted by name by her patients and community members who now know her. Today is a day off work, and Charlotte is in the hardware store trying to find a few supplies for some home renovations. As she is leaving the store, she meets Ted, whose adult daughter Maggie is one of Charlotte's patients. Maggie has depression and anxiety, and over the past year has been struggling with an addiction to painkillers after a fall and ankle surgery. Ted greets Charlotte and thanks her for the care she has provided to Maggie. He goes on to say to Charlotte, "You know, you've done a lot for Maggie, but she's really having a hard time. I think things are worse for her actually—I don't think she's off the pills. Have you seen her? Is she still taking the pills? She told me she isn't, but I don't believe her." Now on the sidewalk, Charlotte replies to Ted acknowledging how worried he must be but noting that she can't talk about Maggie with him. Charlotte also knows that Maggie and Ted have had tensions and challenges in their relationship, and Maggie does not want her father—or anyone—to know anything about their care beyond what she herself shares. Ted responds with a chuckle but raises his voice saying, "Hey, Charlotte, I'm not a stranger! It's me, Maggie's dad. You know how much I've done for Maggie and she's living in my house. I don't need to know details—I just need to know if she's in trouble. You can understand that. We both care for her and want the best for her. Come on! It's a matter of trust!"

What would you do if you were Charlotte? What legal concepts and concerns are most relevant in this case?

THE LAW IN CANADA

The law serves as a form of public policy that represents a collective set of values and beliefs that are deemed important and necessary as a way to maintain order and peace within societies. According to Barkan (2016), the law has five basic functions in our societies, which are:

1. To help maintain order in our social lives.
2. To provide ways of resolving conflicts between people and groups.
3. To reflect the social norms and expectations for individuals, groups, and organizations in their social lives.
4. To help create social change and drive necessary changes in accepted behaviours and norms.
5. To describe the civil rights of individuals and outline ways that those rights are protected.

There are many types of laws at a variety of levels—federal, provincial, territorial, and local—and they all serve specific purposes.

Laws typically reflect the moral values and norms of particular societies, and in this role they can overlap with ethical standards. Intentionally harming a child, for example, is viewed by many as legally and ethically wrong—as both immoral and illegal. There are many instances in which the law and ethics overlap, but there may also be situations in which, for example, there is no prevailing law but rather a moral obligation to do "the right thing." Consider a situation in which someone has shared with you a piece of truthful but hurtful gossip about another individual, which if shared widely, would cause embarrassment or emotional harm to the subject of the gossip. There is no law preventing you from spreading the information, but one might hope that you would feel a moral obligation not to do so and thus avoid causing undue harm to another person.

The laws applicable to nurses in Canada originate from multiple sources. Statutory law refers to laws set out by the government through acts, statutes, codes, or legislation. The term legislation refers to law (commonly regarded as "written law") that is constructed and modified by a legislative body. In Canada, the two primary sources of legislation are the federal Parliament, which consists of the House of Commons, the Senate, and the Governor General, along with provincial legislative bodies (e.g., legislative assemblies, provincial parliaments, and Lieutenant Governors). Legislation can be found in the various *acts* or statutes of Canada as well as those in various provinces and territories accompanied by associated regulations.

A hallmark of Canada's democratic system is that law making ultimately rests in legislative bodies, referred to as the *supremacy of Parliament*. Parliament can ultimately take responsibility for making, amending, and repealing all laws. Canada also operates under a federal system of government that divides these legislative powers exclusively between national and provincial governments. This division of powers is outlined in the *Constitution Act* (1867) of Canada and creates an important background to understanding some of the political contexts of the Canadian health care system and its system of public funding and regulation. For example, most matters of health care and hospitals fall under provincial jurisdiction. However, under the *Canada Health Act* (1985) federal authorities use their spending powers to effectively influence the provision of provincial health care and social services by attaching terms and conditions to the transfer of federal funds to provinces. Medicare, our publicly funded national health insurance program, is a value-based approach to making health care available to all Canadians without financial or socio-economic barriers at the point of care. The federal government, by controlling large portions of the monies necessary to fund the provision of care, indirectly exercises substantial influence over health care delivery and policy in Canada (Downie et al., 2011).

In contrast to statutory law, common law, also referred to sometimes as case law, includes those laws that have been derived from the system of courts and judges. These laws are often referred to as "judicial precedent" or "judge-made." Common laws arise from precedent and are recorded through documentation of relevant case law and the decisions of courts. Canada's common law system is derived from the English common law system.

The system is structured with courts that have different levels of authority. Each level of courts must abide by the decision of a more superior court. For example, a decision in a lower court in Ontario may be overturned by a higher court, e.g., the Ontario Court of Appeals. The highest court of appeal is the Supreme Court of Canada, and the Governor General-in-Council makes the decisions on who will be appointed to the court, with the advice of Cabinet. Although provincial and territorial governments have a say in who will be appointed as a judge in their jurisdictions, they are not involved in the appointment of judges in the federal Supreme Court.

Quebec has a slightly different legal system than the rest of Canada, and most of its provincial laws are limited to and contained within a single written civil code based on the French civil code. Quebec does not have a set of common laws like the rest of Canada, and court decisions related to Quebec provincial laws are often restricted to how courts interpret the civil code.

Canadian law is also influenced by expert opinions and scholarly consensus on how to interpret laws, customary practice, and natural laws. Natural laws are those *higher* laws that apply to all persons and thus should override human-made laws. They include matters such as the right to defend oneself from harm as well as concepts of natural justice and the right to be heard. International laws that have been ratified in Canada may also be binding for Canadians. Finally, various activities in the health care system are governed by private laws. Private laws are those laws administered between persons and include agreements that the courts will enforce as a matter of law; contracts are an example of this type of law. Contracts or agreements that are not otherwise illegal in their intent, with a few exceptions, are generally enforceable in Canadian courts, giving them the full effect of law. Contracts play an important part in health care service delivery and employment arrangements. Although much of contract law is common law, some types of contracts, such as insurance and employment contracts, have been given special attention by legislators over time and are subject to specific statutes. More recently, health care issues involving Indigenous populations in Canada have drawn on international laws and rely heavily on private laws and fiduciary and treaty obligations of the federal state. (Fiduciary: A term used in law and ethics referring to a trusting relationship in which there is a clear and binding obligation to act in the best interests of the other.)

Federal statutes relating to nursing include criminal laws and laws regarding human rights, social welfare, copyright, patents, medications, interprovincial matters, health care funding, and the welfare of Indigenous persons in Canada. Provincial and territorial laws may vary in form and name between provinces and territories, but each province and territory has laws that address the regulation of unions, health care providers, employment, insurance, health insurance systems, hospitals, privacy, informed consent, human rights, and access to information. Laws at all levels and of all types are subject to change over time as a result of their interpretation by the courts and as amended or repealed. Legislation is an important instrument for implementing government policy, and it shapes and influences the political and policy environments of health care.

THE REGULATION OF HEALTH CARE WORKERS

In Canada, health care and its workforce are highly regulated, but these regulations differ significantly across provinces and territories. Commonly, health care workers who must be licensed to practice are referred to as "regulated" and health care workers who do not require a licence are referred to as "unregulated." Regulated health care workers are also accountable to an external regulatory professional body. Examples of regulated health care workers include nurses, pharmacists, and occupational therapists. Through their licence to practice, they are authorized to provide and deliver particular health care acts and therapies. Unregulated health care workers include personal support workers, health and personal care aides as well as physician assistants. Simply distinguishing regulated from unregulated workers oversimplifies the regulatory realities of health care workers in Canada and the transitions underway in regulatory frameworks governing professional health care workers and their authorized practices.

The regulation of who may provide designated health care services may involve processes such as *licensure*, *certification*, or *registration*. Traditionally, licensure has effectively granted the right for group of qualified individuals to perform regulated activities and to identify as a member of that group through use of a designation or credential. Nursing is an example of an occupation where licensure is necessary before designated nursing actions can be performed; registered nurse (RN) is one

type of licensed nursing designation. Licensing bodies are often referred to as *colleges*, *associations*, or *professional regulatory bodies*.

Certification is typically viewed as less restrictive than licensure. Certification refers to protection of the title, and only certain persons who meet explicit qualifications and criteria can use that reserved title. Although licensure creates a situation in which only licensed members may provide certain services with certification, others may still provide the same services but may not use the professional title linked to the certification. This means that members of the public seeking those services must use a degree of caution and care when choosing a provider (Zarzeczny, 2017). As Zarzeczny notes, in a number of provinces, the title of psychologist is restricted for use by anyone other than a person who is a registered psychologist; however, there are not the same limitations on providing counselling or mental health services.

Registration is a means of identifying persons who belong to a group, and may simply require individuals to register to obtain membership (Zarzeczny, 2017). As you can imagine, registration alone offers the least regulatory protection to the public.

Under evolving regulator schema in provinces such as British Columbia, Alberta, and Ontario, health profession regulation is being re-conceptualized to accommodate changing scopes of practice and the realities of practice. Although a full description of these new regulatory frameworks is beyond the scope of this chapter, umbrella legislation governing all health care providers covers the making of regulations that authorize or license acts reserved to specific health care providers. An act associated with professional practices may simultaneously be authorized to those holding different professional designations. For example, an authorized nursing act, like injecting a substance subcutaneously, may be part of registered nurse, practical nurse, and psychiatric nursing scopes of practice. Additionally, advanced nursing practice acts can be authorized to those who are "certified" to conduct these acts. These new regulatory frameworks blur the traditional distinctions among designated professional practices (which are considered to be monopolies) and are examples of the evolution of certification and licensing.

The actions and duties that nurses can legally perform are outlined in legislation as well as in "standards, guidelines, policy positions and ethical standards" (Canadian Nurses Association, 2015, p. 14) of provincial

or territorial nursing regulatory bodies. These actions and duties define the nurse's scope of practice. The ability for licensed practical nurses, registered nurses, registered psychiatric nurses, registered practical nurses, and nurse practitioners to use nursing titles and to conduct designated procedures, processes, and actions is generally set out in nursing practice acts or legislation that creates regulatory authorities or regulatory bodies. For example, registered nurses in British Columbia must be registered with the College of Registered Nurses of British Columbia, a regulatory body created under the province's *Health Professions Act* (1996), to be able to practice; other provinces have similar bodies and acts. These legislative acts and their associated regulations create a form of self-regulating profession: they control who can be licensed, the types of actions that are regulated, reserved, or authorized to nurses, and scope of practice; they set out educational and examination requirements for registration and continuing competency requirements; and they establish governing bodies and processes for monitoring professional conduct and acting on misconduct. Within nursing, various designations help distinguish scope of practice and expected competencies. Advanced nursing practice or specialized nursing actions that exceed the basic scope of practice may also need to be authorized through special certification. Additionally, nurses limit their own individual actions based on their scope of practice and their assessment of personal skills, experience, and competencies. Professional regulations, defined scopes of practice, and individual competencies are important in determining legal authority and responsibilities for nursing actions performed by individuals. They are the primary mechanisms for helping ensure that the public are not exposed to incompetence or unethical actions. Moreover, when a health care worker is regulated through licensing, professional sanctions accompany other available legal actions to protect the public from harm.

IMPLICATIONS AND LIABILITY

Liability and professional sanctions may arise from wrongful, inappropriate, or unethical actions. The law also imposes a special duty on health care workers to protect individuals who are considered vulnerable, such as older adults, those who are incapacitated, and children. Liability and deterrence for wrongful actions are mechanisms to ensure compliance. The consequences faced by nurses who perform wrongful actions fall into four basic categories: criminal liability, civil liability, professional sanctions, and employment ramifications.

Criminal Law

Criminal law is an important branch of public law and deals with crime—often an act committed against another individual but with harms that may resonate beyond the individual to broader society. Criminal liability is largely codified in the *Criminal Code of Canada* (1985) as well as other acts, such as the *Firearms Act* (1995) and the *Controlled Drug and Substances Act* (1996). The federal government allows provinces and territories to administer the criminal justice system and enforce applicable laws. Laws are enforced by the police, the courts, and the penal system, at provincial and municipal levels. Crimes such as writing graffiti or trespassing are seen as less serious and are referred to as *summary offences*. More serious crimes, including sexual offences, kidnapping, or murder, are referred to as *indictable offences*. Some types of crime are referred to as *hybrid crimes*, and the law allows the prosecutor to decide whether to treat it as an indictable or summary offence. Crimes such as murder can never be treated as hybrid, but other crimes, such as sexual assault or assault causing bodily harm, may fall into the hybrid category. Criminal law defines offences and categories and outlines the processes and rules for charging or arresting a person, for ensuring due process, given the category of the crime, for court and trial procedures, and for the assignment of punishment.

Criminal actions have a higher standard of proof than do actions involving other liability. In criminal law, people are presumed to be innocent until proven guilty beyond reasonable doubt. There are thought to be two elements to a crime—the criminal act (also known as *actus reas*) and the intention to commit a crime (also known as *mens rea*). To find an individual guilty of a crime, it is generally accepted that there must be both a criminal act and some intention to commit a criminal act, or knowledge that actions (or lack of action, in some cases) might necessarily lead to a crime. We assume that most conscious, rational persons have the ability to perceive and foresee the natural consequences of their acts, but for those who may be unable to perceive or foresee consequences of their actions (e.g., sufficiently intoxicated, very young children, significant cognitive impairment) *mens rea* can serve to prevent criminal liability.

The following acts are examples of those that are subject to criminal investigation and potential prosecution:

- Certain forms of negligence, assault, and nuisance.
- Actions that result in the spread of communicable diseases.
- Actions that intentionally, wantonly, or recklessly bring about death.

Civil Liability

In contrast to criminal liability, civil liability is a legal obligation that arises when a private wrong, such as a **tort** or breach of contract, is committed, damages or injuries result, and another person can be considered legally responsible. Civil law allows an injured person to bring a lawsuit to claim for damages, commonly referred to as *suing for damages*. Damages are generally reduced to a monetary payment for a wrongful act as compensation to the injured party, but civil lawsuits may also result in a declaratory remedy (such as when a decision regarding ownership is made by the court) or an injunction, in which a court restrains the actions of others as a remedy (e.g., an injunction that prevents a person from making contact with another person).

The wrong or injury that happens to a person or their property as a result of the actions of another person is typically refers to as a tort. A tort may be intentional or unintentional. Examples of intentional torts include assault, battery, trespassing, fraud, or intentional infliction of mental distress. **Negligence** is a common type of unintentional tort and requires that there be an existent duty of care that was breached in a particular way by a person who was expected to uphold a standard of care and who could reasonably foresee that their actions might result in the wrongful act or injury.

In civil liability cases, the standard of proof is based on *a balance of probabilities* rather than the stricter *beyond a reasonable doubt* burden of proof required in criminal law; for example, liability may be found where it was judged *more probable than not* that an action caused the damage. Civil liability claims typically require a person (the plaintiff) to bring a legal action against another (the defendant). Different from criminal prosecutions, which are brought by the state), civil liability cases can be initiated by a person or a business who has suffered a wrong.

Professional Sanctions

Nursing is a self-regulated profession. This means that the government delegated authority to the profession "to regulate itself for the purpose of protecting the public" (College of Nurses of Ontario, 2017, p. 3). Nursing regulatory bodies assume responsibility for ensuring public trust in nurses and for administrative and profession-specific decisions, such as setting minimum educational requirements, setting clinical standards and practice competencies, carrying out quality assurance activities, engaging in patient relations, and addressing ethical, investigative, and disciplinary matters (Zarzeczny, 2017). Most health professions in Canada are regulated in this manner, and the relevant provincial or territorial legislation may be either specific to the profession or "umbrella legislation" (Zarzeczny, 2017, p. 168) in which a number of regulated professions and acts that can be carried out by designated professionals are outlined. Umbrella legislation may be considered as a more modern approach to health professions legislation and as a way to provide more choice for consumers of health care (Zarzeczny, 2017). An example of umbrella legislation is Ontario's Regulated Health Professions Act (RHPA, 1991). Unlike professional membership-based organizations, such as the Ontario Nurses Association, which take on advocacy for the profession, the primary role of professional regulatory bodies is professional self-regulation and ongoing maintenance of public trust and protection (Zarzeczny, 2017).

Disciplining members is the primary mechanism by which professional bodies enforce their standards, and enforcement is an important part of protecting the general public. Professional sanctions and disciplinary actions generally arise from a variety of behaviours that are felt to be unacceptable for members of the profession. Misconduct is a broad category and may include categories of behaviours and actions, such as failing to maintain the standards of practice, working while impaired, theft, breach of **confidentiality**, or poor documentation (College of Nurses, 2018a). Professional sanctions may include loss of licence or any one or a combination of reprimand, fine, remediation requirements, further education, or practice restrictions. Professional sanctions do not restrict other legal actions and remedies, for instance in cases of serious misconduct.

To protect the public interest, professional regulatory bodies have powers of inquiry into member practices and conduct that can be initiated by the regulatory body or that may be initiated upon receiving a complaint from a member of the public. Nurses should be aware of the mechanisms and procedures that may be undertaken by their respective regulatory bodies in response to a public complaint or inquiry. The powers of a regulatory body may also extend to investigation, inspection of records, search and seizure, sanction, and the ability to charge back the costs of these actions to the registrant if wrongdoing is found. Inquiries contested by a registrant, or those of a particularly serious nature, may advance to a disciplinary hearing open to the public. These approaches are consistent with principles of transparency and a public mandate to act in the public's best interest.

Regulatory bodies must follow administrative law procedures in processes to investigate allegations of wrongdoing and in imposing professional sanctions on their members. Professional sanctions have potentially serious consequences for people's careers and lives, and the more serious the consequence proposed, the more important it is that there is due diligence in the process. Regulatory bodies must act only within their legal authority, demonstrate principles of fairness in dealing with complaints and disciplinary matters, and apply principles of natural and administrative justice. Regulatory bodies must also act without bias and discrimination in investigating complaints or allegations. A disciplinary hearing, usually conducted by a disciplinary committee that typically includes members of the public, is the most serious practice review mechanism available to regulatory bodies. A nurse who is responding to a disciplinary hearing may be represented by legal counsel, and some jurisdictions permit representation by a union representative or other advocate. Additionally, a nurse undergoing disciplinary proceedings will have an opportunity to present evidence, make submissions, cross-examine witnesses, and receive written reasons for decisions within a reasonable period of time. Nurses do not always have legal representation during investigative and sanctioning proceedings and, arguably, principles of natural justice would require that options for legal representation be made available to nurses at these times. Decisions of regulatory body disciplinary proceedings may be appealed to the superior court in the province or territory of the proceeding.

EXERCISE 7.1 Think about how self-regulation of professions is an example of good public policy and public protection. Consider the ultimate aims and objectives of regulating health professions and then also consider what might be some current criticisms of professional regulatory bodies.

Employment Ramifications

Employment ramifications may be imposed directly by an employer or may flow indirectly from sanctions imposed by a professional body. Failure to meet employment obligations permit an employer to take various forms of action. Common law, labour law, and employment law regulate the employer–employee relationship and the remedies that employers may take. Collective agreements associated with unionized workplaces are special types of agreements that outline collectively negotiated terms of employment between employers and employees and often have detailed processes for discipline that must be followed. Depending on the employment breach, direct consequences may be punitive in nature and include loss of employment, suspension or reprimand, performance management, increased monitoring, or additional conditions related to continued employment. By contrast, the consequences may be more supportive in an effort to remediate unacceptable practices and include increased mentorship, professional development, education, and support for change. Indirect consequences generally arise from licensing or practice restrictions imposed by professional bodies that affect the registrant's ability to meet employment requirements and expectations. Employment may be difficult to maintain if the limitations placed on a licence are restrictive. Consider a nurse who has a new limitation or restriction on their licence that precludes them handling narcotics. Continuing work on a busy postoperative unit may not be feasible, given that narcotics for post-operative pain are given to almost every patient, several times daily. That same nurse, could, however, work in a unit, such as an outpatient or pre-operative assessment unit, where narcotics are not in use.

NURSING AND THE LAW

Nurses should have a good working knowledge of the law and the key areas of legal concern that apply to nursing practice. Whether you are a new graduate nurse, an ICU nurse, or a nurse manager with many years of practice in a community setting, the law affects you, your patients, and your practice. Entire books are devoted to laws relevant to nursing, and even they do not fully encompass the legal issues that nurse leaders may face. What follows is a brief outline of some key areas of legal concern for nurse leaders. All nurses have a responsibility to learn about the full range of legal concerns and constructs related to their practice areas and responsibilities.

Duty of Care and Standards of Practice

Duty of care is an important overarching legal principle in nursing, and it refers to the legal and professional obligation to act beneficently toward another person or refrain from acting in a way that would cause potential or actual harm. The standards of care owed by health care providers to patients are largely derived from the standards of practice of respective health professions. For example, in nursing in all provinces and territories, standards of practice guide and direct nursing practice and outline levels of competency that nurses are expected to achieve and maintain in practice (College of Registered Nurses of British Columbia, 2018). Management decisions that create work overloads, designate tasks to improperly trained or equipped personnel, fail to adequately orient staff to work environments, or fail to provide adequate resources to allow professionals to meet expected standards of care may shift liability to managers or institutions (Dickens, 2011). Hospitals, for example, may also be negligent and owe their patients and communities duties to "(1) select and maintain competent, adequate staff, (2) provide proper instruction and supervision to staff, (3) provide and maintain proper and adequate equipment and facilities to staff, and (4) establish systems necessary for the safe operation of the hospital" (Dickens, 2011, p. 147).

Duty to Report

Some recent nursing regulations impose new statutory duties on nurses to report other nurses or health care providers to their registration bodies where concern exists that a professional is dangerous to the public or demonstrates sexual misconduct. Of concern here is an individual health care provider's fitness to practise and the protection of the public. In addition, medical practitioners who treat other health care providers who have been admitted to a psychiatric hospital or drug or alcohol addiction treatment facilities may be required to report this to the relevant regulatory body and may also need to include information about the person's condition, treatment, prognosis, and fitness to practise. The British Columbia *Health Professions Act* (1996) is an example of legislation that imposes reporting duties on health care providers across the province. Statutes similar to

the British Columbia *Health Professions Act* create relatively new legal requirements to report the inappropriate conduct of another health care provider when they are potentially dangerous to the public. Failure to report where a requirement exists may invite inquiry into one's own practice. In British Columbia, the statutory duty to report extends to all health care professions, but this statutory duty does not exist in all provinces and territories; however, nurses may also be ethically bound or required under standards of practice to make such reports even without statutory requirements.

Provinces and territories may have statutes that require reporting of certain events of abuse witnessed by nurses in the course of duty. The aim is to protect people in care from abuse, whether they be in residential care, psychiatric treatment facilities, nursing homes, or hospitals (see, e.g., Alberta's Protection for Persons in Care Act, 2009). Statutes may require that individuals and managers report abuse and alleged abusers to external agencies, which may include the police. Other examples of reporting obligations are considered in a subsequent section in this chapter, *Protective and Reporting Laws*. Nurses may be affected by a variety of laws that require reporting, and many statutes provide whistle-blower provisions to protect those who report from reprisals or retaliatory actions by employers or others as a result of the reporting. The intent is to advance the protection of the public and those who take action to safeguard it.

Legal Aspects of Documentation

The requirement for accurate, readable, and timely charting and record keeping has multiple legal sources. Institutional policies and procedures provide the first point of guidance for nurses, but additional documentation may be required to meet practice standards, practice expectations, and changes in patient condition. The timeliness of charting is critical to patient care and well-being. Medical charts are part of interdisciplinary communications that must be up-to-date to ensure proper patient care and to avoid potential legal liability. Charting alerts everyone to potential changes and developments in patient condition. Nursing notes entries are required with minimum frequency as dictated by patient condition, as necessary for quality care, and as directed by institutional policies and procedures. Well-written and appropriately detailed nursing notes can be admitted by courts as part of legal proceedings to establish objective accounts of events. As with all health records, entries should be clear, based on facts, as precise as possible, written as close to the timing of an event as possible, permanent (i.e., not written in pencil), and dated. Additionally, the writer should be clearly indicated with the appropriate nursing or professional designation (e.g., RN, RPN, LPN). Single lines drawn through deletions help ensure that there is no appearance of an attempt was made to hide a portion of the record, but merely to correct the record of clerical error. Corrections made at the time of entry should clearly indicate the change and should include the initials of the original entry maker. All attempts should be made to avoid alteration after the record is made and to avoid any suggestion of alterations to an entry. Any aspect of the entry that raises doubt on behalf of the reader regarding the veracity, legitimacy, or accuracy of what is recorded (such as a questionable alteration, more than a single line through a deletion) may result in the record being questioned as representing the true and accurate representation of events. Legal proceedings involving medical incidents do not often surface for a period of time after the event. Memories of the necessary details of the medical events that are the subject of the proceedings will have faded, so clarity of charting notations is important to reconstructing events and helping refresh memories.

Electronic Records

The now widely accepted use of electronic records and data systems continues to raise new privacy concerns for patients, clinicians, and health systems. Access to information by those unauthorized to view and use it is of great concern, as is the possibility of information being released or shared without permission. The portability—and ever-decreasing size—of laptops, tablets, and mobile devices makes the possibility of identities, personal health information, or data being stolen more realistic. Cloud-based data storage systems give rise to additional security concerns about privacy, access, and security. Concerns about electronic data are related not only to privacy, security, and access but also to ensuring accuracy of records and avoiding errors in entry or records maintenance (Ozair et al., 2015).

As Canada continues to use electronic health records systems that are portable across provinces and territories and health care professions, concerns about protection of personal health information remain. The *USA Patriot Act* (2001) provides a salient example of how individual health data may unintentionally be accessible to state authorities in the United States if the data are stored in or transmitted through the United States. Canadian health authorities have been careful to ensure that data storage, transmission, and processing remain in Canada, but with increasing popularity of cloud-based storage and databanks with servers in multiple countries, hospitals and agencies responsible for data collection and storage must ensure due diligence in protecting data and access only to those who are authorized.

MAINTAINING CONFIDENTIALITY AND PROTECTING PRIVACY

Canadians take their privacy seriously, and they expect that health care professionals will both ensure their privacy and maintain confidentiality. Privacy may be defined as "the right of the individual to determine when, how, and to what extent he or she will release personal information" (*R. v. Duarte*, 1990), and confidentiality relates to holding in private any information provided and protecting the exchange of information with an obligation to prevent release of information to those who are unauthorized (Gibson, 2017). In other words, simply stated, privacy is what we expect as individuals and confidentiality is what we owe others. Nurses, in all kinds of roles, have access to significant personal and confidential information regarding patients, their families, their health, and life experiences. Disclosure of confidential information, particularly in health care settings, can have significant, sometimes life-changing consequences to individuals and their families, and patients trust that, within the limits of the law, what they tell a nurse or allied health care provider, in confidence, will remain so. They also trust that any documentation of their confidential information will be managed securely and appropriately—whether that documentation is in a nursing note or an electronic health record. As we noted, the increasing use of electronic health records to store confidential information and the vulnerability of those technologies, along with the concerns over multiple users requiring access to an individual's personal information, raise additional concerns about how best to protect confidential patient information in health care settings (Gibson, 2017). Laws relating to the legal responsibilities of users of confidential personal information continue to undergo significant changes, and those who fail in those responsibilities can be subject to serious legal and professional actions.

As part of their day-to-day work nurses use, document, and access confidential personal health information of patients. Part of maintaining confidentiality and trust is the treating of all information carefully, including the nurse's decisions about what information should be accessed. Part of the responsibilities of a nurse involves not accessing patient information that is not part of usual nursing care or accessing information about a person not within the circle of care.

EXERCISE 7.2 Most institutions have explicit policies and procedures for who may access patient information and how it can be accessed, as well as monitoring mechanisms to help protect patient confidentiality. Consider an example of a nurse, Talia, working in a cardiac unit in a hospital, whose cousin Robert is a patient on the oncology ward. Robert's wife, Amy, comes to see Talia and tells her that they are anxiously waiting for results from Robert's biopsy. Amy asks Talia to "just check his chart" so they can find out the results and decrease their anxiety and worry "about the unknown." Talia could easily see Robert's results through her electronic record access, but Robert is not her patient, and accessing that information for Amy would be a clear breach of her legal and ethical responsibilities.

In this case, what are Talia's professional and legal responsibilities? If Talia wasn't sure what to do, what types of resources should she access for guidance?

Nurses are likely to encounter legal issues with privacy and confidentiality frequently in the workplace and may find themselves under personal scrutiny for actions performed or neglected regarding patient information. Legal duties to protect the confidentiality of patient information arise out of the duty of health care practitioners to act in their patients' best interests and, as part of those duties, they are considered to be trustees of personal information obtained from patients. With these trusting relationships come clear fiduciary duties regarding acting in the best interest of patients, which involves, among other things, protecting the confidentiality of patient information. Although nurses have legal obligations to maintain confidentiality appropriately, they also have ethical obligations to preserve confidentiality, often incorporated in professional codes of ethics, along with professional obligations. The common law duties respecting confidentiality have been modified by various statutory provisions. The legal landscape of this legislation is complex, by virtue of a number of

factors. First [and] is the division of legislative powers between provinces and territories and the federal government, and the reality that information often flows across provincial borders. Second, some provinces have general privacy and information protection acts only, whereas others have also included health-information-specific acts. The nature of information handled by health care institutions and nurse managers may therefore fall under consideration of more than one specific privacy and information act. For example, in Ontario, employment data on a nurse working at a hospital is not considered health information and is covered under the *Freedom of Information and Protection of Privacy Act (FIPPA)* (1990), but if that nurse were admitted or treated as a patient at the hospital, all health information related to that employee would be covered under the *Personal Health Information Protection Act (PHIPA)* (2004). It is necessary for nurses, managers, and leaders to understand under which acts information is governed to discharge the appropriate legal obligations and duties respecting the treatment of that information.

Health information legislation, like the *Personal Health Information Protection Act* (2004) in Ontario, aims to "balance individuals' right to privacy with respect to their own personal health information with the legitimate needs of persons and organizations providing health care services to access and share this information" (Personal Health Information Protection Act, 2004).

A list of some major information protection statutes in force in Canadian jurisdictions is outlined in Table 7.1. These statutes address the custody, access, disclosure, and use of health information obtained by health care practitioners and the institutions for which they work. Those who access health data are often referred to as *custodians* of health information in the legislation. A careful read of some of the definitions of who is a custodian of information and what information is deemed personal health information may surprise you. For example, Ontario legislation includes the expected list health care providers as "information custodians" but excludes faith healers, traditional Aboriginal healers, and midwives.

The general duty of custodians and trustees of personal health information is to protect the information from disclosure *except where such disclosure is authorized by the information provider*. There are, however, exceptions to this general duty. Typically, information

TABLE 7.1	Select Statutes Relating to Privacy, Confidentiality, and Information Access in Health Care	
Jurisdiction	**Name of Act**	**Common Acronym**
Canada	*Personal Information Protection and Electronic Document Act*, SC 2000, c. 5	PIPEDA
	Privacy Act, RSC 1985, c. P-21	
	Access to Information Act, RSC 1985, c. A-1	
Alberta	*Personal Information Protection Act*, SA 2003, c. P-6.5	PIPA
	Health Information Act, RSA 2000, c. H-5	HIA
	Freedom of Information and Protection of Privacy Act, RSA 2000, c. F-25	FOIP
British Columbia	*Personal Information Protection Act*, SBC 2003, c. 63	PIPA
	Freedom of Information and Protection of Privacy Act, RSBC 1996, c. 165	FOIPPA
	Privacy Act, RSBC 1996, c. 373	
Manitoba	*The Personal Health Information Act*, SM 1997, c. 51, CCSM, c. P33.5	PHIA
	The Privacy Act, RSM 1987, c. P125, CCSM, c. P125	FIPPA
	The Freedom of Information and Protection of Privacy Act, SM 1997, c. 50, CCSM, c. F175	
Ontario	*Personal Health Information Protection Act*, 2004, SO 2004, c. 3, Sch. A	PHIPA
	Freedom of Information and Protection of Privacy Act, RSO 1990, c. F.31	FIPPA
New Brunswick	*Personal Health Information Privacy and Access Act*, SNB 2009, c. P-7.05	PHIPAA
	Right to Information and Protection of Privacy Act, SNB 2009, c. R-10.6	
Newfoundland and Labrador	*Personal Health Information Act*, SNL 2008, c. P-7.01	PHIA
	Access to Information and Protection of Privacy Act, SNL 2002, c. A-1.1	ATIPPA
Northwest Territories	*Access to Information and Protection of Privacy Act*, SNWT 1994, c. 20	
Nova Scotia	*Freedom of Information and Protection of Privacy Act*, SNS 1993, c. 5	FOIPOP
	Hospitals Act, RSNS 1989, c. 208	
Nunavut	*Access to Information and Protection of Privacy Act*, SNWT (Nu) 1994, c. 20, as duplicated for Nunavut by s. 29 of the *Nunavut Act*, SC 1993, c. 28	ATIPP
Prince Edward Island	*Freedom of Information and Protection of Privacy Act*, RSPEI 1988, c. F-15.01	FOIPP
Quebec	*An Act Respecting the Protection of Personal Information in the Private Sector*, RSQ 1993, c. P-39-1	
Saskatchewan	*Health Information Protection Act*, SS 1999, c. H0.021	*HIPA*
	Freedom of Information and Protection of Privacy Act, SS 1990–91, c. F-22.01	*FOIP*
Yukon	*Access to Information and Protection of Privacy Act*, RSY 2002, c. 1	

may be shared within the patient's "circle of care," unless the patient has specifically instructed the trustee of the information not to make such a disclosure. A circle of care may be specifically defined by the relevant legislation but is generally understood as referring to the individuals and institutions directly connected to an individual's health care (Kosseim & Brady, 2008).

Incident reports contain information that may be legally significant—even though that information is not focused on individual care. Incident reports typically collect information on adverse events, near misses, or incidents that potentially place patients or staff at risk. Usually, these reports are not referred to in patient health records but are still considered important and official documentation. Incident reports and the related procedures and follow-ups are important to continuous quality improvement, staff development, and patient and staff safety. These documents would likely fall outside of most health-information-specific protection acts, although they may contain references to individual patients. Procedures around documenting incident reports often strip or remove patient-identifying information from the data at some stage, but procedures for completing these forms, the type of information they should contain, and how the data are handled require clear institutional policy and procedures to minimize unwanted legal use of this information.

Privacy can also relate to the more physical aspects of patient care; for example, intimate aspects of nursing care that, if made public, might result in what we would label as social or psychological harms, and may cause a patient embarrassment or distress. Nurses are ethically bound to preserve dignity in patients and treat patients with respect and compassion—ensuring that patients are not embarrassed or distressed as a result of disclosure of information is naturally a key part of that ethical obligation. Careless or inappropriate actions of nurses who fail to protect the dignity and privacy of patients may result in disciplinary action and legal liability. Such actions have been cast as a type of invasion of privacy tort, but Ontario courts have raised doubt on the success of such a legal precedent, whereas British Columbia, Manitoba, Saskatchewan, and Newfoundland and Labrador have privacy acts that authorize the courts to award damages for invasion of privacy (Peppin, 2011).

Generally, personal information laws provide for the protection of personal health information and impose obligations and responsibilities on health care institutions and their employees. Privacy laws have made the collection, storage, exchange, and disclosure of personal health information more regulated and, accordingly, more complex. Health care employers need clearly developed policies and procedures that follow privacy laws within their jurisdiction to help staff manage these complex laws and guard against liability. Nurses in all areas and contexts are advised to review the personal information protection acts that apply in their jurisdiction of practice, and fully regard themselves as trustees of patient information with all the legal standards required of those standing in positions of trust. The standards to which nurses are held in protecting the personal information of patients are—appropriately—high.

Nurses should be aware of the unique privacy issues associated with electronic medical records (EMRs). In one of its *InfoLaw* information sheets for nurses, the Canadian Nurses Protective Society (2009) addressed unique issues of access, accuracy, theft, and disposal of electronic records. With the growing presence of and reliance on electronic records in health care, these issues are highly relevant to practising nurses.

As noted earlier in the chapter, inappropriate access—that is, accessing a patient's personal information for which you have no legitimate use in the performance of your duties and care of your current patients—may be subject to sanctions. Development and enforcement of clear policies, strong password protections, audit trails, and periodic audit procedures should form part of an organization's plan to guard against improper access to electronic medical records.

In another case, a patient who had requested a copy of his own medical record was inadvertently provided with information on other patients because the data were not appropriately separated, a situation that arose from the inclusion of multiple patients' data in one file or on one DVD. Clear policies to ensure logical separation of different patients' data, to ensure ongoing education, and establish careful checks for patient information should be in place before use or disclosure of that information.

Theft of electronic devices containing protected patient information is a problem that seems to appear regularly in media reports. Similarly, wireless communications and transfers of data, although they enable improvements to patient care through use of portable devices at the bedside or at patients' homes, raise new data security issues. Risk management procedures typically include strong password protection and encryption of storage media if personal health information is permitted to be stored on portable devices. Most health care institutions require use of secure and local servers to store any kind of patient information and discourage providers from using portable devices to store or transport personal health information.

The disposal of electronic records is also problematic. For example, data deleted on an electronic device may not actually be erased from the storage device, but marked as available for overwriting. Policies and practices must address how data can be wiped from storage devices and how storage devices can be destroyed or rendered inoperable in ways that do not allow data retrieval of any residual information. It is equally important to understand that personal information may automatically be stored on devices containing memory or storage capacities, such as fax machines, photocopiers, and personal data devices; this type of storage requires management to avoid inadvertent disclosure. To protect patient information from inappropriate disclosure, nurses must be aware of privacy protection laws, where confidential data exists, and policies and procedures for data access and destruction, audits, and due care.

> **EXERCISE 7.3** Portable devices, such as phones and tablets, are ubiquitous in today's world. Most nursing students and new graduates come to work with their mobile phone or device with them and often use them to look up information, carry out calculations, and even record temporary notes about their patients. Based on what you know about legal and professional expectations regarding portable device use and privacy, what are some guidelines you would highlight for your nursing colleagues regarding use of devices, and for protecting privacy and security of information?

Health Records

Record keeping is generally part of the professional standards of regulated health care professions, but it is also part of the tasks of health care workers who are unregulated. Moreover, health care institutions may be regulated by specific legislative acts to collect and maintain certain types of records on patients. For example, in British Columbia, the *Continuing Care Act* (1996) requires that records be maintained on patients receiving continuing care in areas such as home oxygen supply, home support, meal programs, adult day care services, and continuing care respite services. Special records, such as narcotic control documentation, may also be necessary, and failure to follow legal requirements for such records can result in prosecution. Good-quality health records are important not only in meeting legal requirements but also in providing quality health care to patients. From a nurse leader's perspective, record keeping must meet professional standards, fulfill legal requirements, benefit patients, and help establish or protect legal claims.

Access to Health Records

Relatively recent case law from the Supreme Court of Canada has helped clarify ownership and access issues surrounding patient health records. It is important to keep in mind that this case law may be specifically modified by health record legislation in individual provinces and territories. However, most jurisdictions in Canada have closely followed the court's direction on the issue. As a general rule, the patient does not own the actual health record housed by the health care institution, physician's office, or record keeper. Although ownership rests with the maker and holder of the record, patients ordinarily have the legal right to access the record, subject to some limitations (*McInerney v. MacDonald*, 1992). Patients may not be entitled to immediately access their record, or see portions of it, while they are in active treatment in the hospital, where a physician believes that it is not in their best interests or where disclosure may put a third party at risk. Additionally, patients may require supervision, interpretative assistance, and professional explanation of their records to avoid harmful misinterpretation. Hospitals should develop and maintain clear policies and protocols regarding patient access to their own health records and patient ability to photocopy them (*McInerney v. MacDonald*, 1992). Under many health information privacy acts, patient requests to access their health records must be tracked by an information officer if the records are kept by a custodian under the relevant legislation. This makes it that much more important that procedures and policies are in place and known by all staff. Staff also need to be fully cognizant of who may ultimately view health records when contemplating making entries into them. In a changed era of patient–health care provider relationships, the law makes health care providers and institutions trustees of personal health information; this trusteeship recognizes that liberal access to one's own health record is part of a "philosophy of openness and candour better suited to cultivating mutual trust between patients and their healthcare providers" (Irvine et al., 2013, p. 262).

Patient Safety

In recent years, the emphasis on patient safety and quality care has grown. Creating and maintaining environments that promote patient safety means fostering and developing cultures of safety that move from finding individual blame to looking at how systems can contribute to safety. Fears of liability and cultures of blame associated with revealing adverse events have hampered movement to improved cultures of safety that serve to benefit patients. New legislation in Canada (see, e.g., Manitoba's *Apology Act*, 2007) that prevents apology letters to patients for adverse events being entered into evidence in courts to substantiate wrongdoing and legal liability is one step signalling a movement away from a culture of blame and liability to one that looks for a systematic approach to enhancing patient safety (Robertson, 2008). Moving to cultures of safety that incorporate blamelessness and understanding encourages the reporting of errors and harm to patients so that environments of safety can develop and additional education and training can be offered to avoid harmful recurrence.

PROTECTIVE AND REPORTING LAWS

In certain circumstances, it may be deemed in the public interest for privacy and confidentiality not to be protected, such as when health care providers need to report information to other public authorities. Some laws place a positive duty (a responsibility or burden), on nurses and nurse managers to act to protect an identified subgroup of the Canadian population, often a group who are felt to be vulnerable. All provinces and territories have acts, for example, that make reporting mandatory when an individual reasonably suspects a child is subject to neglect, physical or sexual abuse, or is in need of protection. Laws like the *Child Youth and Family Services Act* (2017) in Ontario outline specific duties to report that apply to all persons, including those, like nurses, who have professional responsibilities towards children and youth. Some provinces have extended this duty to report to include individuals who, by virtue of a disability, are incapable of protecting themselves from such abuse, regardless of age. Reporting in these cases does not require consent to disclose, and the disclosure may contain information that would otherwise be confidential.

Other types of laws also impose duties to report. For example, in the interests of public health protection and promotion, all provinces and territories have public health acts that require health care providers to report patients with communicable diseases, such as hepatitis and tuberculosis, to public health authorities. Several Canadian provinces and territories also require that health care facilities report gunshot wounds to the local police authorities, and in many jurisdictions, this requirement to report also includes stab wounds (e.g., Ontario's *Mandatory Gunshot Wounds Reporting Act*, 2005 and Alberta's *Gunshot and Stab Wound Mandatory Disclosure Act*, 2009). Duties to report without the consent of the information provider or patient also include situations in which a patient is at risk of doing serious bodily harm to self or others, and disclosure may help mitigate this potential risk (e.g., see *Personal Health Information Protection Act*, 2004).

LABOUR AND EMPLOYMENT

Within any facility, employment and labour laws can be complex. Some employees will be covered under collective agreements and some will not. Employees in different occupational categories may be covered under different collective agreements. As a result, health care providers need to know the common laws respecting their employment situation, statutory laws that outline minimum standards of employment, and employment-specific collective agreements and related legislation. Specialists in human resources departments in large organizations can be particularly helpful to nurses, nurse leaders, and nurse managers in sorting through the array of employment and labour laws that are relevant to their workplace and their daily activities and decisions.

Basic employment law is found in common law and includes a duty for employees to follow legitimate employer commands related to their work. These commands may take the form of a manager's direct request and are also contained within institutional rules, policies, and procedures. Common law also provides for reasonable notice for termination of employment, unless it is for just cause. Failure to provide adequate notice is commonly the subject of wrongful dismissal lawsuits claiming money in lieu of such notice. Determining the nature of appropriate notice is not always straightforward and depends on a number of factors, including the nature of the work, seniority, and the ability to find similar work at similar compensation. Common laws are modified by employment standards legislation. Employment standards legislation provides details on minimum wage requirements, prohibition regarding the employment of minors, pay periods, when overtime is to be calculated, maternity and parental leave, minimum notice periods for termination, and vacation entitlements.

A substantial portion of the health care and nursing workforce is unionized. Specific labour relations legislation both permits and protects employee ability to create unions and negotiate collective agreements that displace employment standards legislative provisions. Collective agreements are a special type of employer–employee contract and cover a group of employees who are members of the union. Collective agreements outline the terms and conditions of employment along with "the rights, privileges and duties of the employer, the union and the employees" (Ontario Ministry of Labour, 2017). Collective advocacy, a key foundation of the development of collective agreements, is discussed more in Chapter 21. Collective agreements often contain guidance regarding procedural, grievance, and appeal procedures in dealing with employee concerns or employment conditions. Collective agreements cover a wide range of employment situations, including wages, benefit entitlement, job protection, graduated procedures for terminating an employee for cause, duties to accommodate employees with disability, employment leaves, and procedures in matters affecting employment status or disciplinary actions, including employee rights to union representation. It is important to remember that collective agreements refer to "the collective" rather than individuals and individual situations. Interests of individuals are considered within the context of the interests of the group as a whole in collective agreements and the processes, protections, and benefits outlined therein. Just as individual nurses must be informed about collective agreements that apply to their employment, nurse managers and leaders must also be knowledgeable and skilled in dealing with the provisions of collective agreements within their workplace.

Related to employment laws, and often augmented by collective agreements, health care institutions have duties to staff and patients around issues of safety and ability to practice. Duties extend to ensuring that staffing is sufficient to permit patient safety and safe clinical practice, that staff are provided with adequate orientation to the work environment, that policies and procedures are in place to provide a safe workplace, and that adequate equipment, tools, supplies, resources, and systems exist to maintain safety. Employers must also ensure to adequately train, instruct, and supervise employees, which includes instruction in and training on the proper use of equipment and devices so that employees remain safe (Morris & Clarke, 2011). We know that nurses consider safety of their working environments to be a key factor in decisions to remain or to leave a workplace (Abualrub et al., 2012, Liang et al., 2016). Health care facilities, for example, have some of the highest rates of violence toward nurses, and employers have a duty to reduce risk to employees. Occupational health and safety legislation gives employees the right to refuse to work where that

work, including the operation of equipment, machines, or devices, poses a danger to themselves or others. However, this right is not absolute. Health care workers do not have the right to refuse work where the perceived danger is within their usual or inherent scope of work. So, for example, nurses may not refuse to treat someone with a contagious disease, as this is within the normal and expected scope of nursing work. Additionally, health care workers cannot refuse to work where refusal would directly endanger the life, health, or safety of another person.

Other miscellaneous laws affect nurse leaders' and managers' interactions with employees and employment-related matters. Examples include reporting and record-keeping requirements under employment standards acts, the *Employment Insurance Act* (1996), and Canada's *Pension Act* (1985). Human rights legislation and the *Canadian Charter of Rights and Freedoms* (1982) outline many of the provisions that prohibit discrimination in the workplace based on national origin or ethnicity, race, religion, age, skin colour, gender, sexual orientation, or mental or physical disability. Additionally, there are provincial and territorial laws that outline obligations to protect workers in all work environments from situations that may involve sexual harassment, sexual violence, discrimination, or workplace violence. Some of these laws, such as Ontario's Bill 132 (*Sexual Violence and Harassment Action Plan Act [Supporting Survivors and Challenging Sexual Violence and Harassment]* 2016), describe processes that workplaces must follow, including investigations and reporting obligations, in cases of alleged sexual harassment or incidents of workplace violence.

Mental Health Laws

Mental health acts create special legal considerations in dealing with individuals undergoing treatment for mental health illness. For those living with mental illness or mental health challenges, the law may have a significant impact upon their lives. All provinces and territories have legislation that specifically addresses this subgroup of patients, such as the Mental Health Acts of Nova Scotia (2004) and Manitoba (1998). These acts contain special provisions for the protection of the dignity and rights of persons with mental health disorders. These statutes also provide for involuntary detention of patients and define when consent for medical treatment is and is not necessary. Nurses are often at the front line of ensuring that patients have been afforded the correct legal protections and rights under the mental health acts. Familiarity with the provisions of these acts and how to discharge one's legal and professional obligations to patients in care is not always as straightforward as one might believe. As an example, differences in statutory provisions exist between provinces and territories regarding whether involuntary patients can be forced to take antipsychotic medications believed to benefit their condition. Professional and ethical duties to advocate on behalf of the patient may at times seem to contradict the provision of mental health acts. It is fundamental to understand that even involuntary patients under mental health acts have all the rights and privileges of other patients and Canadians, except where specifically limited by legislation. This may mean, for example, that an involuntary patient cannot refuse to take antipsychotic medication but may have the right to refuse to take a prescribed multivitamin or validly withhold consent to surgery not considered emergency surgery. Interpretation of laws that restrict individual freedoms and rights will favour the least limiting approach.

DRUG LAWS

Access to and the use of drugs is heavily regulated by law and institutional procedures and includes the regulation of those who may prescribe and dispense medications to patients. Nurses must understand their legal capacities to handle, administer, and dispense various drugs and drug types, and legal requirements for accountability and documentation, as well as best practices. Criminal and civil liability may result if drug laws are contravened. In addition to drug laws and policies, there are also a significant number of published guidelines and policy guidance documents for nurses on topics ranging from legalization of marijuana, to harm reduction and opioid use in situations of chronic pain (Canadian Nurses Association, 2017; College of Nurses of Ontario, 2018b; College of Registered Nurses of Nova Scotia, 2017; Dowell et al., 2016).

CONSENT TO TREATMENT

Consent to treatment is grounded in ethical principles of respect for autonomy and in the legal right to be informed about any treatment, and to either accept or refuse an intervention or medical treatment or contact by another person (Nurses Association of New Brunswick,

2015; Peppin, 2011; Robertson, 2008). Patients have the right to provide or withhold consent to medical treatment, and this right is situated within the principle of treating people as ends in themselves and respecting their autonomous choices. To make autonomous choices, patients must have an opportunity to engage in providing informed consent. Health care providers must provide a process of informed consent for patients for almost everything we do "to patients" or involving patients. "The process of informed consent assures the legal protection of a patient's right to personal autonomy with regard to specific treatments and procedures. The concept of informed consent is one that has come to mean that patients are given the opportunity to autonomously choose a course of action in regard to plans for medical care" (Burkhardt et al., 2018). In many cases informed consent is obtained through a formal process. Failure to obtain informed consent before performing an act or intervention on a patient, or when an act exceeds the consent given, may result in what is termed a *battery* in tort law. Battery takes place when someone intentionally touches another without consent (Peppin, 2011). Two important points should be remembered: first, intent to touch is generally inferred by the physical act, regardless of the good intention of the person touching; and second, a person who has legal capacity to grant consent maintains the right to refuse treatment no matter how unreasonable it may seem to others.

Consent laws have been modified by statutory provisions that vary between provinces and territories. Nurses should be aware of the consent laws in the jurisdiction of their practice to avoid legal entanglements. Importantly, legislation dealing with matters of informed consent specifically address when someone has the legal capacity to grant consent; who may make substitute decisions when an individual is unable to make decisions on their own; and what legal process is available for obtaining consent. Comprehensive consent acts have been implemented in British Columbia, Ontario, Prince Edward Island, and Yukon (e.g., see Yukon's *Adult Protection and Decision-Making* Act, 2003). Issues of consent are also considered under statutes that deal with persons without legal capacity to make these decisions; for example, statutes that address adult guardianship, mental illness, substitute decision making, health care directives, powers of attorney, and care facility legislation. It is beyond the scope of this chapter to provide a complete listing of the statutes involved in considering consent or the details of these statutes. The basic information necessary for informed choice as part of valid consent is outlined in Box 7.1 and must be considered in the circumstances of individual patients and procedures. Mental incapacity, temporary or otherwise, is the most common reason why a patient may be legally incapable of providing informed consent. The known wishes of a patient and any consents given before a loss of this capacity are important starting points in determining whether a medical or nursing procedure has been authorized by a patient.

BOX 7.1 Elements of Informed Consent

- The condition for which the patient is being treated and the nature of the treatment or intervention along with expected outcomes.
- The expected or potential benefits of the treatment or intervention.
- The known, anticipated, or foreseeable risks of harm and any possible side effects or discomforts of treatment.
- Previous experiences with the treatment or intervention and incidences of side effects or potential harms.
- Alternative options for treatment and the existing standard of care, as well as possible outcomes if no treatment or intervention were to be provided.
- Who will be responsible for administering the treatment or intervention.
- Information should be provided at an appropriate and accessible level, always considering the patient's age and developmental stage as well as any contextual situations that may relate to cognition or the ability to engage in the consent process (examples might include delirium or untreated serious depression).
- Medical jargon and technical terms must be avoided in consent documents and discussions and if necessary that they are used, they must be defined and explained.
- Patients should be reminded that consent is dynamic and that if they agree to something, there are opportunities to change their mind or revisit their decisions.
- Patients should be given time to consider the information provided to them, including the potential risks and benefits, as well as an opportunity to ask questions and identify gaps in their knowledge and where they may require additional information or clarification to be fully informed.
- Ideally patients should also always have an opportunity to reflect upon the consent process or discuss the options with someone close to them—a friend or family member.

MALPRACTICE

Malpractice, in strict legal terms, encompasses a number of professional wrongdoings and liability (Irvine et al., 2013), but it is commonly understood as a type of medical or nursing negligence. Negligence that has caused suffering or injury may be legally actionable as a claim for damages (and reduced to a claim for money) as a result. Malpractice is a type of tort that has been established in common law and requires an injured person to prove, on balance of probabilities, the following:

- They were owed a duty of care.
- The duty of care was not met or was breached.
- There was reasonable foreseeability.
- Injury or damages were suffered because of the breach.
- The damages or injury would not have occurred but for the negligence (Dickens, 2011).

Reasonable foreseeability means that injuries and damages resulting from some action or failure to act are not simply accidents or errors in judgement (Dickens, 2011; Irvine et al., 2013). Table 7.2 outlines a practice case and the possible elements of malpractice.

Medical Assistance in Dying

As of June 2016, providing medical assistance in dying (MAID) is now legal in Canada. Before the passing of this legislation, assisting someone to end their life was deemed to be illegal according to the Criminal Code of Canada. After a number of challenges to this, one case, *Carter v. Canada (Attorney General)*, resulted in the Supreme Court of Canada declaring that the prohibition on assisted suicide for those competent adults with grievous and irremediable medical conditions was unconstitutional. Bill C-14, *An Act to amend the Criminal Code and to make related changes to other Acts (medical assistance in dying)* passed Royal Assent in 2016 and provides an exemption from criminal charges for those medical and nursing practitioners, as well as pharmacists, who may be involved in

TABLE 7.2	**Elements of Malpractice**
Elements	**Example**
Duty owed the patient	Mr. Singh is a 67-year-old patient who has just had a cardiac catheterization. He has returned to the stepdown unit in stable condition, and his postoperative orders include monitoring of vital signs every 15 minutes for 2 hours then every 30 minutes. The orders also require that the left femoral access site be checked at the same time, along with assessment of distal pulses and any chest pain or shortness of breath.
Breach of the duty owed	At the end of hour 2 of their recovery, Mr. Singh awakens from a drowsy state, feeling clammy and cold. He feels wetness under the left leg and pain down into the left thigh. He isn't sure when the nurse last checked him and reaches for the call bell. The nurse arrives quickly, telling Mr. Singh they let him sleep for half an hour and didn't want to bother him. When the nurse lifts the sheets to examine Mr. Singh, there is a significant amount of blood on the sheets and patient's leg and groin through the bandages. Mr. Singh is also hypotensive and tachycardic.
Foreseeability	One of the most common complications post cardiac catheterization with access at the groin are bleeding and formation of a hematoma. Frequent monitoring of vital signs and the access site is a confirmed method of preventing these complications and catching them early if they do occur.
Causation	Failure to provide adequate and timely monitoring of the femoral access site and vital signs resulted in significant bleeding and formation of a hematoma at the site.
Injury or damages	Mr. Singh has a significant bleed from the femoral access site through the bandage and into his leg. While he dozed, the sandbag providing pressure slipped off his leg and Mr. Singh's access site began to bleed heavily. He has a very large painful hematoma with now additional restrictions on his recovery, including additional bedrest and the need for a transfusion.

providing assistance in dying, as well as clarity on eligibility for MAID. All publicly funded institutions are required to provide access to medical assistance in dying for those who are eligible. As this is a federal Act, each province and territory has outlined specific processes and obligations for those seeking assistance in dying and those health care professionals who may be involved in providing assistance and counsel. Across Canada, provincial regulatory bodies and colleges have published guidelines and policies to help inform scope of practice for those professionals who may be involved in providing MAID and provide more information on the legal and professional contexts. Currently, MAID is available to those 18 years of age or older, who are eligible to receive health services in Canada, who are capable of making decisions related to their health and who have a "grievous and irremediable medical condition" (*Bill C-14*, 2016). This latter criterion is described in more detail—as having a serious and incurable disease or illness that results in being in a state of irreversible decline in capability and functioning. This decline in capability should be demonstrated to cause what can be categorized as intolerable suffering that cannot be relieved or remediated with acceptable treatments or under reasonably acceptable conditions. Finally, there must be

evidence that death is reasonably foreseeable. With these conditions met, a person can make a voluntary request for MAID and provide voluntary consent for such, after being provided with full and complete information about all options available to them, including treatments and palliative care. Currently, MAID is not available to those under age 18, to those with mental health diagnoses or addictions, or as part of an advance directive. MAID is legal and possible via two methods in most provinces and territories: as administered by a health care provider (a physician or a nurse practitioner) and by self-administered ingestion. Both methods require assistance and guidance from a regulated health care professional, and there are safeguards (e.g., waiting periods, opportunity to withdraw consent at any time, strict reporting requirements) built into both processes to ensure that patient choice and dignity are respected and that informed consent and voluntariness are attended to at each step in the process. Reports on MAID in Canada show that, in most provinces and territories, health care providers who are involved in providing medical assistance in dying strongly prefer health care professional–provided assistance rather than self-administration, citing concerns about complications, accurate administration, and procedures

(Health Canada, 2017). Although the law does not require or compel health care providers to take part in any aspect of medically assisted death, it is imperative that health care providers have a comprehensive and clear understanding of the legal and professional aspects of MAID. For nurse practitioners, this requires being consistently up to date on all scope of practice and legal aspects of medical assistance in dying. To date, Canada is the only jurisdiction in which nurse practitioners are permitted to directly take part in providing MAID (Health Canada, 2017). For nurses working across a variety of contexts, this means understanding MAID from both a patient-centred and a professional nursing perspective. Nurses should also have a good understanding not only of the legal aspects of MAID but also of the ethical dimensions of providing assistance at the end of life, and their own values and principles that guide practice and ethical, compassionate care in any situation. Nurses who may have an objection to MAID must still be able to provide holistic and comprehensive nursing care, and in a situation in which a nurse feels that standard of care cannot be provided, another caregiver must be put in place without abandoning the patient. Of course, this applies in all types of ethically charged situations, not only MAID.

LITERATURE PERSPECTIVE

Resource: Thiele, T & Dunsford, J. (2017). Nurse leaders' role in medical assistance in dying: A relational ethics approach. *Nursing Ethics*. 26(4), 993–999. http://dx.doi.org/10.1177/0969733017730684.

Although much of the focus in discussions of MAID is on the legal aspects, concerns, and processes, the implementation of MAID has implications and considerations beyond those only in the legal realm. Many nurses who are involved in direct care of patients who are requesting MAID may find themselves not only faced with learning about a new and ethically complex patient care situation but, for many, questioning their own beliefs and values as well as their professional obligations. In this article, the authors explore the role of nurse leaders in ensuring that nurses are supported in engaging in any and all aspects of MAID, and that they can ensure nurses feel that they have the knowledge of processes and practices, and have also been provided with an opportunity to reflect upon the salient ethical concerns and professional obligations when providing care for patients who are requesting MAID. Noting that, currently, many nurses are balancing the challenge of fulfilling their duty to provide care with ethical concerns and reservations about being involved in medical assistance in dying, the authors identify the important role of nurse leaders in supporting nurses in this and other difficult challenges in ethically charged situations. The authors are clear that, by nurse leaders, they are identifying those in both formal and informal leadership positions, and that the obligation to create a "morally supportive environment" (p. 2) is an obligation for any nurse with a position of influence in an organization. Fulfilling this obligation is most important when direct care nurses find themselves struggling with difficult patient care situations, and MAID is a key example of a patient care situation that many nurses may find challenges

their own beliefs and values. Given that MAID is still a new concept and practice for many nurses and settings, and the processes and policies are still in the beginning stages of implementation in many organizations, this is a time for change and adjustments and, for some nurses, also a time of professional uncertainty.

Implications for Practice

The authors discuss the use of a relational ethics approach to nursing leadership to fulfill the obligation of creating an open and supportive environment. The focus of a relational ethics approach is on building and maintaining relationships and on developing an awareness of how difficult ethical decisions are navigated within the context of relationships, rather than considering decisions or actions simply in isolation. When thinking about MAID being provided in a health care context, we must consider the relationships between the nurse providing direct care, the patient, family and support networks, other members of the health care team, and nurse leaders. Within the boundaries of these relationships, MAID can have a profound effect on the individuals involved, including the nurse. The role of nurse leaders, in this case, is to ensure support for individual nurses in exploring their own values and beliefs, and ensuring that there is both awareness and consideration of the "individual contexts and circumstances that influence the ability to provide effective nursing care in ways that protect nurses' moral agency" (p. 3). This kind of supportive leadership can help engage individual nurses and protect their well-being as well as ensure that they can enact their moral agency in a complex work environment that is ever-changing. A relational ethics framework for understanding MAID and the resultant implications for the practice of individual nurses helps provide support for nurses involved in direct patient care and guidance for nurse leaders.

RISK MANAGEMENT

Portions of risk management fall under the practice of most nurse managers. Risk management is the systematic identification, assessment, and prioritization of risks and the development and implementation of strategies to reduce adverse events and liability associated with these risks. Chapter 22 provides additional information on risk management. Risk management not only reduces losses but also enhances quality outcomes in health care delivery.

Institutional Liability and Insurance

Policy and procedures help improve the safety of staff and patient care and also help limit institutional liability and personal liability in managers. Contributing to the development and implementation of well-developed policy and procedures is an important management function.

Managers have a duty to their employer to manage exposure to liability risks where assessment of this risk is possible and insurance coverage may be adversely affected without proper management actions. Where the potential for liability exists, it is incumbent on managers to notify the institution's insurance company. Larger health care institutions often have a risk manager, a legal officer, or an institutional lawyer to whom a manager can turn for advice and guidance about potential legal risks. However, the task of recognizing and appropriately documenting the events that lead, or potentially lead, to a liability risk often rests with managers.

Workers' compensation programs exist in all provinces and territories and are a form of employment-based, mandatory insurance that managers must know about. These programs offer compensation and rehabilitation support to employees injured at the workplace. Failure to comply with policies, procedures, and workplace orders originating from workers' compensation boards can result in various forms of liability.

Occupational health and safety legislation and associated regulations address general workplace safety issues as well as the use of hazardous materials, radiation, and chemicals. Additionally, this legislation addresses issues such as workplace violence and harassment and imposes obligations on employers for the development of policies, procedures, safety programs, reporting, and documentation (see, e.g., Part III of Ontario's *Occupational Health and Safe Act*, 1990).

> **EXERCISE 7.5** Laws, policies, and regulations exist in every type of institution and social context, guiding behaviours, actions, and processes. There are many policies that affect your life as a student nurse, as a new graduate nurse, or even as an experienced nurse leader. Review a policy that affects you today. Is the policy current, and does it note that it has been regularly reviewed and revised? Does it reflect other overarching laws or guidelines? Think about how you would revise it, or how you might ensure it reflects current practice and context. Where would you look to find out if the policy is relevant and responsive? Consider ways in which you would aim to engage other stakeholders who are affected by such a policy to provide feedback, revise, and ensure relevance to practice.

CONCLUSION

Although laws are often rooted in ethical and moral principles, laws and ethics differ and may offer different, complementary, or contradictory solutions to individual situations. As a result, there is value in considering legal and ethical concerns and situations separately in health care decision making but remaining attentive to where there is overlap. In the last two chapters, legal and ethical concerns in nursing have been highlighted. It is important to keep in mind that legal and ethical issues do not only arise in acute care settings or situations of *life and death*. There are ethical and legal implications in much that nurses and nurse leaders do as part of their professional roles in complex health care environments. Nurses at all stages of their careers must be attuned to both ethically charged and legally relevant situations across all types of practice settings and know where to seek sound advice and additional resources.

? A SOLUTION

The concerns raised in "A Challenge" are not unusual. For nurses in rural or community settings, notions of privacy and confidentiality are often not as straightforward as they may be, for example, in a large acute care centre where you might encounter a patient during one visit or hospital stay and then never again. Nurses who live and work in smaller communities and rural settings often find that they have patient care interactions in both the formal workplace and in the broader community as they move through the typical activities of their day. In their communities, they describe feeling more visible, and this visibility can create obligations and expectations, especially in regard to being approachable and accessible at all times (Kulig et al., 2009; Zibrik et al., 2010; Burkhardt et al., 2018). Nurses working in rural settings often describe being approached to talk about, or disclose, patient care information outside of the workplace and often in public and social settings. In turn, nurses in these situations must balance their clear professional and legal duty of maintaining patient confidentiality with a desire not to be seen as rude or standoffish. For many nurses, achieving this balance can be challenging. In Charlotte's case, she clearly has a duty to Maggie to protect her privacy. Although Ted, Maggie's father, appears to be well-intentioned, Charlotte cannot simply disclose information about Maggie to appease him. Ted tries to compel Charlotte by telling her that this is a matter of trust, meaning that Charlotte should trust that he has Maggie's best interests in mind as Charlotte also does. Although that may be true, Charlotte cannot breach the trust that Maggie has placed in her, as a health care provider, based on an assumption. Legally, Maggie is an adult and has not provided clear consent for her information to be shared with anyone, even her father. To meet her obligation to her patient, and as a way to maintain a positive and professional image in the moment, Charlotte can empathize with Ted's voiced concern for his daughter. She can also remind Ted of her professional and legal obligations to maintain confidentiality and encourage Ted to have a caring conversation with Maggie directly.

If you were in a similar situation, how might you approach the situation, as you try to balance your legal and professional obligations with a desire to sustain a positive and professional public image?

▌ THE EVIDENCE

Being a professional nurse in a rural setting can extend "beyond the physical boundaries of the workplace" (Zibrik et al., 2010. p. 24). Given that, defining what professionalism looks like in such a setting can be challenging, and experiences of nurses in rural settings are often described in terms of not only the formal work setting but also the broader community. In the work of Zibrik and colleagues examining the experiences and ideas about professional practice of nurses working in rural settings in Alberta and British Columbia, rural nurses often spoke about their role and experiences not in the workplace per se but in the community and in interactions outside of the workplace. Maintaining confidentiality was one challenge rural nurses often discussed, and the nurses in this study identified that their professional obligations regarding confidentiality is even more important in close-knit and smaller communities where family connections, social ties, or friendships often overlap with professional roles. Although Kulig et al. (2009) note that communities play an important role in how many rural nurses' sense of professionalism is developed and sustained, there are aspects of that unique relationship that can be both rewarding and challenging. The entrenchment of rural nurses in their communities can have positive effects that help promote and reinforce professionalism (Zibrik et al., 2010). That same entrenchment does mean, though, that confidentiality is often a concern outside the workplace—and that this can result in a feeling of being "constantly engaged" (p. 31) as a professional nurse, even when outside of work and in personal or social interactions. Although most standards of practice and professional guidelines regarding legal and ethical expectations maintaining confidentiality pertain to the nurse in the workplace, for nurses in rural settings, these professional obligations extend well beyond into all aspects of their lives in smaller communities.

✳ NEED TO KNOW NOW

- Understand the legal ramifications of all nursing roles, in terms of federal, provincial, and territorial laws. Query legal staff and privacy officers at your employer, administration, and the nursing regulatory agencies and associations as needed.
- Understand where liability for your own actions may occur; particularly, understand your personal obligations toward protecting patient privacy and confidentiality, your duty to practise in accordance with nursing standards, acting within your scope of practice and personal practice competencies.
- Consult with your regulatory or professional association if you have questions about insurance issues that protect you against personal liability for errors and omissions occurring in the course of your professional practice. Know what activities may not be covered by your insurance policy, such as independent practice and volunteer board work.
- Consult your nursing union for assistance in navigating legal issues and legal questions you may have related to your employment. Many nursing workplace environments are unionized, and benefits include access to lawyers familiar with nursing and health law.
- Your regulatory body or nursing association may offer assistance with assessing and avoiding legal issues with your professional practice.
- Understand the laws in your province or territory that address informed consent and substitute decision making to help inform and keep your practice person-centred and respectful of the best interests and wishes of your patients.
- Ensure that your documentation is accurate, precise, and timely, as warranted by patient condition. Focus on objective facts and be accountable for your entries.
- Expect that laws affecting your practice will evolve and change and ensure that you keep current with any changes that may affect your practice.
- Keep in mind that there may be overlap between legal and ethical responsibilities and ensure you can differentiate between them in critical situations.

▌ CHAPTER CHECKLIST

This chapter explores multiple legal issues as they pertain to nursing and nursing leadership.

Legal areas that all nurses must understand include the following:
- The sources of law (federal, provincial, territorial, and common law).
- The regulatory and licensing frameworks that are relevant to health care.
- Sources of legal liability and practice implications:
  - Criminal liability
  - Civil liability, including malpractice, duty of care, and practice standards
  - Professional sanctions
  - Employment ramifications.
- Privacy, confidentiality, and access to information laws that vary across provinces and territories and are generally outlined in statute law.
- Laws that govern duty to report and protective laws that are aimed at protecting individuals viewed as vulnerable.
- Leadership in nursing includes having knowledge of what laws and legal constructs can have an effect upon your practice and keeping informed of changes

to these relevant laws. Some important areas that are evolving include:
- Medical assistance in dying
- Duty to report
- Documentation and the importance of protecting privacy and confidentiality
- The impact of electronic record keeping and related law

Nurses in management roles must have enhanced understanding of the following:
- Labour and employment laws.
- Duty of care owed by employers to others.
- Patient rights and patient decision making.

Although management may require enhanced knowledge, all nurses and nurse managers have a part to play in risk management and mitigation, including roles in addressing the following:
- Health records maintenance by those not governed by professional standards.
- Multiplicity of health care providers and access to health records.
- Patient safety and quality of care.
- Interprofessional teams and medical assistance in dying.

TIPS FOR INCORPORATING LEARNING ABOUT LEGAL CONCERNS INTO NURSING PRACTICE SETTINGS

- Locate and review the relevant scope of practice documents and nursing standards of practice within your jurisdiction.
- Apply legal principles (such as protecting privacy and ensuring informed consent) in all health care settings and situations.
- Legal concerns can be complex and often do not involve simple solutions. Know when you are faced with a situation that has legal implications

and seek additional expert opinion before acting.
- Continue to look for ways to influence policy and procedures in your work area that support evidence-based practice, promote patient best interests and safety, and that contribute to ongoing quality improvement.
- Locate and read your local policies on patient information, protection, and disclosure.

Visit the Evolve website for Suggested Readings, Internet Resources, and additional resources related to the content in this chapter: http://evolve.elsevier.com/Canada/Yoder-Wise/leading/.

REFERENCES

Statutes

Adult Protection and Decision-Making Act, SY. (c. 21)., (2003). Sch. A (Yukon).

An Act to amend the Criminal Code and to make related changes to other Acts (medical assistance in dying,) 2016

Apology Act, SM 2007, c. 25, CCSM c. A98 (Manitoba).

Canada Health Act, RSC 1985, c. C-6 (Canada).

Canadian Charter of Rights and Freedoms, Part I of the Constitution Act, 1982, being Schedule B to the Canada Act 1982, (UK), 1982, c. 11.

Child Youth and Family Services Act,2017, SO 2017, c. 14, Schedule 1 (Ontario).

Constitution Act, 1867 (U.K.), 30 & 31 Vict, c. 3.

Continuing Care Act, RSBC 1996, c. 70 (British Columbia).

Criminal Code, RSC 1985, c. C-46 (Canada).

Employment Insurance Act, SC 1996, c. 23 (Canada).

Freedom of Information and Protection of Privacy Act, RSO 1990, c. F-31 (Ontario).

Gunshot and Stab Wound Mandatory Disclosure Act, SA 2009, c. G-12 (Alberta).

Health Professions Act, RSBC 1996, c. 183 (British Columbia).

Mandatory Gunshot Wounds Reporting Act, 2005, SO 2005, c. 9 (Ontario).

Pension Act, RSC 1985, c. P-6 (Canada).

Personal Health Information Protection Act, 2004, SO 2004, c. 3, Sch. A (Ontario).

Protection for Persons in Care Act, SA 2009, c. P-29.1 (Alberta).

USA Patriot Act of 2001, 115 USC Stat. 272 (2001).

Case Law

Carter v. Canada (Attorney General) 2015 SCC 5 [2015] 1 SCR 331.

R. v. Duarte, [1990] 1 SCR 30.

Texts

Abualrub, R. F., Gharaibeh, H. F., & Bashayreh, A. E. (2012). The relationships between safety climate, teamwork and intent to stay at work among Jordanian hospital nurses. *Nursing Forum, 47*(1), 65–75.

Barkan, S. (2016). *Law and society: An introduction.* New York: Routledge.

Burkhardt, M., Walton, N., & Nathaniel, A. (2018). Rural, remote and Indigenous nursing in Canada. In *Ethics and Issues in Contemporary Nursing* (3rd ed., pp. 462–484) Toronto: Nelson.

Canadian Nurses Association. (2015). *Framework for the practice of registered nurses in Canada* (2nd ed.). Ottawa, ON: Author. https://www.cna-aiic.ca/~/media/cna/page-content/pdf-en/framework-for-the-pracice-of-registered-nurses-in-canada.pdf.

Canadian Nurses Association. (2017). *Harm reduction and illicit substance use. Implications for nursing.* Ottawa, ON: Author. https://www.cna-aiic.ca/-/media/cna/page-content/pdf-en/harm-reduction-and-illicit-substance-use-implications-for-nursing.pdf?la=en&hash=5F5BBCDE16C7892D9C7838CF62C362685CC2DDA7.

Canadian Nurses Protective Society. (2009). Privacy and electronic medical records. *InfoLaws* (1), 18. https://www.cnps.ca/upload-files/pdf_english/privacy_emr.pdf.

College of Nurses of Ontario. (2018a). *Professional conduct, Professional Misconduct.* Toronto, ON: Author. https://www.cno.org/globalassets/docs/ih/42007_misconduct.pdf.

College of Nurses of Ontario. (2018b). *Controlled substances – resources and references*. Toronto, ON: Author. http://www.cno.org/en/trending-topics/nps-and-prescribing-controlled-substances/controlled-substances---resources-and-references/.

College of Registered Nurses of Nova Scotia. (2017). *Medication guidelines for registered nurses*. Halifax, NS: Author. https://crnns.ca/wp-content/uploads/2015/05/Medication-Guidelines.pdf.

College of Registered Nurses of British Columbia. (2018). *Practice Standards*. Vancouver, BC: Author. https://www.crnbc.ca/Standards/PracticeStandards/Pages/Default.aspx.

Dickens, B. (2011). Medical negligence. In J. G. Downie, T. A. Caulfield, & C. M. Flood (Eds.), *Canadian health law and policy* (4th ed., pp. 115–151). Markham, ON: LexisNexis Canada.

Downie, J. G., Caulfield, T. A., & Flood, C. M. (Eds.). (2011). *Canadian health law and policy* (4th ed). Markham, ON: LexisNexis Canada.

Dowell, D., Haegerich, T. M., & Chou, R. (2016). Centre for Disease Control Guideline for prescribing opioids in chronic pain—United States, 2016. *Recommendations and Reports*, 65(1), 1–49. https://www.cdc.gov/mmwr/volumes/65/rr/rr6501e1.htm.

Gibson, E. (2017). Health information: Privacy, confidentiality and access. In J. Erdman, V. Gruben, & E. Nelson (Eds.), *Canadian health law and policy* (5th ed.). (pp. 207–227). Markham, ON: LexisNexis Canada.

Health Canada. (2017). 2nd *Interim Report on Medical Assistance in Dying*. Ottawa, ON: Author. https://www.canada.ca/en/health-canada/services/publications/health-system-services/medical-assistance-dying-interim-report-sep-2017.html.

Irvine, J. C., Osborne, P. H., & Shariff, M. (2013). *Canadian medical law: An introduction for physicians, nurses, and other health care professionals* (4th ed.). Scarborough, ON: Thomson Carswell.

Kosseim, P., & Brady, M. (2008). Policy by procrastination: Secondary use of electronic health records for health research purposes. *McGill Journal of Law & Health*, 2(1), 5–46.

Kulig, J. C., Stewart, N., Penz, K., Forbes, D., Morgan, D., & Emerson, P. (2009). Work setting, community attachment, and satisfaction among rural and remote nurses. *Public Health Nursing*, 26(5), 430–439.

Liang, H., Tang, F., Wang, T., Lin, K., & Yu, Sh. (2016). Nurse characteristics, leadership, safety climate, emotional labour and intention to stay for nurses: A structural equation modelling approach. *Journal of Advanced Nursing*, 72(12), 3067–3080.

Morris, J. J., & Clarke, C. D. (2011). *Law for Canadian health care administrators* (2nd ed.). Markham, ON: Butterworths.

Nurses Association of New Brunswick. (2015). *Guidelines for consent*. Fredericton, NB: Author. http://www.nanb.nb.ca/media/resource/NANB-GuidelinesForConsent-E.pdf.

Ontario Ministry of Labour. (2017). *Collective bargaining: Agreements and Negotiations: FAQ*. Ontario: Author. https://www.labour.gov.on.ca/english/lr/faqs/lr_faq1.php#what2.

Ozair, F. F., Jamshed, N., Sharma, A., & Aggarwal, P. (2015). Ethical issues in electronic health records: A general overview. *Perspectives in Clinical Research*, 6(2), 73–76.

Peppin, P. (2011). Informed consent. In J. G. Downie, T. A. Caulfield, & C. M. Flood (Eds.), *Canadian health law and policy* (4th ed., pp. 153–194). Markham, ON: LexisNexis Canada.

Robertson, G. B. (2008). A view of the future: Emerging developments in health care liability. *Health Law Journal (Special edition)*, 1–12.

Zarzeczny, A. (2017). The role of regulation in health care - professional and institutional oversight. In J. Erdma, V. Gruben, & E. Nelson (Eds.), *Canadian health law and policy* (5th ed., pp. 161–182). Markham, ON: LexisNexis Canada.

Zibrik, K. J., MacLeod, M. L. P., & Zimmer, L. V. (2010). Professionalism in rural acute-care nursing. *Canadian Journal of Nursing Research*, 42(1), 20–36.

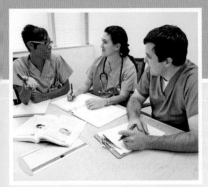

8

Making Decisions and Solving Problems

Janet L. McCabe

This chapter presents an overview of problem solving and decision making. It examines the intellectual processes involved in problem solving and decision making, including rational thinking, critical thinking, creative thinking, and intuition, as well as individual and group decision biases. Approaches to problem solving, decision making, group decision making strategies, and decision-making support tools are identified.

OBJECTIVES

- Distinguish between the terms *problem* and *decision* and understand the relationship between problem solving and decision making.
- Identify the intellectual processes involved in problem solving and decision making within the health care context.
- Describe how the scientific method, critical thinking, nursing process, creative thinking, and intuitive thinking relate to decision making.
- Explain the effect of decision biases, fallacies, and personal attributes on the quality of decisions.

- Understand how problem-solving skills apply to nursing practice.
- Compare three models of decision making: the rational decision-making model, the bounded rationality model, and the Clinical Judgement Model.
- Describe the group decision-making process and understand its importance for interdisciplinary health care teams.

TERMS TO KNOW

availability bias
confirmation bias
creative decision making
critical thinking
decision bias
decision making
fallacies

group invulnerability
group polarization
groupthink
heuristics
hindsight bias
intuition
nominal group technique

optimizing decision
problem solving
prudence trap
satisficing decision making
six thinking hats
SWOT analysis
team dynamics

❓ A CHALLENGE

Shyanne, a recently hired nurse at a youth walk-in clinic, was thrilled about starting her first full-time job. As team leader of the Youth Engagement program, she would be working with a staff of three experienced mental health workers to develop and deliver workshops on health and wellness, social interaction, and leadership skills to local youth. Shyanne had previous experience working at the clinic during the summer for the past two years and was comfortable with her co-workers and supervisor. She was eager to start planning youth development workshops that would help her young patients develop the tools they need to address problems they were experiencing, become more confident, and learn basic life skills. Her co-workers were supportive and very interested in Shyanne's new ideas for youth skill development. The only problem was that Shyanne did not feel she was supported by her supervisor, Rhea, to implement the new program. Although Rhea was responsive to Shyanne's ideas and seemed to accept them, she did not share her enthusiasm about advancing the plan. Rhea's response to Shyanne's request to move forward was "let's wait and see." Shyanne was discouraged at first, and the more Rhea stalled, the more frustrated Shyanne became.

What is the problem that Shyanne is facing? What advice would you give to Shyanne to help solve this problem?

INTRODUCTION

Problem solving and decision making are essential skills for nurse managers, nurse leaders, and staff nurses. According to Mintzberg (1973), managers have three key roles: interpersonal contact, information processing, and decision making. Problem-solving skills are universal and can be applied in any situation. Numerous technological, social, political, and economic changes have dramatically increased the need for problem solving in health care, and specifically within the context of nursing. Consider these recent and continuously evolving changes in the health care landscape: increased patient acuity, shorter hospital stays, a shortage of health care providers, interprofessional and patient-centred care, an increase in the use of technology by providers and patients, greater emphasis on quality and patient safety, diverse patient populations, and the continuing shift from inpatient to community. These examples are only a few of the changes that require nurses to be able

to problem solve effectively and make sound decisions. The complexities and problems that result from rapid changes strain the abilities of nurses to process large quantities of information, understand the interrelationships among elements in the organization, and keep pace with new developments. Keeping pace requires a good knowledge of traditional and contemporary approaches to problem solving and decision making.

PROBLEM SOLVING AND DECISION MAKING

The Difference Between a Problem and a Decision

Effective problem-solving and decision-making skills are essential for dealing with ambiguity and uncertainty in work environments. Although problem-solving and decision-making skills are accepted core functions of nursing, many nurses are often too busy to apply these skills in a purposeful way. However, by using problem-solving and decision-making skills on a regular basis, nurses will be able to perceive difficult clinical issues as intellectual challenges that develop their critical-thinking skills and good judgement. Sound knowledge of the core concepts and skills related to problem solving and decision making begins with a good understanding of the associated terminology, processes, and models.

A *problem* is a recognized difference between current and desired conditions or a gap between "what is" and "what should be" with an accompanying perception that something should be done to resolve it. Some problems demand immediate attention, for example, a patient with chest pain and blood pressure of 180/100. Other problems can be resolved over time: for example, improving ineffective communication processes between departments. A *decision* is a choice between alternative courses of action or interventions that are selected for implementation to solve a *problem*.

The Relationship Between Problem Solving and Decision Making

Although often thought of as the same process, decision theorists distinguish between problem solving and decision making. Problem solving is a comprehensive, sequential, cognitive process used to solve a problem by reducing the difference between current and desired conditions. A review of the literature on problem solving and decision making shows a difference of opinion about these concepts, which may partly explain the variety of models that exist. Some see the problem-solving process as an integrated process, with decision making dispersed throughout (Huitt, 1992). Others argue that the two concepts are interchangeable. Certain scholars question the value of defining a structured problem-solving or decision-making process because structured and purposeful processes do not appear to reflect what people actually do when they solve problems or make decisions (Tanner, 2006). Others see problem solving as a comprehensive, overarching process with decision making as "a process within a process," taking place at a distinct point or step in the problem-solving process and as a recurring activity (Kepner & Tregoe, 1965), which is the perspective presented in this chapter. Figure 7.1 helps illustrate where decision making occurs within the problem-solving process. Regardless of the theoretical perspective, the two elements essential to solving any problem are problem analysis and decision making. Problem analysis includes identifying, clarifying, and verifying a problem, while decision making focuses on developing cognitive strategies to solve a problem.

Decision making is "a process that chooses a preferred option or a course of actions from among a set of alternatives on the basis of given criteria or strategies" (Wang & Ruhe, 2007, p. 73). Decision making in risky situations involves estimating the probability of success of alternatives, given the complexity, level of risk, and the certainty of outcome of each alternative (Riabacke, 2006). Decision making is most often associated with the rational decision-making model (Lunenburg, 2010), which will be discussed later in the chapter. According to *Principles of Management* (2015), there are different levels of decisions that occur within all organizations (including health care) these being the following:

- Strategic decisions.
- Tactical decisions.
- Operational decisions.

Strategic decisions are focused on the organization as a whole, such as determining the vision and mission of a health care institution, and the scope of care provided. Tactical decisions are intended to determine how things will be accomplished. They are typically made by managers; in the case of the vision/mission example, managers may need to determine how to implement a new focus. Finally, operational decisions are those made by every employee on a daily basis. Decision-making skills

are also applicable to nursing practice. From a patient care perspective, patients and health care team members are increasingly engaging in shared decision making. In addition, nursing managers and leaders use decision making to guide decisions on staffing mixes. For example, the College of Nurses of Ontario (2011) has developed a framework designed to help nurses make effective decisions regarding which category of nurse (registered nurse or registered practical nurse) matches patient needs.

INTELLECTUAL PROCESSING IN PROBLEM SOLVING AND DECISION MAKING

Intellectual processes are mental operations that enable one to acquire new knowledge, apply that knowledge in both familiar and unique situations, and control the mental processing that is required for knowledge acquisition and use. These processes are reflected in the problem-solving and decision-making models presented below. The use of different decision-making models will be driven by the nature of the decision to be made, the context that the decision is being made within, and the experiences of those involved. Many of the models discussed below represent a sequential critical-thinking process that outlines the mental operations (e.g., conceptualizing and synthesizing) used to generate new knowledge or solve problems. Within the following section four general models of decision making are discussed: the scientific method, the nursing process, the problem-solving process, and the decision-making process. This is followed by more explicit situational decision-making models: ethical decision making, creative decision making, and shared decision making. Lastly, the roles of critical thinking and intuition in decision-making models are discussed.

Scientific Method

The scientific method is a rational and logical approach to problem solving that is widely used and has proven to be effective over time. It is the foundation of many models of decision making, and is especially useful when testing hypotheses. It is a familiar process that reflects the cognitive behaviours that occur in a predictable order when conducting experiments or solving problems. The six steps in the scientific method are as follows:

1. Identify and clarify a problem.
2. Determine the problem's significance and relevance.

3. Gather data about the problem and its causes.
4. Generate hypotheses and choose alternatives to solve the problem.
5. Test selected alternatives.
6. Plan, implement, and evaluate the effects of the selected alternatives.

The scientific method is often used within the context of research.

Nursing Process

The five-step, systematic nursing process is based on the scientific method; however, it is tailored to the field of nursing. The steps in the process are:
1. Assessment.
2. Diagnosis.
3. Planning.
4. Implementation.
5. Evaluation.

The steps are sequential, interactive, and cyclic. The nursing process is goal-directed and guides nurses in problem solving for health conditions. Problem identification typically occurs in the assessment and evaluation steps, whereas decision making is particularly evident in the diagnosis and planning steps.

Problem-Solving Process

The problem-solving process is based on the scientific method. Various models are described in the literature, but most include essential cognitive components. The traditional seven-step problem-solving process is cyclic: steps in the process are repeated to solve a problem (Fig. 8.1). Feedback from failed attempts to solve a problem reactivates the problem-solving process, using different alternatives.

Decision-Making Process

The decision-making process is an integral component of the problem-solving process and is mainly associated with making choices among alternatives for action. Two commonly used models of decision making are the rational decision-making model and the bounded rationality model. These models will be compared later in this chapter. The rational decision-making model consists of five steps that are similar to the problem-solving process:
1. Define a problem or opportunity.
2. Set goals (outcomes) and identify evaluation criteria.
3. Identify alternatives for each outcome.

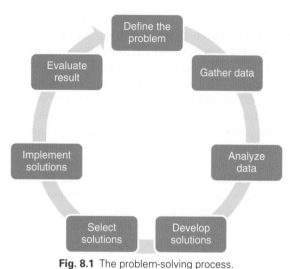

Fig. 8.1 The problem-solving process.

4. Evaluate alternatives for each outcome.
5. Choose the preferred alternative.

Ethical Decision Making

The steps in ethical decision making are similar to those in the rational decision-making model. However, ethical principles and arguments are applied throughout the intellectual-reasoning process to help determine ethically sound alternatives or options for action. These principles are highly relevant for trying to address today's complex health care problems. Ethics and ethical decision making are discussed in Chapter 6. Ethical decision making is used when there is no clear right or wrong answer within a situation.

Creative Decision Making

Creative decision making is the generation of new and imaginative ideas to solve problems (*Principles of Management*, 2015). Creative decision making is a combination of divergent thinking and rational decision making. The decision-making process involves the use of brainstorming and other techniques, such as "mind tools," to generate innovative and novel ideas. Creative decision making may be utilized when a team is attempting to explore or generate alternatives to the current norm. For example, a nurse manager may be attempting to explore options for addressing shift scheduling on the ward or communication strategies to inform nurses of policy changes. There is also evidence that suggests creative decision making can be used during times of crisis, especially within a team that has a high level of trust (Sommer & Pearson, 2007).

Shared Decision Making

Within health care, another approach to decision making that is increasingly gaining traction is *shared decision making*. Shared decision making has been described as an approach that lies between the health care provider (or team of providers) making a decision independently (often viewed as paternalistic decision making) and an informed approach in which the patient alone, provided with information, makes a decision (Friesen-Storms et al., 2015). Shared decision making may be used in supporting patients to make decisions about a variety of treatment options available to them while also considering their personal values.

Critical Thinking

Effective problem solving and decision making are based on an individual's ability to think critically. Although critical thinking has been defined in numerous ways, Scriven and Paul (2007) describe it as "the intellectually disciplined process of actively and skillfully conceptualizing, applying, analyzing, synthesizing, and/or evaluating information gathered from, or generated by, observation, experience, reflection, reasoning, or communication, as a guide to belief and action" (para. 1). Glaser (1941) asserted that critical thinking is based on critical inquiry (logic and argumentation). Using this perspective, critical thinking is associated with a thoughtful and orderly approach to considering problems, knowledge of methods of logical inquiry and reasoning skills, and the ability to apply them. In practice, critical thinking involves recognizing problems and finding ways to solve them by gathering pertinent information, appraising evidence, and evaluating arguments. It requires an examination and testing of beliefs, assumptions, and relationships among propositions in light of evidence to reach valid conclusions. Glaser's view of critical thinking is particularly valuable for ethical decisions and other complex problems and exposes the various personal elements of decision making.

Intuition and Decision Making

Intuition is "using or based on what one feels to be true even without conscious reasoning; instinctiveness" (Oxford Dictionary, n.d.). Intuition provides instantaneous access to this information, without conscious thought. People tend to rely on intuition primarily when in stressful situations where information is limited, and the problems are unclear. For example, Cork (2014) discovered that within the emergency department, nurses working triage used their intuition to prioritize patient care. This demonstrates how people respond to cues in the situation and draw from stored information (tacit knowledge that is hard to describe) in the subconscious to make rapid decisions instead. The alternative would be to take an incremental, analytical approach, such as that found in the rational decision-making model. Rational thinking and intuitive thinking are complementary, and successful decision making is a balance between the two approaches. The role of intuition in nursing has been supported by Benner and Tanner (1987). It is most commonly used in the decision making of expert practitioners. In nursing, "gut feeling" responses are associated with intuition, and themes that emerge from intuition are referred to as "knowing or understanding" (Smith, 2007, p. 16). Intuition can be enhanced through decision-making strategies, such as brainstorming and group discussions (Smith, 2007). Nurses must always be vigilant that their intuition does not lead to the identification or imposition of suboptimal decisions.

Putting It All Together

Figure 8.2 illustrates the relationships among the foregoing intellectual processes. The scientific method is at the core of rational, systematic models of critical thinking, problem solving, and the nursing process. Creative decision making and intuitive decision making are not regarded as rational-thinking approaches. Although both include sequential steps, the intellectual processes differ. Creativity and intuition feed rational-thinking processes and therefore can be seen as complementary thinking processes. Similarly, ethical decision making is a systematic, values-oriented approach to reasoning that complements the scientific method.

FACTORS THAT AFFECT THE QUALITY OF DECISIONS

Individual Decision Biases

Many factors, such as past experiences, personal attributes, and cognitive biases, interfere with the quality of a decision (Henriksen & Dayton, 2006). People tend to make decisions based on heuristics, which are educated

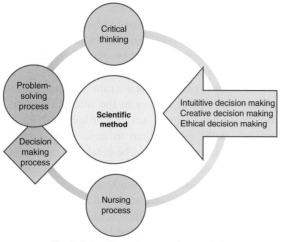

Fig. 8.2 Intellectual processing models.

guesses or "rules of thumb." Heuristics are based on experience and general knowledge about how things work, as opposed to specific information about the situation at hand. Mostly they are helpful, especially when time is not available to collect and assess relevant information. However, they can lead to decision bias, or error in judgement, when relevant information is omitted. A number of individual decision biases have implications for nurses and other health care providers. Confirmation bias is the tendency for people to seek information that reaffirms an idea rather than information that contradicts the idea (McAllister, 2003). Availability bias is the tendency for people to base their judgement on a preceding and memorable event that is readily recalled rather than complete information on the present situation. Hindsight bias is the tendency for people to overestimate their ability to predict an event after the fact, which the phrase "I knew it all along" suggests. Hindsight bias interferes with people's ability to learn from the past because it leads them to be overconfident in their predictive skills, which can interfere with their ability to make good judgements. Another individual bias is the prudence trap; the tendency for people to be too cautious and avoid risks that may be justified. Nurse managers and nursing leaders need to be alert to individual decision biases and address how to avoid them in in making decisions and when interacting with individual professionals and patients.

Group Decision Biases

Decision biases can also affect the group decision-making process and its outcomes. Groupthink, the most common group decision bias, is a phenomenon in which group members are so concerned with avoiding conflict and supporting their leader and other members that important facts, concerns, and differing views are not raised that might indicate an alternative decision. Recall from a discussion in Chapter 1 how being a good follower may require you to raise important overlooked facts and concerns. Failure to bring up options, explore conflict, or challenge the status quo results in ineffective group functioning and decision outcomes. Group polarization is the tendency for groups to make decisions that are more extreme (risky or conservative) than the privately held beliefs of individual group members. When groups polarize toward one extreme or the other, their decisions could lead to negative outcomes, such as financial loss or failed projects. The reasons for such radical shifts in decisions vary. One explanation is that groups are more confident than individuals because of strength in numbers and a sense that responsibility for the decision is shared. Group invulnerability is the perception of group members that the group cannot be wrong, which can lead the group to make overly optimistic or overly risky decisions. Nurse managers and leaders need to monitor group processes for group decision biases to maintain the quality of group decisions.

Fallacies

Fallacies are beliefs that appear to be correct but are found to be false when examined by logical reasoning rules. Logical reasoning uses syllogisms to make valid arguments. A *syllogism* is "a formal argument consisting of a major and a minor premise and a conclusion" (*Merriam-Webster's online dictionary*, n.d.). The major premise states a general rule, followed by a minor premise, which includes statements of fact about a person, thing, or group. The conclusion connects the premises, sequentially, into a general principle. The premises, when true, support the conclusion. For example, "All humans have brains; Dan is human and therefore Dan has a brain" is a syllogism, and the conclusion is true. "All humans have brains; Bugsy has a brain and therefore Bugsy is human" has some logical pattern, but it contains a fallacy because Bugsy is a dog.

Fallacious arguments can result in wrong decisions and actions. Numerous types of fallacies exist, and a complete discussion of each of these fallacies is beyond the scope of this chapter. Examples help demonstrate the importance of recognizing fallacies. The *gambler's fallacy* is a common fallacy related to probabilities. With a fair coin, the probability of getting heads or tails on a single toss is ½ (one in two). If we have tossed 20 heads in a row, we might believe that the chance of the next coin toss being tails has increased. However, each coin toss has the same probability, regardless of the previous toss, so an equal chance (i.e., 50–50) remains that the next toss will be tails. Another common fallacy is the *hasty generalization*, which is a broad claim based on assumptions and insufficient facts. A *post hoc error* occurs when it is quickly and incorrectly assumed that an event was caused by the one that preceded it. Time constraints, interruptions, heavy workloads, and other factors interfere with logical reasoning and effective decision making. Awareness of fallacies is the first step in learning how to avoid them.

Personal Attributes

Certain personality factors, such as self-esteem and self-confidence, affect whether one is willing to take risks in solving problems or making decisions. Keynes (2008) stated that individuals may be influenced by social pressures. For example, one may be inclined to make decisions to satisfy people to whom they are accountable and from whom they feel social pressure.

Personal internal and external factors can influence how a decision-making situation is perceived. Internal factors include variables such as the decision maker's physical and emotional state, personal philosophy, biases, values, interests, experience, knowledge, attitudes, and risk-seeking or risk-avoiding behaviours. External factors include environmental conditions, time, and resources. Decision-making options are externally limited when time is short or when the environment is characterized by a "we've always done it this way" attitude. For example, addressing a practice intervention on a ward that is solidified in policy can be challenging, even if there is existing evidence-based practice literature to change the practice.

EXERCISE 8.1 Describe a decision-making situation in which your decision failed because of a personal decision bias. What barriers did you encounter? What strategies could you have used to avoid the error? If faced with the same decision now, knowing what you know, would you make a different decision?

APPLYING THE PROBLEM-SOLVING PROCESS

As noted in Fig. 8.1, the problem-solving process involves seven steps: (1) define the problem, (2) gather data, (3) analyze the data, (4) develop solutions, (5) select solutions, (6) implement the solutions, and (7) evaluate the result. People adopt different approaches to problem solving and decision making, ranging from intuition to in-depth logical processing. Often, the approach used depends on the circumstances and the individual's level of problem-solving expertise. The nursing process is the most commonly used formal problem-solving process in nursing. In the problem-solving example that follows, a generic seven-step model of problem solving, which incorporates the nursing process, illustrates how the steps in the process apply to nursing practice. The problem-solving steps that rely heavily on decision-making processes are indicated.

Problem Solving in Nursing Practice
Step 1:
Define the Problem. Problem analysis begins with an investigation of the presenting problem. Patients who enter the health care system often have a number of interrelated problems. On admission, a complete intake history and patient assessment is conducted to identify and clarify any problems. Identifying a problem entails collecting preliminary data from as many sources as possible to describe fully the patient's problem or problems. The most common cause of failure to resolve a problem is the improper identification of the problem; therefore problem recognition and identification are considered the most vital steps. The quality of the patient outcome depends on accurate identification of the problem, which is likely to recur if the true underlying causes are not targeted.

Step 2:
Gather Data. Once the preliminary investigation is completed and the problem is identified, nurses can focus on in-depth data collection to resolve the issue using relevant and evidence-based resources. The data gathered should consist of objective (facts) and subjective (feelings) information. Facts that are gathered should be valid, accurate, relevant to the issue, and timely. Data collection is influenced by many factors, including the amount and accuracy of available information,

the values, attitudes, and experiences of those involved, and time. Sufficient time should be allowed for the collection and organization of data. Data collection tools, such as the five Ws—who, what, when, where, why— can be used to improve the quality of information. A list of questions could include the following:

- Who is affected by the problem?
- Who is responsible for addressing the problem?
- What is the nature of the problem?
- When did the problem start?
- Where did the problem originate?
- Why did the problem occur?

Step 3:

Analyze the Data. Data should be carefully analyzed to explore the full extent of the problem, root causes, and contributing factors. Nurses can refer to clinical reasoning guides and a compendium of nursing diagnoses for this purpose. This analysis should lead to a nursing diagnosis and potential solutions to the problem.

Step 4:

Develop Solutions (Decision Making). Patient outcomes are linked to nursing diagnoses. By linking outcomes to nursing diagnoses, nurses can discover which solution would be most appropriate for a patient. Not all possible solutions can be applied, but it is important to consider the advantages and disadvantages of each, based on a set of priorities. One source of outcomes is evidence-informed best practices that have been formulated for clinical use through decision analyses, such as systematic reviews (see Khan, 2010). Systematic reviews involve extensive research analyses of previous problems to identify, select, and validate best practices. Nurses should use their professional judgement, assessment information, and collaboration with the patient to determine the outcomes that might have the most value for the patient as an individual.

Step 5:

Select Solutions (Decision Making). After possible patient outcomes have been generated, decisions are made about which alternatives are most appropriate. This involves a deliberate process of determining the alternatives to meet each outcome, establishing priorities among alternatives, and choosing the most appropriate patient outcome for implementation. An outcome for a patient in pain after surgery might be "to achieve a level

of pain that the patient can reasonably tolerate." Alternatives for pain control might be assessed, using general knowledge or decision rules about how to assess pain and the appropriate interventions for each level of pain.

If the investigation indicates that no action should be taken because the problem is beyond the nurse leader's control or the problem is likely to resolve itself spontaneously, a *purposeful inaction* or a "do nothing" approach might be taken (Burrow et al., 2007). For example, in certain instances, a nurse manager may decide to leave things as they are by being indifferent. This indifference could be focused on a particular issue or a chronic pattern of problems. If the response is to a chronic pattern, the nurse leader's behaviour might be construed as a lack of caring, which could have a negative effect on staff and patients. It is important for nurse leaders to communicate the underlying reasons for purposeful inaction.

Step 6:

Implement the Solutions. Implementing a plan of action to solve a problem requires attention to details. If the plan introduces an innovation, the adjustment to it may create problems. If the intervention does not address root causes, it may be ineffective. Any deviations in the patient's condition or unexpected responses should be monitored and decisions should be made to adapt the care plan. The implementation phase should include a contingency plan to deal with negative consequences if they arise.

Step 7:

Evaluate the Result. An evaluation of patient outcomes reflects the quality of problem analysis, decision making, and interventions. Feedback that is obtained from the health care team and the patient is assessed and used to revise or continue with the plan. Considerable time and energy are usually spent on identifying the problem or issue, generating possible solutions, selecting the best solution, and implementing the solution. In the past, evaluation and follow-up were often neglected. Today, health care organizations have to meet stringent quality control standards. It is important to delegate responsibility for evaluation and monitoring of outcomes early in the problem-solving process. Typically, health care teams assume this responsibility and continuously monitor practices to identify areas for improvement. Deviations from quality control standards usually occur to maintain high quality of care. This topic is addressed in Chapter 22.

EXERCISE 8.2 Find a case description of a patient's condition in a journal. Use a five Ws approach (described in Step 1 of "Problem Solving in Nursing Practice") to generate questions for gathering data from the case. What information did you obtain in response to your questions? What gaps did you identify in the case description?

DECISION-MAKING MODELS

For health care providers, decision making in health care settings has become increasingly challenging. As a result, the trend in health care has been to adopt well-established business models of decision making and decision support tools. A decision-making model is a guide to decision making for individuals or groups. The rational decision-making model, the bounded rationality model, and the Clinical Judgement Model are common approaches to decision making. These models will be explored in this section, together with decision support tools that complement them.

Rational Decision-Making Model

The rational decision-making model (sometimes called the *rational choice model*) originated in the field of economics and has been adopted by many other fields, including nursing and management. The model holds that patterns of rational decision are based on minimizing risk while maximizing profit (Simon, 1979). In health care, at a clinical level, we see much discussion on the concept of "rational decision making," perceptions of risk, and decision making. One good example of this is within adolescence (Reyna & Rivers, 2008). However, the traditional perspective of rational decision making involves the individual, or organization, choosing a rational action, based on individual preferences. Three assumptions are made about individual's preferences: (1) all actions can be ranked according to preference, (2) all actions can be compared with other actions, and (3) alternatives are independent. These assumptions explain the structure and content of the rational decision-making model. In applying this model, goals are set first, and then the criteria are stated and weighted according to importance. Finally, alternatives are generated and compared to determine which best satisfies the criteria (Box 8.1). Although this model appears to be reliable, it is not always easy to use to make good decisions (Korte, 2003; Lunenburg, 2010).

BOX 8.1 A Six-Step Rational Model for Decision Making

1. Define the problem and identify goals to solve it.
2. Identify decision criteria that must be met to achieve each goal.
3. Weight (rank) the criteria according to level of importance.
4. Generate alternatives or courses of action to solve the problem.
5. Rate each alternative in its ability to satisfy each criterion.
6. Evaluate each alternative against the weighted criteria to determine the alternative with the highest total score, which is the optimal choice.

Typically, most people apply less stringent models to ill-defined problems and uncertain situations. Although these models appear to be prescriptive, they are usually not applied deliberately or in logical order. Experienced decision makers tend to be flexible in their approach to decision making, moving back and forth through the steps or applying several steps simultaneously.

A Rational Decision-Making Tool

Decision-making tools help visualize options under consideration and allow the comparison of options using common criteria. Criteria, which are determined by the decision makers, may include time required, ethical or legal considerations, equipment needs, and cost. The relative advantages and disadvantages should be listed for each option. For example, the nurse manager of a hospital education department is assessing whether it is better to retain the services of an outside consultant to coordinate an advanced cardiac life support (ACLS) course in the hospital, pay the per-person fees to send the staff to another hospital for training, or train staff as ACLS instructors who can then provide training in-house. The type of information this nurse manager might compile includes a breakdown of the costs for the three options, equipment needs, the benefits of each option, the number of nurses who need the course, and future training needs.

A weighted decision matrix, illustrated in Fig. 8.3, is commonly used to calculate preferred alternatives when using the rational decision-making model (Borysowich, 2006). The matrix uses the following steps:

1. Identify a desired outcome.
2. Enter criteria that can fulfill the desired outcome in the left column.

Outcome: ACLS Instruction		ALTERNATIVES (Options)					
		Consultant		Send off site		Train trainer	
Criteria	Weight	Rating	Score	Rating	Score	Rating	Score
Time	4	2	8	5	20	3	12
Workload issues	3	3	9	3	9	1	3
Cost	2	3	6	3	6	2	4
Total			23		35		19
Preferred option					35*		

Fig. 8.3 Weighted decision matrix on how to train nurses in ACLS (Advanced Cardiac Life Support).

3. In column 2, rank each criterion (e.g., 0–5 scale, with 5 being most important) in order of importance.
4. Generate different options that might meet all of the criteria and enter them in the second row from the top.
5. In the rows, rank (e.g., 0–5 scale) each criterion on how well the alternative meets that criterion (e.g., satisfaction level).
6. Multiply the weight for each criterion by its rating for each alternative and enter the result in the score columns (weight × rating = score).
7. Total the scores for each alternative. The highest score indicates the preferred option.

> **EXERCISE 8.3** You are trying to decide which of three job offers to accept. Each role involves being a registered nurse on an acute medical ward. However, each job is in a different city. The first is within a small northern hospital, the second is in a major city centre, and the third is an international role, within an urban facility. Discuss the value and application of the rational decision-making tool for selecting which position to accept.

Bounded Rationality Model

The bounded rationality model was proposed by Nobel Prize winner Herbert Simon, who observed that the rational (choice) decision-making model did not fit with observations of behavioural psychologists (Jones, 1999). Simon argued that people were constrained or "bounded" by personal and environmental factors that limited their abilities to make rational decisions. In addition, individuals may not evaluate all of the existing alternatives. The bounded rationality model then is a model for making practical decisions. Limits

on important factors, such as knowledge, capacity to process information, expertise, resources, and unfavourable or uncertain environment conditions prevent people from making, what others may consider, an optimal decision. In fact, in such cases, people are most likely to engage in satisficing decision making, the selection the option that is acceptable but not necessarily the best, when an optimizing decision is not feasible. An *optimizing decision* is the act of selecting the ideal solution or option to achieve goals. An example of a satisficing approach is the tendency of a decision maker to rely on heuristics (defined earlier) to select the solution that meets the minimal objective or standard for a decision. It allows for quick decisions and may be most appropriate when time is an issue. To illustrate, a nurse practitioner may rely on a reliable, short questionnaire to decide whether to place a patient with chest pain on an observation unit or on a low-intensity medical unit upon admission. The trend toward standardizing decision making by modelling and testing such heuristics can improve decision making in the health care environment. Some decisions are based on firmly established criteria in health care, such as traditions, values, doctrines, culture, and the policies of the organization. While every leader or manager should understand and strive towards organizational mandates, the limitations of standardizing decision making should also be considered. For example, while best-practice guidelines are an example of standard guidelines for decision making, nurses must have advanced decision-making skills to make independent judgements on problems that are not readily solved through clinical guidelines.

Tools for Making Practical (Bounded Rationality) Decisions

The tools commonly associated with practical (bounded rationality) decisions in health care are heuristics, medical algorithms, and portable digital instruments, especially when decisions are being made in clinical settings. The tools used to make bounded rationality decisions should match the situation. They should be easy to use, practical, and not require in-depth analyses because of time constraints. They should be able to capture essential data that will be sufficient, rather than the optimum data. A fishbone diagram, commonly used in quality improvement programs and sometimes referred to as a cause-and-effect diagram, can be used to identify the potential causes of problems quickly. The fishbone diagram is a good example of a tool that is effective in unstructured work environments.

The fishbone diagram identifies the effect of a problem first and the causes of a problem second (Embury, 2014). The head of the fish states the problem, and the ribs of the fish outline potential causes. The ribs of the fish are labelled by category. The major categories can be the four Ms (methods, machines [equipment], manpower [people], and materials), the four Ps (place, procedure, people, and policies), or the four Ss (surroundings, suppliers, systems, and skills). One particular set of categories may be more relevant to a particular problem. Applying the four Ps category to nursing, *place* could be the location or facilities for holding wellness clinics, *procedures* could include communication problems or lack of protocols, *people* could include inadequate staffing or staff mix and knowledge or skills deficits, and *policies* could include rules or guidelines that relate to activities such as training programs and equipment.

An example of a fishbone diagram based on the four Ms appears in Fig 8.4.

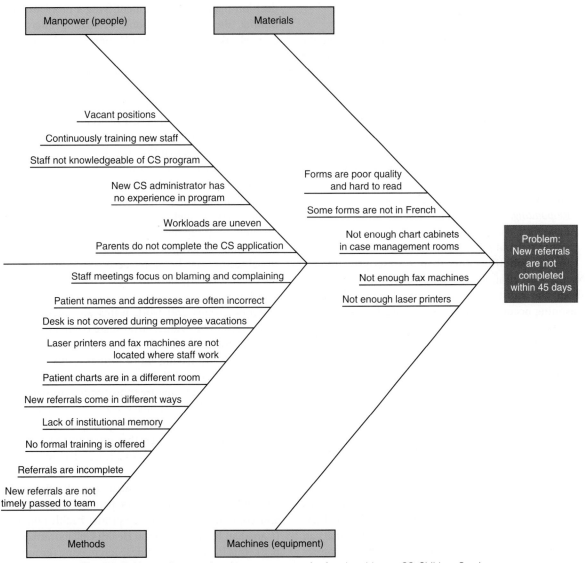

Fig. 8.4 Fishbone diagram showing root causes of referral problems. *CS,* Children Services.

EXERCISE 8.4 Use a fishbone diagram and the four Ps category to identify all the factors (causes) that might explain low attendance at monthly unit meetings you are conducting for the nursing staff of your general medicine unit. The meetings are held once a month, on a Friday, at 1900 shift change. List as many issues or root causes as possible. Discuss your diagram with a classmate. Brainstorm together for additional causes to determine the most important causes of low attendance. Give some examples of actions that you could take for each cause to increase attendance at your monthly meetings.

Clinical Judgement Model

The Clinical Judgement Model described by Tanner (2006) in the Literature Perspective box emphasizes the role of intuition in decision making by nurses, particularly expert nurses (Tanner, 2006, p. 204). This model is systematic and similar in its sequence of steps to other models, although the thinking processes involved differ. Tanner identified four decision making phases:

1. *Noticing*: responding to cues based on knowledge and experience.
2. *Interpreting*: reasoning and sense making.
3. *Responding*: deciding on the best options.
4. *Reflecting*: examining one's own actions, patient responses, and subsequent learning.

It is an intuitive rather than a prescriptive model. Nurses use clinical reasoning to reach judgements about the most appropriate interventions. Clinical reasoning occurs in transitions and during reappraisal as situations unfold. Intuition is used when problems are complex, the decision maker has the expertise for solving similar complex problems, subtle changes are difficult to detect, information is unclear or confusing, factors in the external environment are challenging, and changes in the patient's condition are occurring rapidly.

Clinical Judgement Support Tool for Students

Clinical journalling is prescribed for students who use the Clinical Judgement Model. This established teaching tool can be used to assess students' knowledge, skills, and affective development. By regularly recording their thoughts in a journal, students can capture data that can be interpreted for specified reasons, such as comprehension, skill development, and cognitive reflection on

the meanings and implications of experiences. Tanner's (2006) Clinical Judgement Model can be used to guide retrospective reflection on decision making.

GROUP DECISION MAKING

More frequently in health care environments and nursing education, the concept of interprofessional practice and education is highlighted as a means to improve patient outcomes. This requires the use of group decision making (as would shared decision making—discussed earlier). Like individual decision making, group decision making involves identifying a problem, determining alternative solutions, evaluating alternatives, and selecting a solution. For unpredictable problems, satisficing or intuition may apply. In groups, decision making is accomplished through collaboration among group members who share common goals and are mutually supportive. Groups tend to make better decisions than individuals because of accumulated expertise and resources, and because members are likely to commit to alternatives that they develop. In deciding to use the group process for decision making, it is important to consider group composition. Homogeneous groups may be more compatible; however, highly cohesive groups may be ineffective in decision making if they succumb to group biases, such as group polarization or groupthink. Heterogeneous groups, such as interprofessional teams, may be more successful in problem solving because divergent thinking is useful in creating best decisions.

Work groups and work teams are interdependent collections of individuals who share common goals and specific outcomes for their organizations, with work teams typically having more formal status than work groups (Nielsen, 2012). In health care, loosely organized work groups and teams are transitioning from multidisciplinary to interdisciplinary teams (see Chapter 25). With a growing emphasis on quality care and workplace safety, it is expected that interprofessional teams will become more involved in clinical decision making. In health care, interprofessional collaboration involves the development and maintenance of relationships among "learners, practitioners, patients/clients/families and communities to enable optimal health outcomes" (Canadian Interprofessional Health Collaborative, 2010, p. 8). This involves shared decision making (group decision making) as well as trust and respect. Furthermore decision making within this type of team "is based on an integration of the knowledge and expertise of each professional, so that solutions to complex problems can be proposed . . . in an open-minded way" (D'Amour et al., 2005, p. 120). Generally, interprofessional teams have authority and accountability for planning, decision making, and implementing goals. Increasingly, management decisions are being assigned to these types of teams when problems are complex, information is needed from many sources, a quality decision is required, and commitment to the decision is necessary for implementation of the decision.

LITERATURE PERSPECTIVE

Resource: Tanner, C. A. (2006). Thinking like a nurse: A research-based model of clinical judgment in nursing. *Journal of Nursing Education*, 45(6), 204–211.

Tanner engaged in an extensive review of 200 studies focusing on clinical judgement and clinical decision making to derive a model of clinical judgement that can be used as a framework for instruction. The first review summarized 120 articles and was published in 1998. The 2006 article reviewed an additional 71 studies published since 1998. Based on an analysis of the entire set of articles, Tanner proposed five conclusions, which are listed below. The reader is referred to the article for detailed explanation of each of the five conclusions.

The author considers clinical judgement as a "problem solving activity." She notes that the terms *clinical judgement*, *problem solving*, *decision making*, and *critical thinking* are often used interchangeably. For the purpose of aiding in the development of the model, Tanner defined *clinical judgement* as actions taken based on the assessment of the patient's needs. Clinical reasoning is the process by which nurses make their judgements (e.g., the decision-making process of selecting the most appropriate option):

1. Clinical judgements are more influenced by what nurses bring to the situation than the objective data about the situation at hand.
2. Sound clinical judgement rests to some degree on knowing the patient and their typical pattern of responses, as well as an engagement with the patient and their concerns.
3. Clinical judgements are influenced by the context in which the situation occurs and the culture of the nursing care unit.
4. Nurses use a variety of reasoning patterns alone or in combination.
5. Reflection on practice is often triggered by a breakdown in clinical judgement and is critical for the development of clinical knowledge and improvement in clinical reasoning. (Tanner, 2006)

The Clinical Judgement Model developed through the review of the literature involves four phases that are similar to the problem-solving and decision-making steps described in this chapter. The model starts with a phase called *noticing*. In this phase, the nurse comes to expect certain responses resulting from knowledge gleaned from similar patient situations, experiences, and knowledge. External factors influence nurses in this phase, such as the complexity of the environment and values, and typical practices within the unit culture.

The second phase of the model is *interpreting*, during which the nurse understands the situation that requires a response. The nurse employs various reasoning patterns to make sense of the issue and to derive an appropriate action plan.

The third phase is *responding*, during which the nurse decides on the best option for handling the situation. This is followed by the fourth phase, *reflecting*, during which the nurse assesses the patient's responses to the actions taken.

Tanner emphasized that "reflection-in-action" and "reflection-on-action" are major processes required in the model. Reflection-in-action is real-time reflection on the patient's responses to nursing action with modifications to the plan based on the ongoing assessment. On the other hand, reflection-on-action is a review of the experience, which promotes learning for future similar experiences. Nurse educators and leaders or managers can employ this model with new and experienced nurses to aid understanding of the thought processes involved in decision making.

Implications for Practice

Nurse educators, managers, and leaders can employ this model with new and experienced nurses to aid in understanding the thought processes involved in decision making. For example, students and practising nurses can be encouraged to maintain reflective journals to record observations and impressions from clinical experiences. In clinical-post conferences or staff development meetings, the nurse educator, manager, or leader can engage staff in applying the five phases Tanner proposed to their lived experiences. The ultimate goal of analyzing their decisions and decision-making processes is to improve clinical judgement, problem solving, decision making, and critical-thinking skills.

Leadership and Team Development for Decision Making

Teams share decision making in order to meet their goals and are successful when members have the necessary decision-making and group-interaction skills to perform as a team. Shared decision making involves important elements of leadership and followership. Understanding and appreciating professional roles and responsibilities, and communicating effectively, are among the most valued group-member competencies in shared decision making (Suter et al., 2009).

Kozlowski and Ilgen (2006) identified key cognitive and behavioural processes that enable group members to achieve their goals. These are coordination, cooperation, and communication; group member competencies; regulations; and group performance dynamics. The group leader is the most important facilitator of these processes. The Research Perspective supports the importance of leadership in shared decision making. Morgeson et al. (2010) identified the specific leadership support needs of team members from a meta-analysis of studies on team leadership. They developed a taxonomy of these needs, which includes leadership functions for team building (transition phase) and team performance (action phase). Team building needs to include competent, motivated members; clear goals and expectations; training; help with sense making; and feedback. Leadership functions needed for team performance are team monitoring; management of team boundaries; assistance with tasks; help with solving problems; resources; encouragement for self-management; and support for the social climate. This taxonomy focuses on followers in a group or team and the leadership support that they need, regardless of source, to help them fulfill goals such as effective group decision making.

RESEARCH PERSPECTIVE

Resource: MacPhee, M., Wardrop, A. & Campbell, C. (2010). Transforming work place relationships through shared decision making. *Journal of Nursing Management*, 18, 1016–1026.

The shared decision-making model is a professional practice model that promotes nurses' control over and accountability for decisions that affect themselves and their patients. It is facilitated by access to information, resources, supports, and informal or formal lines of power. The authors examined the effect of shared decision making between nurses and nurse leaders around workload issues. Specifically, they examined the relationships within project teams (members and front-line leaders) and the relationships between project teams and mid-level leaders.

Four nurse-led project teams participated in the study to learn how to work together in a new nursing workload project. The study used participatory action research as its methodological approach. Participatory action research is a dynamic, collaborative process for helping people address social issues influencing their lives. The approach involves cycles of planning, acting, and reflecting, giving people the opportunity to bring about change and social improvement. Data were collected through observation, field notes, interviews, and focus groups. The participant observers also acted as facilitators of the project to enable nurses to gradually assume control over practice.

Shared decision making led to a number of successful outcomes, including team pride, the team's ability to engage in discussions with the nurse leader about work issues, and team involvement in shared decision making. Conflict and communication issues surfaced related to history, power dynamics, hierarchical differences, and roles and responsibilities. The study concluded that leadership has a critical role in transforming workplace relationships through shared decision making. It also confirmed the importance of leadership competencies related to communication, team building, conflict resolution, and change management.

Implications for Practice

This study provides nurse managers and leaders with insight into the complexity of team building, which occurs simultaneously with changing team members' roles and relationships. In reflecting on the process, the authors commented on the importance of strategic planning for future programs and the need for nurse managers and leaders to have strong team-building, communication, and conflict-resolution skills. Conflict is inevitable in group development, particularly in the early stages of development. Differences in goals, values, attitudes, role expectations, role changes, communication barriers, and historical issues all contribute to team conflict. In this study, conflict took place in the early stage of group development. It would be interesting to compare these observations with those at a later stage of group development.

Team Development

In most organizations, team leaders are responsible for team development and team performance. As coaches, team leaders are expected to provide guidance and direction to individuals to help them fulfill their roles. They take responsibility for their own development and serve as models to their followers. Leadership is discussed further in Chapters 1, 2, 17, and 18. The competencies described here include some of the important learning needs identified by team members and leaders.

Coordination, Cooperation, and Communication

Coordination involves synchronizing tasks among other health care providers and agencies to deliver patient care in different health agencies. In health care, work is streamlined in an orderly way to ensure completion of tasks on schedule and to reduce the incidence of omissions and errors. However, the coordination of services in health care is challenging when patients require multiple services from different agencies and health care providers (Khan, 2010). Effective nurse managers and leaders build efficient teams that can integrate and organize work as well as liaise with networks outside the team's boundaries to ensure continuity of care. Computer technology and standardized protocols and guidelines can enhance coordination and delivery of services. These support tools also facilitate decision making at different points in the care continuum. Students are involved in work coordination across departments and agencies, which gives them many opportunities to study and promote coordination.

Cooperation is the voluntary effort on the part of individuals to work with others to achieve common goals in a noncompetitive manner. When people cooperate willingly, more positive work outcomes can be expected. Cooperation in teams involves sharing goals, information, expertise, and resources for task completion. Effective nurse managers and leaders promote cooperation between individuals and teams by setting clear goals, delegating tasks appropriately, monitoring workflow, and providing assistance for resolving conflicts that are related to joint task performance and decision making.

Effective *communication* is vital for group decision making. Poor communication, which can cause conflict and misunderstandings, can reduce team effectiveness. In health care teams, communication problems have been associated with hierarchical differences among team members, differences in expertise, the complexity of care, rapid decision making, role conflict, blocked

upward communication, and interpersonal power issues (Suter et al., 2009). These factors present challenges for group function, group decision making, and patient care, which means that training in communication and decision-making skills is essential for nurse managers and leaders.

Team Competencies

Competencies are task-related knowledge, skills, and attitudes that reflect a task and can be measured. It is difficult to measure competencies for the team as a whole, but individual team members are accountable for their own task performance. Team building requires clear goals and expectations, task training, and feedback on performance. Decision making is a challenging task in interdisciplinary teams and one that is not easily managed. Advances in training resources, such as virtual team-building programs, can be used to promote effective decision making and team building and assist nurse managers and leaders to gain these requisite competencies for team building. Other resources, including professional programs, can enhance skill development in leaders. Feedback provided by leaders to team members on their performance is important for motivation and continuous learning.

Team Performance Dynamics

Team dynamics is defined as the way team members interact and react to changing circumstances. Positive team dynamics are conducive to shared decision making (Morgeson et al., 2010).

Persistent problems, such as group polarization, groupthink, conflicts of interest, and different perspectives, can lead to team dysfunction. Conflicts within the team may be related to task, relationships, or behaviours. For example, disagreements can arise about team decision-making tasks (Jehn et al., 2008). Research has shown that moderate amounts of conflict may be helpful for motivating team members, but in general, conflict can interfere with work satisfaction, cognitive processes, and the willingness of group members to work together. By carefully monitoring the team's progress, team leaders can detect and address conflict before it escalates. Conflict resolution strategies are discussed in Chapter 24.

A competency-based training program for effective team dynamics can be used by nurse managers and leaders to set standards for behaviour. The following competencies can help foster positive team performance dynamics:

- Establish ground rules for the team climate (ethical behaviour, work ethic, trust, shared decision making).
- Work with team members to set strategic goals for the team.
- Promote effective team communication (listening, encouraging participation, negotiating).
- Manage dysfunctional conflict in the team (conflict resolution strategies).
- Manage dysfunctional communication in the team (jargon, interruptions).
- Provide coaching for tasks and give constructive feedback.
- Use decision tools to help solve complex problems.
- Engage team members in reflection on team performance.

Team Decision Support Tools

Making decisions in a team can be challenging, particularly in interdisciplinary teams. Professional differences and independent focus of practice can make it difficult for team members to cross boundaries and negotiate to reach consensus on patient-care outcomes. Collaborative decision tools can help minimize some of these barriers and assist the team in reaching a consensus to resolve issues.

Brainstorming

Brainstorming is a useful technique for stimulating the creative, spontaneous, and free-flowing thoughts of individuals and teams. It is important for generating novel ideas and focusing attention on specific issues. To ensure that creativity is not stifled, participants are asked to state whatever comes to mind when responding to questions. Responses should not be censored or ridiculed. Many ideas can be generated quickly and at minimal cost through brainstorming. The quantity of responses is not as important as the quality, which is achieved through a process of categorizing and evaluating content at the end of a brainstorming session. This method is useful for teams who get stalled in the problem analysis phase of decision making or when generating alternatives for interventions to solve problems. It also helps relieve tensions among members who are locked into a particular position that others are unable to accept. However, brainstorming does have some disadvantages that limit its success. For example, it is difficult to sort content into useful categories for analysis, some people are intimidated by sharing ideas that pop into their heads, and facilitators may not have the needed skills for the task. The introduction of electronic brainstorming has transformed this process. Content can be captured anonymously so that inhibited members can participate, and people's ideas are instantly visible and can be sorted into manageable categories for analysis. Some disadvantages of electronic brainstorming limit its appeal, such as cost, limited accessibility, information overload, and difficulties with evaluating data.

Six Thinking Hats

Six thinking hats is a powerful decision-making tool that can be used by groups to look at problems laterally from six different perspectives (De Bono, 2009). Cioffi (2017) discussed the use of the six thinking hats techniques to aid collaborative decision making within patient family meetings, specifically as a means to aid communication. The hats have different colours, and each represents a different style of parallel thinking or role that a wearer assumes in a group. As participants switch from one hat to another, they are able to examine and reconsider their own style of thinking and how it affects their decision making. The six thinking hats are as follows:

- *Black hat:* negative, critical
- *Blue hat:* rational, decisive
- *Green hat:* creative, innovative
- *Red hat:* intuitive, emotional
- *Yellow hat:* positive, optimistic
- *White hat:* objective, factual

This decision tool is highly rated for critical thinking, communication, collaboration, and creativity. It has a positive effect on group dynamics when everyone has a chance to participate and can be objective in their approach to decision making.

Nominal Group Technique

Nominal group technique is used to identify a problem, generate solutions, and establish priorities by obtaining views on a topic and arriving at a consensus (Harvey & Holmes, 2012). Typically, this is accomplished through the use of a structured, mediated, approach. This technique is efficient and useful for controlling negative group behaviours (such as discussion domination by a few members) and increasing the participation of all group members in the problem-solving process.

In the nominal group technique, the process begins by presenting a problem. Participants are given a period of approximately 10 minutes of silence to generate and record their ideas on how to address the problem. Then, all ideas are shared with the group using a chalkboard, flip chart, or computer screen. After the ideas have been shared, the group discusses the ideas for clarity and evaluates the merits of each idea. Next, each member silently and independently ranks each idea. The solution chosen is the one that receives the highest ranking by the majority of participants.

This technique is most useful when in-depth thinking from a variety of perspectives about options and strategies is needed to reach a quality decision. However, some members may feel that the process involved is too formal and may not like the restricted social interaction during decision making.

SWOT Analysis

SWOT analysis is a study of an organization's internal strengths and weaknesses, as well as its external opportunities and threats (Pearce, 2007). It is commonly used in strategic planning or marketing efforts but can also be used by individuals and groups in decision making. During a SWOT analysis, team members list the Strengths, Weaknesses, Opportunities, and Threats related to the situation under consideration. Table 8.1 shows how SWOT analysis can be used to facilitate a nursing decision to transfer a nurse who has worked in a medical–surgical unit for five years to a critical care unit (CCU). SWOT analysis is an efficient tool for scanning the internal and external environments of an organization so that it can minimize and correct its weakness and threats, and to build on strengths and opportunities. However, the knowledge gained about the state of the internal and external environment may be too costly to change or impossible to change. The cost of equipment and supplies may escalate internally, and external policies and mandated programs may increase costs.

SOAR Analysis

SOAR is a creative planning process, rooted in appreciative inquiry (a creative approach to problem

TABLE 8.1 **SWOT Analysis**	
Internal	
Strengths	*Weaknesses*
• Familiar with the health care system	• Has not attended the critical care class
• Clinically competent and has received favourable performance appraisals	• Has had a prior unresolved conflict with one of the surgeons who frequently admits to the critical care unit (CCU)
• Good communication skills; well-liked by her peers	• Is uncertain whether she wants to work full-time, 12-hour shifts
• Recently completed 12-lead electrocardiogram (ECG) interpretation class	
External	
Opportunities	*Threats*
• Anticipated staff openings in the CCU in the next several months	• Possible bed closures in another CCU may result in staff transfers, thus eliminating open positions
• Critical care course will be offered in 1 month	• Another medical–surgical nurse is also interested in transferring
• Advanced cardiac life support (ACLS) course offered four times a year	
• A friend who works in CCU has offered to mentor her	

solving). Appreciative inquiry "seeks out the best of 'what is' to help ignite the collective imagination of 'what might be', with the aim of generating new knowledge that expands the 'realm of the possible' and helps people envision a collectively desired future" (Kaminski, 2012).

A SOAR analysis includes identifying Strengths, Opportunities, Aspirations, and Results, and is a more positive alternative to the traditional SWOT analysis (Stavros & Hinrichs, 2009). Importantly, a SOAR approach is different from a SWOT analysis in that it is action oriented and focuses on innovation and breakthroughs by engaging all levels, rather than SWOT, which is rooted in analysis, small improvements, and tends to be implemented from a top down approach (Stavros & Hinrichs, 2009).

EXERCISE 8.5 SWOT analysis is a practical tool for decision making. Use the example in Table 8.1 to conduct a SWOT analysis of a hospital discharge plan for a patient to decide if the plan is appropriate. When you are finished, discuss if this analysis would have had a different outcome had a SOAR approach been utilized.

EXERCISE 8.6 Use the Research Perspective box to generate options for managing group conflict in the shared decision-making program between nurses and nurse leaders around workload issues.

Which decision-making tool would be most helpful to guide the selection of a best option? Explain your answer.

CONCLUSION

Problem-solving and decision-making skills are essential for nurse managers, formal nurse leaders, and informal nurse leaders. However, problems in the health care setting are often complex and difficult to solve. Decision-making models and tools are helpful but can be limited by flaws in decision making, interpersonal conflict, and unpredictable conditions, such as crises. Continuous skill development and self-reflection will improve the ability of nurse managers and leaders to think critically and solve complex problems.

⚡ A SOLUTION

On the surface, it appears that Shyanne's supervisor, Rhea, made a conscious decision to avoid implementing the project, which confused and frustrated Shyanne. Rhea's passive but not indifferent response made it challenging for Shyanne, a new employee, to confront the issue. Shyanne decides to ask Rhea why she feels the project should not be implemented, and Rhea shares that she doesn't feel the current program needs adapting, and that she is concerned about cost. Shyanne asks Rhea if it would be all right to spend some time looking at the current and alternative programs, to which Rhea agrees. Using the problem-solving process, Shyanne prepares a short brief to present to Rhea. She begins by summarizing the approach and impact of the existing programs and then clearly defines the problems faced by the youth utilizing the walk-in clinic and supports this with data from the community. Shyanne then works with colleagues to develop a few different solutions to the problem (creative problem solving), outlines how they would be implemented and the costs involved and evaluation schemes for each. In comparison to the existing program. This exercise helps Shyanne take a more objective view of the problem, through which her understanding of the complexity of the issue is widened, and the report provides a starting point for looking at alternatives as a team.

Would this be a suitable approach for you? Why or why not?

▎ THE EVIDENCE

Penz and Bassendowski (2006) examined barriers to evidence-based nursing in clinical practice. They observed that while nurse educators and clinical nurse educators have a mandate to model and facilitate evidence-based practice, barriers in clinical settings make it difficult for nurses to apply their evidence-based knowledge and skills. The current emphasis on evidence-based practice comes from concerns within medicine about deficits in the quality of medical practice. Defined by Sackett et al. (1996) as "the conscientious, explicit, and judicious use of current best evidence in making decisions about the care of individual patients" (p. 71), evidence-based practice has become a requirement in many health care disciplines. Different definitions of evidence-based nursing practice exist, but most definitions address the importance of basing practice decisions on recent research that is validated through nurses' knowledge and systematic reviews. Other elements, such as nurse's intuition and sound judgement, are associated with definitions of evidence-based nursing practice. Some of the barriers to evidence-based practice in the current study were lack of time; insufficient access to libraries near clinical settings, current research journals and the Internet; inadequate research knowledge and learning opportunities; and unsupportive clinical cultures. Based on previous research, the authors emphasized the importance of helping nursing students develop critical-thinking skills and independent thinking to guide systematic investigations. Developing intellectual curiosity is necessary to help students explore beyond the traditional approaches to practice. In practice settings, clinical educators should know how to search for and evaluate evidence. The authors recommended journal clubs to facilitate analysis of emerging research, critical inquiry, and increased accessibility to research evidence.

The authors drew on accumulated research to emphasize the value of clinical educators as change agents for evidence-based practice to mitigate some of the barriers to implementation of evidence-based practice. Clinical educators can be role models for practitioners and set the tone for change in the clinical setting. Using their sound foundation in evidence-based research, they can establish orientation programs that promote evidence-based practice and ensure that valid practices are incorporated into policies, procedures, and practice guidelines. An evidence-based nursing approach will improve patient outcomes and decision making by clinical nurses.

✳ NEED TO KNOW NOW

- Know how to distinguish a problem from its symptoms.
- Know how to use diagnostic tools to gather and analyze data about problems.
- Know how to use decision-making models to guide the decision-making process and determine best alternatives for action.
- Understand the importance of evidence-informed literature for nursing practice.
- Understand the importance of creativity, intuition, and shared decision making.
- Understand the importance of effective problem solving and decision making for health care providers.

CHAPTER CHECKLIST

The ability to make good decisions and encourage effective decision making in others is a hallmark of nursing leadership and management. A nurse manager or leader is in a good position to facilitate effective decision making by individuals and groups. Doing so requires good communication, conflict resolution, and mediation skills; knowledge of group dynamics; and the ability to foster an environment conducive to effective problem solving, decision making, and creative thinking.

- Problem solving is a comprehensive, sequential, cognitive process used to solve a problem by reducing the difference between current and desired conditions.
- Decision making is a phase of problem solving, which includes a reasoning process to analyze proposed alternatives (options) for action to determine the most appropriate choice.

- The scientific method is a rational, logical, and widely used problem-solving approach. It is the foundation for many models of decision making.
- Creativity and intuition feed rational-thinking processes and therefore can be seen as complementary thinking processes.
- Decision bias, or error in judgement, is a concern when relevant information is omitted. Groupthink is an example of a group decision bias.
- Decision-making styles and personal factors, such as self-esteem and self-confidence, influence decision making.
- Decision-making tools support decision making, especially in groups.
- The situation and circumstances should dictate the leadership style used by a nurse manager or leader to solve problems and make decisions.

TIPS FOR DECISION MAKING AND PROBLEM SOLVING

- Be conscious of personal influence on problem situations and decision-making processes; use safeguards against known biases.
- Research journal articles and relevant sections of textbooks to increase your knowledge base.

- Examine new approaches to problem resolution through experimentation and calculate the risk to self and others.
- Become skilled in using decision-enabling tools.

Visit the Evolve website for Suggested Readings, Internet Resources, and additional resources related to the content in this chapter: http://evolve.elsevier.com/Canada/Yoder-Wise/leading/.

REFERENCES

Benner, P., & Tanner, C. (1987). Clinical judgment: How expert nurses use intuition. *American Journal of Nursing, 1*, 23–31.

Borysowich, C. (2006). *Constructing a weighted matrix.* http://it.toolbox.com.

Burrow, J. L., Kleindl, B., & Everard, K. E. (2007). *Business principles and management* (12th ed.). Mason, OH: Thomson South-Western.

Canadian Interprofessional Health Collaborative. (2010). *A National Interprofessional Competency Framework.* Vancouver: Canadian Interprofessional Health Collaborative.

Cioffi, J. M. (2017). Collaborative care: Using six thinking hats for decision making. *International Journal of Nursing Practice, 23* n/a. https://doi.org/10.1111/ijn.12593.

College of Nurses of Ontario. (2011). *RN and RPN practice: The client, the nurse and the environment.* Toronto, ON: Author. http://www.cno.org/learn-about-standards-guidelines/standards-and-guidelines/.

Cork, L. L. (2014). Nursing intuition as an assessment tool in predicting severity of injury in trauma patients. *Journal of Trauma Nursing, 21*, 244–252.

D'Amour, D., Ferrada-Videla, M., San Martin Rodriguez, L., & Beaulieu, M. D. (2005). The conceptual basis for interprofessional collaboration: Core concepts and theoretical frameworks [Review]. *Journal of Interprofessional Care, 19*(Suppl. 1), 116–131. https://doi.org/10.1080/13561820500082529.

De Bono, E. (2009). *Six thinking hats.* London, UK: Penguin.

Embury, D. C. (2014). Fishbone Diagram. In D. Coghlan, & M. Brydon-Miller (Eds.), *The SAGE Encyclopedia of Action Research.* London: SAGE Publications. https://doi.org/10.4135/9781446294406.

Friesen-Storms, J., Bours, G., van der Weijden, T., & Beurskens, A. (2015). Shared decision making in chronic care in the context of evidence based practice in nursing. *International Journal of Nursing Studies, 52*, 393–402.

Glaser, E. M. (1941). *An experiment in the development of critical thinking.* New York, NY: Teachers College, Columbia University.

Harvey, N., & Holmes, C. A. (2012). Nominal group technique: An effective method for obtaining group consensus. *International Journal of Nursing Practice, 18*, 188–194.

Henriksen, K., & Dayton, E. (2006). Organizational silence and hidden threats to patient safety. *Health Services Research, 41*(4, Pt2), 1539–1554.

Huitt, W. (1992). Problem solving and decision making: Consideration of individual differences using the Myers-Briggs Type Indicator. *Journal of Psychological Type, 24*, 33–44. http://www.edpsycinteractive.org/papers/prbsmbti.htm.

Jehn, K. A., Greer, L. L., Levine, S., et al. (2008). The effects of conflict types, dimensions, and emergent states on group outcomes. *Group Decision and Negotiation, 17*, 465–495. http://www.academia.edu/2094806.

Jones, B. D. (1999). Bounded rationality. *Annual Review of Political Science, 2*, 297–321.

Kaminski, J. (2012). Theory applied to informatics—Appreciative inquiry. *Canadian Journal of Nursing Informatics, 7*(1). http://cjni.net/journal/?p=1968.

Kepner, C. H., & Tregoe, B. B. (1965). *The rational manager: A systematic approach to problem solving and decision making.* New York, NY: McGraw-Hill.

Keynes, M. (2008). Making good decisions: Part 1. *Nursing Management, 14*(9), 32–34.

Khan, E. (2010). Team-based care interventions involving nurses and primary care or community pharmacists improve hypertension control. *Evidence Based Nursing, 13*, 47–48. https://doi.org/10.1186/s12872-017-0472-y.

Korte, R. F. (2003). Biases in decision making and implications for human resource development. *Advances in Developing Human Resources, 5*(4), 440–457. https://doi.org/10.1177/1523422303257287.

Kozlowski, S. W. J., & Ilgen, D. R. (2006). Enhancing the effectiveness of work groups and teams. *Psychological Science in the Public Interest, 7*(3), 78–124. https://doi.org/10.1111/j.1529-1006.2006.00030.x.

Lunenburg, F. C. (2010). The decision making process. *National Forum of Educational Administration and Supervision, 4*(1), 1–12.

MacPhee, M., Wardrop, A., & Campbell, C. (2010). Transforming work place relationships through shared decision making. *Journal of Nursing Management, 18*, 1016–1026.

McAllister, M. (2003). Doing practice differently: solution-focused nursing. *Journal of Advanced Nursing, 41*, 528–535.

Mintzberg, H. (1973). *The nature of managerial work.* New York, NY: Harper & Row.

Morgeson, F. P., DeRue, D. S., & Karam, E. P. (2010). Leadership in teams: A functional approach to understanding leadership structures and processes. *Journal of Management, 36*(1), 5–39. https://doi.org/10.1177/0149206309347376.

Nielsen, T. M. (2012). The evolving nature of work teams: Changing to meet the requirements of the future. In C. Wankel (Ed.), *21st century management: A reference handbook* (pp. 3–14). Thousand Oaks, CA: Sage. http://sk.sagepub.com/reference/management/n50.xml.

Oxford Dictionary (n.d.). Intuition. http://en.oxforddictionaries.com

Pearce, C. (2007). Ten steps to carrying out a SWOT analysis. *Nursing Management, 14*(2), 25.

Penz, K. L., & Bassendowski, S. L. (2006). Evidence-based nursing in clinical practice: Implications for nurse educators. *The Journal of Continuing Education in Nursing, 37*(6), 250–254.

Principles of Management. (2015). Minnesota: University of Minnesota. https://doi.org/10.24926/8668.1801.

Reyna, V. F., & Rivers, S. E. (2008). Current theories of risk and rational decision making. *Developmental Review, 28*(1), 1–11.

Riabacke, A. (2006). Leader or managerial decision making under risk and uncertainty. *IAENG. International Journal of Computer Science, 32*(4). http://www.iaeng.org/IJCS/issues_v32/issue_4/IJCS_32_4_12.pdf.

Sackett, D. L., Rosenberg, W. M. C., Gray, J. A. M., et al. (1996). Evidence-based practice: What it is and what it isn't. *BMJ, 312*(13), 71–72.

Scriven, M., & Paul, R. (2007). *Defining critical thinking.* http://www.criticalthinking.org/.

Simon, H. A. (1979). Rational decision making in business organizations. *The American Economic Review, 69*(4), 493–513.

Smith, A. J. (2007). Embracing intuition in nursing practice. *Alabama Nurse, 34*(3), 16–17.

Stavros, J. M., & Hinrichs, G. (2009). *The thin book of SOAR: Building strengths-based strategy.* Bend, OR: Thin Book Publishing.

Suter, E., Arndt, J., Arthur, N., et al. (2009). Role understanding and effective communication as core competencies for collaborative practice. *Journal of Interprofessional Care, 23*(1), 41–51. https://doi.org/10.1080/13561820802338579.

Syllogism. (n.d.). (In Merriam-Webster's online dictionary. http://www.merriam-webster.com/dictionary/syllogism.

Sommer, A., & Pearson, C. M. (2007). Antecedents of creative decision making in organizational crisis: A team-based simulation. *Technological Forecasting and Social Change, 74*(8), 1234–1251.

Tanner, C. A. (2006). Thinking like a nurse: A research-based model of clinical judgment in nursing. *Journal of Nursing Education, 45*(6), 204–211.

Wang, Y., & Ruhe, G. (2007). The cognitive process of decision making. *International Journal of Cognitive Informatics and Natural Intelligence, 1*(2), 73–85. http://www.ucalgary.ca/icic/files/icic/67-IJCINI-1205-DecisionMaking.pdf.

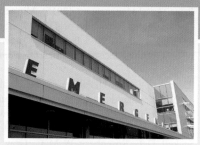
© Can Stock Photo Inc. / blondsteve

9

Health Care Organizations

Karen Spalding

Nurses need to understand the basic framework and operations of the Canadian health care system as the context for their health care organization and their own work. This chapter presents the key elements of the Canadian health care system—such as its funding structure and the organization of health care services—that affect the provision of health care services. It also considers health care organizations within their dynamic context and the primary forces that influence how they operate. Finally, this chapter explores the health human resources that sustain health care, including the education, type of practice, and scope of practice associated with key health care provider roles.

OBJECTIVES

- Describe the Canadian health care system and the five criteria established by the *Canada Health Act* for federal government financial support of health care in the provinces and territories.
- Describe the current challenges faced by the Canadian health care system.
- Identify the roles and responsibilities of the federal, provincial, and territorial governments in funding, organizing, and delivering health care services.

- Describe the types and classifications of health care services.
- Analyze health care organizations from an open-systems perspective, and describe the influence of external forces.
- Identify the education, type of practice, and scope of practice associated with key health care provider roles.

TERMS TO KNOW

Canada Health Act
primary care
primary health care (PHC)

private funding
public funding
secondary health care

social determinants of health
strength-based nursing
leadership

ⓘ A CHALLENGE

Alex, a nurse manager of an inpatient general surgery unit, was reviewing the number of planned surgeries for the next week that would lead to patient admissions onto the unit. She was very concerned as she realized in reviewing the current inpatients that the unit would be over capacity by Thursday. In addition, this forecasting did not take into account any emergency surgeries of patients admitted through the Emergency Department (ED) needing an inpatient. The ED was constantly calling her unit to take patients because patients were sometimes waiting days on stretchers in hallways and alternative spaces across the hospital (i.e., large storage rooms were being used as patient areas as were unoccupied offices). This situation was not unusual; however, the government had recently imposed stricter guidelines for hospitals to report if patients stayed in the ED for more than 24 hours. This was placing extreme pressure on their nursing colleagues in the ED as it had funding implications for the hospital overall. Therefore Alex wanted to discharge patients in their unit to support the ED.

The plan was to implement an improved process to discharge patients to home and community care, as they found that physicians had very frequently cleared the patient to leave hospital, but there was not the support they needed at home. Thus many discharges were unduly delayed, and patients were staying on the general surgery unit longer then they needed.

What would you do if you were Alex to help improve the discharge process for patients from the general surgery unit?

INTRODUCTION

Health care is one of the largest and most complex industrial and service sectors in Canada. Services are delivered by a multitude of health care organizations that differ in size, type, structure, and internal complexity. Furthermore, the funding models and legislation differs between the health care sectors, so it is important for student and registered nurses to understand what the implications of this are for how care is organized and delivered. While each organization and sector is different, all share common features: a collection of people oriented towards achieving established health care goals; work that is divided into specialized functions; and work that is coordinated to maintain the stability and continuity of the organization over time (Johns &

Saks, 2001). Understanding these features makes it possible to study the nature of the health care organization, identify its components, and determine how tasks and responsibilities are divided to provide evidence-based interventions and coordinated to achieve good patient outcomes. It is also important to know how health care organizations are affected by external forces (legislation, accreditation standards, government) and internal forces, such as input from health care providers, nurse managers, patients, and others who have a stake in the organization. These forces, along with external forces, such as government legislation and funding, together help explain why health care organizations fail or remain stable and productive.

Although many books and articles talk about "the" Canadian health care system, in fact there is not one system across the country. Rather, each province and territory in Canada is responsible for delivery of health and social care services for its citizens (Health Canada, 2018a). The organization of Canada's health care system is largely determined by the Canadian Constitution, in which roles and responsibilities are divided between the federal and provincial and territorial governments. The provincial and territorial governments have most of the responsibility for delivering health and other social services. The federal government's role in health care includes setting and administering national principles for the system under the Canada Health Act (1984), financial support to the provinces and territories, and several other functions, including funding and/or delivery of primary and supplementary services to certain groups of people. These groups include: First Nations people living on reserves; Inuit; serving members of the Canadian Forces; eligible veterans; inmates in federal penitentiaries; and some groups of refugee claimants (Health Canada, 2018b).

HISTORY OF MEDICARE

Before World War II, health care in Canada was, for the most part, privately delivered and funded. In 1947, the government of Saskatchewan introduced a province-wide universal hospital care plan. By 1950, both British Columbia and Alberta had similar plans. The federal government passed the *Hospital Insurance and Diagnostic Services Act* in 1957, which offered to reimburse, or cost share, one-half of provincial and territorial costs for specified hospital and diagnostic services. This Act provided for publicly administered universal coverage for a specific set of services under uniform terms and conditions. All provinces had implemented full insurance coverage for medically necessary hospital and physician services by 1971; this coverage is commonly referred to as Medicare.

FUNDING

From 1957 to 1977, the federal government's financial contribution in support of health care was determined as a percentage (50%) of provincial and territorial expenditure on insured hospital and physician services. In 1977, under the *Federal-Provincial Fiscal Arrangements and Established Programs Financing Act*, cost sharing was replaced with a block fund, in this case, a combination of cash payments and tax points. This new funding arrangement meant that the provincial and territorial governments had the flexibility to invest health care funding according to their needs and priorities. Federal transfers for post-secondary education were also added to the health transfer. From 1977 there have been ongoing changes to the funding formula. The most significant change arose in 1984 with the establishment of the *Canada Health Act* (CHA). This legislation replaced the federal *Hospital and Medical Insurance Acts*, and consolidated their principles ensuring all Canadians, no matter their financial circumstances, would have reasonable access to medically necessary hospital and physician services. Federal funding is transferred to the provinces and territories so that they can provide these basic services, assuming that the provinces and territories meet specific criteria and conditions. The terms and conditions the provinces and territories must adhere to to receive federal funding, are referred to as the five principles of the Canada Health Act as follows:

1. Public administration (provincial and territorial health insurance plans must be administered on a not-for-profit basis by public authorities that are accountable to the governments).
2. Comprehensive (provincial and territorial health insurance plans must cover all insured health care services, which include physician services, hospital care, and medically required dental procedures performed in a hospital).
3. Universality (all residents of a province or territory must have access to public health care insurance and insured health care services on uniform terms and conditions).
4. Portability (provinces and territories must cover insured health care services provided to their citizens when temporarily absent from their province or from Canada, and services must be uninterrupted when citizens move from one province or territory to another).
5. Accessibility (insured persons must have reasonable and uniform access to insured health care services, free of financial or other barriers). Contributions by patients through user charges or extra billing are prohibited (Health Canada, 2018b).

Over the years, other than funding, the role of the federal government in the overall design of the provincial/territorial health care "system" has eroded. The last time there was an agreement on standards or benchmarks of care was in 2004 with the Health Accord. At this time, a First Ministers' conference (ministers from each province/territory that are in charge of health) focused on developing an action plan for health system renewal, and the First Ministers agreed to work in partnership with health care providers and citizens to reform the health care system. Three years later, they passed the *2003 First Ministers' Accord on Health Care Renewal* and presented *A 10-Year Plan to Strengthen Health Care* (Motiwala et al., 2005).

As part of the renewal efforts, the Health Council of Canada was established to monitor the progress and health outcomes of these accords (Dobrow et al., 2014). Included in the 10-year plan were recommendations to decrease wait times for certain procedures; increase funds for home care, Indigenous health, and the supply of health care providers; introduce electronic health records; and develop primary care. However, the outcomes related to the Health Accord were not strictly enforced or tracked, and by the time it expired, a new federal political party (Progress Conservatives) had been elected to power, and although they adhered to the agreed funding formula, they did not engage actively with provinces or territories on health care related matters. In keeping with this attitude, in 2014 the federal government under Stephen Harper stopped funding the Health Council of Canada (Dobrow et al., 2014).

Since 2015, with Justin Trudeau's Liberals in power at the federal level, there has been direct engagement with the First Ministers, and although unable to negotiate a nationwide Health Accord, in August 2017 all provinces agreed to what they referred to as "Common Statement of Principles on Shared Health Priorities" (Health Canada, 2018c).

Even though there were separate agreements made with each province and territory, the common priorities across all jurisdictions included home and community care and mental health and addictions. For example, in February 2017, British Columbia signed on to the health care deal with the federal government with an agreement that was to provide more than $1 billion for home care and mental health. The province also received an additional $10 million in emergency management funds to help deal with BC's opioid crisis. Under the deal, Ottawa will also provide BC $1.4 billion for home care and mental health over the next 10 years. Saskatchewan signed a deal in January 2017 with the federal government where the province will receive $190.3 million for home care and $158.5 million for mental health services over the next 10 years. Nunavut, Yukon, and the Northwest Territories also signed bilateral deals with the federal government on health-care transfers.

The deal means that the territories will together get an additional $36.1 million in new financial funding for mental health and home care over the next 10 years, that began in the 2017–2018 fiscal year (Health Canada, 2018c).

Although Canada ensures that its citizens are guaranteed to receive hospital and doctor services deemed to be medically necessary, medical advances, along with consumer demands and requirements, have resulted in the need for significant health care reforms (Picard, 2017). Health care costs continue to rise, and the current state of the global economy suggests that funding health care at its present level will be difficult in the future. Public demands for better quality of care and access to care are still major concerns, especially for home and long-term care (LTC) services. For the most part, home and continuing care services are not covered by the Canada Health Act; however, all the provinces and territories provide and pay for certain home and LTC services. The success of reform efforts requires capable nurse managers and leaders who understand how their health care organization functions and how to influence others in increasing organizational effectiveness within the context not only of the organization but also within their jurisdiction.

THE CANADIAN HEALTH CARE SYSTEM

There are a number of different elements to health care systems that are important to understand to comprehend the features of the models that exist in different jurisdictions across Canada. It is therefore important to discuss what is meant by public and private and to distinguish between financing and delivery, and indicate possible combinations of these two dimensions. Different models may exist in different jurisdictions, and may vary across such services as hospital care, physician services, pharmaceuticals, diagnostic imaging, long-term care, rehabilitation, primary care, and home care.

The terms public and private apply to both how care is financed and how it is delivered, and can be divided as follows. *Public* can refer to different levels of government, including national, provincial, regional, and local (municipal). *Private* can include: *corporate for-profit* business (which has a responsibility to maximize return to shareholders); for-profit small business (which also might include health care professional practices, such as physician or physiotherapist offices; not-for-profit (NFP) organizations (both large and small organizations, including hospitals and home care/community agencies); and individuals and their families (who may pay for and provide many services) (Evans, 1984). There is also a growing number in the quasi-public category, which are legally private, but heavily regulated, and span the boundary between public and private. This would include many of the Canadian regional authorities, such as the Local Health Integration Networks (LHINs) in Ontario.

It is also important to distinguish between how care is paid for (*financing*) and how it is *delivered*. A range of models exist, reflecting the different roles for public and private provision outlined above. The OECD identifies four main types of funding for health services, these being:

- Public payment through government taxation/general revenues.
- Public/quasi-public payment through social insurance.
- Private insurance.
- Direct out-of-pocket payments.

These different funding models reflect different philosophical and political views about which costs should be born collectively (i.e. by government) and which should be the responsibility of individuals and their families (OECD, 2015).

With respect to the delivery of services, providers may fall into a variety of these public–private categories. For example, a government-owned hospital would be classified as public delivery; this is a common model in England, Australia or Sweden. Most hospitals in Canada fall in the private, not-for-profit category as they receive funding from governments; however, they each have their own board of governors and their employees are hospital employees, not government employees. Physician offices (standalone general practitioners or specialists, such as dermatologists) in most jurisdictions across Canada are private, for-profit small businesses. Pharmaceutical companies are usually private, for-profit, investor-owned corporations, as are some home-care agencies and retirement and long-term care homes throughout Canada.

Therefore health care systems represent various combinations of public/private financing and public/private delivery (see Table 9.1). These different models of care are used not only in different jurisdictions but also across different sectors of care. For example, acute care sector hospitals in Ontario would fall within public financing and private delivery. However, for the home-care sector in Canada there are examples of public financing and public delivery (public health nurses); private financing and private insurance (recipients of nursing home care services can purchase directly with a home care agency); and public financing and private delivery (a for-profit home-care agency is contracted out to provide nursing services to individuals in their homes).

HEALTH CARE SERVICES FUNDING

Federal Funding

The federal government fulfills its fiscal responsibility to the provinces and territories mainly through transfer

TABLE 9.1   Classifications of Health Systems

	Public Financing	Private Financing
Public Delivery	UK – National Health Service	User fees for government (public) services
Private Delivery	Public insurance (Medicare) (Canada)	Private Insurance (USA)

Adapted from Toth, F. (2016, May). Classification of healthcare systems: Can we go further? *Health Policy*. 120(5):535–543; Böhm, K., Schmid, A., Götze, R., Landwehr, C., Rothgang, H. (2013). Five types of OECD healthcare systems: Empirical results of a deductive classification. *Health Policy*. 113(3): 258–269.

payments. Table 9.2 shows the amount of transfer and equalization payments made from 2012 to 2019. The amount of individual transfer payments for health care services is determined by a formula that is based on the financial capacity of each jurisdiction to deliver services. Equalization payments are distributed to those provinces and territories that do not have sufficient capacity to provide necessary services. Additional federal health care allocations, such as funding to reduce wait times, or to increase home-care services, are made at the discretion of the federal government.

In addition, the federal government directly funds services to groups such as First Nations and Inuit, military personnel, prisoners in federal penitentiaries, and recent immigrants (Health Canada, 2018b). It also has criminal law powers to protect Canadians through control of possible hazards from products or materials, such as food and drugs, controlled substances, medical devices, industrial and consumer products, cosmetics, tobacco, radiation-emitting devices, and pest control products (Public Health Agency of Canada, 2018).

Provincial and Territorial Funding

Health care spending represents the largest single budget item for provincial and territorial governments

TABLE 9.2   Federal Support to Provinces and Territories: Major Transfers, 2014–2019

	2014–2015	2015–2016	2016–2017	2017–2018	2018–2019
(IN $ MILLIONS)					
Canada Health Transfer	32 114	34 026	36 068	37 150	38 584
Canada Social Transfer	12 582	12 959	13 348	13 748	14 161
Equalization Payments	16 669	17 341	17 880	18 254	18 958
Per capita allocation (In dollars)	1832	1900	1959	1988	2031

Adapted from Department of Finance Canada. (2018). Federal support to province and territories. Retrieved from http://www.fin.gc.ca/fedprov/mtp-eng.asp. Reproduced with the permission of the Minister of Finance Canada, 2014.

and is therefore a constant concern. Spending on health care varies across jurisdictions in Canada, but on average, provinces spend approximately 38% of their total budgets on healthcare (Canadian Institute for Health Information [CIHI], 2018). Figure 9.1 provides a snapshot of how each province and territory compares in their health care spending. All governments make efforts to contain health care costs while maintaining quality care. Total health spending was forecast to reach $6,604 per Canadian in 2017, almost $200 more per person than in 2016 ($6,419). Total health expenditure per person was expected to vary across the country from $7,378 in Newfoundland and Labrador and $7,329 in Alberta, to $6,367 in Ontario, and $6,321 in British Columbia. Internationally, Canada's health spending per person in 2015 (CA$5,782) was similar to spending in France (CA$5,677), Australia (CA$5,631), and the United Kingdom (CA$5,170).

The most recent report by CIHI (2018) estimates that a total of $253.5 billion was spent on health care in Canada in 2016. This represents about 11.3% of Canada's GDP, or roughly $6,839 per Canadian. Since 1997, hospitals have accounted for the most significant share of health spending, followed by drugs and physician services. Hospitals (28.3%), drugs (15.7%), and physicians (15.1%) are expected to continue to use the largest share of health care dollars in 2018. Data show that the country's health spending was forecast to grow by almost 4.2% in 2018, a slight increase in the rate of growth compared with earlier in the decade. *National Health Expenditure Trends, 1975 to 2018* found that health costs were expected to represent 11.3% of Canada's GDP in 2018, similar to 2017 at 11.5% (CIHI, 2018).

These rising costs are important constraints on the ability of Canadian health care organizations to deliver safe and effective health services. To carry out their health care responsibilities within the mandate of the *Canada Health Act*, the provinces and territories make up the remaining health budget with revenues from taxation (Health Canada, 2018b). Since 1997, the public-sector (government) share of total health expenditures has remained relatively stable at around 70% (CIHI, 2018). The private sector has three components, the largest of which is out-of-pocket spending (15%), followed by private health insurance (12%). The public/private split has been fairly consistent since the

early 2000s, with the public-sector share of total health spending remaining relatively stable at around 70% (CIHI, 2018).

Each provincial and territorial government has its own public health insurance plan. The plan's funds are used to deliver a broad range of services, such as those in large tertiary/quaternary care health science centres; small community hospitals; drug benefits; laboratory/imaging and other diagnostic services; and the services of health care providers. Most plans also provide coverage for medications for people over 65 years of age and for people requiring social assistance.

An increase in private funding in the Canadian health care system has raised concerns that this will compromise the public health care system. The growth rates of private health expenditure has been fairly consistent since the early 2000, with the public-sector share of total health spending remaining relatively stable at around 70%. In 2000, 2005, and 2015, the split was 70% public and 30% private. Only in 2010 was it slightly different at 71% and 29% (CIHI, 2018). Private funding primarily comprises out-of-pocket payments and private health insurance payments. Other industrialized countries also have a mix of public–private health funding (Table 9.3). The *Canada Health Act* does not specifically prohibit private funding, but some provinces prevent private insurance plans from covering services that are identified in the *Canada Health Act* as medically necessary.

ORGANIZING THE DELIVERY OF CARE

As well as allocating funds to meet health care needs, the provinces and territories are responsible for hospital care and the primary care provided by physicians, nurses, physiotherapists, and allied professionals (Health Canada, 2018c). The health care system consists of many services and health care providers, including hospitals, ambulatory clinics, and community health programs, such as home care, mental health care services, and public health programs. It also includes many support services, such as diagnostic services, regulatory bodies, and professional associations. Each province has legislation that regulates the health professions. Most of these health professionals are self-regulated by governing bodies, often called professional colleges or boards. These governing bodies are responsible for registration, protection of the public, complaints, and maintenance

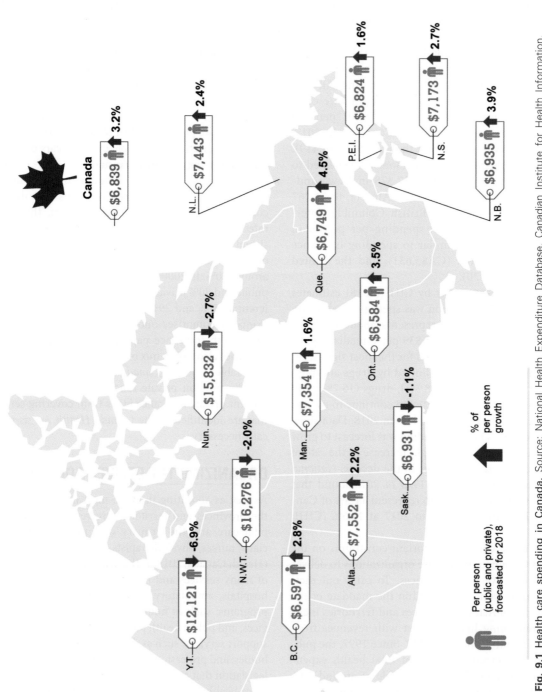

Fig. 9.1 Health care spending in Canada. Source: National Health Expenditure Database, Canadian Institute for Health Information. Retrieved from https://www.cihi.ca/sites/default/files/document/nhex-trends-narrative-report_2016_en.pdf

TABLE 9.3   Health Care Spending in OECD Countries Ranked by GDP, 2015

Country	Per Capita ($US)	% of GDP	% Public Spending	% Private Spending
United States	11 916	16.9	51	49
Netherlands	6639	10.7	81	19
France	5677	11.1	79	21
Germany	6709	11.2	84	16
Canada	5782	10.4	70	30
Sweden	6601	11.0	70	16
New Zealand	4443	9.3	80	20
United Kingdom	5170	9.9	80	20
Australia	5631	9.4	67	33
OECD Average	4826	8.9	72	28

Adapted from Canadian Institute for Health Information. (2017). *National health expenditure trends 1975 to 2013.* Ottawa, ON: Author. Retrieved from https://www.cihi.ca/en/how-does-canadas-health-spending-compare-internationally

of competency that is based on the provincial legislation. The precise professions that are registered vary by province. For example, in Ontario, traditional Chinese medicine practitioners and acupuncturists are regulated, but this is not the case in Alberta or Saskatchewan. Paramedics are a regulated profession in Alberta but not in Ontario, British Columbia, or Manitoba. Ontario's Regulated Health Professionals Act (RHPA), 1981, sets a framework that regulates the scope of practice of 29 colleges governing health professions in Ontario. In Nova Scotia, under the Nova Scotia Regulated Health Professions network (http://www.nsrhpn.ca/), there are 22 regulated professions. Alberta has 31 regulated health professions. The majority of these are regulated by self-governing colleges under Alberta's Health Professions Act (HPA).

Figure 9.2 illustrates how the health care system is organized in Canada. In such a complex system, management and leadership skills are needed to motivate people, coordinate work, and produce quality outcomes. Governments accomplish these and other objectives by sharing responsibility with regulatory bodies, such

as **Regional Health Authorities (RHAs)** that oversee health care delivery, and self-regulatory authorities called "colleges" or "boards" that regulate health care provider groups.

A variety of trained professionals are required to deliver health care services. Some, but not all, are health professionals. The Canadian Institute for Health Information (CIHI) tracks data for many health occupations, including their level of education, employment rates, and demographics such as age and years in practice. They devote particular attention to physicians, nurses, and (since 2005) such professionals as occupational therapists, pharmacists, physiotherapists, medical radiation technologists, and medical laboratory technologists.

APPROACHES TO DELIVERING CARE

Regional Health Administration

The equitable and efficient allocation of health care resources dominates public discussion in many Western countries. In the late 1980s, most provincial health ministries created regional branches based on geographical boundaries called *health regions* and made them responsible for the local delivery and administration of health care services. Health regions offer some localized control over health care services delivery. Health ministries also determined that delegating provincial responsibilities for service delivery to regional bodies would be useful in containing costs and improving efficiencies in health care delivery while being responsive to local needs. Provinces have revised the size and structures of health regions over time, and these regions may have different names from one province to another. For example, in many provinces, health regions are called *Regional Health Authorities*, but Ontario has a system of *Local Health Integration Networks* (LHINs) that plan, integrate, and fund health care services. Health regions are responsible for governing, planning, prioritizing, budgeting, and allocating funds to health agencies and delivering and managing health care services within predetermined regional areas (Ronson, 2006). The regional health administration system is consistent with population health and wellness approaches to health care and reflects the primary care goals of reducing exclusion and social disparities, organizing health care services around people's needs, integrating health into all

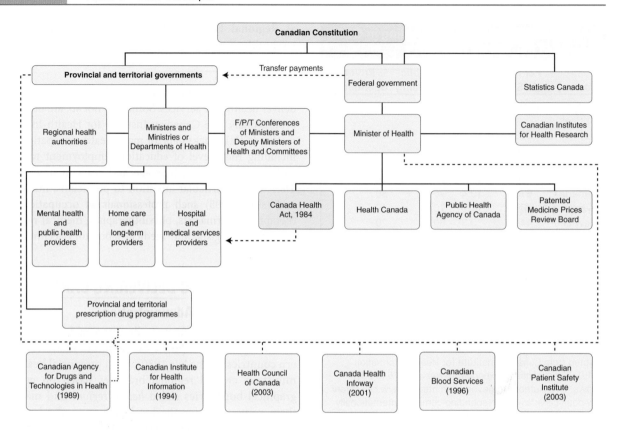

Note: Solid lines represent direct relationships of accountability while dotted lines indicate more indirect or arm's length relationships.
Fig. 9.2 Organization of the Canadian health care system. *F*, federal; *P*, provincial; *T*, territorial.

sectors, pursuing collaborative models of policy dialogue, and increasing stakeholder participation (World Health Organization, 2014a).

Typically, health regions are governed by a board made up of local health care providers and community stakeholders. The idea behind regionalization of health care is based on the idea that by devolving resource allocation decisions to local entities they will be more effective and efficient, since their mandate is to understand the specific region's health care needs. For example, British Columbia had five geographically based Regional Health Authorities. However, given the unique health needs of their First Nations people, they added a sixth regional authority.

BC's First Nations Health Authority is the first province-wide health authority of its kind in Canada. In 2013, the First Nations Health Authority assumed the programs, services, and responsibilities formerly handled by Health Canada's First Nations Inuit Health Branch—Pacific Region. The First Nations Health Authority is part of a unique health governance structure that includes political representation and advocacy through the First Nations Health Council, and technical support and capacity development through the First Nations Health Directors Association. In Ontario, LHINs have slightly less authority for decision making than do other health region organizations in other provinces. This is because Ontario is the only province in which hospitals continue to have their own boards and therefore are private, albeit not-for-profit, entities.

Over time, the challenges in organizing and funding the delivery of health services have motivated some provinces to reduce the number of health regions and contemplate and trial other cost-saving initiatives. For example PEI and Alberta originally split their provinces into multiple regional authorities; however, as of 2018, each province only has one region. Efforts to reduce health care services to regions may be divisive if they are perceived to distribute funds unfairly or inequitably among similar regions within a province. Drawing similarities across health regions is also considerably complex because of the vast geographical areas and the diversity of populations. Knowledge and skill will be needed to determine the metrics to use in determining the right mix of services and providers required for the populations in each region and/or province.

TYPES AND CLASSIFICATIONS OF HEALTH CARE SERVICES

Health care delivery can be classified in various ways. Conceptual divisions that consider the sequencing and classification of health care services offer an understanding of the roles of different organizations, the way in which they relate to one another, and the overall provision of health care services. In Canada, health care services are classified based on the sequence in which they are delivered:

1. Primary health care services (what happens first)
2. Secondary health care services (what happens next)
3. Additional (supplementary) health care services (Health Canada, 2018a).

These health care services can be further classified based on types of care:

1. Public health services/prevention services
2. Community care services
3. Hospital care services.

Community care services are further divided into residential care, community mental health and addiction services, and home care services. Hospital care services are further divided into primary, secondary, tertiary, and quaternary health care. Table 9.4 presents the basic framework of health care services and service classifications in Canada. The distinction between types of services is not always clear-cut, especially from the patients' or users' perspective, but the framework presented in Table 9.4 can serve as a guide to health care delivery in Canada.

Basic Framework of Services
Primary Health Care Services

Terminology related to primary health care can be confusing. In Health Canada documents, as in Table 9.4, *primary health care services* are generally the first point of contact for individuals with the system; at this point of care, health care providers also help coordinate health care services and ensure continuity of care for patients across the system (Health Canada, 2011). However, this terminology has not been universally adopted. Primary health care (PHC) and primary care are often used interchangeably, but they are distinct concepts. *Primary care* is the first point of entry in the Canadian health care system and deals with the majority of health issues. Primary care comprises the assessment, diagnosis, and treatment of an individual by a general practitioner or family physician, nurse practitioner, or other authorized health care provider; it is considered part of the

TABLE 9.4 Types and Classifications of Health Care Services	
Type	**Description**
Basic Framework of Services	
Primary health care services	• First-contact services for routine problems and emergencies • Provision of coordination of patients' health care services to ensure continuity of care and ease of access across the health care system • Holistic approach to health promotion and disease prevention
Secondary health care services	• Referrals to specialized care in hospitals, long-term care, or in the community • Services that may be provided in the home, community, or institution (mostly long-term care facilities)
Additional health care services	• Prescription drugs, dental care, vision care, and other therapies not usually covered by public health insurance • Sometimes part of first-contact services, sometimes part of secondary services
Service Classifications	
Public health services/ prevention services	• Service to individuals and communities to promote health, prevent disease, and control infectious diseases

Continued

TABLE 9.4   Types and Classifications of Health Care Services—cont'd

Type	Description
Community Care Services	
Continuing care and rehabilitation	• Complex continuing care (CCC) and rehabilitation services care for ill, medically complex, and disabled patients • Services that are sometimes attached to or within close proximity of hospital services
Residential care	• Care provided in residential settings (e.g., long-term care, supportive housing, and retirement homes)
Community mental health and addiction services	• Care provided in nonacute care institutions, community settings, and group homes to promote health, support recovery from mental illness, and provide programs and resources
Home care services	• Care delivered in community settings, including private homes, to people needing health care supports to remain independent, and community dwelling • Sometimes used temporarily to aid patients with acute and chronic conditions recovering at home • Mental health services often have a component of home care services for those living in private homes • Palliative care services or end-of-life health services that are provided at home
Hospital care services (primary, secondary, tertiary, quaternary care)	• Primary care: generally offered by a general practitioner, family physician, or nurse practitioner outside of hospital • Secondary care: the starting point of hospital inpatient care, it is treatment by specialists to whom a patient has been referred by a primary care provider or been admitted through urgent care services located at the hospital (typically community hospitals) • Tertiary care (or tertiary hospital): highly specialized services (e.g., academic teaching hospital) • Quaternary care: centres for treatment of extremely rare medical conditions (generally part of a large, tertiary care hospital)
Ambulatory care	• Care provided to outpatients, ranging from primary care to urgent care in clinics or emergency departments • Care provided by hospitals for special health care needs that cannot easily be offered through home care services; patients do not stay at the hospital overnight
Emergency care	• Treatment of urgent to life-threatening problems
Acute care	• Treatment for a disease or severe episode of illness or surgery for a short period of time
Specialized services	• Treatment for trauma, specified injuries, joint replacements, organ replacements • The classification often used to help monitor service provision goals

Based on Canadian Institute for Health Information. (2014). Information about health care. Health Canada. (2011). Canada's health care system. Retrieved from https://www.canada.ca/en/health-canada/services/canada-health-care-system.html

larger concept of primary health care. This year marks the 40th anniversary of the Declaration of Alma-Ata, which was adopted at the International Conference of Primary Care in 1978. According to the World Health Organization (WHO, 1978), *primary health care* is a community-based health care service philosophy that is focused on illness prevention, health promotion, treatment, rehabilitation, and identification of people at risk. Through access to resources and education, people

are empowered to be responsible, self-reliant, and participate in their health care. Health care services are provided by teams of health care providers (e.g., physicians, nurses, midwives, other practitioners, community members) close to where people live and work. Practical, affordable, scientifically sound methods and technologies are encouraged to maintain quality care and manage costs (Canadian Nurses Association [CNA], 2015). "Primary health care is a philosophy and approach that is integral to improving the health of all Canadians and the effectiveness of health service delivery in all care settings. PHC focuses on the way services are delivered and puts the people who receive those services at the centre of care" (CNA, 2015). The essential principles of PHC are set out in the WHO's Declaration of Alma-Ata.

Secondary Health Care Services

Secondary health care services take place after the initial patient contact with primary health care services. For example, a patient may be referred for specialized care to a hospital or other facility. Secondary health care services can also be provided in the home, community (e.g., community clinics), or long-term care or chronic care facility. Referrals to this type of care can be made by primary health care providers, community-based health organizations, families, and patients themselves (Health Canada, 2011). The "secondary" in *secondary health care services* refers only to the timing and referral of these services after primary health care services have occurred.

Additional Health Care Services

Additional health care services are not usually covered by public health insurance. For example, prescription medications (with some exceptions), dental care, vision care, and acupuncture therapies are not usually covered by public health insurance. Typically, supplemental health insurance (available from some employers) or private purchases are used to cover such costs. Moreover, the escalating costs of drugs has led a number of governments to decide to subsidize catastrophic drug coverage and engage in deliberations with pharmaceutical corporations on cost control.

Service Classifications
Public Health Services/Prevention Services

The mandate of the Public Health Agency of Canada is to: promote health; prevent and control chronic diseases and injuries; prevent and control infectious diseases; prepare for and respond to public health emergencies; serve as a central point for sharing Canada's expertise with the rest of the world; apply international research and development to Canada's public health programs; and strengthen intergovernmental collaboration on public health and facilitate national approaches to public health policy and planning (Public Health Agency of Canada [PHAC], 2011). While predominantly funded by the federal government in the past, the costs and responsibilities for public health services are now shared among all levels of government. In Ontario, for example, much of the funding for public health comes from provincial and municipal governments. The public health system encourages good health in Canadians by helping prevent injuries and chronic diseases, promoting a healthy lifestyle, and preventing the spread of infectious diseases. Public health nurses and community nurses take on a wide range of educational and support roles in the community, manage communicable diseases in the community, and are among the first responders to public health crises.

Home and Community Care Services

Home and community care services include a large range of services delivered in private homes, long-term residential care settings, retirement communities, and community clinics, excluding those services related to public health and prevention services. The Canadian Home Care Association (CHCA, 2013, p. xi) definition of home care is used by most of the provincial and territorial home care programs although the scope of services that are publicly funded varies by each province. The CHCA defines home care as "an array of services for people of all ages, provided in the home and community setting, that encompasses health promotion and teaching, curative intervention, end-of-life care, rehabilitation, support and maintenance, social adaptation and integration, and support for family caregivers" (CHCA, 2013, p. xi). Community care services include continuing care and rehabilitation services for individuals with medically complex conditions or disabilities. These services assist people who have chronic and acute illnesses receive the care they need in their home or community. Home and community care may include nursing care; personal care, such as bathing and foot care; home support, such as meal preparation; and in-home respite care, that is, caring for someone while family members have a rest.

Long-term care includes the care provided in nursing homes, personal care facilities, and assisted-living arrangements. Many long-term care facilities are privately owned, and some receive public funding for certain care services. For example, provincial and territorial plans usually cover the costs of the medical services provided in long-term care facilities, while individuals remain responsible for their room and board costs (in some cases, individuals receive subsidies for room and board) (Government of Canada, 2018). The operation of long-term care facilities is governed by provincial or territorial legislation.

Community care services are delivered by independently practising health care providers, professional groups, multidisciplinary teams, and private for-profit and not-for-profit organizations. The regional authorities in each jurisdiction determine the eligibility and processes for assessing an individual's need for home care. Because services in the community are outside the CHA, citizens have a legal right to be assessed; however, there is no legislated guarantee that they will be provided with publicly funded home care services. Therefore the level and type of services provided in home and community not only vary by province and territory; they also vary within each jurisdiction (CHCA, 2013). The roles for nurses in home and community care are very diverse, ranging from providing direct patient care to managing a team of providers case coordination or running home care agencies. Home service coordinators also manage long-term care placements for those deemed unable to return to their own home for care. Most community care case managers are nurses, but other health care providers in these roles include social workers, physiotherapists, and occupational therapists. Mental health services are provided in the community by case managers, independently practising health care providers, or multidisciplinary teams that include physicians, psychiatrists, nurses, psychologists, social workers, recreational and occupational therapists, and other support staff. Clinics and special programs for addictions are available throughout Canada.

Hospital Care Services

Hospitals play a major role in the delivery of acute health care services. "Hospital services" are outlined in the *Canada Health Act* and include the following:

1. Standard or public ward accommodation and meals.
2. Nursing service.
3. Diagnostic procedures, such as blood tests and X-rays.
4. The administration of medications.
5. The use of operating rooms, case rooms, and anaesthetic facilities.

Hospitals that are described as private, not-for-profit entities receive public funds for their services. Some hospitals are governed by boards that make decisions about the hospital's operations and its priorities, but increasingly this decision-making responsibility is being delegated to Regional Health Authorities (see above; Ontario has standalone hospitals remaining). Provincial and territorial governments have authority over the amount of public money that will be allocated to a hospital, the services that it provides, and incentives for hospitals to meet budget and quality care metrics (i.e. quality improvement plans for hospitals in Ontario are tied to salary for the hospital CEOs). Hospitals are represented by professional associations that lobby on behalf of their constituents in the best interests of their organizations and influence government health care policy.

Hospital care ranges from ambulatory to highly specialized services. Community hospitals typically provide general and comprehensive care that does not require specialists or advanced diagnostic and treatment facilities. Tertiary hospitals provide acute and complex care, such as consultation, diagnostics, intensive care, and emergency care to patients who are referred to them. In larger centres, tertiary hospitals may form networks. Hospital stays are usually short, but treatment may be transferred to home care. Highly specialized care (quaternary care) is provided in Academic Health Science Network hospitals in urban settings or specialized and specialized units in other health centres.

> **EXERCISE 9.1** Visit the Ministry of Health websites for two provinces and/or territories and compare their organizational structure related to health regions/authorities. What types of services and which professions are included within the scope of the health regions and which are not included? What are the expectations of the organizations and professionals with regard to yearly reporting to their local regional board related to funding, quality, and outcomes?

A THEORETICAL PERSPECTIVE

Strengths-Based Leadership

As discussed in this chapter, the future of the health care system includes focuses on health promotion, primary care, and community-based home care, with hospitals still being a core pillar of the health care system, but not its primary service (Institute of Medicine, 2012). In addition, there is a movement towards individuals and local communities having a greater responsibility for their own health care and the related health care decisions.

Gottleib (2012) discusses key principles of nursing leadership that are founded upon the theoretical underpinnings of strengths-based nursing care. This approach is about expanding the imaginary horizons of nurse managers, nurse leaders and the nurse at the bedside.

Although not explicitly identified as strengths-based, the nursing leaders who created the magnet hospitals were in effect practising elements of strengths-based nursing leadership. Magnet hospital nursing leaders created positions and a workplace environment that gave nurses the opportunities, resources, power, and status to shape and control their own practice (Kramer et al., 2007). More recently, the concepts of empowerment and transformational leadership have some strengths-based elements as their underpinnings (Laschinger et al., 2006; White & O'Brien-Pallas, 2010).

The eight principles of strengths-based nursing leadership are:

- Principle #1: Works with the whole while appreciating the interrelationships among its parts.
- Principle #2: Recognizes the uniqueness of staff, nurse leaders, and the organization.
- Principle #3: Creates work environments that promote nurses' health and facilitate their development.
- Principle #4: Understands the significance of subjective reality and created meaning.
- Principle #5: Values self-determination.
- Principle #6: Recognizes that person and environment are integral and that nurses function best in environments where there is a "goodness of fit" that capitalizes on their strengths.
- Principle #7: Creates environments that promote learning and recognizes the importance of readiness and timing.
- Principle #8: Invests in collaborative partnerships. (Gottlieb et al., 2012, pp. 42–47)

Given the fast-paced demands of health care organizations, nursing assessments of patients are often made from a deficit model. Nurses are expected to assess the "problems" or issues and then determine appropriate nursing interventions. While determining the interventions suited to a patient, it is beneficial to identify the strengths the individual currently has and then build upon those to address the health "deficits" or "problems" the assessment brings to light. As discussed above, it has been shown that taking into account the strengths of a patient can be very beneficial to their recovery.

Reflecting on the principles of strengths-based nursing leadership and a patient you recently cared for—how would you, as a nurse/nursing student approach interactions with patients differently to ensure that you are taking a strengths-based approach?

Furthermore, when working with co-workers, challenges may arise in team-based interactions, and it is critical to step back and not just focus on all the "challenges" that a difficult situation provides. Instead it is important to determine what strengths that individual brings to your team and focus on those first rather than the negative aspects.

EXTERNAL FORCES INFLUENCING HEALTH CARE ORGANIZATIONS

Organizations are strongly influenced by many changes, events, and conditions in their surrounding environments. These external forces are typically grouped into distinct categories, such as economic, legal–political, sociocultural, accreditation, technology, professional associations and unions, and regulatory bodies. These forces affect health care organizations separately and in combination. Although an organization's internal forces interact with and influence the external environment, the effect of external forces on the organization is greater.

Legal–Political Forces

The components of the Canadian health care system are shaped primarily by public policy and therefore are heavily influenced by legal–political forces. The federal, provincial, and territorial levels of government enact laws and set policies to regulate health care delivery. These directives have a major effect on the governance of health care organizations. Provinces and territories have most authority over the organization, management, and delivery of health care. However, the *Canada Health Act* is the most influential legislation in health care. As mentioned earlier, the Act established five criteria that the provinces and territories must meet to receive federal funds for health care. These criteria encourage the provinces and territories to support and adhere to the principles of the *Canada Health Act*. Health Canada, a federal department, is responsible for administering provisions of the *Canada Health Act* and has either total or partial responsibility for other health-related acts, such as the *Controlled Drugs and Substances Act*, *Department of Health Act*, *Financial Administration Act*, and *Quarantine Act*. These Canadian statutes can be accessed at http://laws-lois.justice.gc.ca/eng/acts/.

Health Canada has a Strategic Policy Branch that plays a key role in health policy, communications, and consultations. It includes the Health Care Policy Directorate and the Office of Nursing Policy. The Health Care Policy Directorate is responsible for improving the access, quality, and integration of health care services to better meet the health needs of Canadians, wherever they live or whatever their financial circumstances. This oversight ensures that the *Canada Health Act* will be implemented as it was intended. The Office of Nursing Policy was created in 1999 with the intent of strengthening the focus of nursing issues within Health Canada and provides advice on the nursing perspectives of policies, issues, and programs. It works closely with the nursing community to fulfill its role through liaison with provincial/territorial level nursing officers and relevant national nursing associations, such as the Canadian Nurses Association. The Office of Nursing Policy has been a partner in the development of national policies, such as healthy workplaces and the sustainability of the health care system.

Economic Forces

Scarce resources, increasing costs, a variable economy, an anticipated increase in the number of older adults who will require care, and pace of technological change (requiring substantial investments) place considerable strain on the Canadian health care system (Health Canada, 2015). Since 1997, hospitals have accounted for the most significant share of health spending, followed by drugs and physician services. Hospitals (28.3%), drugs (15.7%), and physicians (15.1%) are expected to continue to account for the largest shares of health dollars (close to 60% of total health spending). Over the past couple of years, the pace of drug spending growth has increased. Drug expenditures grew by approximately 4.2% in 2018. Spending on hospitals in 2018 will grow by approximately 4%, while physician spending growth will be at 4.1%. It is anticipated that, overall, health expenditure will represent 11.3% of Canada's gross domestic product in 2018. The trend over the last 40-plus years shows that when there is economic growth, there is more health care spending (CIHI, 2018).

Hospitals have been associated with high costs and inefficient management, and recent years have seen most hospitals go through processes such as LEAN to improve efficiencies. Work inefficiency has been linked to poor quality of care and high costs. Integrated health care systems (Health Canada, 2011) and interprofessional clinical teams (Reeves et al., 2017) are viewed as solutions to rationalizing health care costs and improving patient outcomes in hospitals. Strengthening primary health care is a proposed solution for controlling costs while improving access to community-based care. By focusing on chronic disease prevention and health promotion, the goal is to reduce chronic diseases, assist people to better manage their health, and avoid hospitalization for conditions that can be managed through community-based care.

Sociocultural Forces

Sociocultural forces—such as customs, values, beliefs, education, level of income, and patterns of behaviour—influence lifestyle and well-being. Attitudes towards health and patterns of accessing health care may be shaped by these factors. For example, compared with affluent people, those of lower socioeconomic status are more likely to have poor health and to require more care. In 2005, WHO identified the **social determinants of health**, which are the conditions in which people are born, live, and work; these conditions are shaped by economics, social policies, and politics. According to WHO (2014b), "the social determinants of health are mostly responsible for health inequities." The social determinants of health are listed in Box 9.1. In 2013, the Canadian Nurses Association (CNA) published a position paper confirming that nurses have an integral role in acting on all the social determinants of health. Social determinants of health involve both macro economic policies and broad social agendas of government. Part of the role of nurses is to influence these agendas through advocacy and political action. Nurse managers and leaders also need to consider how the social determinants of health affect the patient population in their health care organizations to best facilitate organizational planning and operations.

Accreditation

Many health care organizations participate in accreditation, which is "a process of assessing health services against standards, to identify what is being done well and what needs to be improved" (Accreditation Canada, 2013). The accreditation process is ongoing and involves the periodic evaluation of the extent to which

BOX 9.1   Social Determinants of Health

Determinants of health are the broad range of personal, social, economic, and environmental factors that determine individual and population health. The main determinants of health include:

1. Income and social status.
2. Employment and working conditions.
3. Education and literacy.
4. Childhood experiences.
5. Physical environments.
6. Social supports and coping skills.
7. Healthy behaviours.
8. Access to health services.
9. Biology and genetic endowment.
10. Gender.
11. Culture.

the organization is meeting the set standards. Accreditation evaluations by external reviewers (surveyors) often require accredited hospitals and other accredited health care organizations to implement changes. Thus for organizations seeking to maintain accreditation, the need to achieve the minimum standards set for accreditation effectively becomes an external force for change. Chapter 22 provides more details on accreditation.

ISO international standards (http://www.iso.org) may also apply to select ancillary and supply organizations in the health care sector.

Technology

In the health care field, technological advances can influence the ability of health care providers to improve clinical practice and communication (Naylor, 2017). They are also essential to improving quality of life and life expectancy (see also Chapter 13). Consider the advances made in joint replacements, diagnostic imaging, and coronary procedures as examples. Some might argue that these innovations are not cost effective and that their costs will likely increase in the future because of the demands of a large, aging population. Less expensive and effective innovations may reduce costs in the short term, but as the population of older adults grows, the high demand for these innovations will increase and so too will their costs.

Information technology, now regarded as an essential investment for health care delivery, has the capacity to improve the efficiency of work processes in health care organizations. Electronic health records, for example, can improve the accuracy of information and accelerate the flow of a patient's information to all those who are directly involved in the patient's care (Lee et al., 2017). Manual errors, such as the duplication of tests, and errors in recording, can be reduced. Ordering and dispensing medications can be streamlined and controlled. Tracking systems can be used for storage and retrieval of information that can be recalled for treatment and research purposes. Videoconferencing networks, such as the Ontario Telestroke Program, facilitate emergency neurological consultations and provide timely access for patients in areas that do not have access to specialists.

In Canada, the drive to implement electronic health records (EHR) and other health information technology as widely as possible has been strong. The implementation of EHRs requires skilled leadership and management to negotiate best uses. Canada Health Infoway was established in 2001 as a not-for-profit organization funded by the federal government to work with health care organizations and others to foster and "accelerate the development, adoption and effective use of digital health innovations across Canada . . . [to] help deliver better quality and access to care and more efficient delivery of health services for patients and clinicians" (Canada Health Infoway, 2014, p. 1). Early stages of development will require training and vigilance in developing this technological system.

> **EXERCISE 9.2** Identify sociocultural patient-care needs that you have observed in health care organizations. Give examples to show what you would do to address these needs.

Professional Associations and Unions

Professional associations are not-for-profit, voluntary organizations that act in the interests of their members and their patients (see Chapters 7, 12, 19, and 20). They promote the advancement of the discipline by facilitating continuing education and research; mentoring in career development; advocating on issues relevant to the discipline; promoting interaction among members through conferences and networking; and providing access to personal or career-related benefits. Unions are not-for-profit organizations that have significant influence on the organization of health human resources (the labour force) in health care. Those employed in a position covered by a collective agreement are normally required to join the union and contribute financially to union operations through the payment of union fees. Like professional associations, union organizations also support advancement of the nursing discipline, continuing education, research, mentorship, advocacy, healthy work environments, and networking. In Canadian health care organizations, professional associations and unions have a major influence on policymaking, organizational structures, work, and professional practices that affect health care organizations.

Influence on Policy

Many health care provider associations and unions lobby governments on behalf of their disciplines and members. National organizations, such as the Canadian Medical Association and the Canadian Nurses Association, lobby governments to influence policy development or changes to advance the interests of patients, the community, and their profession. Each province and territory has its own professional health associations and regulatory bodies that may lobby parliamentary committees for changes in policy or new policy directions to improve the status of a group or deal with its issues (Chapter 21) provides a complete list of nursing regulatory bodies). The Canadian Nurses Association is a federation of provincial and territorial nursing associations, and therefore represents a national voice when seeking to influence policymakers. Similarly, unions from across the provinces and territories often have associated national federations to bring a national voice to important issues. They use a variety of media to gain support for a proposal, including press releases, position papers, campaigns, radio or television interviews, and posters. Access to politicians and government officials can be helpful to influence change. Nurses have successfully influenced policies on entry to practice, scope of practice, work environments, and health promotion initiatives. Large organizations have the ability, time, and resources to be successful in lobbying, but some issues require sustained lobbying effort over years to achieve results.

RESEARCH PERSPECTIVE

Resource: Laschinger, H. K., & Read, E. A. (2016). The effect of authentic leadership, person-job fit, and civility norms on new graduate nurses' experiences of coworker incivility and burnout. *Journal of Nursing Administration*, 46(11), 574–580.

The authors suggest that the nurse leaders who have an authentic leadership style can be key in improving the working environment for New Graduate Nurses (NGNs) as they report a better job fit and experience less workplace incivility. Research has shown that because of NGNs' inexperience and cultural acceptance of incivility in nursing, they are at a high risk of experiencing incivility from coworkers. The objective of this study was to survey NGNs across Canada to ask them about their experiences with incivility in the workplace, as well as ask about the leadership traits of their nurse managers and whether they established positive work environments. The leadership traits of an authentic leader and the importance of establishing a positive and healthy work environment are in line with the strengths-based nursing leadership principles discussed earlier in this chapter. In Laschinger's study, 993 NGNs across 10 Canadian provinces were surveyed about incivility in their workplaces as well asked about their nurse leaders' behaviours relevant to authentic leadership traits and behaviours. The authors found that new graduate nurses' perceptions of their managers' authentic leadership behaviours were positively related to person-job fit, leading to higher perceptions of civility norms in the workplace.

Implications for Practice

The authors suggested that it is important for nurse leaders to develop a strong rapport with NGNs so they can have open and honest conversations about their work-related needs and expectations. This helps build a positive work environment and helps nurse leaders understand what person-job fit means to NGNs. One strategy that nurse leaders can use is the creation of civility norms in their workplace, as this will help improve satisfaction and retention of NGNs. In addition, NGNs need to consider the manager's leadership style and workplace environment/culture in making career decisions.

The authors suggested that when leaders develop organizational structures that empower nurses to deliver optimal care, they promote a greater sense of fit between nurses' expectations of work life quality and organizational goals and processes. This greater sense of fit can create a stronger work engagement and lower burnout. Reforms in health care delivery may lead to greater empowerment of nurses.

Influence on Practice and Research

The influence of professional associations and unions on practice and research is significant. For example, the Canadian Nurses Association has a long history of providing continuing professional developmental programs to build nursing practice with the goal of sustaining excellence in all areas of nursing, including practice, education, research, policy making, and innovation. In addition specialty practice groups facilitate professional development of their members by preparing them for certification and helping them gain research skills. Members are encouraged to share their practices and research at conferences and professional gatherings. Some groups provide scholarships for graduate work, such as the Registered Nurses Foundation of Ontario (RNFOO). The Canadian Federation of Nurses Unions lobbies governments to improve all aspects of nurses' work life.

Many nonprofessional specialty organizations influence health care organizations. Not-for-profit volunteer groups run by members of the community and supported by health care providers manage organizations such as the Canadian Diabetes Association and the Heart and Stroke Foundation of Canada. These organizations raise funds to support research, education, personal care, and disease control. They also lobby governments.

> **EXERCISE 9.3** Visit the website of the nurses' association or college that licenses nurses in your province or territory. Examine the processes for licensing nurses and monitoring nursing care. What processes are in place to ensure the public's safety? What regulatory processes are in place to support the interests of the public?

Regulatory Bodies

Health care organizations are regulated and monitored by external organizations. Chapter 7 also presents some of the regulations that affect health care organizations. Most health care organizations are legally accountable to federal and provincial or territorial ministries of health and are mandated to protect the health and safety of the patients and the communities they serve. In addition, individuals who belong to professional groups, such as nurses, are accountable to the professional regulatory organizations that license and monitor them. As the number of policy-driven interventions increases in response to changing circumstances, organizations will have to become more involved with government agencies to plan, implement, and evaluate projects.

Managing regulatory changes can be challenging. As new regulations are applied to policies and practices in response to health care concerns, people often experience information overload, a steep learning curve, and, in some instances, a resistance to change. The demands on individuals will likely increase as the integration of health care providers and organizations increases.

The following examples illustrate how regulatory changes impact health care organizations.

The recent emphasis on patient safety and quality care emerged from an international concern about troubling data on medication errors, drug-resistant infections within hospitals, and other negative indicators. Canada, together with a number of other industrialized countries, instituted programs and measures to change practices within health care organizations. In Canada, two agencies were established to guide improvements in education, system innovation, communication, regulatory affairs, and research that influence improved safety practices: the Canadian Patient Safety Institute (CPSI; http://www.patientsafetyinstitute.ca) and the Institute for Safe Medication Practices (ISMP; http://www.ismp-canada.org). ISMP, CIHI, and Health Canada developed the Canadian Root Cause Analysis Framework for health care organizations to analyze contributing factors that led to a critical incident or close-call medication error. Consistent with other countries, health care organizations responded by implementing health promotion programs, such as an intensive hand-washing campaign to control the spread of infection. Cooperation and adherence with policy was encouraged, and work was monitored closely to ensure good results.

In 2010, Ontario passed the *Excellent Care for All Act* to strengthen quality care, safety, and accountability in all Ontario health care organizations. The Act requires that health care providers set up quality committees to guide and report on specific quality initiatives, prepare quality improvement plans, make results of interventions available to the public, conduct patient satisfaction surveys, and develop ways to improve public relations. The Act mandated a more rigorous approach to quality control, called quality improvement (QI). QI achieves quality through an "incremental change" to solving persistent and elusive problems in the workplace. In 2016, Ontario passed the Patients First Act, which builds upon the 2010 legislation to create a more patient-centred health care system in the province. The major change with this legislation focused on home and community care, one of the fastest growing health care sectors. The Local Health Integration Networks (the name of the health regions in Ontario) became responsible for home care and primary care planning to ensure the patients are getting better coordinated care, and the health system is more integrated and responsive to local needs.

HEALTH HUMAN RESOURCES

The large workforce that sustains health care delivery in Canada comprises many health care providers, including regulated and unregulated health care providers. The focus in this chapter is on the regulated nursing workforce. Canada's regulated nursing workforce continues to grow, but the annual growth rate from 2016 to 2017 was the slowest in 10 years. Canada experienced 0.7% growth in the regulated nursing workforce in 2017, compared with an annual growth rate of 1.3% to 2.8% over the past decade. This slowed growth is attributed to the declining number of new nursing graduates, the growing number leaving the profession late in their careers and an increase in part-time and casual positions (CIHI, 2017). In 2016, there were 421 093 regulated nurses with an active licence in Canada, and 298 743 were RNs (4832 NPs), and 116 491 LPNs (LPN here includes all practical nurses as in some provinces they are called Licensed Practical Nurses and others they are called Registered Practical Nurses, but RPN in BC, for example, stands for Registered Psychiatric Nurses) and 5859 Registered Psychiatric Nurses (CIHI, 2017). Monitoring the trend in the supply of internationally educated nurses (IENs) is another important factor in understanding changes in the supply of regulated nurses. While the proportion of IENs increased slightly from 2007 (6.7%, 23 764) to 2016 (8.1%, 33 789), the average annual growth over the same period declined to 4.0% in 2016, from a high of 8.2% in 2008. A 15-year percentage growth rate report on 16 health care provider groups (1997 to 2011) ranked the top three growth areas as social workers

(163%), dental hygienists (102%), and occupational therapists (102%); it ranked the bottom three growth areas as medical laboratory technologists (15%), registered nurses (18%), and dentists (28%) (growth rates of practical nurses and psychiatric nurses were not reported because of data variations) (CIHI, 2013a). Each health care provider group and professional designation has specific educational requirements and is associated with a type and scope of practice based on regulation. These factors influence decisions made by managers and leaders about the availability of nurses and the mix of skills required in various organizations (see Chapter 15).

Education

Most professional disciplines require a minimum of four years of undergraduate education to enter practice and some require a graduate degree (i.e. physiotherapy and occupational therapy) (CIHI, 2013a). Registered nurses require a baccalaureate degree (except in Quebec) to enter practice, and practical nurses and psychiatric nurses require a diploma to enter practice. National exams are required for all regulated nurses entering practice in Canada. Master's degrees in nursing can generally be completed in two years, and a Doctor of Philosophy (PhD) in nursing can generally be completed in four to six years. A master's degree for entry to practice as a nurse practitioner is not required in most, but not every province or territory. The number of nurse practitioners grew by 96% between 2008 and 2012 and reached a total of 3286 (CIHI, 2013b).

Type of Practice

Health care in Canada has traditionally focused on episodic and responsive primary care delivery models, with a focus on hospitals (Health Canada, 2011). However, with changing demographics and the focus on finding sustainable solutions to maintaining a top-rated health care system shifting to more distributed, community-based care, health promotion and prevention are modifying the emphasis on types of health care provider practices (Health Canada, 2011). Nurses practise in most areas of health care, at different levels of care, as generalists and specialists, and along the full continuum of care. Most nurses are employed by organizations, but nurse practitioners and some specialty nurses may maintain independent practices. Funding cuts in the past decade have influenced the ratio of regulated nursing staff to unregulated staff assisting in the delivery of nursing services, which has raised concerns among nurses about the quality of care and safety of the work environment in which they work.

Scope of Practice

Expanding the scope of practice for nurses is expected to alleviate the costs of delivering care, improve access to care, and increase work efficiency. In Canada, unregulated health care providers have been assigned some traditional nurse tasks, such as administering routine medication and obtaining routine vital signs. Additionally, the roles and responsibilities of licensed practical nurses (LPNs) and registered practical nurses (RPNs) have expanded to help meet the needs of nursing staff and cost management. LPNs and RPNs are practical nurses that have the same scope of practice however, their title changes depending on the province. For example Efforts continue within health care organizations to best match or rationalize qualifications and competencies to essential health provision tasks. New roles, such as physician's assistant, navigator in case management, and program manager have also been introduced. Several provinces and territories have expanded the scope of practice for a number of health care providers; for example, in some jurisdictions, nurse practitioners are authorized to set broken bones, dentists can write prescriptions, pharmacists can write refills for medications, give flu vaccinations and physiotherapists can order X-rays and treat injuries. Fricke (2005) provided a rationale for extending physiotherapy into a primary care role as first contact or consultant for musculoskeletal conditions. A study of the effectiveness of advanced practice nurses in long-term care has shown to contribute to staff skill development and fewer individuals being transferred from long-term care homes to acute care hospital emergency departments (Klassen et al., 2009). Leaders will have roles in both influencing and responding to changing landscapes around scope of practice in health care providers.

> **EXERCISE 9.4** Ask a public health nurse and a community nurse who provide direct patient care about their roles. How do their roles differ?

CONCLUSION

Knowledge of the contexts in which health care organizations operate is important to understanding the potential effects of various forces on organizational goal achievement. External forces such as legal–political, economic, sociocultural, accreditation, technology, professional associations and unions, and regulatory bodies will continue to shape health care delivery in Canada. The key principles of the *Canada Health Act*, continued emphasis on advancing reform in primary health care access, and emphasis on patient safety, patient engagement and quality improvement remain paramount. Nurses represent a significant portion of the health human resources necessary for health care organizations to reach their goals, and all nurses—whether in formalized leadership roles or not—benefit from an increased understanding of the context in which health care organizations operate. With this knowledge, nurses can better understand organizational structures, planning, operations, and responses to change as organizations attempt to achieve their goals. Savvy nurse managers and leaders assess the internal and external forces that influence their health care organization when planning and before acting.

❓ A SOLUTION

Alex found that many patients remained in the emergency department after their medical issues were resolved because of emotional or mental health issues. Therefore he contacted the Mental Health Assessment Group to get their help in prioritizing these patients' management and discharge. He also found that a number of patients were waiting for nursing, physiotherapy, and other support staff services to coordinate plans for discharge. Alex also alerted administration about the need for a more rapid patient assessment and management plan. Often patients await consultation with physicians who are otherwise occupied with other patients. Alex raised the problematic emergency department overcrowding issue with the physicians and asked for their help in accelerating patient discharge.

Would these solutions work for you? Why or why not?

THE EVIDENCE

A study by Edwards et al. (2007) set out to describe the impact of implementing six nursing Best Practice Guidelines (BPGs) on nurses' familiarity with patient referral resources and referral practices.

Although referring patients to community care services is important for optimum continuity of care, referrals between hospital and community sectors are often problematic. A pre- and post-study design was used. For each BPG topic, referral resources were identified. Information about these resources was presented at education sessions for nurses. Pre- and post-questionnaires were completed by a random sample of 257 nurses at seven hospitals, two home visiting nursing services, and one public health unit. Average response rates for pre- and post-implementation questionnaires were 71% and 54%, respectively. Chart audits were completed for three BPGs (n = 421 pre- and 332 post-implementation). Post-hospital discharge patient interviews were conducted for four BPGs (n = 152 pre- and 124 post-implementation). Statistically significant increases occurred in nurses' familiarity with resources for all BPGs, and they self-reported referrals to specific services for three guidelines. Higher rates of referrals were observed for services that were part of the organization where the nurses worked. There was almost a complete lack of referrals to Internet sources. No significant differences between pre- and post-implementation referral rates were observed in the chart documentation or in patients' reports of referrals. Implementing nursing BPGs, which included recommendations on patient referrals, produced mixed results. Nurses' familiarity with referral resources does not necessarily change their referral practices. Nurses can play a vital role in initiating and supporting appropriate patient referrals. BPGs should include specific recommendations on effective referral processes, and this information should be tailored to the community setting where implementation occurs.

NEED TO KNOW NOW

- Understand that the Canadian health care system faces ongoing challenges.
- Know the role of federal and provincial or territorial governments in funding, organizing, and delivering care.
- Know the role of Regional Health Authorities and public–private partnerships.
- Be able to describe the types and classifications of health care services.
- Identify the trends and impact of health human resources on health care organizations.

CHAPTER CHECKLIST

- The health care organization, related governmental structures, and funding arrangements that support Canadian health care services are key to understanding health care organizations in their contexts.
- According to the *Canada Health Act*, to qualify for federal health care funding, provinces and territories must meet five criteria:
  - Public administration
  - Comprehensiveness
  - Universal coverage
  - Portability
  - Accessible
- Canadian health care is funded through federal taxation and provincial or territorial taxation, with most revenue coming from income taxes and consumption taxes.
- Contemporary health care organizations have adopted a more flexible, responsive, team-oriented approach to management, consistent with the principles of open-systems theory.
- As part of health care reform, most provincial health ministries have delegated the responsibility for the delivery and administration of health services to Regional Health Authorities.
- Health care services in Canada can be divided into a framework based on the sequence of access: primary care services, secondary care services, additional health care services:

- Primary health care services are first-contact services for routine problems and emergencies. They are also the point of referral and coordination of patient care through the continuum of care. Primary care and primary health care are distinct. *Primary care* is the first point of contact with a general practitioner, and *primary health care* is a community-based health care service philosophy that is focused on illness prevention, health promotion, treatment, rehabilitation, and identification of people at risk.
- Secondary health care services take place after the initial patient contact with primary health care services. The primary care practitioner refers the patient to specialized care, which may be provided in a hospital, the home, community, or long-term care or chronic care facility.
- Additional health care services are those services not usually covered by public health insurance (e.g., prescription medications [with some exceptions], dental care, and vision care).

- Health care services can also be classified by type of service:
  - Public health services/prevention services
  - Community care services
  - Continuing care and rehabilitation
    - Residential care
    - Community mental health and addiction services
  - Home care services
  - Hospital care services (primary, secondary, tertiary, quaternary)
  - Ambulatory care
  - Emergency care
  - Acute care
  - Specialized services
- Health human resources represent a mix of regulated and unregulated health care providers. Nurse shortages, the educational requirements of nurses, and type and scope of practice affect health care organization performance.

TIPS FOR NURSE MANAGERS AND LEADERS

- Understand the contexts and large organizational frameworks in which health care organizations work to better understand the influences that act upon health care organizations and are critical to effective organizational leadership and management.
- Understand that nurses represent a significant portion of the health human resources necessary for health care organizations to reach their goals. All

nurses, whether leaders or followers, benefit from an increased understanding of the contexts in which health care organizations operate.
- Research new health care delivery models, such as integrated primary care, to continually acquire new knowledge and skills in leadership for managing integrated teams.

Visit the Evolve website for Suggested Readings, Internet Resources, and additional resources related to the content in this chapter: http://evolve.elsevier.com/Canada/Yoder-Wise/leading/

REFERENCES

Statutes
Canada Health Act. (1985). *RSC* c. C-6 (Canada).
Excellent Care for All. (2010). *SO* c. 14 (Ontario).

Texts
Accreditation Canada. (2013). *Accreditation basics*. Retrieved from: http://www.accreditation.ca/accreditation-basics.
Canada Health Infoway. (2014). *2014–2015 Summary corporate plan: Improving health care through innovation*. Retrieved from: https://www.infoway-inforoute.ca/index.php.

Canadian Home Care Association (CHCA). (2013). *Portraits of home care in Canada 2013*. Author.
Canadian Institute for Health Information. (2013a). *Canada's health care providers, 1997–2011—A reference guide*. Ottawa, ON: Author. Retrieved from: https://secure.cihi.ca/estore/productFamily.htm?pf=PFC2161&lang=en&media=0.
Canadian Institute for Health Information. (2013b). *Regulated nurses, 2012—Summary report*. Ottawa, ON: Author. Retrieved from: https://secure.cihi.ca/estore/product Family.htm?locale=en&pf=PFC2385.

Canadian Institute for Health Information (CIHI). (2017). *National health expenditure trends 1975 to 2017*. Ottawa, ON: Author. Retrieved from: https://secure.cihi.ca/free_products/nhex2017-trends-report-en.pdf.

Canadian Institute for Health Information (CIHI). (2018). *National health expenditure trends, 1975–2018*. Ottawa, ON: Author.

Canadian Nurses Association. (2015). *Primary health care*. Ottawa, ON: Author. Retrieved from: https://www.cna-aiic.ca/~/media/cna/page-content/pdf-en/primary-health-care-position-statement.pdf.

Department of Finance Canada. (2018). *Federal support to provinces and territories*. Retrieved from: http://www.fin.gc.ca/fedprov/mtp-eng.asp.

Dobrow, M. J., Abbott, J. G., & Kitts, J. (2014, March). *What the loss of the health council of Canada means for Canadians. Longwoods.com*. Health Services Publishing.

Edwards, N., Davies, B., Ploeg, J., et al. (2007). Implementing nursing best practice guidelines: Impact on patient referrals. *BMC Nursing, 6*(4). https://doi.org/10.1186/1472-6955-6-4.

Evans, R. G. (1984). *Strained Mercy. The Economics of Canadian Healthcare*. Toronto: Butterworths.

Fricke, M. (2005). *Physiotherapy and primary health care: Evolving opportunities*. Winnipeg, MB: Manitoba Branch of the Canadian Physiotherapy Association, the College of Physiotherapists of Manitoba and the Department of Physical Therapy, School of Medical Rehabilitation. University of Manitoba.

Gottlieb, L. (2012). *Strengths based nursing care: Health and healing for person and family*. New York: Springer Publishing Company.

Gottlieb, L. N., Gottlieb, B., & Shamian, J. (2012, July). Principles of strengths-based nursing leadership for strengths-based nursing care: A new paradigm for nursing and healthcare for the 21st Century. *Nursing Leadership, 25*(2), 51–55. https://doi.org/10.12927/cjnl.2012.22961.

Government of Canada. (2018). *Federal/provincial/territorial ministers responsible for seniors forum*. Retrieved from: https://www.canada.ca/en/employment-social-development/corporate/seniors/forum.html.

Health Canada. (2011). *Canada's health care system*. Retrieved from: http://www.hc-sc.gc.ca/hcs-sss/pubs/system-regime/2011-hcs-sss/index-eng.php.

Health Canada. (2018a). *About primary health care*. Retrieved from: https://www.canada.ca/en/health-canada/services/health-care-system/reports-publications/health-care-system/canada.html#a12.

Health Canada. (2018b). *Canada's health care system*. Retrieved from: https://www.canada.ca/en/health-canada/services/canada-health-care-system.html#a21.

Health Canada. (2018c). *Shared health priorities*. Retrieved from: https://www.canada.ca/en/health-canada/corporate/transparency/health-agreements/shared-health-priorities.html.

Health Canada. (2015, July). *Unleashing innovation: Excellent healthcare for Canada. Report of the advisory panel on healthcare innovation*. Author.

Institute of Medicine. (2012, September). Roundtable on Value & Science-Driven Health Care. In M. B. McClellan (Ed.), *(Chair), Institute of Medicine of the National Academies. Meeting conducted at The National Academy of Science* Washington, DC. Retrieved from: https://nam.edu/wp-content/uploads/2017/12/Briefing-Book_Combined.pdf.

Johns, G., & Saks, A. M. (2001). *Organizational behaviour*. Toronto, ON: Pearson Education.

Klaasen, K., Lamont, L., & Krishnan, P. (2009). Setting a new standard of care in nursing homes. *Canadian Nurse, 105*(9), 24–30.

Kramer, M., Maguire, P., Schmalenberg, C., Andrews, B., Burke, R., Chmielewski, L., et al. (2007). Excellence through evidence: Structures enabling clinical autonomy. *Journal of Nursing Administration, 37*(1), 41–52.

Laschinger, H. K. S., Wong, C. A., & Greco, P. (2006). The impact of staff nurse empowerment on person–job fit and work engagement/burnout. *Nursing Administration Quarterly, 30*(4), 358–367.

Lee, T. Y., Sun, G. T., Kou, L. T., & Yeh, M. L. (2017, October 23). The use of information technology to enhance patient safety and nursing efficiency. *Technology Health Care, 25*(5), 917–928. https://doi.org/10.3233/THC-170848.

Motiwala, S. S., Flood, C. M., Coyte, P. C., & Laporte, A. (2005). The first ministers' accord in health renewal and the future of home care in Canada. *Longwoods Review, 2*(4), 2–9.

Naylor, D., et al. (2017). *Investing in Canada's future: strengthening the foundations of Canadian research. Canada's Fundamental Science Review*. Retrieved from: http://www.sciencereview.ca/eic/site/059.nsf/vwapj/ScienceReview_April2017.pdf/$file/ScienceReview_April2017.pdf.

OECD. (2015). *Fiscal sustainability of health systems: Bridging health and finance perspectives*. Paris: OECD Publishing. https://doi.org/10.1787/9789264233386-en.

Picard, A. (2017). *Matters of life and death: Public health issues in Canada*. Madeira Park, BC: Douglas and McIntyre.

Public Health Agency of Canada (PHAC). (2011). *About the agency*. Retrieved from: https://www.canada.ca/en/public-health/corporate/mandate/about-agency/mandate.html.

Public Health Agency of Canada. (2018). *Home page*. Retrieved from: https://www.canada.ca/en/public-health.html.

Reeves, S., Xyrichis, A., & Zwarenstein, M. (2017). Teamwork, collaboration, coordination, and networking: Why we need to distinguish between different types of interprofessional practice. *Journal of Interprofessional Care, 32*(1), 1–3. https://doi.org/10.1080/13561820.2017.1400150.

Ronson, J. (2006). Local health integration networks: Will "made in Ontario" work? *Healthcare Quarterly, 9*(1), 46–49. https://doi.org/10.12927/hcq.2006.17903.

White, S., & O'Brien-Pallas, L. (2010). *The healthy work environments best practice guidelines pilot evaluation final report: Degree of presence of recommendations in action in nursing practice and nursing work settings.* Toronto: RNAO.

World Health Organization. (1978). Declaration of Alma-Ata. In *International Conference on Primary Health Care* (pp. 6–12). Alma-Ata, USSR. Retrieved from: http://www.who.int/publications/almaata_declaration_en.pdf.

World Health Organization. (2014a). *Primary health care.* Retrieved from: http://www.who.int/topics/primary_health_care/en/.

World Health Organization. (2014b). *What are social determinants of health?* Retrieved from: http://www.who.int/social_determinants/sdh_definition/en/.

10

Understanding and Designing Organizational Structures

Terri Stuart-McEwan

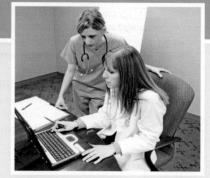

This chapter explains key concepts related to organizational structures and provides information on designing effective structures. This information can be used to help new managers function in an organization and to design structures that support work processes. An underlying theme is designing organizational structures that will respond to the continuous changes taking place in the health care environment.

OBJECTIVES

- Analyze the relationships among mission, vision, and philosophy statements and organizational structure.
- Analyze factors that influence the design of an organizational structure.
- Compare and contrast the major types of organizational structures.
- Evaluate the forces that are necessitating the reengineering of organizational systems.

TERMS TO KNOW

bureaucracy
chain of command
flat organizational structure
functional structure
hierarchy
hybrid organizational structure
line function
matrix structure
mission

organization
organizational chart
organizational culture
organizational structure
organizational theory
philosophy
redesign
re-engineering
restructuring

service-line structure
shared governance
span of control
staff function
system
systems theory
vision

❓ A CHALLENGE

A new hospital was created by the merger of two small former community hospitals. This new organization has experienced two different leadership structures since the merger over five years ago. Attempting to combine these two leadership structures contributed to at least two sets of conflicting operating policies that served to direct care. As a result, the standard of care was also driven by two different sets of policies. Laurie, a registered nurse, has been appointed as director of Patient Care Programs and is responsible for leading the implementation of a new organizational plan. However, implementation of the plan has been hindered, as several of the nurse manager and supervisor positions are vacant. Sometimes no nurse manager is available to clarify which practice should be followed or to recognize any major clinical conflicts that could lead to significant patient-care problems.

What are some strategies you would use to begin to lead the implementation of the new plan? What should Laurie keep in mind, at this point?

INTRODUCTION

The term organization has multiple meanings. It can refer to a business structure designed to support specific business goals and processes, or it can refer to a group of individuals working together to achieve a common purpose. Regardless of how the term is used, learning to determine how an organization accomplishes its work, how to operate productively within an organization, and how to influence organizational processes is essential to a successful professional nursing practice.

Organizational theory (sometimes called *organizational studies*) is the systematic analysis of how organizations and their component parts act and interact. Organizational theory is based largely on the systematic investigation of the effectiveness of specific organizational designs in achieving their purpose. Organizational theory development is a process of creating knowledge to understand the effect of identified factors, such as organizational culture, organizational technology—which is defined as all the work being carried out—and organizational structure or organizational development. A purpose of such work is to determine how organizational effectiveness might be predicted or controlled through the design of the organizational structure.

Specific organizational theories provide insight into areas such as effective organizational structures,

motivation of employees, decision making, and leadership. Systems theory is commonly used in health care to analyze how various independent parts interact to form a unified whole or to disrupt a unified whole. A system is an interacting collection of components or parts that together make up an integrated whole. The basic tenet of systems theory is that the individual components of any system interact with each other and with their environment. To be effective, professional nurses need to understand the specific part—role and function—they play within a system and how they interact, influence, and are influenced by other parts of the system.

An organization's mission, vision, and philosophy form the foundation for its structure and performance as well as the development of the professional practice models it uses. An organization's mission states the reason for the organization's existence and will influence the design of the structure (e.g., to meet the health care needs of a designated population, to provide supportive and stabilizing care to an acute care population, or to provide high-quality end-of-life care). The vision is the articulated goals to which the organization aspires. A vision statement conveys an inspirational view of how the organization wishes to be described at some future time. It suggests how far to strive in all endeavours. Another key factor influencing structure is the organization's philosophy. A philosophy expresses the values and beliefs that members of the organization hold about the nature of their work, about the people to whom they provide service, and about themselves and others providing the services.

EXERCISE 10.1 Consider how you might use the information in the Introduction to:
1. Analyze an organization that you are considering joining to determine whether it fits your professional development plans.
2. Assess the functioning of an organization of which you are already a member.
3. Assess and redesign the structure or philosophy to better accomplish the mission of an organization you are considering joining or of which you are already a member.

MISSION

A mission statement is a formal document that articulates an organization's distinct and enduring purpose. It should answer some really fundamental questions about an organization, such as, "Why do we exist?" "What is our purpose?"

"What do we want to achieve?" In answering these questions, a mission statement becomes the cornerstone of every organization's formal strategy (Bart & Hupfer, 2004).

The mission statement sets the stage by defining the services to be offered, which, in turn, identify the kinds of technologies and human resources to be employed. Mission statements of health care systems typically refer to the larger community the organizations serve as well as the specific patient populations to whom they provide care. In Canada, most provinces provide care to geographic health regions, known as Regional Health Authorities (RHAs), or Local Health Integrated Networks (LHINs) in Ontario. These governance models are used to administer and/or deliver health care to its citizens. Mission statements are generally developed for each RHA. Individual hospitals and other health care agencies that link to that RHA may or may not have their own mission statements. For example, in the Southwest Ontario Local Health Integration Network (LHIN), the vision statement is, "a healthier tomorrow for everyone" and the mission statement is, "working with our communities to deliver quality care and transform the health care system" (South Ontario LHIN, 2014). Within the LHIN, the Southwest Ontario Aboriginal Health Access Centre (SOAHAC) has created its own vision, mission, and values to address the unique needs of the community. Their vision is, "a healthy balanced life through mental, physical, spiritual and emotional well-being" and their mission is, "to empower Aboriginal families and individuals to live a balanced state of well-being by sharing and promoting wholistic health practices" (SOAHAC, 2014). The same Aboriginal Health Access Centre articulates a set of values that are core to the mission including respect, compassion, quality and the honouring of all traditional values (SOAHAC, 2014). RHAs and LHINs are primarily focused on population and primary health, whereas hospitals are typically focused on treatment and acute services. The missions of long-term care facilities are primarily oriented towards maintenance, social support, and quality of life; and the missions of health centres are oriented towards promoting optimal health status for a defined group of people. The definition of services to be provided and the implications for technologies and human resources greatly influence the design of the organizational structure (i.e., how work is divided within an organization). Hospitals or health care organizations may also have vision, mission, and values statements specific to particular clinical services or professional departments, such as nursing.

In Canada, the Canadian Nurses Association (CNA) is the national voice of nursing and serves to advance the practice of nursing and the profession across provincial and territorial associations. Each provincial association, in turn, provides professional standards of care and regulatory scope of practice guidelines that organizations must use for nurses practising within the organization. Thus, nursing, as a profession, often formulates its own mission statement, which describes its contributions that are aligned to national/provincial standards and achieve the organization's overall mission. An example of a mission statement for nursing professionals appears in Box 10.1.

One of the purposes of the nursing profession is to provide nursing care to patients. The nursing mission statement helps describe why nursing exists within the context of the interprofessional team and organization. It is typically written so that others within the organization can know and understand nursing's role in achieving the employer's mission. The mission should be the guiding framework for decision making and should be known and well understood by other health care providers, by patients and their families, and by the community. It helps underpin the important relationships among nurses and patients, employer personnel, the community, and health and illness. This statement should provide direction for the evolving statement of values and beliefs or philosophy and the organizational structure and it should be reviewed for accuracy and updated routinely by professional nurses providing care.

BOX 10.1   Example of a Nursing Mission and Vision Statement

An example of a mission and vision statement for nursing was created at a hospital that clearly outlines the unique contributions of nursing within an organization

The vision statement states:

Nurses are healthcare leaders that strive to empower patients, caregivers and communities to optimize health care and outcomes across the continuum of care. Our nurses provide a holistic, inter-professional delivery of care that is focused on high quality, excellence and best clinical evidence that promotes and support the unique needs of our patients and families.

In addition their Mission Statement states:

Our Nurses are committed to patient-centred care that is provided in a safe, compassionate and healing environment.

VISION

Various definitions of vision exist; however, they all portray a future picture of the organization and stress the need for goals and strategies to be directed towards achievement of this envisioned future. Vision statements are future-oriented, purposeful statements designed to identify the desired future of an organization. They serve to unify all subsequent statements towards the view of the future and to convey the core message of the mission statement. Typically, vision statements are brief, consisting of only one or two phrases or sentences. An example of a vision statement for nursing appears in Box 10.1.

PHILOSOPHY AND VALUES

A philosophy is a written statement that articulates the values and beliefs held about the nature of the work required to accomplish the mission and the nature and rights of both the people being served and those providing the service. For example, the mission statement may incorporate the provision of patient-centred care as an organizational value. The philosophy statement would then support this value through an expression of a belief in the responsibility of nursing staff to act as patient advocates and to provide quality care according to the wishes of the patient, family, and significant others.

Values are evolutionary in that they are shaped both by the social environment and by the stage of development of professionals delivering the service. Nursing staff reflect the values of their time. The values acquired through research and education are reflected in the nursing philosophy. For example, research regarding patient safety and nurse outcomes ensures that nursing practice is focused on achieving and enhancing patient-centred care. Values often help guide organizational obligations and rights. In dynamic and ever-changing organizations, value statements may require updating and revising on a regular basis to ensure that they reflect the extension of rights brought about by such changes.

Many health care organizations focus primarily on short and succinct descriptions of their core values, which are the foundation for their mission and goals, rather than extended descriptions of philosophy. A review of Canadian hospital mission statements by Williams et al. (2005) found that values predominated other types of content and that the primary values included commitment to patient care, respect and esteem for staff, teamwork, commitment to community, education and research, trust,

caring, and compassion. For example, Eastern Health in Newfoundland and Labrador describe values including Respect, Integrity, Fairness, Connectedness, and Excellence, but that above all, Eastern Health values the delivery of quality programs and services in a caring manner (Eastern Health, Newfoundland and Labrador, 2017).

EXERCISE 10.2

1. Take a few minutes to develop a personal philosophy statement based on your own vision, values, and beliefs for your nursing practice.
2. Obtain a copy of the vision and philosophy statement of an organization you are familiar with or one you could see as your future employer. How do the vision, values, and beliefs in these documents compare with your own philosophy about nursing practice? Is there a fit or a mismatch for you?
3. Search the websites of your local regional health authority or health care agencies, such as hospitals, nursing homes, or public health units, and examine how they have described their missions, visions, values, and beliefs or philosophy for the services they provide. What similarities and differences can you identify by employer?

ORGANIZATIONAL CULTURE

An organization's mission, vision, and philosophy shape and reflect its organizational culture. Organizational culture is the implicit knowledge or values and beliefs within the organization that reflect the norms and traditions of the organization. It is exemplified by rituals and customary forms of practice, such as dress policy, the celebration of promotions, and professional performance. Examples of norms that reflect organizational culture are the characteristics of the people who are recognized as heroes by the organization and the behaviours—either positive or negative—that are accepted or tolerated within the organization.

Culture within organizations is demonstrated in two ways that can be either mutually reinforcing or conflict producing. Organizational culture is typically expressed in a formal manner via mission, vision, and philosophy statements; job descriptions; and policies and procedures. Beyond formal documents and verbal descriptions given by administrators and managers, organizational culture is also represented in the day-to-day experience of staff and patients. To many, it is the lived experience that reflects the true organizational culture. Do the decisions made within the organization consistently demonstrate that the organization values its patients and keeps their needs at the forefront? Are the employees treated with trust and respect, or are the words used in recruitment ads simply empty promises with little evidence to back them up? When there is a lack of congruity between the expressed organizational culture and the experienced organizational culture, confusion, frustration, and poor morale often result (Casida, 2008; Laschinger et al., 2016; Melnick et al., 2009).

Organizational culture can be effective and promote success and positive outcomes, or it can be ineffective and result in disharmony, dissatisfaction, and poor outcomes for patients, staff, and the organization. A number of workplace variables are influenced by organizational culture (Chen, 2008). A recent study demonstrated the positive influence of two key aspects of organizational culture, collective perceptions of unit leadership and workplace empowerment, on individual nurses' organizational commitment in acute care hospitals (Laschinger et al., 2009). Workplace empowerment at the unit level can be construed as an aspect of unit or organizational culture. Similarly, culture may include the values and norms that influence how supportive the unit or workplace is as a learning environment for students or new staff members during orientation. The manner and degree to which students and new orientees are respected, welcomed, and supported by members of the unit or organization may be determined by the culture (Engle et al., 2017; Henderson et al., 2012; Wong, 2012). In addition, a culture that encourages seeking new ways of improving practice and also promotes professional development of members is more likely to also improve care outcomes.

When seeking employment or advancement, nurses need to assess the organization's culture and develop a clear understanding of existing expectations as well as the formal and informal communication patterns. Various techniques and tools can help nurses perform a cultural assessment of an organization, such as the Denison Organizational Culture Survey described by Casida (2008) or Cooke's Organization Culture Inventory used in the systematic review of organizational culture research in health care by Bellot (2011). With a solid understanding of organizational culture, nurses will be better able to be effective change agents and help transform the organizations in which they work. The Research Perspective below presents a qualitative study that explored the organizational attributes that best support the work of Canadian public health nurses. One of the major attributes was the local organizational culture (Meagher-Stewart et al., 2010).

RESEARCH PERSPECTIVE

Resource: Meagher-Stewart, D., Underwood, J., MacDonald, M., et al. (2010). Health policy: Organizational attributes that assure optimal utilization of public health nurses. *Public Health Nursing*, 27(5), 433–441.

This Canada-wide project included an investigation of the salient organizational attributes necessary to promote optimal use of public health nurses (PHNs). Considerable knowledge exists about work environment conditions that best support acute care nursing practice, but less is known about the organizational conditions that support public health nursing. As part of a pan-Canadian research program examining community nursing workforce capacity, this project used focus group methodology to identify the organizational attributes that best support PHNs to work effectively. Qualitative data were collected from 156 participants in 23 focus groups in six geographically diverse regions of Canada over a six-month period in 2007–2008. The focus groups included 12 groups of 85 front-line PHNs (from urban or rural/remote settings) and 11 groups of 71 policymakers or managers involved with public health nursing practice (from urban or rural/remote settings). Values and effective leadership were identified as key organizational attributes at all levels of the public health system. Three subthemes of attributes relevant to organizational culture were as follows:

A shared vision—participants stressed that effective organizations maintained a clear vision, mission, and goals for public health.

A culture of creativity and responsiveness to community needs at both the front-line and management levels.

Effective leadership, which participants identified as showing respect, trust, and support for PHNs working to their optimal capacity.

Implications for Practice

Findings from this study highlight the relevance of organizational culture and leadership to optimizing nursing outcomes in Canadian public health. The diversity of practice settings (rural or remote and urban) represented in the study increased the potential for application to other public health settings. Moreover, the consistency of findings across positions highlighted the importance of shared responsibility for creating organizational culture and vision. The need for effective and positive leadership at all levels is key to facilitating optimal work environments and practice outcomes.

FACTORS INFLUENCING ORGANIZATIONAL DEVELOPMENT

To be most effective, organizational structures should reflect the organization's mission, vision, philosophy, goals, and objectives. Organizational structure defines how work is organized, where decisions are made, and the authority and responsibility of workers. It provides a map for communication and outlines decision-making paths. As organizations change through restructuring and other types of processes (including, for example, mergers of hospitals, government mandates, and specific losses or additions of care programs), it is essential that structures change to accomplish revised missions.

One of the best theories to explain today's nursing organizational development is chaos (complexity, nonlinear, quantum) theory. In essence, chaos theory suggests that lives—and organizations—are really web-like. Pulling on one small segment rearranges the web, a new pattern emerges, and yet the whole remains. This theory, applied to nursing organizations, suggests that differences logically exist between and among various organizations and that the constant environmental forces continue to affect the structure, its functioning, and its services. Brafman and Beckstrom (2008), in their aptly named book *The Starfish and the Spider*, identified how organizations differ and yet are successful. Spider organizations are built like a spider, and when the head is destroyed, the spider dies. The starfish, on the other hand, can lose an appendage, and it just grows another one. In fact, a starfish, when cut in half, creates two starfish. Organizations that are controlled in a heavily centralized way can diminish quickly without the strong, central figure. Organizations that are self-generating quickly share leadership as needed and often continue to thrive. The important point for any organization is to find what is the best or most adaptive balance between centralization and decentralization.

The issues in health care delivery, with their concomitant changes such as increases or decreases in government funding with new regulations and the development of networks for delivery of health care, have profound effects on organizational structure designs. Canadian health care organizations must be responsive to changes in government (provincial, territorial, and federal) policy, financing, and organization-level structural or policy changes that cause individual organizational units to be concerned with efficiencies in service delivery, redeployment of existing resources, reorganization, restructuring, and realignment of services through various redesign processes. In addition, patients and families expect that care will be individualized to meet their needs, which means that more decision making must be done where the care is delivered. Increased public knowledge about health issues and care programs has resulted in patients expecting immediate access to care.

Information from internet sources is significantly altering the expectations and behaviours of health care professionals and users. For example, many provinces have health quality councils that maintain websites where members of the public can access a searchable database that aims to provide public reporting about patient care and system indicators, such as hospital-associated infections, hand hygiene adherence, and hospital mortality rates. For example, Health Quality Ontario (2018), Health Quality Council Alberta (2018), and Saskatchewan Health Quality Council (2018) monitor quality indicators, such as provincial wait times (e.g., emergency, surgery) and appropriateness of care recommendations from Choosing Wisely (n.d.). These websites are designed to assist the public to become informed users of their provincial health care system. Changes in both facility design and care delivery systems are likely to continue as efforts are made to increase access, reduce wait times and costs, and enhance efficiencies while still striving to improve patient outcomes.

In Canada, rising health care costs, demands for quicker access to care, changes in government policy, and technological and research innovations are key factors influencing organizational structure design. These factors necessitate the re-engineering of health care structures. Whereas redesign is a process of analyzing tasks to improve efficiency (e.g., identifying the most efficient flow of supplies to a nursing unit) and restructuring entails fundamental changes to an organization to achieve greater efficiency or profit (e.g., identifying the most appropriate type and number of staff members for a particular nursing unit), re-engineering involves a total overhaul of an organizational structure. It is a radical reorganization of the totality of an organization's structure and work processes. In re-engineering, fundamentally new system and organizational expectations and relationships are created. An example of where re-engineering is required is the area of technological change—particularly in clinical information systems that provide a means of creating a comprehensive health care record for patients. The potential for making information concerning a patient immediately accessible to both the interprofessional team and patient can have a profound positive impact on health care structures and decision making.

For example, in chronic disease management, such as diabetes or heart failure, the convergence of patient access to health care technology and information has created the opportunity for nurses to practice with a high degree of interprofessional collaboration. Research has demonstrated that structural empowerment, authentic leadership, and professional nursing practice environments are all significant, independent predictors of nurses' confidence to actively participate in interprofessional collaborative practice. This is evident when they are in environments that support and recognize their professional role (Regan et al., 2016). Therefore re-engineering chronic disease management structures that enable nurses to practice at their full scope will support improved patient care and health care outcomes.

Regardless of the level of changes made within an organization—redesign, restructuring, or re-engineering—health care professionals and patients alike, will inevitably feel the effects. Some of the changes result in improvements, whereas others may not; some of the effects are expected, whereas others may be surprising. It is critical therefore that nurse leaders as well as staff nurses be vigilant for both anticipated and unanticipated results of organizational changes. Nurses need to position themselves to participate in change discussions and evaluations. Ultimately, it is their day-to-day work with their patients that is affected by the decisions made in response to a rapidly changing environment (Cormack et al., 2007; Martin et al., 2007; Murphy & Roberts, 2008). The Evidence section at the end of this chapter describes the impact of organizational restructuring on nurses.

EXERCISE 10.3 Reflect on your own experiences of changes that have necessitated re-engineering. These may include changes associated with implementation of new emergency department wait-time reduction strategies, development of policies to carry out legislative regulations related to patient information and confidentiality, or development of new community primary health care centres. Identify examples of how systems of communication and decision making were either adequate or inadequate to cope with these changes.

CHARACTERISTICS OF ORGANIZATIONAL STRUCTURES

The characteristics of different types of organizational structures provide a catalogue of options to consider in designing structures that fit specific situations. Knowledge of these characteristics also helps managers understand the structures in which they currently function.

Organizational designs are often classified by their characteristics of complexity, formalization, and centralization. *Complexity* concerns the division of labour in an organization, the specialization of that labour, the number of hierarchical levels, and the geographical dispersion of organizational units. *Division of labour* and *specialization* refer to the separation of processes into tasks that are performed by designated people. The horizontal dimension of an organizational chart, the graphical representation of work units and reporting relationships, relates to the division and specialization of labour functions attended by specialists. Hierarchy connotes lines of authority and responsibility. Chain of command is a term used to refer to the hierarchy depicted in vertical dimensions of organizational charts. Hierarchy vests authority in positions on an ascending line away from where work is performed and allows control of work. Staff members are often placed on a bottom level of the organization, and those in authority, who provide control, are placed in higher levels. Span of control refers to the number of individuals a supervisor manages. For budgetary reasons, span of control is often a major focus for organizational restructuring. Although cost implications arise when a span of control is too narrow, when a span of control becomes too large, supervision can become less effective. The Literature Perspective describes the effect of span of control on unit performance and outcomes.

LITERATURE PERSPECTIVE

Resource: Wong, C. A. (2015). Examining the relationships between span of control and manager job and unit performance outcomes. *Journal of nursing management*, 23(2), 156–168.

Multiple studies have shown that managers are critical to creating environments that empower nurses for professional practice. There is significant evidence that demonstrates that span of control (SOC) has an impact upon front-line managers (FLM), and increased awareness SOC affects issues such as nurse satisfaction and unit outcomes. Using a non-experimental predictive survey design, Wong examined FLM SOC in 14 Canadian academic hospitals with 121 managers completing an online survey of work characteristics and The Ottawa Hospital SOC tool. Unit turnover data was collected from organizational databases. There was significant evidence that as SOC increased, so did manager role overload and the unit frequency of adverse outcomes, and there was decreased job satisfaction and work control.

Implications for Practice

During times of organizational change, leaders need to be aware of the relationship between a manager's span of control and staff and unit effectiveness. Organizations that ensure that FLM have adequate SOC will have a positive effect on patient and staff outcomes, such as frequency of medication errors, nosocomial infections, staff work-related injuries, and other safety outcomes.

Organizational size is closely related to the complexity of the organization. The stability and viability of an organization requires a certain essential base of resources. Efficiencies are often achieved when organizations increase in size, and this is often part of the rationale behind mergers of health care facilities (Smith et al., 2006). When organizations grow larger with more units or subdivisions and levels of decision making, they become more complex.

Geographical dispersion refers to the physical location of units. Units of work may be in one building, in several buildings in one location, spread throughout a city, or in different towns, provinces, territories, or even countries. The more dispersed an organization is, the greater are the demands for creative designs that place decision making related to patient care close to the patient and, consequently, far from the central office. A similar type of complexity exists in organizations that deliver care at multiple sites in the community; for example, RHAs usually have multiple sites and types of health care facilities that previously may have been independent organizations, each with unique identities and cultures. It then becomes challenging to create a new overall culture and garner the commitment of employees, managers, and other stakeholders to the new organization (Smith et al., 2006).

Formalization is the degree to which an organization has rules, stated in terms of policies that define a member's function. The amount of formalization varies among institutions. It is often inversely related to the degree of specialization and the number of professionals within the organization.

EXERCISE 10.4 Review a copy of a nursing department's organizational chart and identify the divisions of labour, the hierarchy of authority, and the degree of formalization.

Are the relationships clear? Is there anything in the organization chart that is different from what you would expect?

Centralization refers to the location where a decision is made. Decisions are made at the top of a centralized organization. In a decentralized organization, decisions are made at or close to the patient-care level. As organizations grow larger, they sometimes increase centralization of decision making. Highly centralized organizations often delegate *responsibility* (the obligation to perform the task) without the *authority* (the right to act, which is necessary to carry out the responsibility). For example, some hospitals have delegated both the responsibility and the authority for admission decisions to the clinical managers (decentralized), whereas others require the nurse supervisor or clinical directors to make such decisions (centralized).

EXERCISE 10.5 Review nursing policies in a public health department, a primary health care centre, a community care access centre, and a hospital.

Are there common policies? Does one of the organizations have more detailed policies than the others? Is this formalization consistent with the structural complexity of the organization?

BUREAUCRACY

Many organizational theories in use today find their basis in the works of early twentieth-century theorists: Max Weber, a German sociologist who developed the basic tenets of bureaucracy (Weber, 1947); and Henri Fayol, a French industrialist who crafted 14 principles of management (Fayol, 1949). Initially, bureaucracy referred to the centralization of authority in administrative bureaus or government departments. The term has come to refer to an inflexible approach to decision making or an employer encumbered by "red tape" that adds little value to organizational processes.

Bureaucracy is an administrative concept imbedded in how organizations are structured. It arose at a time of societal development when services were in short supply, workers' and patients' knowledge bases were limited, and technologies for sharing information were undeveloped. Characteristics of bureaucracy arose out of a need to control workers and were centred on the division of processes into discrete tasks. Weber proposed that organizations could achieve high levels of productivity and efficiency only by adherence to what he called "bureaucracy." Weber believed that bureaucracy, based on the sociological concept of rationalization of collective activities, provided the idealized organizational structure. Bureaucratic structures are formal and have a centralized and hierarchical command structure (chain of command). Bureaucratic structures have a clear division of labour and well-articulated and commonly accepted expectations for performance. Rules, standards, and protocols ensure uniform actions and limit individualization of services and variance in workers' performance. In bureaucratic organizations, as shown in Fig. 10.1, communication and decisions flow from top to bottom. Although it enhances consistency, bureaucracy, by nature, limits employees' autonomy.

In developing his 14 principles of management, Fayol outlined structures and processes that guide how work is accomplished within an organization. Consistent with theories of bureaucracy, his principles of management include division of labour or specialization, clear lines of authority, appropriate levels of discipline, unity of direction, equitable treatment of staff, the fostering of individual initiative, and the promotion of a sense of teamwork and group pride (Fayol, 1949). More than 60 years after they were described, these principles remain the basis of most organizations. Therefore to be effective organizational leaders, nurses need to be familiar with the theory and concepts of bureaucracy.

EXERCISE 10.6 Develop a list of decisions that you, as a nurse or student nurse, would like to make to optimize family involvement in the care of one your patients. Think about *where* decisions regarding family involvement and visiting are made in your nursing organization and unit.

For example, who designs unit visiting schedules and do they meet the needs of the patient, the family and the staff providing care? What types of decisions can you make regarding this patient's family's involvement? Are these decisions made at the level of nurse–patient, at the level of management, at a unit or organizational level? What challenges do you see you may face as you try to enact the decisions you have outlined?

At the time that bureaucracies were developed, these characteristics promoted efficiency and production. As the knowledge base of the general population and employees grew and technologies developed, the bureaucratic structure no longer fit the evolving situation. Increasingly, employees and patients or patients functioning in bureaucratic situations complain of "red tape," procedural delays, and their own resultant frustration.

The characteristics of bureaucracy can be present in varying degrees. An organization can demonstrate bureaucratic characteristics in some areas and not in others. For example, nursing staff in critical care units may be granted autonomy in making and carrying out direct patient care decisions, but they may not be granted a voice in determining work schedules or financial reimbursement systems for hours worked.

One method to determine the extent to which bureaucratic tendencies exist in organizations is to assess the organizational characteristics of the following:
- Labour specialization (the degree to which patient care is divided into highly specialized tasks).

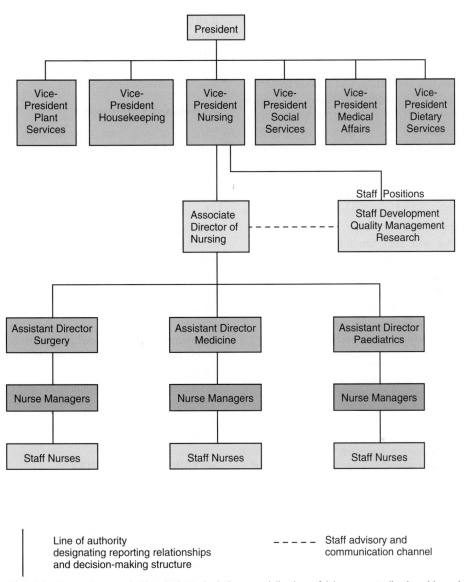

Fig. 10.1 A bureaucratic organizational chart depicting specialization of labour, centralization, hierarchical authority, and line and staff responsibilities.

- Centralization (the level of the organization on which decisions regarding carrying out work and remuneration for work are made).
- Formalization (the percentage of actions required to deliver patient care that is governed by written policy and procedures).

EXERCISE 10.7 Analyze the decisions identified in Exercise 10.6 from a nurse manager's perspective. Is that perspective similar to or different from the original perspective you identified?

Decision making and authority can be described in terms of line and staff functions. **Line functions** are those that involve direct responsibility for accomplishing the objectives of a nursing department, service, or unit. Line positions may include registered nurses, registered psychiatric nurses, registered practical nurses, and unregulated care providers who have the responsibility for carrying out all aspects of direct care. **Staff functions** are those that assist those in line positions in accomplishing the primary objectives. In this context, the term *staff positions* should not be confused with specific jobs that include "staff" in their names, such as "staff nurse" or "staff physician." Staff positions include staff development personnel, researchers, and special clinical consultants who are responsible for supporting line positions through activities of consultation, education, role modelling, and knowledge development, with limited or no direct authority for decision making. Line personnel have authority for decision making, whereas personnel in staff positions provide support, advice, and counsel. Organizational charts usually indicate line positions through the use of solid lines and staff positions through broken lines. Line structures have a vertical line, designating reporting and decision-making responsibility. The vertical line connects all positions to a centralized authority (see Fig. 10.1).

To make line and staff functions effective, decision-making authority is clearly spelled out in position descriptions. Effectiveness is further ensured by delineating competencies required for the responsibilities, providing methods for determining whether personnel possess these competencies, and providing means of maintaining and developing the competencies.

EXERCISE 10.8 Organizational structures vary in the extent to which they have bureaucratic characteristics. Using observations from your current practice, tick the "Present" column beside the bureaucratic characteristics that you believe apply to the organization. What does this analysis indicate about the bureaucratic tendency of the organization? Do the environment and technologies fit the identified bureaucratic tendency? (Consider the state of development of information systems, method of care delivery, patients' characteristics, workers' characteristics, and regulatory status.)

Characteristic	Present
Hierarchy of authority	
Division of labour	
Written procedures for work	
Limited authority for workers	
Emphasis on written communication related to work performance and workers' behaviours	
Impersonality of personal contact	

TYPES OF ORGANIZATIONAL STRUCTURES

In health care organizations, the most common types of organizational structures are functional, service line,

matrix, or flat. Nursing organizations often combine characteristics of several of these structures to form a hybrid structure. Shared governance is an organizing structure designed to meet the changing needs of professional nursing organizations.

Functional Structures

Functional structures arrange departments and services according to specialty. This approach to organizational structure is common in health care organizations. Departments providing similar functions report to a common manager or executive (Fig. 10.2). For example, a health care organization with a functional structure would have vice-presidents for each major function: nursing, support services, finance, human resources, and information technology.

This organizational structure tends to support professional expertise and encourage advancement. It may, however, result in discontinuity or fragmented patient-care services. Delays in decision making can occur if a silo mentality develops within groups. In fact, Lencioni (2006) points out the pitfalls of departments that work within silos. For example, patient care issues that depend on interdepartmental collaboration and communication (e.g., medication administration that require pharmacy and nursing input) typically must be raised to a senior management level before a decision can be made.

Service-Line Structures

In service-line structures (sometimes called *product lines*), the functions necessary to produce a specific service or product are brought together into an integrated organizational unit under the control of a single manager or executive (Fig. 10.3). For example, a cardiology service line at an acute care hospital might include all professional, technical, and support personnel providing services to the cardiac patient population. The manager or administrator in this service line would be responsible for any cardiac services situated within the emergency department, the coronary care unit, the cardiovascular surgery critical care unit, the telemetry unit, the cardiac catheterization lab, and the cardiac rehabilitation centre. In addition to managing the budget and the facilities for these areas, the manager typically would be responsible for coordinating services for the physicians and other providers who admit and care for these patients.

The benefits of a service-line approach to organizational structure include coordination of services, an

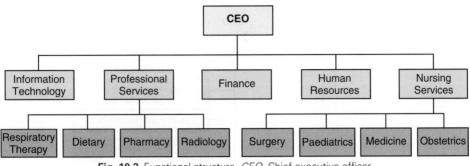

Fig. 10.2 Functional structure. *CEO*, Chief executive officer.

expedited decision-making process, and clarity of purpose. The limitations of this model can include increased expense associated with duplication of services, loss of professional or technical affiliation, and lack of standardization.

Matrix Structures

Matrix structures are complex and designed to reflect both function and service in an integrated organizational structure. In a matrix organization, the manager of a unit responsible for a service reports to both a functional manager and a service- or product-line manager. For example, a director of pediatric nursing could report to both a vice-president for pediatric services (the service-line manager) and a vice-president of nursing (the functional manager) (Fig. 10.4).

Matrix structures can be effective in the current health care environment. The matrix design enables timely response to forces in the external environment that demand continual programming, and it facilitates internal efficiency and effectiveness through the promotion of cooperation among disciplines. However, such a structure can lead to some dispersion of accountability and potential conflict as some employees may report to more than one supervisor. Another disadvantage is that a matrix structure may lead to an increase in bureaucracy, in the form of more meetings or slower decisions where too many people are involved.

A matrix structure combines both a bureaucratic structure and a flat structure; teams are used to carry out specific programs or projects. A matrix structure superimposes a horizontal program management over the traditional vertical hierarchy. Personnel from various functional departments are assigned to a specific program or project and become responsible to two supervisors—their functional department head and a program manager. This creates an interdisciplinary team. Matrix structures permit better cross-communication among various organizational units or departments and may serve to flatten or simplify decision-making structures and allow for timely and quality responses to changes initiated by factors outside the control of the organization. Organizations that operate in a dynamic environment and need to make decisions more quickly (often bringing higher-level decision makers in contact with front-line activities) while including a broad cross-section of the organization's functional units, often create structures that are reflective of matrix structures.

A line manager and a project manager must function collaboratively in a matrix organization. For example, in nursing, there may be a chief nursing executive, a nurse manager, and staff nurses in the line of authority to accomplish nursing care. In the matrix structure, some of the nurse's time is allocated to project or committee work. Nursing care is delivered in a teamwork setting or within a collaborative model. The nurse is responsible to a nurse manager for nursing care and to a program or project manager when working within the matrix overlay. Well-developed collaboration and coordination skills are essential to effective functioning in a matrix structure. The nature of a matrix organization, with its complex interrelationships, requires workers with knowledge and skill in interpersonal relationships and teamwork.

One example of the matrix structure is the patient-focused care delivery model that is being implemented in some facilities. Another example is the program focused on specialty services, such as geriatric services, women's services, and cardiovascular services. A matrix model can be designed to cover both a patient-focused care delivery model and a specialty service. Other examples

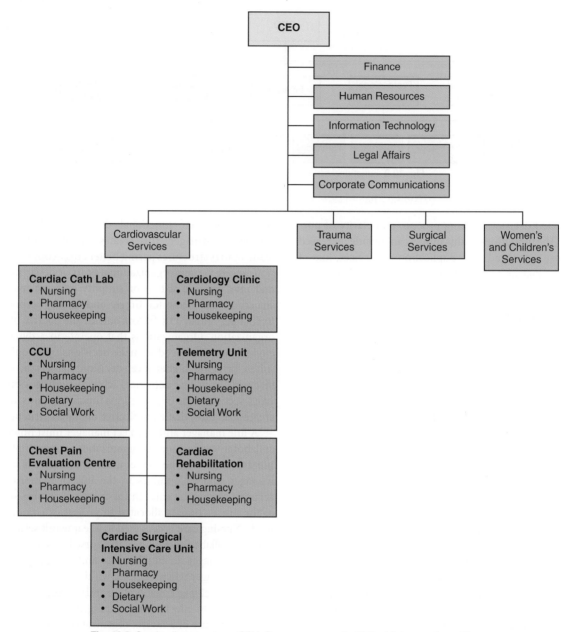

Fig. 10.3 Service-line structure. *CCU,* Coronary care unit; *CEO,* chief executive officer.

are special health care facility programs, such as discharge planning, quality and risk management, and professional practice.

Flat Structures

The primary organizational characteristic of a *flat* structure is the delegation of decision making to the professionals doing the work. The term *flat* signifies the removal of hierarchical layers, thereby granting authority to act and placing authority at the action level (Fig. 10.5). Decisions regarding work methods, nursing care of individual patients, and conditions under which employees work are made where the work is carried out. In a flat organizational structure, decentralized

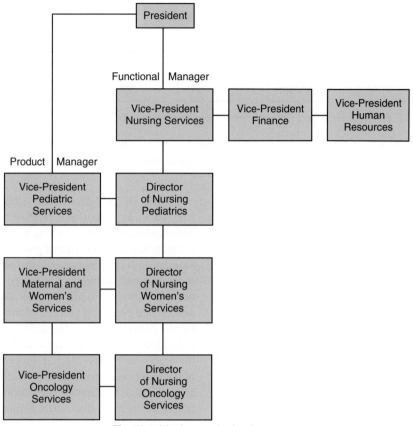

Fig. 10.4 Matrix organizational structure.

decision making replaces the centralized decision making typical of functional structures.

Flat organizational structures are less formalized than hierarchical organizations. A decrease in strict adherence to rules and policies allows employees to make individualized decisions that fit specific situations and meet the needs created by the increasing demands associated with government funding and policy, technological change, and public expectations. For example, work supported by Safer Healthcare Now!, the flagship program of the Canadian Patient Safety Institute (2018), invests in front-line providers and the delivery system to improve the safety of patient care throughout Canada by implementing interventions known to reduce avoidable harm. Safer Healthcare Now! is a resource for front-line health care providers and others who want to improve interventions and patient safety. Interventions such as central line infections, patient falls, management of infection prevention and control are recognized as key initiatives to decrease patient harm within the health care system.

Decentralized structures are not without their challenges, however. These include the potential for inconsistent decision making, loss of growth opportunities, and the need to educate managers to communicate effectively and demonstrate creativity in working within these nontraditional structures (Matthews et al., 2006).

The degree of flattening varies from organization to organization. Decentralized organizations often retain some bureaucratic characteristics. They may at the same time have units that are operating as matrix structures. A hybrid organizational structure has characteristics of several types of organizational structure.

As organizational structures change, some managers are hesitant to relinquish their traditional role in a centralized decision-making process. This reluctance, when combined with recognition of the need to move to a more facilitative role, is partially responsible for the development of hybrid structures. Managers are unsure of what needs to be controlled, how much control is needed, and which mechanisms can replace control.

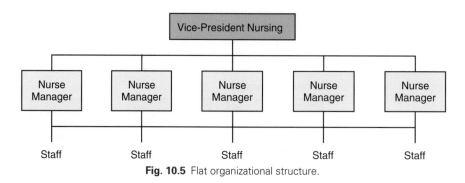

Fig. 10.5 Flat organizational structure.

Fear of chaos without control predominates. Education that prepares managers to use leadership techniques that empower nursing staff to take responsibility for their work is one method of minimizing managers' fears. These fears stem from loss of centralized control as authority with its concomitant responsibilities moves to the place of interaction. The evolutionary development of shared-governance structures in nursing departments demonstrates a type of flat structure being used to replace hierarchical control.

Shared Governance

Shared governance is a flat type of organizational structure with decentralized decision making. It goes beyond participatory management by creating an organizational structure that helps nursing staff have more autonomy to govern their practice. Accountability is the foundation for shared governance. To be accountable, authority to make decisions concerning all aspects of responsibilities is essential. The need for authority and accountability is particularly important for nurses who treat the wide range of human responses to wellness states and illnesses. Organizations in which professional autonomy is encouraged have higher levels of staff satisfaction, enhanced productivity, and improved retention (Moore & Hutchinson, 2007; Ulrich et al., 2007). One longitudinal study found that empowerment and perceived support for professional practice was positively related to perceptions of unit-level effectiveness to meet patient care needs (Spence et al., 2016). There is a large body of evidence indicating that by creating workplace environments that are both structurally and psychologically empowering, health care managers contribute to employee well-being and ultimately higher levels of organizational commitment. Tools to evaluate empowerment can measure and monitor changes, especially in times of organizational change (Laschinger et al., 2016).

Shared or self-governance structures, sometimes referred to as *professional practice models*, go beyond decentralizing and diminishing hierarchies. In an organization that embraces shared governance, the structure's foundation is the professional workplace rather than the organizational hierarchy. Shared governance vests the necessary levels of authority and accountability for all aspects of the nursing practice in the nurses responsible for the delivery of care. The management and administrative level serves to coordinate and facilitate the work of the practising nurses. Mechanisms are designed outside of the traditional hierarchy to provide for the functional areas needed to support professional practice. These functions include areas such as quality management, competency definition and evaluation, and continuing education. Changing nurses' positions from dependent employees to independent, accountable professionals is a prerequisite for the radical redesign of health care organizations that is required to create value for patients. Doing so requires administrators, managers, and staff to abandon traditional notions regarding the division of labour in health care organizations. MacPhee et al.'s (2010) three-year participatory action research project conducted in selected sites in British Columbia showed the importance of staff nurse–nurse leader-shared decision-making teams in addressing workload issues. The structures of shared governance organizations vary. Box 10.2 shows three governance structures in progressive stages of evolution. As shown, evolution is moving structure beyond committees imposed on hierarchical structures to governance structures at the unit level.

Nurse managers who emphasize transparency, balanced processing, self-awareness, and high ethical standards also effectively increase nurses' perceptions of workplace empowerment, which in turn enhances their performance and job satisfaction (Wong & Laschinger, 2012). Additionally, work environments that provide

BOX 10.2   Shared-Governance Structure Evolution

Phase One

Representative staff nurses are members of clinical forums, which have authority for designated practice issues and some authority for determining roles, functions, and processes. Managers are members of the management forums, which are responsible for the facilitation of practice through resource management and location. Recommendations for action go to the executive committee, which has administrative and staff membership that may or may not be in equal proportion. The nurse executive retains decision-making authority.

Phase Two

Representative staff nurses belong to nursing committees that are designated for specific management or clinical functions. These committees are chaired by staff nurses or administrators appointed by the vice-president of nursing/chief nursing officer. The nursing committee chairs and nurse administrators make up the nursing cabinet, which makes the final decision on recommendations from the committees.

Phase Three

Representative staff nurses belong to councils with authority for specific functions. Council chairs make up the management committee charged with making all final operational organizational decisions.

open access to information, resources, support, and opportunities for learning and professional development both empower and enable nurses to accomplish their work (Wong, 2013). Shared-governance structures require new behaviours of all staff, not just new assignments of accountability. Particularly important are the areas of interpersonal relationship development, conflict resolution, and personal acceptance of responsibility for action. Education, conflict management, and experience in group work are essential for successful transitions.

ANALYZING ORGANIZATIONS

When an organization is analyzed, it is important to scrutinize the various systems that exist to accomplish the work of the organization. This includes delineating the processes or procedures that have been developed to coordinate the work to be done. To conceptualize how the organization functions, it is imperative to know the

recruitment procedures, the method of selecting individuals for positions, the reporting relationships, the information network, and the governance structure for nurses. In a positive organization, the mission, vision, and philosophy fit with the structure and practices. Organizational strategies that create manageable spans of control for frontline managers are essential to ensure they are able to achieve exemplary job and unit outcomes while having the necessary time and energy to facilitate staff work engagement and to participate in proactive future system developments (Wong, 2013). Professional standards in Canada, the Canadian Nurses Association (http://www.cna-nurses.ca), provincial and territorial professional nursing associations, and nurse licensing agencies set standards and guidelines for quality nursing services in organizations. Provincial nurse licensing bodies set mandatory standards of practice. Professional associations at the provincial and territorial or national levels represent nurses and work to advance the practice and profession of nursing, improve health outcomes, and influence health policy. For example, the Registered Nurses' Association of Ontario (http://www.rnao.org) has developed Best Practice Guidelines for healthy work environments on a number of topics, including nursing leadership, staffing and workload, managing workplace violence, cultural diversity, and workplace health and safety. In addition, Accreditation Canada (http://www.accreditation.ca) is a not-for-profit, independent organization that provides health care organizations with an external peer review process to assess and improve the services they provide to their patients based on standards of excellence. The accreditation program covers diverse health care services, and standards are based on research and best practices. It also addresses the management function across and throughout all levels of the organization, rather than individual or position-specific competencies. The organization's standards clarify the requirements for effective operational and performance management supports, decision-making structures, and the infrastructure needed to drive excellence and quality improvement in health care service delivery in all departments and programs, including nursing.

EMERGING FLUID RELATIONSHIPS

Under the continuum of care, when health care services occur outside of institutional parameters, different skill sets, relationships, and behavioural patterns will be required. Organizations are beginning to lose their traditional boundaries. Old boundaries of hierarchy, function, and geography are disappearing. Vertical integration aligns dissimilar but related entities, such as the hospital, home care employer, rehabilitation centre, long-term care facility, insurance provider, and medical office or clinic. New technologies, fast-changing public demands for service, changes in government policy, and global competition are revolutionizing relationships in health care, and the roles that people play and the tasks that they perform have become blurred and ambiguous.

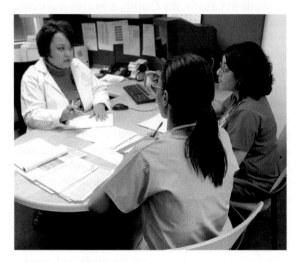

Nurses must have the ability to work with other members of the organization to design organizational models for care delivery that meet patient needs and priorities.

In the future, nurses will no longer practise in geographically limited settings, but rather in systems of care that have extended boundaries. Reframing or changing current static organizations into vibrant learning organizations will require significant effort (Garvin et al., 2008). A learning organization is an organization that is continually expanding its capacity to create its future and provide opportunities and incentives for its members to learn continuously over time (Senge, 2006). To be successful, nurses need to be able to participate as active members in these living-learning organizations. Nurses, whether leaders, managers, or staff, must have the ability to work with other members of the organization and with society at large to design organizational models for health care delivery that meet patient needs and priorities. It is essential to take a new look at the nature of the work of nursing and propose innovative models for nursing practice that consider emerging technologies, patient engagement, and rapidly changing health care needs. Employee participation and learning environments go hand in hand, and work redesign needs to be regarded as a continuous process. It is essential that nurses value their and others' autonomy to deal successfully in these new structures.

? A SOLUTION

Laurie's first task was to determine and establish the management structure, including how the scope of responsibility had changed for individual managers. The next step was to actively recruit for the vacant positions and ensure that effective retention strategies were implemented so that those who were already members of the team were committed to the new direction. Laurie also created a staff development coordinator position to involve nurse managers in the development of a vision for clinical management.

After establishing the management team, Laurie's next priority was to articulate core competencies for the clinical staff. Staff participated in identifying and designing the initial set of competencies through staff representatives from each major clinical department. At the same time, the management team has been developing a second set of competencies that are unit-specific. The interest and enthusiasm the nurses have shown in meeting this challenge has been very gratifying. Also, the staff development coordinator has been an asset, with previous university teaching experience, the coordinator appreciates the importance of high standards and consistency in staff education. The staff development coordinator has also been using already-existing connections to help develop a solid recruitment program.

Would this be a suitable approach for you? Why or why not?

THE EVIDENCE

Organizational culture plays an important role in creating a positive work environment and enhancing employee commitment and intent to stay after major organizational changes. Gregory et al. (2007) invited 1173 front-line registered nurses working in acute care settings in Newfoundland and Labrador to participate in a survey following a restructuring and regionalization of health services in 2005. Changes in health care services included moving from a facilities-based structure to a functional-based structure with multidisciplinary teams, a change to program-based management, a 40–50% reduction of management and support personnel, the closure and merger of hospitals and facilities, and the dislocation of approximately 50% of nursing staff. Of the nurses surveyed, a final sample of 343 was obtained for a response rate of 29.4%. *Organizational culture* in this study was defined as satisfaction with the emotional climate of the workplace, practice issues, and collaborative relations with management and other disciplines. Although nurses were moderately satisfied with their jobs, they reported negative effects from the restructuring on organizational culture, trust in their employers, and their commitment to stay with their organization. Study findings supported the connection and impact of organizational culture on nurses' trust in their employer and job satisfaction and, ultimately, on nurses' commitment to the organization and their intent to stay.

The study also provided evidence of the impact of organizational changes on the attitudes of nurses. The researchers made recommendations on how managers might reduce the negative impact of restructuring activities. They suggested that positive leaders who are present, visible, and accessible to all staff were necessary to renew and revitalize supportive organizational cultures. Moreover, they also suggested that managers who focus on developing and implementing strategies to enrich culture (in particular, the emotional climate), control practice issues, encourage collaborative relationships, and rebuild trusting relationships with nurses could positively influence reorganizational changes. Creating a more supportive work environment requires a partnership approach with all levels of health care providers to identify and implement interventions and policies that are responsive to employee needs. Research results suggested that it is advantageous for managers to emphasize transparency, balanced processing, self-awareness, and high ethical standards to increase nurses' job satisfaction and performance (Wong, 2013).

✴ NEED TO KNOW NOW

- Know the mission, vision, values, and philosophy of your organization and work unit.
- Identify the expected lines of communication as presented on the formal organizational chart.
- Analyze actual workplace practices for opportunities to streamline decision making.

CHAPTER CHECKLIST

The mission, vision, and values of the organization determine how nursing care is delivered in a health care organization. Changes occurring in the organization's mission affect both the culture of the workplace and the philosophies regarding the work required to accomplish the mission. Actualizing new missions and philosophies requires re-engineered organizational structures that place decision-making authority and responsibility where care is delivered. Decision-making responsibility requires staff to understand the organization's mission and to participate in the development of mission and philosophy statements.

- Five factors influencing design of an organization structure are the following:
  1. The types of service performed or the product produced.
  2. The characteristics of the employees performing the service or producing the product.
  3. The beliefs and values held by the people responsible for delivering the service concerning the work, the people receiving the services, and the employees.
  4. The technologies used to perform the service and produce the product.

5. The needs, desires, and characteristics of the users of the product or service.

- Re-engineering, the complete overhaul of an organizational structure, is driven by the following forces:
  - Changes in government policy and funding.
  - Public demand for services.
  - Enhanced technology and research evidence.
- Bureaucratic structures are characterized by the following:
  - A high degree of formalization.
  - Centralization of decision making at the top of the organization.
  - A hierarchy of authority.
- Structures can be organized along the following lines:
  - Functional.
  - Service-line.
  - Matrix.
  - Flat.
- Functional structures are characterized by the following:
  - Departments and services organized according to specialty.
  - Discontinuity of patient services because of silo mentality, even when structure supports professional expertise and encourages advancement.
- Service-line structures are characterized by the following:
  - Functions necessary to provide a specific service brought together under a single line of authority.
- Matrix structures are characterized by the following:
  - Dual authority for product and function.

- Mechanisms, such as committees, to coordinate actions of product and function managers.
- Success that depends on recognition and appreciation of each other's missions and philosophies and commitment to the organization's mission and philosophy.
- Flat organizations are characterized by the following:
  - Decision making concerning work performed, decentralized to the level where the work is done.
  - Authority, accountability, and autonomy, as well as responsibility, provided to staff performing care.
  - Low level of formalization in relation to rules, with processes tailored to meet individual patients' needs.
- Mission, vision, and values determine the characteristics of the organizational structure by doing the following:
  - Describing patient needs and services as a prescription for the technologies and human resources needed to accomplish the defined purpose (mission).
  - Creating an ultimate state of existence (vision).
  - Citing values and beliefs that shape and are shaped by the nature of the work and the rights and responsibilities of workers and patients.
  - Designing characteristics that support the service implementation to fulfill the mission and philosophy (structure).
- Shared governance is characterized by the following:
  - The creation of organizational structures that allow nursing staff more autonomy to govern their practice.
  - Recruitment and retention of nursing staff while meeting patient needs in an effective and efficient manner.

TIPS FOR UNDERSTANDING ORGANIZATIONAL STRUCTURES

- Professional nurses in staff or followership positions need to understand the mission, vision, philosophy, and structure at the organization and unit level to maximize their contributions to patient care.
- The overall mission of the organization and the mission of the specific unit in which a professional nurse is employed or is seeking employment provide information concerning the major focus of the work to be accomplished and the manner in which it will be accomplished.
- Understanding the philosophy of the organization or unit where work occurs provides knowledge of the

behaviours that are valued in the delivery of patient care and in interactions with persons employed by the organization.
- Formal organizational structures describe the expected channels of communication and decision making.
- Matrix organizations usually have two persons responsible for the work, and therefore it is important to know to whom you are responsible for what.
- For a shared-governance structure to function effectively, the professionals providing the care must put mechanisms in place to promote decision making about patient care.

Visit the Evolve website for Suggested Readings, Internet Resources, and additional resources related to the content in this chapter: http://evolve.elsevier.com/Canada/Yoder-Wise/leading/.

REFERENCES

Bart, C. K., & Hupfer, M. (2004). Mission statements in Canadian hospitals. *Journal of Health Organization and Management, 18*(2), 92–110. https://doi.org/10.1108/14777260410538889.

Bellot, J. (2011). Defining and assessing organizational culture. *Nursing Forum, 46*(1), 29–37. https://doi.org/10.1111/j.1744-6198.2010.00207.x.

Brafman, O., & Beckstrom, R. A. (2008). *The starfish and the spider: The unstoppable power of leaderless organizations.* New York, NY: Penguin Books.

Canadian Patient Safety Institute. (2018). *Safety healthcare now.* Ottawa, ON: Author. http://www.saferhealthcarenow.ca/EN/Pages/default.aspx.

Casida, J. (2008). Linking nursing unit's culture to organizational effectiveness: A measurement tool. *Nursing Economic$, 26*(2), 106–110.

Chen, Y. C. (2008). Restructuring the organizational culture of medical institutions: A study of a community hospital in the I-Lan area. *Journal of Nursing Research, 16*, 211–219. https://doi.org/10.1097/01.JNR.0000387308.42364.34.

Choosing Wisely Canada. (n.d.). Recommendations. https://choosingwiselycanada.org/.

Cormack, C., Hillier, L. M., Anderson, K., et al. (2007). Practice change: The process of developing and implementing a nursing care delivery model for geriatric rehabilitation. *Journal of Nursing Administration, 37*(6), 279–286. https://doi.org/10.1097/01.NNA.0000277719.79876.ec.

Eastern Health, Newfoundland and Labrador. (2017). *Foundations Statements of Vision and Mission.* http://www.easternhealth.ca/AboutEH.aspx?d=1&id=709&p=73.

Engle, R. L., Lopez, E. R., Gormley, K. E., Chan, J. A., Charns, M. P., & Lukas, C. V. (2017). What roles do middle managers play in implementation of innovative practices? *Health Care Management Review, 42*(1), 14–27.

Fayol, H. (1949). *General and industrial management.* London, UK: Pitman.

Garvin, D. A., Edmondson, A. C., & Gino, F. (2008). Is yours a learning organization? *Harvard Business Review, 86*(3), 109–116.

Gregory, D. M., Way, C. Y., LeFort, S., et al. (2007). Predictors of registered nurses' organizational commitment and intent to stay. *Health Care Management Review, 32*(2), 119–127. https://doi.org/10.1097/01.HMR.0000267788.79190.f4.

Health Quality Ontario. (2018). *Public reporting: Patient safety.* http://www.hqontario.ca/public-reporting/patient-safety.

Health Quality Council Alberta. (2018). *Health Outcomes.* http://www.hqca.ca/studies-and-reviews/health-outcomes-measurement/.

Henderson, A., Cooke, M., Creedy, D. K., et al. (2012). Nursing students' perceptions of earning in practice environments: A review. *Nurse Education Today, 32*, 299–302. https://doi.org/10.1016/j.nedt.2011.03.010.

Laschinger, H. K., Finegan, J., & Wilk, P. (2009). Context matters: The impact of unit leadership and empowerment on nurses' organizational commitment. *Journal of Nursing Administration, 39*, 228–235. https://doi.org/10.1097/NNA.0b013e3181a23d2b.

Laschinger, H. K., Read, E., & Zhu, J. (2016). 23. Employee empowerment and organizational commitment. *Handbook of Employee Commitment, 319.*

Lencioni, P. (2006). *Silos, politics and turf wars: A leadership fable.* San Francisco, CA: Jossey-Bass.

MacPhee, M., Wardrop, A., & Campbell, C. (2010). Transforming work place relationships through shared decision making. *Journal of Nursing Management, 18*, 1016–1026. https://doi.org/10.1111/j.1365-2834.2010.01122.x.

Martin, S. C., Greenhouse, P. K., Merryman, T., et al. (2007). Transforming care at the bedside: Implementation and spread model for single-hospital and multihospital systems. *Journal of Nursing Administration, 37*, 444–451. https://doi.org/10.1097/01.NNA.0000285152.79988.f3.

Matthews, S., Spence Laschinger, H. K., & Johnstone, L. (2006). Staff nurse empowerment in line and staff organizational structures for chief nurse executives. *Journal of Nursing Administration, 36*(11), 526–533.

Meagher-Stewart, D., Underwood, J., MacDonald, M., et al. (2010). Organizational attributes that assure optimal utilization of public health nurses. *Public Health Nursing, 27*(5), 433–441. https://doi.org/10.1111/j.1525-1446.2010.00876.x.

Melnick, G., Ulaszek, W. R., Lin, H. J., et al. (2009). When goals diverge: Staff consensus and the organizational culture. *Drug and Alcohol Dependence, 103*, S17–S22. https://doi.org/10.1016/j.drugalcdep.2008.10.023.

Moore, S. C., & Hutchinson, S. A. (2007). Developing leaders at every level: Accountability and empowerment actualized through shared governance. *Journal of Nursing Administration, 37*, 556–558. https://doi.org/10.1097/01.NNA.0000302386.76119.22.

Murphy, N., & Roberts, D. (2008). Nurse leaders as stewards at the point of service. *Nursing Ethics, 15,* 243–253. https://doi.org/10.1177/0969733007086022.

Regan, S., Laschinger, H., & Wong, C. (2016). The influence of empowerment, authentic leadership, and professional practice environments on nurses' perceived interprofessional collaboration. *Journal of nursing management, 24*(1), E54–E61. https://doi.org/10.1111/jonm.12288.

Saskatchewan Health Quality Council. (2018). *Health System Performance.* https://hqc.sk.ca/health-system-performance/how-our-health-care-system-is-doing.

Senge, P. M. (2006). *The fifth discipline: The art & practice of the learning organization.* Random House Digital.

Smith, D. L., Klopper, H. E., Paras, A., et al. (2006). Structure in health agencies. In J. M. Hibberd & D. L. Smith (Eds.), *Nursing leadership and management in Canada* (3rd ed.). (pp. 163–198). Toronto, ON: Elsevier Canada.

Southwest Ontario Local Health Integration Network (LHIN). (2014). *About our LHIN.* http://www.southwestlhin.on.ca/aboutus.aspx.

Southwest Ontario Aboriginal Health Access Centre (SOAHAC). (2014). *Mission and overview.* https://soahac.on.ca/mission-overview-2016/.

Spence Laschinger, H. K., Zhu, J., & Read, E. (2016). New nurses' perceptions of professional practice behaviours, quality of care, job satisfaction and career retention. *Journal of nursing management, 24*(5), 656–665. https://doi.org/10.1111/jonm.12370.

Ulrich, B. T., Buerhaus, P. I., Donelan, K., et al. (2007). Magnet status and registered nurse views of the work environment and nursing as a career. *Journal of Nursing Administration, 37*(5), 212–220. https://doi.org/10.1097/01.NNA.0000269745.24889.c6.

Weber, M. (1947). *The theory of social and economic organization.* Parsons, NY: Free Press.

Williams, J., Smythe, W., Hadjistavropoulos, T., et al. (2005). A study of thematic content in hospital mission statements: A question of values. *Health Care Management Review, 30*(4), 304–314. https://doi.org/10.1097/00004010-200510000-00004.

Wong, C. A., & Laschinger, H. (2012). Authentic leadership, performance, and job satisfaction: The mediating role of empowerment. *Journal of advanced nursing, 69*(4), 947–959. https://doi.org/10.1111/j.1365-2648.2012.06089.x.

Wong, C. A., Elliott-Miller, P., & Laschinger, H. (2013). Examining the relationships between span of control and manager job and unit performance outcomes. *Journal of nursing management, 23*(2), 156–168. https://doi.org/10.1111/jonm.12107.

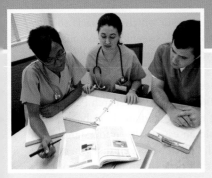

11

Cultural Diversity in Health Care

Yolanda Babenko-Mould

This chapter focuses on the importance of cultural considerations for patients and staff. Although it does not address comprehensive details about any specific culture, it does provide guidelines for actively incorporating cultural competence into the roles of leading and managing. This chapter also presents the concepts and principles of cultural safety and emphasizes the importance of respecting diverse lifestyles. It includes scenarios and exercises that promote an appreciation of cultural richness.

OBJECTIVES

- Understand the concepts of culture, cultural diversity, cultural sensitivity, cultural competence, and cultural safety in leading and managing in nursing.
- Understand how cultural diversity affects leading and managing in health care organizations.
- Describe how prejudice can interfere with quality patient care.

- Identify theoretical models that can help health care providers deliver culturally competent patient care.
- Understand individual and societal factors related to cultural diversity.
- Consider how nurse managers and leaders can design services and programs to meet the needs of culturally diverse staff and patients.

TERMS TO KNOW

cross-culturalism
cultural competence
cultural diversity
cultural imposition

cultural marginality
cultural safety
cultural sensitivity
culture

ethnocentrism
multiculturalism
transculturalism

⚡ A CHALLENGE

Dwayne is a newly graduated nurse practitioner from London, Ontario, who has been assigned to practice in an outpost community in the Northwest Territories. In addition to providing nursing care to a population of approximately 1 500 individuals (most of whom are Indigenous peoples), part of Dwayne's role will be to manage the small community health clinic, which is staffed by two nurses and an administrative assistant who are of Indigenous origin. This will be Dwayne's first experience working in the Northwest Territories and in the role of a nurse manager. Given that they will work in a community with a rich heritage, Dwayne wants to ensure that their nursing practice reflects cultural safety so that their associations with clinic personnel and patients are respectful.

If you were Dwayne, how might you enhance your understanding of cultural safety so that you relate well to staff members and the community you will serve?

INTRODUCTION

Concepts and Principles

What is *culture*? Does it exhibit certain characteristics? What is *cultural diversity*, and what do you think of when people refer to *cultural sensitivity, cultural competence*, and *cultural safety*? Are *culture* and *ethnicity* the same? Some answers to these questions appear in this chapter. Nurse managers and leaders are concerned with culture, particularly as it relates to patient care and diversity in the workplace. Culture, a social determinant of health, has historically been defined broadly as "shared patterns of learned behaviours and values transmitted over time, and that distinguish the members of one group from another" (Canadian Nurses Association [CNA], 2004, p. 2). This view recognizes that culture helps shape us but does not define who we are as individuals; culture is dynamic and changing, and people come to understand culture by interacting with one another and developing relationships. In this chapter, culture is viewed from this constructivist perspective (Gray & Thomas, 2006), which is an understanding of culture that aligns with that of the Aboriginal Nurses Association of Canada (ANAC) (2009, p. 1) as noted in *Cultural Competency Framework for Nursing Education.*

The constructivist perspective moves away from a historical or *essentialist* perspective of culture. The essentialist perspective holds that culture is not changeable, that people are simply a product of their culture, and that the "norm" culture in Canada is white and moderately affluent. Any culture outside of this supposed norm is "different." The essentialist perspective can lead groups who are considered "different" to be devalued, which reinforces imbalanced power relationships. By contrast, a constructivist perspective of culture recognizes that various social, political, historical, and economic forces have influenced or shaped an individual to a certain moment in time. As Racine (2014) argues, without recognizing that culture is not about a "norm of the majority group" (p. 7), cultural stereotypes that equate difference with "othering" will continue to proliferate. Thus each person's individual experience of culture varies and cannot be easily categorized. What this means for nurse managers, nurse leaders, and staff nurses is that they need to dedicate time to building relationships with colleagues and patients to become aware of their particular cultural beliefs, practices, values, and ways of being to avoid erroneous assumptions. It is also important for nurse managers and leaders to engage health care staff in

discussions about the ways in which culture is socially constructed, so as to avoid sweeping generalizations and cultural stereotypes. Discussion should focus on the "agents and forces contributing to such construction as well as consequences resulting from these processes" (Gray & Thomas, 2006, p. 78). The Research Perspective below illustrates that nursing students have been found to predominantly hold an essentialist understanding of culture. Gregory et al. (2010) proposed that when nurse leaders and nursing staff develop an awareness of their assumptions and beliefs about culture, they are better prepared to learn about how culture shapes themselves, their colleagues, and perceptions about care practices. However, as Gray and Thomas (2006) propose, a critical lens needs to be used to push awareness further to explore the processes that have led to such values and beliefs and to continually question who is disadvantaged by an essentialist conceptualization of culture. Such awareness and knowledge can open up pathways for discussion about factors impacting care, such as power, colonialism, and racism to ultimately create a space for relational care practices with patients and their families (Hartrick et al., 2005).

Language clarity among nurse managers, nurse leaders, staff nurses, and nursing students is important so that everyone uses common points of reference in practice. Language clarity is also important to nurse leaders and staff nurses in relation to quality patient-care practices. When a message communicated to or by a patient is translated from one language to another, it is important to ensure linguistic equivalence, which means that the message must have the same meaning in both languages. Achieving an equivalent translation involves interpretation, which extends beyond a "word-for-word" translation. When providing care to a patient from another culture whose first language is not English, the nurse must realize that the process of translation of illness or disease conditions and treatment can be complex. Thus, a nurse who values cultural safety should advocate for and retain a translator for the patient. By doing so, the principles of equity and justice for the patient are at the forefront of how the nurse engages in the care experience.

As role models, nurse managers and leaders can demonstrate a constructivist perspective of cultural diversity through their everyday actions. It is vital to explore the idea of cultural diversity at an individual level. The International Council of Nurses (ICN) (2013) notes that diversity in nursing "means understanding

RESEARCH PERSPECTIVE

Resource: Gregory, D., Harrowing, J., Lee, B., Doolittel, L., & Sullivan, P. S. (2010). Pedagogy as influencing nursing students' essentialized understanding of culture. *International Journal of Nursing Education Scholarship, 7*(1), 1–17.

In a study by Gregory et al. (2010), 14 nursing and 8 non-nursing student participants were asked to define *culture* and write narratives regarding specific cultural encounters. The researchers found that of the 14 nursing students, 13 viewed culture from an essentialist perspective and only one viewed culture from a constructivist perspective. The researchers also found that of the eight non-nursing students, three viewed culture from an essentialist perspective and five viewed culture from a constructivist perspective. According to these findings, most nursing students perceived culture as something unchanging, passed down from gener-

ation to generation, and associated with defined behaviours. Such a view limited participants' abilities to consider culture as dynamic, related to context, and unique to each individual. By contrast, the nursing student who framed culture from a constructivist perspective wrote narratives that recognized culture as temporal or ever-evolving and not solely able to define who patients are as individuals.

Implications for Practice

Based on the study findings, nursing student participants predominantly reflected essentialist rather than constructivist perspectives of culture. The researchers affirmed that nurse educators should be aware of their perspective on culture and how culture is taught to nursing students to be able to move away from the limiting essentialist perspective.

that each individual is unique, and recognizing individual differences. These differences may span the dimensions of race, ethnicity, gender, sexual orientation, socio-economic status, age, physical abilities, religious beliefs, political beliefs or other ideologies" (p. 2). The Registered Nurses' Association of Ontario (2007) proposes a similar definition, in that cultural diversity "is used to describe variation between people in terms of a range of factors such as ethnicity, national origin, race, gender, ability, age, physical characteristics, religion, values, beliefs, sexual orientation, socio-economic class, or life experiences" (p. 70). Further, Burnard and Gill (2009) suggest that culture reflects an individual's identity or sense of self. However, as Hartrick et al. (2005) note, given that culture is a socially constructed perspective, context (historical, social, political) must be taken into account when considering individual difference (p. 32). When considering culture and cultural diversity, a constructivist perspective "makes visible the fluid processes involved as one's cultural identity is constantly being defined, re-defined, negotiated and managed through individual and societal processes. A critical constructivist viewpoint helps make these processes visible and invites exploration of the consequences of such processes—again, establishing opportunities for connection and understanding between nurse and patient. Practically speaking, having an appreciation for the lived experience of mediating multiple identities is consistent with nursing's commitment to respect and appreciation for people" (Gray & Thomas, 2006, p. 80).

Cultural sensitivity has been understood to be the capacity to recognize and be sensitive to differences between cultures. However, Hartrick et al. (2005) argue that the term *cultural sensitivity* does not include "sensitivity to context and the structural determinants of health" (p. 310) and requires no formal action by the nurse to create any form of change around factors contributing to inequities and injustice. Movement toward a constructivist perspective on cultural sensitivity involves recognizing one's own biases and judgements and understanding how such factors impact relationships among colleagues in practice settings, and the delivery of care, and take action to un-learn Eurocentric values and beliefs to advance quality of care.

The *Code of Ethics for Registered Nurses* (CNA, 2017) sets out primary nursing values (see Chapter 6) that should be applied in a way that respects the cultural diversity of health care staff, patients, and their families. For instance, the nursing value—promoting justice— requires that "nurses uphold principles of justice by safeguarding human rights, equity and fairness and by promoting the public good" (p. 15). Applying this value to nursing practice, if a nurse manager or leader does not support a nurse who seeks to provide an interpreter for a patient who cannot speak English, then the patient is not being treated fairly or equally, and the patient's human rights are essentially violated. This ethical value helps nurses recognize that health care must be provided to culturally diverse populations in Canada and globally.

Effective leaders shape their organization in a way that demonstrates cultural competence in action. *Cultural competence* is the process of integrating values, beliefs, and attitudes different from one's own perspective to render effective nursing care. "Culturally competent practices are a congruent set of workforce behaviours, management practices and institutional policies within a practice setting resulting in an organisational environment that is inclusive of cultural and other forms of diversity" (Pearson et al., 2007, p. 55). According to Noone (2008): "Nursing leaders at all levels are calling for a nursing workforce able to provide culturally competent patient care. Our commitment to social justice and the practical demands of the workplace call for nursing to take strong, sustained, and measurable actions to produce a workforce that closely parallels the population it serves" (p. 133). It is important to acknowledge that cultural competency does not mean becoming an expert in every form of culture, but it is aligned with learning about how to engage in respectful relationships (Indigenous Health, 2017) with patients, families, communities, and nursing colleagues.

Cultural safety relates to the acknowledgement that power difference and inequities exist in systems, including health care (ANAC, 2009). It refers to what is experienced by a patient when health care providers communicate in a respectful and inclusive way, empowering the patient in decision making and ensuring maximum effectiveness of care (National Aboriginal Health Organization, 2008). Nurse managers, nurse leaders, and staff nurses have a vital role to play in addressing issues of power and inequity through collaborative advocacy efforts and by uncovering practices that can lead to inequitable access to care or to forms of discrimination or racism that can ultimately affect the provision of care (Varcoe, 2004, as cited in ANAC, 2009). A lack of mutual understanding between people from different cultures can lead to cultural marginality, which has been defined as "situations and feelings of passive betweenness when people exist between two different cultures and do not yet perceive themselves as centrally belonging to either one" (Choi, 2001, p. 193). Therefore, it is imperative for nurse managers, nurse leaders, and staff nurses not to make assumptions about culture, and to initiate a dialogue with individuals to explore what culture means for them.

> **EXERCISE 11.1** If you were to provide care to a patient from another culture in an acute care setting, in what ways could you ensure cultural safety?
>
> How would these actions be different from how you have provided care in the past or have seen care provided by others in the past?

CULTURAL DIVERSITY IN HEALTH CARE ORGANIZATIONS

The demographics of the nursing profession have historically not matched general demographics related to gender and ethnic diversity. The numbers of men recruited into the profession have risen but not to the point of creating gender equality. According to the Canadian Institute of Health Information (CIHI) (2018), approximately 8% of all registered nurses in Canada were male in 2017. Although stereotypes (e.g., "not smart enough for medical school") have diminished over the years, the number of men in nursing still does not approach the proportional number of men in Canada. In terms of ethnic diversity, according to the Statistics Canada 2016 Census, there were 1 673 785 individuals identifying as Indigenous peoples in Canada (2018). The Canadian Indigenous Nurses Association (CINA) (2018) notes there are 9 695 Indigenous nurses in Canada, which reflects 3% of the overall Registered Nursing population in Canada. However, Indigenous peoples account for 4.9% of the Canadian population (CINA, 2018; Exner-Pirot, 2016). According to the CIHI, as of 2017, approximately 34 101 Registered Nurses (including Nurse Practitioners) in Canada received their original nursing education in a country other than Canada. Although these numbers suggest diversity among nurses in practice, it is critical for nurse managers and leaders to consider cultural diversity in terms of the many layers of contextual issues that have shaped each nurse, and what that means for the provision of a culturally safe working environment for all nurses.

Given that "cultural safety is not about cultural practices but the recognition of social, economic, and political positions of groups in society" (Richardson et al. 2017, p. 2), it is vital that nurse leaders and nurses have opportunities for professional development to learn about the concept and how to enact it in practice to create culturally safe practice settings. By extension, staff nurses require ongoing education about how to provide culturally safe care to patients while also supporting a culturally safe work environment. Such environments are fundamental to advancing quality patient care.

> **EXERCISE 11.2** On the accompanying Evolve site under Additional Resources, complete the Cultural Competence Self-Assessment Tool for Primary Health Care Providers.
> What did you learn from using the tool? In what ways might you develop additional cultural competence?

Managing in a Culturally Diverse Environment

Managing in a culturally diverse environment means managing personal thinking and helping others think in new ways. Managing issues that involve culture—whether institutional, ethnic, gender, religious, or any other kind—requires patience, persistence, and much understanding. One way to promote this understanding is through shared stories that have symbolic power.

> **EXERCISE 11.3** Think of a recent event in your learning environment or workplace, such as a project, task force, or celebration. What meaning did people give to the event? What quality of the learning environment or workplace did it symbolize (e.g., effectiveness, values and beliefs, innovation)? How is cultural diversity considered?

A health care organization with a straightforward mission and clear goals, rewards, and acknowledgement of efforts leads to greater productivity and work effort from a culturally diverse staff who aspires to unity, while recognizing that assimilation is not a goal to attain unity in the practice setting. When assessing staff diversity, the nurse manager can ask these questions:

- What is the cultural representation of individuals in the workplace?
- What kind of team-building activities are needed to create a cohesive workforce for effective health care delivery?
- How can management and staff further enhance cultural competence and cultural safety in the workplace?

Nurse managers and leaders who have a positive view of culture and its characteristics effectively acknowledge cultural diversity among staff and patients. This includes providing culturally sensitive care to patients while simultaneously balancing a culturally diverse staff. On a larger organizational scale, Baumann et al. (2017) recommend the following actions for leaders to promote and support cultural diversity in the practice setting: "demonstrate senior leadership commitment to diversity, communicate the importance of diversity across the organization, create and update inclusive policies and procedures, develop and implement a diversity and inclusion strategy, orient new staff and provide ongoing training for all staff, and recruit, retain, and promote a culturally diverse workforce" (p. 6).

To show their understanding and value of cultural diversity, nurse managers and leaders need to approach every staff person as an individual. More specifically, in the practice setting, nurse managers can promote inclusion and communication in relation to performance where a nurse manager can make sure messages about patient care are received. This might be accomplished by sitting down with a staff nurse and analyzing the situation to ensure that understanding has occurred. In addition, the nurse manager might use a communication notebook that allows the nurse to have time to "digest" information by writing down communication areas that may be unclear.

Although staff members may have different cultural origins and may be diverse in appearance, values, beliefs, communication patterns, and mannerisms, they have many things in common. For example, staff members want to be accepted by others and to succeed in their jobs. With fairness and respect, nurse managers and leaders should openly support the competencies and contributions of staff members from all cultural groups with the goal of achieving quality patient care. For effective staff interaction, the nurse manager can also make a special effort to pair mentors and mentees who have different ethnic backgrounds.

Sullivan and Decker (2009) described the importance of communication and how cultural attitudes, beliefs, and behaviour affect communication. Body movements, gestures, verbal tone, and physical closeness in communication tend to be determined by a person's culture. For the nurse manager or leader, understanding culturally specific behaviours is imperative in accomplishing effective communication in a diverse workforce.

For nurse managers and leaders, attending to cultural diversity requires being sensitive to, or being able to, embrace the emotions of a large multicultural group comprising staff and patients. It might mean acknowledging and respecting choices related to faith. For instance, Muslims are one of the fastest-growing populations in North America and worldwide. El Gindy (2004) addressed the need to show respect for and accommodate Muslim nurses' dress requirements and to understand the role of Islam in their lives. For example, one Muslim nurse wore her hijab and became frustrated because the infection control staff consistently asked her to wear short sleeves or to roll up the sleeves. El Gindy stated that for Muslim women, following the Islamic dress code is necessary to obey the diktat that their body must be covered in the presence of males who are not family. Regardless of organizational setting, health care providers should be made aware of religious beliefs, whether they exist among staff or patients, and respond to them in a positive way.

A nurse manager's or leader's choices, decisions, and behaviours reflect learned beliefs, values, ideals, and preferences. A nurse manager or leader who shows respect for culturally diverse individuals and groups supports the best interests of both staff and patients.

Cultural Diversity and Patient Care

In Canada, many patients in health care settings are new to this country. According to the 2011 National Household Survey, 6.8 million people, or 20.6% of the total Canadian population, were born outside the country (Statistics Canada, 2013). This was the highest proportion since 1931, when foreign-born people made up 22.2% of the population (Statistics Canada, 2003, p. 4). Further, of the 1.2 million immigrants who arrived between 2006 and 2011, 56.9% were from Asia, including the Middle East; 13.7% from Europe; 12.3% from the Caribbean, Central and South America; 12.5% from Africa; and 3.9% from the United States (Statistics Canada, 2013). New immigrants to Canada might have varied understandings about the Canadian health care system, their rights to health care through Canada's national health insurance plan, and how to navigate the health care system. Often, issues of accessibility to health care influence whether care is ever sought or provided.

Accessibility to health care in Canada is based on the *Canada Health Act* principles of universality and accessibility (Health Canada, 2014). However, such principles are not always adequately upheld. For instance, individuals living in rural or remote areas might not have ready access to health care or might have access to limited amounts and types of care. Further, individuals who do not speak English or French as their first language may find it challenging to know how or where to access health care. Such discrepancies in Canada's health care system challenge nurse managers and leaders who seek to value, respect, and provide individualized attention to patients and staff regardless of their culture, education, geographical location, or socioeconomic status. Novice nurse managers and leaders may feel that they lack "real-life" experience that could help them address staff and patient needs. In reality, although a lack of experience may be a slight drawback, it is by no means an obstacle to addressing individual staff and patient issues. If nurse managers and leaders understand people and their needs, they can advocate for and gain access to health care for all Canadians.

Communication and Patient Care

Nurse leaders need to ensure that clear and understandable communication takes place between health care providers and patients. Ineffective communication by staff with patients and others can lead to misunderstandings and eventual alienation. The use of a health professional interpreter can be an effective strategy when caring for non–English-speaking or limited–English-speaking patients. The current practice seems to be one of using these interpreters rather than translators when speaking with non–English-speaking patients. Why? Purnell and Paulanka (2008) advocate that trained health care providers who act as interpreters can decode words and provide the right meaning of the message. However, Purnell and Paulanka also state that interpreters might affect the reporting of symptoms if they apply their own ideas or omit information. It is important to allow time for translation and interpretation and to clarify information as needed. When patients and health care providers cannot communicate effectively, inequities in accessing needed health care services might translate into negative health outcomes.

CULTURAL DIVERSITY AND PREJUDICE

Canadian society is considered to be a "cultural mosaic" because it includes people of different ethnicities who maintain their culture and language. Given that Canada's population includes Indigenous peoples, immigrants from all over the world, and refugees from war-torn areas, cultural diversity is the norm and ought to be respected and valued as contributing to the unique and non-homogeneous character of the country.

Based on the College of Nurses of Ontario (2009) ethical framework, nurses have an obligation to care for all patients, regardless of differences—whether they are related to culture, economic status, or gender. Providing care for a person or people from a culture other than one's own is a dynamic and complex experience. The experience according to Spence (2004) might involve "prejudice, paradox and possibility" (p. 140). Prejudices "enable us to make sense of the situations in which we find ourselves, yet they also constrain understanding and limit the capacity to come to new or different ways of understanding. It is this contradiction that makes prejudice paradoxical" (Spence, 2004, p. 163). Although it may seem incongruent with prejudice, paradox describes the dynamic interplay of tensions between individuals or groups. It is our responsibility to acknowledge the "possibility of tension" as a potential for new and different understandings derived from our communication and interpretation. Possibility, therefore, presumes a condition for openness with a person from another culture (Spence, 2004). Using hermeneutic interpretation, Spence conducted a study that consisted of accounts from 17 New Zealand nurses who delivered nursing care to patients in acute medical and surgical wards, public health centres, mental health settings, and midwifery specialties. Spence found that prejudice was a condition that enabled or constrained interpretation based on one's values, attitudes, and actions. By talking with people outside their "circle of familiarity" the nurses enhanced their understanding of personally held prejudices. As such, the provision of patient care also became a learning opportunity, which detracted from prejudice and opened up the potential for new understanding and awareness of culture from an individual or family perspective.

EXERCISE 11.4 In a group, discuss the values and beliefs of justice and equality. As a nurse, you may have strong values and beliefs, but you may never have observed their application in health care. Consider language, skin colour, dress, and gestures of patients and staff from various cultures. How will you learn and value what individual differences exist?

CULTURE AND THEORETICAL FRAMEWORKS AND MODELS

How do managers, leaders, and followers take all of the expanding information on cultural diversity in health care and give it a useful organizing structure that can be applied to practice? The Aboriginal Nurses Association of Canada (2009), Purnell (2002), Campinha-Bacote (1999, 2002), and Giger and Davidhizar (2002) provide theoretical models to guide health care providers in delivering culturally competent patient care.

The Aboriginal Nurses Association of Canada (2009) identifies six core competencies that reflect a curriculum framework about cultural competence and cultural safety for First Nations, Inuit, and Metis nursing. They note that this framework can be applied to non-Indigenous learners and faculty as well in the academic and practice setting. The six competencies cover: postcolonial understanding, communication, inclusivity, respect, indigenous knowledge, and mentoring and supporting students for success. Each competency statement is supported by a number of outcomes that learners should be able to achieve to demonstrate competency for engaging in culturally safe nursing practice.

The Canadian Research Institute for the Advancement of Women (CRIAW) developed a model reflecting intersectional identities in the form of a wheel image with the core representing unique aspects of an individual, which is encircled by elements representing one's identity, and further circled by types of "discrimination/isms/attitudes that impact identity" (Simpson, 2009, p. 5). The "outermost circle represents larger forces and structures that work together to reinforce exclusion" (Simpson, 2009, p. 5). This model can be used to help learners become more self-aware of their own multi faceted identities, while also enabling them to transpose the model to consider how it applies to individuals and groups in society that they will be working with as colleagues or caring for in the practice setting. The model can also be used to help learners engage in discussion about social and economic injustices, about policies that perpetuate injustice (Simpson, 2009), and each nurse's role in advocating and leading change to enable culturally safe practice environments and patient care. More recently, in its *Guide for Working with Indigenous Students* (2018), Western University in London, Ontario, adapted the CRIAW (2009) intersectionality model to the context of Indigenous students' intersectional identities (Clark, 2012). This model varies from the original as it

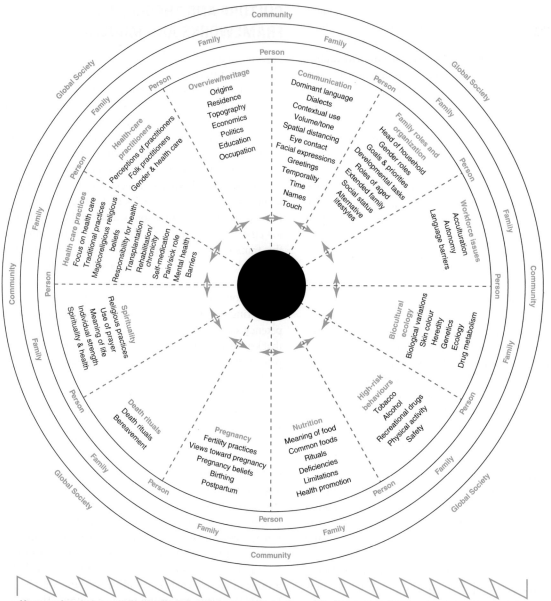

Unconsciously Incompetent - Consciously incompetent - Consciously competent - Unconsciously competent

Variant cultural characteristics: age, generation, nationality, race, colour, gender, religion, educational status, socioeconomic status, occupation, military status, political beliefs, urban versus rural residence, enclave identity, marital status, parental status, physical characteristics, sexual orientation, gender issues, health literacy, and reason for migration (sojourner, immigrant, asylee, undocumented status)

Unconsciously incompetent: not being aware that one is lacking knowledge about another culture
Consciously incompetent: being aware that one is lacking knowledge about another culture
Consciously competent: learning about the client's culture, verifying generalizations about the client's culture, and providing culturally specific interventions
Unconsciously competent: automatically providing culturally congruent care to clients of diverse cultures

Fig. 11.1 Purnell model for cultural competence. (Copyrighted by Larry Purnell, PhD, RN, FAAN.)

focuses on the "unique realities of Indigenous students, including students' relationship to their homelands, their relationship to community and family histories, the effects of colonial violence and intergenerational trauma, and students' struggle against and resistance to the dominant educational system" (Western University, 2018, p. 26).

Purnell's (2002) Model for Cultural Competence provides an organizing framework (Fig. 11.1). The model uses a circle with the outer zone representing global society, the second zone representing community, the third zone representing family, and the inner zone representing the person. The interior of the circle is divided into 12 pie-shaped wedges delineating cultural domains and their concepts (e.g., workplace issues, family roles and organization, spirituality, and health care practices). The innermost centre circle is black, representing unknown phenomena. Cultural consciousness is expressed in behaviours from unconsciously incompetent (being unaware of one's lack of cultural knowledge), consciously incompetent (being aware of one's lack of cultural knowledge), consciously competent (providing culturally specific interventions), to unconsciously competent (automatically providing culturally congruent care to patients). The usefulness of this model is derived from its concise structure, applicability to any setting, and wide range of experiences that can foster inductive and deductive thinking when assessing cultural domains.

Campinha-Bacote's (1999, 2002) model of cultural competence in health care delivery comprises five constructs: cultural awareness, cultural knowledge, cultural skill, cultural encounters, and cultural desire. These constructs have an interdependent relationship, and health care providers must address or experience each of them. In doing so, health care providers cultivate greater cultural competence. Cultural awareness is the self-examination and in-depth exploration of one's own cultural and professional background. It involves the recognition of one's bias, prejudices, and assumptions about individuals from other cultures (Campinha-Bacote, 2002). "One's world view can be considered a paradigm or way of viewing the world and phenomena in it" (Campinha-Bacote, 1999, p. 204). Cultural knowledge is the process of seeking and obtaining a sound educational foundation about diverse cultural and ethnic groups. Further, obtaining cultural information about the individual patient's health-related beliefs and values will help explain how they interpret their illness and how it guides their thinking, doing, and being (Campinha-Bacote, 2002). The skill of conducting a cultural assessment is learned while assessing one's values, beliefs, and practices to provide culturally competent services. Cultural encounters are direct engagement with individuals from other cultures. This process allows the person to validate, negate, or modify their existing cultural knowledge. It provides culturally specific knowledge bases from which the individual can develop culturally relevant interventions. Cultural desire requires the intrinsic qualities of motivation and genuine caring of the health care provider to want to engage in becoming culturally competent (Campinha-Bacote, 1999).

The Giger and Davidhizar (2002) Transcultural Assessment Model identifies phenomena to assess the provision of care to patients from different cultures. Their model is based on the idea that each individual is distinct and can be assessed using six cultural phenomena: communication, space, social organization, time, environmental control, and biological variations. The model is also based on several premises related to culture: culture is a patterned behavioural response that develops over time; is shaped by values, beliefs, norms, and practices; it guides our thinking, doing, and being; and implies a dynamic, ever-changing, active, or passive process.

INDIVIDUAL AND SOCIETAL FACTORS

Nurse managers must work with staff to foster respect of different cultures. To do this, nurse managers need to accept three key principles. Multiculturalism refers to a society characterized by ethnic or cultural heterogeneity; it is an important part of Canadian identity that is recognized in the *Canadian Charter of Rights and Freedoms* ("Multiculturalism," n.d.). However, debates exist about the ways in which Canadian policy and laws have traditionally not been inclusive of Indigenous peoples' rights, as historical paternalistic and assimilation practices were ongoing in Canada through the later part of the twentieth century, and where Indigenous peoples' land rights only began to be recognized in law in the 1970s (Queen's University, 2018). Cross-culturalism refers to mediating between or among cultures. Transculturalism refers to bridging significant differences in cultural practices. In some instances, *transculturalism* has been defined narrowly as a comparison of health beliefs and practices of people from different countries or geographical regions. However, culture can be construed more broadly to include differences in health beliefs and practices by gender, race, ethnicity, economic status, sexual orientation, and disability or physical challenge. Thus, when transcultural care is discussed, we should consider differences in health beliefs and practices not only between and among nationalities but also between genders, and between and among individuals of different races, ethnic groups, and socioeconomic levels. As a consequence, nurses need to consider multiple factors about all individuals.

EXERCISE 11.5 Consider doing a group exercise to enhance cultural sensitivity. Ask each group member to write down four to six beliefs that they value in their culture. When everyone has finished writing, have the group members exchange their lists and discuss why these beliefs are valued. When everyone has had a chance to share lists, have a volunteer compile an all-encompassing list that reflects the values of your workforce. (The key to this exercise is that many of the values are similar or perhaps even identical.)

Ethnocentrism and cultural imposition are two practices that do not support a cohesive workforce or quality patient care. Ethnocentrism "refers to the belief that one's own ways are the best, most superior, or preferred ways to act, believe, or behave" (Leininger, 2002, p. 50). Cultural imposition is defined as "the tendency of an individual or group to impose their values, beliefs, and practices on another culture for varied reasons" (p. 51). Such practices constitute a major concern in nursing and "a largely unrecognized problem as a result of cultural ignorance, blindness, ethnocentric tendencies, biases, racism or other factors" (p. 51).

Although the literature has addressed the multicultural needs of patients, it is sparse in identifying effective methods for nurse managers to use when dealing with multicultural staff. Differences in education and culture can influence patient care, and uncomfortable situations may emerge from such differences. For example, staff members may be reluctant to admit language problems that hamper their written communication. They may also be reluctant to admit their lack of understanding when interpreting directions. Psychosocial skills may be problematic as well, because some non-Western cultures encourage emotional restraint. Staff may have difficulty addressing issues that relate to private family matters. The lack of assertiveness and the subservient physician–nurse relationships of some cultures are other issues that provide challenges for nurse managers. Nurse managers can help prepare staff to handle cultural work situations in two ways: by arranging unit-oriented workshops to address effective techniques and by involving family to better understand cultural differences as they apply to patient care.

Giddens (2008) has encouraged the use of multi-contextual learning environments to enhance the learning of diverse students. She created a Web-based virtual community called The Neighborhood as an exemplar of such a learning environment. The Neighborhood features 30 fictional characters from different cultural and socioeconomic backgrounds with different health issues and their interactions with health care providers in various health care settings. It is designed to promote conceptual learning and offer an alternative approach to learning about diversity in undergraduate nursing programs. According to Giddens, "The Neighborhood presents nursing concepts in a rich personal and community context through stories and supplemental multimedia" (p. 78). Nurse managers can also use this innovative teaching tool to expand staff members' understanding of how to interact with diverse patients. In addition, this learning tool helps address the Institute of Medicine's (2004) finding that the lack of cultural diversity in the nursing workforce affects the quality of health care delivery.

EXERCISE 11.6 As a small group activity, reflect on previous or current clinical practice settings where you have had a clinical placement. Do these settings have professional development programs or policies related to cultural diversity in the workplace? If yes, why is that the case? What do the programs cover? What do the policies propose in regard to staff and patients? If there are no programs or policies, why do you think they have not been implemented?

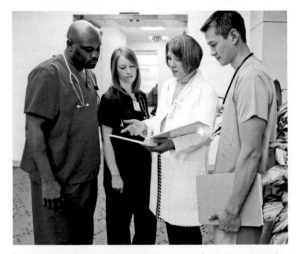

Respecting cultural diversity in the team fosters cooperation and supports sound decision making.

DEALING EFFECTIVELY WITH CULTURAL DIVERSITY

Nurse managers and leaders are the key people who must address cultural diversity in the health care workplace. They must give unwavering support to embracing diversity in the workplace rather than use a standard "cookie cutter" approach. Creating a culturally safe workplace involves a long-term vision and both financial and health care provider commitment. Nurse managers and leaders need to make the strategic decision to design services and programs to meet the needs of culturally diverse staff and patients.

Nurse managers hold the key to making cultural diversity an asset. They have the position of power to create activities and programs that enrich the cultural knowledge of staff. For example, they can capitalize on the staff's personal cultural beliefs and knowledge to achieve better quality care outcomes. One way to do so is to allow staff to verbalize their feelings about particular cultures in relationship to personal beliefs. Another is to have two or three staff members of different ethnic origins present a patient-care conference, giving their views on how they would care for a specific patient's needs based on their own ethnic values.

Mentorship programs should be established so that all staff can expand their knowledge of cultural diversity. Mentors have specific relationships with their mentees. The more closely aligned a mentor is with the mentee (e.g., similar age group, ethnicity, and primary language), the more effective the relationship. Programs that address the staff's cultural diversity should not try to make people of different cultures pattern their behaviour after the prevailing culture. Nurse managers must carefully select those mentors who ascribe to transcultural, rather than ethnocentric, values and beliefs.

A much richer staff exists when nurse managers build on the valuable culture of all staff members and when diversity is rewarded. Nurse managers are aware of the increasing shortage of nurses, the demanding work environment with its external influences, and studies indicating that new nurses have a high rate of intention to leave during their first professional nursing position because of job dissatisfaction and level of stress (Lavoie-Tremblay et al., 2008). The first year of a nursing position may be even more challenging for individuals whose culture differs from the predominant unit culture.

The National Quality Forum (NQF) (2009) created a comprehensive framework for measuring and reporting cultural competency in health care settings. The 45 preferred practices the NFQ endorses fall within the following domains: leadership; integration into management systems and operations; patient–provider communication; care delivery and supporting mechanisms; workforce diversity and training; community engagement; and data collection, public accountability, and quality improvement. The NQF framework provides nurse managers, leaders, and staff with preferred practices that can enhance the delivery of culturally competent patient care.

Continuing-education programs can also help nurses learn about the care of different ethnic groups. For example, professional organizations related to cultural groups and institutions might develop or sponsor a workshop or conference on cross-cultural nursing for nursing service staff and faculty in schools of nursing who have had limited preparation in cultural care or cultural beliefs in healing.

> **EXERCISE 11.7** Identify a situation in which working with culturally diverse staff had positive or negative outcomes. If a negative outcome resulted, what could you have done to make it a positive one? If a positive outcome resulted, share lessons learned on how to make future interactions positive.

> **EXERCISE 11.8** Identify a situation involving a staff member or student nurse colleague requesting additional days of leave that required a culturally sensitive decision. What cultural practices did you learn about in regard to this request and decision?

> **EXERCISE 11.9** Holiday celebrations have cultural significance. Select a specific holiday, such as the Chinese Lunar New Year, Araw ng mga Patay (Philippines), or Diwali (India). What is the cultural meaning of the holiday? How do staff members or students of the respective culture celebrate the festive day? Does the nursing unit or academic environment engage in recognition of special holidays?

The two scenarios described in Box 11.1 illustrate how problem-solving communication can promote mutual understanding and respect. The first scenario

BOX 11.1   Problem-Solving Communication: Honouring Cultural Attitudes

Scenario 1: A Nurse Manager and Another Staff Member

Eastern Catholics celebrate a loved one 40 days after their death. The nurse manager needs to recognize that time off for a nurse involved in this celebration is imperative. Such an occurrence had to be addressed by a nurse manager of Asian descent. The nurse manager quickly realized that the nurse, whose mother died in India, did not ask for any time off to make the necessary burial arrangements but, rather, waited 40 days to celebrate their mother's death. The celebration included formal invitations to a church service, as well as a dinner after the service. One day, during early morning rounds, the nurse explained how death is celebrated by many Eastern Catholics. The Bible's description of the Ascension of the Lord into heaven 40 days after his death served as the conceptual framework for the loved one's death. The grieving family believed their loved one's spirit would stay on earth for 40 days. During these 40 days, the family held prayer sessions meant to assist the "spirit" to prepare for its ascension into heaven. When the 40 days have passed, the celebration previously described marks the ascension of the loved one's spirit into heaven. Because this particular unit truly espoused a multicultural concept, the nurses had no difficulty in allowing the Indian nurse two weeks of unplanned vacation so that their mother's "passage of life" celebration could be accomplished in a respectful, dignified manner.

Scenario 2: A Nurse, a Patient, the Family, and the Community

Bourque Bearskin (2011), a Cree/Métis nurse from a First Nations community, tells the story of Nicole, a 19-year-old First Nations member of a northern community, who was seriously injured in a car accident while she was the passenger of a vehicle with a drunk driver. Her injuries included a serious brain stem injury that required she be transferred from her community to a tertiary hospital in the south. The nurses in the intensive care unit (ICU) cared for her for two days before Nicole's family were able to travel to the hospital from their northern community. Her parents and extended family, including the community Elder, arrived and requested permission to integrate traditional approaches to care with the other aspects of nursing care for Nicole. Bourque Bearskin describes what happened:

The Elder requested permission from the nursing staff to perform a ceremony that would include smudging (ritual cleansing) and the use of traditional medicines. However, because of the concern for the safety of other patients in the ICU, the staff denied the request, and the family members were disappointed; the deep despair on their faces was evident. They continued to make requests and incorporate their traditions in caring for Nicole. They pin a medicine pouch to the inside of the nursing gown close to the body and near the heart. They believed that the contents would protect her and guide her to the spirit world. With clear directions to the staff not to touch or remove the pouch, the family returned on numerous occasions to find that it had been removed and pinned to the wall. The staff contended that the pouch impeded their ability to provide safe care; because in their view the risk of infection was a serious concern, they had removed the pouch. Upset, the family members approached the nurses with harsh words, but the nurses labeled them difficult, uncooperative, and disrespectful of hospital policies. After several discussions the staff permitted the family to tie the pouch to Nicole's left ankle. However, on another occasion the family found the pouch tied to Nicole's left big toe. Distressed and feeling helpless, the family said nothing though they were extremely angered by the situation. To help ease the tensions with the family, the staff scheduled an interdisciplinary meeting during which the physician informed the family that Nicole would recover and that, as soon as she was stable, she would be transferred home. With this renewed hope, the family began the necessary preparations to return home to the north. They left the next day, and a day later Nicole died alone. (p. 550)

Bourque Bearskin's description of Nicole's care in the ICU highlights the importance for nurses to understand the unique cultural needs of patients and their families and illuminates the importance of honouring cultural approaches to health care. How might the nurses have incorporated cultural competence and cultural safety into their approach to Nicole's care?

involves a nurse manager and a staff member from a different culture, and the second scenario involves a nurse, an individual coping with a terminal illness, and the connectedness of community.

CONCLUSION

Nurses are called upon to provide quality care for a growing number of culturally diverse patients. Nurse managers and leaders who embrace diversity inspire others to do the same. They make clear that staff are valued as individual people, not as representatives of some group. By showing respect for all patients, regardless of their cultural background, nurse managers and leaders demonstrate to staff nurses that their cultural differences are also valued. It is key for nurse managers and leaders to attend to diversity issues in the nursing workforce with the same zest as they do patient issues. Promoting cultural awareness and understanding is essential to workplace harmony as well as quality, culturally competent, and safe care.

? A SOLUTION

To increase his cultural competence, Dwayne decided that it was important to strive to learn more about every person—patients and colleagues—encountered in his practice. Dwayne knew cultural safety might be an important part of northern experiences and that being aware of one's own cultural perspective might be the first step to understanding other cultures. Dwayne asked people to talk about themselves and encouraged them to share their life stories. With a genuine interest in learning about northern ways and northern peoples, Dwayne listened for what people valued and how they experienced the health care system. Dwayne realized that the people encountered in the community and in practice held the expertise needed to increase Dwayne's knowledge of northern life and culture. Dwayne also participated in local community events, which offered greater insight into local ideas, beliefs, and values.

Would this be a suitable approach for you? Why or why not?

▎ THE EVIDENCE

1. Acknowledging cultural diversity in patients and staff requires leaders to be proactive.
2. Working with culturally diverse nursing organizations enhances opportunities for successful recruitment and retention.
3. Taking deliberate actions to acknowledge and celebrate culturally related events helps employees from various groups feel valued.

✳ NEED TO KNOW NOW

- Determine what the dominant cultural groups are in your community and know what the implications for care are.
- Be aware that many subcultures exist within cultures and that each individual has their own perspective of culture and how it influences the health and illness experience.
- Recognize that culture is a social construction that is influenced by historical, political, and social contexts.
- Be alert for opportunities to learn about coworkers' cultural backgrounds and practices.
- Know how to retrieve literature and research related to best practices and evidence for cultural topics in health care.

CHAPTER CHECKLIST

All potential or current nurse managers or leaders must acknowledge and address cultural diversity among staff and patients. Culture lives in each of us. It contributes to how we think, what we value, how we behave, and how we communicate with each other. In everyday work activities, the nurse manager must be able to do the following:

- Assess staff diversity and use techniques to manage a culturally diverse workforce and recognize staff members' diverse strengths. Use the strengths to benefit the unit and patients.
- Lead staff with a clear understanding of principles that embrace culture, cultural diversity, and cultural sensitivity.
- Be able to communicate effectively with staff and patients from diverse cultural backgrounds:
- Recognize terms that have different meanings for individuals in different cultures.
- Understand that nonverbal behaviours also carry different connotations depending on one's culture.
- Appraise factors, both individual and societal, inherent in cultural diversity:
- Three key principles foster respect for different lifestyles:

- *Multiculturalism* refers to maintaining several different cultures simultaneously.
- *Cross-culturalism* refers to mediating between or among cultures.
- *Transculturalism* denotes bridging significant differences in cultural practices.
- Ethnicity, national origin, race, gender, ability, age, physical characteristics, religion, values, beliefs, sexual orientation, socioeconomic class, and life experiences are important factors to consider in dealing fairly with all cultures and staff members.
- Use tools that clarify staff cultural diversity effectively:
- Mentoring programs can help staff expand their knowledge of cultural diversity and recognize their own biases as well as better integrate with diverse colleagues.
- Continuing education programs can help nurses learn about caring for different ethnic groups in ways that honour patients' beliefs.
- Appreciate the cultural richness of staff and patients.
- Print and online resources can provide nurses with valuable information on cultural topics.

TIPS FOR DEALING WITH CULTURAL DIVERSITY

Canadian nurse managers practise in a culturally rich country. Thus, nurse managers need to do the following:

- Describe effective techniques for managing a culturally diverse workforce.
- Encourage programs that show appreciation for and build understanding of the cultural diversity of staff and patients.
- Help address the special cultural needs of colleagues and patients.
- Understand that culture does not simply relate to individual values and beliefs, but has been influenced by historical, political, and social forces.

- Recognize how a lack of understanding about cultural safety in the workplace among colleagues and in patient care situations can lead to issues of prejudice and discrimination.
- Commit to engaging in cultural humility, which involves "a lifelong journey of self-reflection and learning. It involves listening without judgement and being open to learning about our own culture and our biases. Cultural humility is a building block for cultural safety" (Northern Health-Indigenous Health, 2018).

Visit the Evolve website for Suggested Readings, Internet Resources, and additional resources related to the content in this chapter: http://evolve.elsevier.com/Canada/Yoder-Wise/leading/.

REFERENCES

Aboriginal Nurses Association of Canada. (2009). *Cultural competence and cultural safety in nursing education*. Ottawa, ON: Aboriginal Nurses Association of Canada. Retrieved from: http://www.anac.on.ca/Documents/Making%20It%20Happen%20Curriculum%20Project/FINALFRAMEWORK.pdf.

Baumann, A., Ross, D., Idriss-Wheeler, D., & Crea-Arsenio, M. (2017). *Strategic practices for hiring, integrating, and retaining internationally educated nurses: Employment Manual*. Hamilton, ON: Nursing Health Services Research Unit (NHSRU), McMaster University.

Bourque Bearskin, R. L. (2011). A critical lens on culture in nursing practice. *Nurse Ethics, 18*(4), 548–559. https://doi.org/10.1177/0969733011408048.

Burnard, P., & Gill, P. (2009). *Culture, communication and nursing*. Harlow, UK: Pearson Education.

Campinha-Bacote, J. (1999). A model and instrument for addressing cultural competence in health care. *Journal of Nursing Education, 38*(5), 203–207.

Campinha-Bacote, J. (2002). The process of cultural competence in a delivery of healthcare services: A model of care. *Journal of Transcultural Nursing, 13*(3), 181–184.

Canadian Indigenous Nurses Association. (2018). *2018 University of Saskatchewan & Canadian Indigenous Nurses Association fact sheet: Aboriginal Nursing in Canada*. Author. Retrieved from: http://indigenousnurses.ca/resources/publications.

Canadian Institute of Health Information. (2018). *Regulated nurses, 2017: Data tables*. Author.

Canadian Nurses Association. (2004). *Position statement: Promoting culturally competent care (retired)*. Canadian Nurses Association. Retrieved from: http://www.cna-aiic.ca/sitecore%20modules/web/~/media/cna/page%20content/pdf%20fr/2013/09/05/18/06/ps73_promoting_culturally_competent_care_march_2004_e.pdf#search=%22culture%22.

Canadian Nurses Association. (2017). *Code of ethics for registered nurses*. Toronto, ON: Author. Retrieved from: https://www.cna-aiic.ca/html/en/Code-of-Ethics-2017-Edition/files/assets/basic-html/page-1.html.

Choi, H. (2001). Cultural marginality: A concept analysis with implications for immigrant adolescents. *Issues in Comprehensive Pediatric Nursing, 24*, 193–206.

Clark, N. (2012). *Perseverance, determination and resistance: An indigenous intersectional-based policy analysis of violence in the lives of indigenous girls*. Learning Circle. Retrieved online: http://learningcircle.ubc.ca/files/2013/10/7_Indigenous-Girls_Clark-2012.pdf.

College of Nurses of Ontario. (2009). *Practice standard: Ethics*. Retrieved from: http://www.cno.org/Global/docs/prac/41034_Ethics.pdf.

El Gindy, G. (2004). Treating Muslims with cultural sensitivity in a post-9/11 world. *Minority Nurse*, 44–46 Winter.

Exner-Pirot, H. (2016). *Aboriginal Nursing Canada fact sheet. Outreach and Indigenous Engagement College of Nurses*. University of Saskatchewan. Retrieved from: https://nursing.usask.ca/documents/aboriginal/AboriginalRNWorkforceFactsheet.pdf.

Giddens, J. F. (2008). Online content: Achieving diversity in nursing through multicontextual learning environments. *Nursing Outlook, 56*, 78–83.

Giger, J. N., & Davidhizar, R. (2002). The Giger and Davidhizar transcultural assessment model. *Journal of Transcultural Nursing, 13*(3), 185–188.

Gray, D. P., & Thomas, D. J. (2006). Critical reflections on culture in nursing. *Journal of Cultural Diversity, 13*(2), 76–82. ISSN:10715568.

Gregory, D., Harrowing, J., Lee, B., et al. (2010). Nursing pedagogy as contributing to essentialized understanding of culture among undergraduate nursing students. *International Journal of Nursing Education Scholarship, 7* Article [On-line].

Hartrick Doane, G., & Varcoe, C. (2005). *Family nursing as relational inquiry: Developing health-promoting practice*. Lippincott Williams & Wilkins.

Health Canada. (2014). *Canada's health care system*. Ottawa, ON: Author. Retrieved from: http://www.hc-sc.gc.ca/hcs-sss/pubs/system-regime/2011-hcs-sss/index-eng.php.

Indigenous Health. (2017). *Cultural safety: Respect and dignity in relationships*. BC: Northern Health: Prince George.

Institute of Medicine. (2004). *In the nation's compelling interest: Ensuring diversity in the health-care workforce*. Washington, DC: National Academies Press.

International Council of Nurses. (2013). *Cultural and linguistic competence: Position statement*. Geneva, Switzerland: Author. Retrieved from: http://www.icn.ch/images/stories/documents/publications/position_statements/B03_Cultural_Linguistic_Competence.pdf.

Lavoie-Tremblay, M., O'Brien-Pallas, L., Gelinas, C., et al. (2008). Addressing the turnover issue among new nurses from a generational viewpoint. *Journal of Nursing Management, 16*(6), 724–733.

Leininger, M. (2002). Essential transcultural nursing care concepts, principles, examples, and policy statements. In M. Leininger, & M. R. McFarland (Eds.), *Transcultural nursing: Concepts, theories, research & practice* (3rd ed.) (pp. 50–130). New York, NY: McGraw-Hill Medical.

Multiculturalism. (n.d.). Historica Canada. Retrieved from: http://www.thecanadianencyclopedia.ca/en/article/multiculturalism/.

National Aboriginal Health Organization. (2008). *Cultural Competency and safety: A guide for health care administrators, providers and educators*. Ottawa. ON: Author. Retrieved from: http://www.naho.ca/documents/naho/publications/culturalCompetency.pdf.

National Quality Forum. (2009). *Endorsing a framework and preferred practices for measuring and reporting cultural competency.* Washington, DC: Author. Retrieved from: http://www.qualityforum.org/Publications/2009/04/A_Comprehensive_Framework_and_Preferred_Practices_for_Measuring_and_Reporting_Cultural_Competency.aspx.

Noone, J. (2008). The diversity imperative: Strategies to address a diverse nursing workforce. *Nursing Forum, 43*(3), 133–143.

Northern Health – Indigenous Health. (2018). *Cultural safety poster series.* Retrieved from: https://www.indigenoushealthnh.ca/sites/default/files/2017-06/Posters-Cultural-Safety.pdf.

Pearson, A., Srivastava, R., Craig, D., et al. (2007). Systematic review on embracing cultural diversity for developing and sustaining a healthy work environment in healthcare. *International Journal of Evidence-Based Healthcare, 5,* 54–91.

Purnell, L. D. (2002). The Purnell model of cultural competence. *Journal of Transcultural Nursing, 13*(3), 193–196.

Purnell, L. D., & Paulanka, B. J. (2008). *Transcultural health care: A culturally competent approach* (3rd ed.). Philadelphia, PA: FA Davis.

Queen's University. (2018). *Multicultural policy index.* Retrieved from: http://www.queensu.ca/mcp/.

Registered Nurses' Association of Ontario. (2007). *Embracing cultural diversity in health care: Developing cultural competence.* Toronto, ON: Author.

Racine, L. (2014). The enduring challenge of cultural safety in nursing. *CJNR, 46,* 6–9. Retrieved from: http://cjnr.archive.mcgill.ca/article/view/2445/2439e.

Richardson, A., Yarwood, J., & Richardson, S. (2017). Expressions of cultural safety in public health nursing practice. *Nursing Inquiry, 24,* 1–10. https://doi.org/10.1111/nin.12171.

Simpson, J. (2009). *Everyone belongs: A toolkit for applying intersectionality.* Ottawa, ON: Canadian Research Institute for the Advancement of Women. Retrieved from: www.criaw-icref.ca/sites/criaw/files/Everyone_Belongs_e.pdf.

Spence, D. (2004). Prejudice, paradox and possibility: The experience of nursing people from cultures other than one's own. In K. H. Kavanaugh, & V. Knowlden (Eds.), *Many voices: Toward caring culture in healthcare and healing* (pp. 140–180). Madison, WI: The University of Wisconsin Press.

Statistics Canada. (2003). *2001 census: Analysis series. Canada's ethnocultural portrait: The changing mosaic (Catalogue no. 96F0030XIE2001008).* Ottawa, ON: Author. Retrieved from: http://www12.statcan.gc.ca/access_acces/archive.action-eng.cfm?/english/census01/products/analytic/companion/etoimm/pdf/96F0030XIE2001008.pdf.

Statistics Canada. (2013). *Immigration and ethnocultural diversity in Canada: National household survey, 2011.* Ottawa, ON: Author. Retrieved from: http://www12.statcan.gc.ca/nhs-enm/2011/as-sa/99-010-x/99-010-x2011001-eng.pdf.

Statistics Canada. (2018). *2016 Census topic: Aboriginal peoples.* Retrieved from: https://www12.statcan.gc.ca/census-recensement/2016/rt-td/ap-pa-eng.cfm.

Sullivan, E. J., & Decker, P. J. (2009). *Effective leadership and management in nursing* (5th ed.). Upper Saddle River, NJ: Prentice Hall.

Western University. (2018). *Guide for working with indigenous students: Interdisciplinary Development Initiative (IDI) in applied indigenous scholarship.* Author. Retrieved from: www.indigenousguide.uwo.ca.

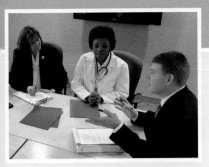

12

Power, Politics, and Influence

Maura MacPhee

This chapter considers how power and politics influence the roles of leaders and how leaders use power and politics to be influential. It also explores contemporary concepts of power, empowerment, types of power exercised by nurses, personal and organizational strategies for exercising power, and the power of nurses to shape health care policy.

OBJECTIVES

- Explore the types of power in relation to nursing.
- Describe the empowerment strategies used by effective leaders.

- Choose appropriate power strategies to influence the politics of the workplace, professional organizations, and government.

TERMS TO KNOW

coalitions	network	power
empowerment	policy	public policy
influence	policy process	stakeholders
lobbying	politics	

❓ A CHALLENGE

Carol is a Bachelor of Science in Nursing student and is excited about becoming a registered nurse. The nurse who helped her during her labour made a positive impact on her, which is why she decided that she wanted to become a nurse. Carol had a difficult pregnancy and labour with her daughter. During labour, the nurse not only skillfully guided Carol through the challenges she was facing but also made Carol feel safe and confident in her care. Carol wanted to provide the same level of care to other moms and dads going through the birth experience. Most of Carol's friends are not nurses, and at a recent birthday party, a long-time friend said that she was surprised that Carol had chosen nursing as a career. She said, "Well, it's not very challenging, is it? You just do what the doctors tell you to do. On all the TV shows I've seen, nurses aren't portrayed in a very flattering way. Aren't you worried about what others will think of you?"

How should Carol respond to this statement?

INTRODUCTION

Many definitions of power are context- or discipline-specific. Power in nursing practice relates to nurses' capacity to empower patients, which can have transformative, healing benefits (Benner, 2001). The most common definition of power used in leadership and management comes from Rosabeth Moss Kanter, a business management expert from Harvard Business School. According to Kanter (1993), power "is the ability to get things done, to mobilize resources, to get and use whatever it is that a person needs for the goals he or she is attempting to meet" (p. 166).

The concept of empowerment depends on the theoretical framework in which it is considered. Three common theoretical perspectives on empowerment are critical social theory, social psychological theories, and organizational and management theories (Trus et al., 2012). *Critical social theory* focuses on power and empowerment in relation to how the nursing discipline is viewed in different social or societal contexts over time. Pervasive stereotypes about nurses are promoted through the media, such as popular TV shows. For example, historically, nurses have been portrayed as sexualized, uneducated handmaidens of physicians. The Truth About Nursing is an international not-for-profit organization that seeks to increase public understanding of nursing. It monitors news articles, TV shows, movies, and songs for their portrayal of nursing. Where problems exist, the organization arranges meetings with major corporations and producers to discuss ways to improve media representation of nurses (Summers, 2014). *Social psychological theories* focus on how individuals are intrinsically motivated by the work they do. When people believe that there is meaning and significance to what they do, they report feeling more psychologically empowered in their workplace (DiNapoli et al., 2016). Positive psychology is one branch of social psychology that strives to understand what factors in different contexts are associated with individual feelings of happiness and engagement which, in turn, may affect how they work. Visit the University of Pennsylvania's authentic happiness website to measure your levels of personal empowerment and happiness (http://www.authentichappiness.sas.upenn.edu). *Organizational and management theories* focus on

the distribution of power in organizations. Organizational empowerment structures in health care have a greater influence on nurses' work attitudes and behaviours than personal characteristics and socialization experiences (Dahinten et al., 2016). Dr. Heather Laschinger devoted her career to studying nurses' workplace empowerment. See a tribute to her life's work at http://www.longwoods.com/content/24987.

Policy is a specifically designated statement to guide decisions and actions. Within health care organizations, nurses are expected to adhere to organizational policies as well as procedures, which are guidelines for nurses to follow to correctly perform a task. In health care settings, policies and procedures are both "power tools," a term coined by Kanter (1993), because they provide nurses with legitimate power to carry out health care interventions.

Another type of policy of importance to nurses is public policy. Public policy is "a course of action that is anchored in a set of values regarding appropriate public goals and a set of beliefs about the best way of achieving those goals" (Bryant, 2009, p. 1). Public policy decisions are shaped by a variety of forces, including political, social, and economic forces. Public policy (enacted through governments' policy decisions) determines the distribution of resources that influence people's health. In Canada, many public policy decisions of importance to nurses involve the social determinants of health, or those factors that significantly influence people's health and wellness. Health Canada is the federal department that oversees the health and well-being of Canadians. Health Canada's website (http://www.hc-sc.gc.ca) has a wealth of information about policy activities related to Canadians' health, including information on policy actions involving the social determinants of health, such as proper housing and nutrition.

In 1999, Health Canada created the Office of Nursing Policy (ONP) to "help Canadians maintain and improve their health through the development of policy which integrates the views of nurses and the nursing profession" (Health Canada, 2009). Some of the ONP's functions include identifying important policy issues based on best evidence, disseminating important policy-related information, and advocating for Canadians—getting them involved in policy activities, such as policy development and consulting with key stakeholder groups. Stakeholders are considered those individuals, groups, or organizations that are influenced by an issue or invested in policy related to an issue. A recent joint publication by the Canadian Foundation for Healthcare Improvement and the Office of Nursing Policy recommended a series of evidence-informed nurse recruitment and retention policy initiatives (McGillis Hall et al., 2013).

Politics involves "using power to influence, persuade, or otherwise change—it is the art of understanding relationships between groups in society and using that understanding to achieve particular outcomes" (McIntyre & McDonald, 2010, p. 70). Influence is the process of using power—from the punitive power of coercion to the interactive power of collaboration. Nurses' lack of involvement in politics is sometimes associated with their discomfort with acknowledging and using power. Nursing has been a predominantly female profession, and women traditionally were not socialized to exert power. Now in the twenty-first century, nurses must exercise their power to create a strong voice for nursing. This is an era of rapid and often unplanned change with dramatic nursing shortages. Nurses must use their collective power and flex their political muscles to create a preferred future for the health care system, health care consumers, and the profession of nursing (Udod & Racine, 2014).

KEY POWERFUL CANADIAN NURSE LEADERS

Canada's first nurse, Jeanne Mance (1606–1673), was an inspirational woman who helped found Montreal's first hospital, a hospital that was under her direction for 17 years. Mance procured funds and resources and recruited workers from France to support her unwavering mission to care for the sick in the New World (Daveluy, 2018).

Many Canadian nurses have received public acknowledgement and awards for their positive contributions to the health and well-being of Canadians. The Order of Canada, awarded through the office of the Governor General, has been presented to over 30 nurses, including Dr. Helen K. Mussallem. Dr. Mussallem received the highest level of the Order of Canada in 1969 for her many contributions to society. She was the first

Canadian nurse to earn a doctoral degree, and she was the first Canadian nurse to address the annual general assembly of the Canadian Medical Association (CMA). She was also a prominent policymaker and advocate as the chair for the World Health Organization Scientific Group on Research in Nursing and the Economic Council of Canada (see the Helen Mussallem biography project at http://drhkm.ca).

Another influential Canadian nurse leader is Dr. Judith Shamian, past president of the Canadian Nurses Association (CNA) and past president and chief executive officer of the Victorian Order of Nurses. Dr. Shamian was elected as president of the International Council of Nurses (ICN) in 2013. Dr. Shamian championed a collaboration between the CNA and the CMA to develop a set of principles to promote primary health care in Canada. The health care principles supported by the CNA–CMA include patient-centred care, quality care, health promotion and illness prevention, equitable care, sustainable care, and accountable care (CNA-CMA, 2013). The CNA–CMA has been lobbying (seeking to influence) government policymakers to have these principles guide policymaking discussions at the provincial, territorial, and federal levels.

TYPES OF POWER

Nurses often view power as if it were totally contradictory to the caring nature of nursing. However, nurses exercise power in many ways in their daily nursing practice. Nurses routinely influence patients to improve their health status, which is an essential element of nursing practice. For example, nurses provide health teaching to patients and their families with the goal of promoting optimal health. Nurses seek to enhance evidence-informed care delivery by instructing their colleagues about new policies or protocols being implemented in their organization. Nurses coach other nurses to improve their performance. The chief nursing officer of a hospital manages a multimillion-dollar budget. All of these examples are exercises of power.

Hersey et al. (1979) developed a classic formulation on the basis of social power. Sullivan (2013) modified these types of power to reflect a nursing perspective. Examples of types of power are given in the Theory Box. These types of power are not mutually exclusive. They

THEORY BOX

Types of Power

Key Contributors	Key Ideas	Application to Practice
Types or bases of social power were formulated by Hersey et al. (1979) to explain the personal use of power. Sullivan (2013) reorganized these types, eliminating much of the overlap in the original categories.	**Personal power:** Based on one's reputation and credibility.	The leader of a provincial or territorial nurses' association may have access to provincial or territorial government leaders based on personal power. This leader has worked with government members for many years and is known for integrity—following through on promises of support and providing useful information on matters related to health.
	Expert power: Results from the knowledge and skills one possesses that are needed by others.	An advanced practice nurse is viewed as the clinical expert on a nursing unit.
	Position power: Possessed by virtue of one's position within an organization or status within a group.	The dean of a school of nursing is viewed on campus as powerful because this dean leads the fastest-growing academic unit on campus.
	Perceived power: Results from one's reputation as a powerful person.	A nursing student seeks out a certain nurse leader as a preceptor during a senior clinical practicum because of the leader's reputation with nurses and students within the organization.
	Connection power: Gained by association with people who have links to powerful people.	At one acute care hospital during a Nurses' Week celebration, nurses take advantage of the opportunity to have extended, informal conversations with the hospital's chief nursing officer.

are often used in concert to exert influence on individuals or groups.

Nurses commonly use all of these types of power while implementing a wide range of nursing activities. Nurses who teach patients use expert power by virtue of the information they share with patients. Nurses also exercise position power because they are accorded a certain status by society. Members of a provincial or territorial nurses' association who lobby members of parliament use expert, perceived, personal, and position power when trying to gain legislators' support for health care legislation. New graduates, employed on probationary status until they demonstrate the initial clinical competencies of a position, may view the nurse leader as exercising both position and expert power related to their evaluation for continued employment. Nursing faculty and skilled clinicians exercise expert and perceived power as students emulate their behaviour. Connection power is evident at any social gathering in the workplace. People of high status (e.g., vice-presidents, directors, deans) within an organization may be sought out for conversation by those who want to move up the organizational hierarchy.

Having a high-status position in an organization immediately provides stature, but power depends on the ability to accomplish goals from that position. Although some may think that *knowledge is power*, acting on that knowledge is where the real power lies. Sharing knowledge expands one's power and, in turn, empowers others, including colleagues and patients (Sullivan, 2013).

EXERCISE 12.1 Part A. Recall a recent opportunity in which you observed the work of an expert nurse. Think about that nurse's interactions with patients, family members, nursing colleagues, and other health care providers. What kinds of power did you observe this nurse using? What did the nurse do and say that told you, "This is a powerful person"?

Part B. Using the Types of Power Questionnaire found on the Evolve website, rate your current level of power for each of the five types of power outlined in the Theory Box (on the previous page). Think of one strategy to increase each type of power. Some people think that power is finite and must be given to them, but in actuality, power is limitless—we choose how to increase our power bases through what we do and say.

	Current Rating
	1----2----3----4----5
Type of Power	1 = powerless,
Questionnaire	5 = very powerful
Personal Power	Current rating: 1—2—3—4—5
Strategy for raising personal power:	
Expert Power	Current rating: 1—2—3—4—5
Strategy for raising expert power:	
Position Power	Current rating: 1—2—3—4—5
Strategy for raising position power:	
Perceived Power	Current rating: 1—2—3—4—5
Strategy for raising perceived power:	
Connection Power	Current rating: 1—2—3—4—5
Strategy for raising connection power:	

EMPOWERMENT THEORIES AND NURSING

Empowerment is essential to nursing. It is the process of exercising one's own power. It is also the process by which we facilitate the participation of others in decision making and taking action so they are free to exercise power (Goedhart et al., 2017). This section focuses on three theoretical perspectives of empowerment and how they relate to nursing.

Critical Social Theories and Empowerment

Critical social theories focus on how society controls access to power based on individual characteristics, such as skin colour, gender, religion, and sexual orientation. The most common critical social theories are critical race theory and feminist theory. Those groups whose freedoms and rights are restricted by socially imposed inequalities are known as *oppressed groups* (Udod, 2008). Sociologists consider nurses an "oppressed group" because of their historical domination by medicine. The traditional health care hierarchy that placed medicine at the top may be related to the fact that nursing has been a predominantly female profession supervised by predominantly male physicians. Gender, class, and status no doubt have contributed to nursing's long-time subordination to medicine. One characteristic of oppressed group behaviour is that the group's inability to realize that powerlessness is socially conditioned—and can be challenged. Individuals within oppressed groups tend to oppress others that they can dominate (consider the notion "nurses eat their young": although it is a very common phrase, it provides a brief context to this description). Bullying and horizontal violence are oppressed group behaviours. The following Literature Perspective provides an example of nursing student oppression and empowerment. The opposite of oppression is emancipation, and critical social theory examines ways in which social activism can be used to end oppression (Purpora et al., 2012; Sauer, 2012; Udod, 2008).

Structural Empowerment Theory

Structural empowerment theory postulates that employees of organizations become empowered when they gain access to opportunities, information, resources, and supports through informal and formal power sources. This theory is based on the ethnographic work of Kanter (1993), who observed that employee attitudes and behaviour were influenced by their access to empowerment structures within their workplaces. *Access to opportunity* refers to having professional advancement opportunities or opportunities to be involved in organizational activities beyond one's job description. *Access to information* refers to having the necessary information about aspects of organizational functioning to be effective in the workplace. *Access to resources* refers to having the resources needed to efficiently and effectively carry out one's work. *Access to support* involves receiving

LITERATURE PERSPECTIVE

Resource: Bradbury-Jones, C., Sambrook, S., & Irvine, F. (2011). Nursing students and the issue of voice: A qualitative study. *Nurse Education Today*, 31: 628–632.

The purpose of this qualitative study was to explore the empowerment of nursing students in clinical practice. Thirteen students were interviewed at annual intervals during their nursing program, from first year to graduation. Many first-year students felt that they were powerless to express their opinions when they had patient-care concerns. In these instances, they psychologically withdrew from these situations as a coping response. As they progressed in the program, "voice" increased among most of the students. They realized that strongly stating their opinions would be counterproductive, so they created "bridges" or "negotiating voices" to carefully craft their statements between a continuum of "exit" (i.e., no voice) to "voice" (i.e., speaking up). Some students said that they had to dampen their voice to avoid labels, such as "cocky." Other research has shown that students are at risk for disciplinary power or ostracism if they appear too confident or assertive—even when a patient's welfare is at stake.

Implications for Practice

Students' voice may be hampered by fear of reprisal in situations where poor patient care conditions exist. Instructors and education programs need to provide safe places for students to express their concerns and collectively discuss options to address these power imbalances. Most organizations have confidential reporting systems where unsafe conditions or inappropriate behaviours can be documented—by students, faculty, and staff. Adequate orientation to clinical teams can also be helpful, and strong practice–academic collaborations between educational institutions and practice settings can help promote team spirit where students are considered important members of clinical teams.

From a critical social theory perspective, nurse empowerment signifies that nurses are aware of the influence of power on them and how power influences their behaviour toward others. However, nurses may exert power over others in unconscious, well-intentioned ways. One UK study found that primary care nurses unknowingly controlled their patients' decisions during asthma teaching sessions. Although the nurses said that they used shared decision making with their patients, the researchers found that the nurses only offered patients opportunities to make decisions about their inhaler devices based on the nurses' preselected recommendations. Rather than empowering patients by treating them as equal partners in decision making, these nurses tightly controlled information to conform decisions to their agenda (Upton et al., 2011).

A Canadian study examined nurses' workplace violence through a critical social theory lens (St-Pierre & Holmes, 2008). According to these researchers, nurses have come to accept violence as a regular occurrence and to doubt their rights with respect to a safer work environment. Nurses are at high risk for workplace violence, even compared with police officers and prison guards. Despite the high risk of nurses' work, nurses tend to under-report violent episodes because they view them as part of their job. Workplace violence can contribute to stress, depression, and workplace injuries and absenteeism. Nurse absenteeism is closely tracked and monitored by supervisors; nurses know they are under surveillance, making them question their own needs versus those of the organization. Nurses are also expected to "normalize" unsafe work conditions for the greater good of the organization. Because of cost efficiencies, everyone within the organization is expected to accept cuts in resources and proper supports. Workplaces need to explore what policies need to be in place to change the culture and empower nurses to report workplace violence (International Council of Nurses, 2017). Because of rising trends in nurses' workplace violence in Canada, the Canadian Nurses' Association and the Canadian Federation of Nurses' Unions issued a joint position statement on workplace bullying and violence (2014).

support to fulfill one's job responsibilities and engage in relevant decision making (Kanter, 1993). *Formal power* comes from an individual's position of formal authority within an organization, and *informal power* is based on networks and alliances with supervisors, peers, and other contacts within and outside the organization. The following Literature Perspective is an example of how Kanter's structural empowerment theory has been applied to theoretical understandings of nursing care (see Table 12.1).

LITERATURE PERSPECTIVE

Resource: Laschinger, H., Gilbert, S., Smith, L., et al. (2010). Towards a comprehensive theory of nurse/patient empowerment: Applying Kanter's empowerment theory to patient care. *Journal of Nursing Management*, 18: 4–13.

These authors argue that a key responsibility of nurses is to empower patients for optimal health and well-being. Very little research has been done that directly links nurse activities to patient empowerment. This conceptual paper proposes a nurse/patient empowerment model that incorporates many empowerment concepts: nurse structural empowerment, nurse psychological empowerment, nurses' use of patient empowering strategies, and patient empowerment. The major proposition is that empowered nurses are better able to empower their patients. Empowered patients have increased capacity to care for themselves, access needed health services, and express satisfaction with health care delivery. The paper provides many examples of patient-empowering nurse behaviours that are related to Kanter's (1993) structural empowerment theory. Examples are presented in the Table 12.1.

Examples of Patient-Empowering Nurse Behaviours

TABLE 12.1	**Components of Kanter's (1993) Theory**
Access to information	• Respond to patients' questions in clear, understandable terms.
	• Always explain your actions before carrying them out.
Access to support	• Ask patients what you can do for them.
	• Offer encouraging remarks for meeting health goals.
Access to resources	• Facilitate access to community resources.
	• Facilitate patients' access to the health care team.
Access to opportunity	• Provide patients with opportunities to practise new skills.
Informal power	• Promote positive, trusting relationships between the patient, their family, and the team.
Formal power	• Refrain from using your formal authority to intimidate or dominate patients' decision making.

IMPLICATIONS FOR PRACTICE

This article provides an excellent overview of important empowerment terms, and it has tables with nurse-empowering behaviours and patient-empowering behaviours. Use this article as a learning resource to gain familiarity and comfort with key empowerment concepts and their applications.

Nurses' perceptions of access to organizational empowerment structures have been associated with numerous positive outcomes, such as organizational commitment, job satisfaction, trust, and low burnout. In Canada, an eminent nurse researcher, Dr. Heather Laschinger, conducted over two decades of research on workplace empowerment (Cicolini et al., 2014). In one study, Laschinger and colleagues examined how access to organizational empowerment structures (i.e., structural empowerment) influenced new nurses' job satisfaction. This study further examined the impact of new nurses' personal resources or psychological capital on job satisfaction. The concept of psychological capital comes from the positive psychology movement, and it represents individuals' positive human strengths. Positive personal resources include self-efficacy or self-confidence to succeed, hope, optimism, and resilience. The researchers found that personal resources and access to workplace empowerment structures both positively influenced new nurses' job satisfaction. The researchers recommended that: "Orientation processes and ongoing management support…will help create positive perceptions of the workplace, enhancing job satisfaction" (Stam et al., 2015, p. 190).

EXERCISE 12.2 Think about a recent clinical experience in which you empowered a patient. What did you do for and/or with the patient (and family) that was empowering? How did you feel about your own actions in this situation? How did the patient (or family) respond to your efforts? How does the Literature Perspective above help you think differently about your role as a nurse in relation to patient empowerment?

Social Psychological Theories and Psychological Empowerment

Psychological empowerment refers to an individual's belief in their empowerment at work. Spreitzer (2007) identified the following four main dimensions of empowerment:

1. *Meaning*, which implies a good fit between the individual's work role and his or her beliefs, values, and behaviours.
2. *Impact*, which is the degree to which an individual can make a significant difference at work.
3. *Self-determination*, which is the degree to which an individual has control over what he or she does at work.
4. *Competence*, which is an individual's belief that he or she can perform work activities successfully.

Empowerment comes from within, but outside catalysts can "spark" people's positive beliefs about themselves. For example, nurse leaders can catalyze nurses' belief in themselves (i.e., psychological empowerment) by providing them with organizational empowerment structures. Early on, Laschinger et al. (2009) found that the quality of nurse–nurse leader relationships and nurses' perceptions of access to empowerment structures influenced nurses' feelings of psychological empowerment that in turn enhanced their commitment to the organization. Organizational commitment is closely tied to actual turnover. This seminal study provided evidence that strong leaders can initiate an empowerment chain reaction among followers: strong leader–follower relationships→ ↑nurse perceptions of structural empowerment→ ↑ feelings of psychological empowerment→ ↑ positive follower outcomes, such as organizational commitment and nurse retention. Strong leaders, especially leaders who use structural empowerment as a major organizational strategy, can raise nurses' psychological beliefs about their capacity to be valued contributors in their workplaces (Cicolini et al., 2014).

Another area of study from social psychology is leaders' use of specific empowerment strategies, known as *leader-empowering behaviours* (LEBs) (Cziraki & Laschinger, 2015; Dahinten et. al., 2013). The five major LEB categories appear in Table 12.2, along with examples of each. Some research has shown that LEBs are important for supporting new graduate nurses (Ulrich et al., 2010).

TABLE 12.2 Leader-Empowering Behaviours

Leader-Empowering Behaviour Category	Nursing Example
Enhancing the meaningfulness of work	Inspiring staff to follow the organization's vision and mission through transformational leadership
Fostering participatory decision making	Providing release time for nurses to participate in shared governance councils
Providing autonomy from bureaucratic restraints	Eliminating unnecessary policies and procedures; supporting nurses to regularly update evidence-informed protocols
Facilitating goal accomplishment	Providing educators and professional development opportunities
Expressing confidence in high performance	Publicly acknowledging nurses' professional accomplishments and contributions to interprofessional teamwork

EXERCISE 12.3 Part A. Observe the first-line nurse leader (manager/nurse in charge) on your clinical unit. Write down examples of leader-empowering behaviours (LEBs) you observed (see Table 12.2). Were you able to find an example of each type of behaviour?

Part B. Because leader-empowering behaviours have a strong influence on nurses, interview a few nurses on your clinical practicum unit. Ask them to provide examples of the leader's LEBs. If the staff and you are able to provide many examples of LEBs, it is likely that the work environment is an empowering one where nurses appear to work well together and to enjoy their work—even in stressful situations. If the staff and you are not able to provide examples of LEB, it is likely that the work environment is less empowering and less satisfactory to staff. Do you see evidence of the link between the leader's use of LEB and staff behaviour on the unit?

An Empowering Professional Identity

Nurses' use of power has implications for nursing practice, politics, and policy.

Power and professionalism are closely related; having a strong professional identity is important because a lack of empowering professional identity means that others can step in and decide what nursing is and what nurses can do (ten Hoeve et al., 2014). Empowered nurses demonstrate a positive and professional attitude about being a nurse to nursing colleagues, patients, and their families, other colleagues in the workplace, the public, and government. This attitude facilitates the exercise of power among colleagues while educating others about nurses and nursing. A powerful image is important because the impressions we make on people influence the way they view us now and in the future, as well as how they value what we do and say.

EXERCISE 12.4 How do you routinely introduce yourself to patients, families, physicians, and other colleagues? A powerful and positive approach involves making eye contact with each individual, shaking hands, and introducing yourself by saying, "I'm Ted Carvalho, a nursing student in the baccalaureate nursing program at University X." If you do not currently use this technique, try it out. Note any difference in the responses of people whom you meet using this technique in comparison with a less formal approach. How are you contributing to a powerful, professional identity for nursing?

Professional identity arises through a socialization process whereby individuals learn the behaviours, attitudes, and values associated with their profession. Professional nursing socialization often begins in nursing programs where students learn about professional standards of practice and codes of ethics (Chapter 6). Entry into the workplace can cause a significant clash between learned ideals and actual nursing practice: "reality shock" is a term originally coined by Kramer (1974) to describe this values clash. Another, more recent term in the literature is "transition shock" (Duchscher, 2009). Transition shock refers to new nurses' feelings of anxiety and insecurity that may happen after graduation during initial professional adjustment.

Transition programs are one way to ease new graduate nurses' entry to practice (Rush et al., 2013). Laschinger and colleagues conducted a Canada-wide study of new nurse graduates, the Starting Out study, to better understand what work environment factors best support new nurses' transition to practice. As noted above, formal transition programs are important to new nurses. In addition, the researchers found that new nurses do best in environments with adequate staffing, a balance of experienced and new nurses, and a culture that fosters curiosity and continual learning (Regan et al., 2017).

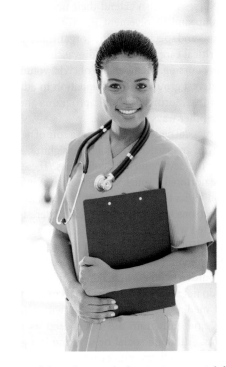

A powerful professional identity is essential for successful political efforts in the workplace, the profession, and the public policy arena.

POWER STRATEGIES

Networking and coalition building are additional power strategies used by nurse leaders that are effective at different levels: from intra-organizational to provincial or territorial and federal levels.

Networking

Networking is an important power strategy and political skill. A network is a result of identifying, valuing, and maintaining relationships with a system of individuals who are sources of information, advice, and support (MacPhee et al., 2009). Many nurses have relatively limited networks within the organizations where they are employed. They tend to interact with the people with whom they work most closely. One way to expand a workplace network is to have lunch or coffee with someone from another department, including individuals from other disciplines, at least two or three times a month. Nurses can also extend their networks through membership and involvement in professional nursing associations and specialty practice organizations in areas such as critical care nursing, cardiovascular nursing, or emergency nursing. Membership of civic, volunteer, and special interest groups and participation in educational programs (e.g., formal academic programs and conferences) are other ways to network.

The successful networker identifies a core of networking partners who are particularly skilled, insightful, and eager to support the development of colleagues. These partners need to be nurtured through strategies such as information sharing on topics that relate to their interests; introducing them to persons who have comparable interests or who are connected with others of influence; staying connected through notes, e-mail, phone calls, or instant messages; and meeting them at important events. Successful networkers are not a burden to others in making requests for support, and they do not refuse the support that is provided.

Social media, such as Facebook, Twitter, LinkedIn, YouTube, and Instagram are often used as networking forums. Although social networking is a great way to connect with others, nurses must adhere to professional principles of social networking (Green et al., 2014). Some well-publicized examples of Facebook gone "afoul" include three US students who were temporarily suspended from their program for posting a picture of themselves with a human placenta and a nurse in the United Kingdom who was professionally investigated by her regulatory body for posting this comment on Facebook: "Euthanasia for gingers, the elderly and those with bad toenails" (Smith, 2012, p. 64). Although the nurse intended this comment to be humorous, other nurses on Facebook were offended by this posting and reported her to the regulatory body (Smith, 2012).

The College of Registered Nurses of Nova Scotia (2012) developed the recommendations outlined in Table 12.3 for the appropriate use of social media by nurses, nursing students, employers, and nurse educators.

The CNA *Code of Ethics for Registered Nurses* (see Chapter 6) provides a framework for ethical decision making, and this framework can provide guidance with respect to nurses' use of social media. Chapter 13 also addresses elements of professional practice in using electronic communications.

Coalition Building

The exercise of power is often directed at creating change. Although an individual can often be effective

TABLE 12.3   Recommendations for the Appropriate Use of Social Media

Registered Nurses and nursing students using social media tools:

Abide by organizational policies concerning personal and professional social media tools.

Protect personal identity by reading, understanding, and using the strictest privacy settings to maintain control over access to personal information.

Maintain privacy and confidentiality of clients and coworkers or fellow students' information and immediately report any breach to their employer or faculty.

Maintain professional nurse–client professional boundaries and avoid engaging in personal social media relationships with clients.

Refrain from posting any client information or image(s) unless it is related to employer expectation for client care.

Never post unprofessional or negative comments about clients, co-workers, other students or employers.

Avoid using social media sites to vent or discuss work/school-related events and refrain from commenting on posts of this nature made by others.

Maintain a professional manner in postings, photos, and/or videos.

Never speak on behalf of a health care organization unless authorized to do so.

Keep work/school-related social media activities separate from personal social media activities.

Create strong passwords and change them frequently. Do not share passwords with others.

Avoid offering health-related advice in response to posted comments or questions; if relied upon, such advice could trigger professional liability (CNPS, 2010) and/or a complaint to the College.

College of Registered Nurses of Nova Scotia, Position Statement: Social Media., Retrieved from https://www.crnns.ca/documents/PositionStatement_SocialMedia.pdf

at exercising power and creating change, certain changes require collective action. Coalition building is an effective political strategy for collective action. Coalitions are groups of individuals or organizations that join together temporarily around a common goal. Coalitions of professionals and consumers can be particularly powerful in influencing public policy related to health care. During the Severe Acute Respiratory Syndrome (SARS) outbreak in Toronto, the Community Coalition Concerned about SARS was formed to quickly disseminate information about the syndrome, fight against potential ethnic group discrimination through advocacy work, and organize fundraising events to support front-line workers and SARS research. The coalition included 63 Chinese-Canadian businesses, as well as community, cultural, religious, and professional organizations. Other Asian ethnic groups worked with the coalition, including Japanese, Korean, Sri Lankan, and Filipino groups. One of the most outstanding coalition actions was the rapid mobilization of user-friendly, linguistically and culturally appropriate telephone support lines. Over 100 volunteers were available to answer calls and provide emotional and informational support (Dong et al., 2010).

Nursing organizations often use coalition building when dealing with government policymakers. As mentioned above, Shamian's CNA–CMA collaboration on the development of health care principles for legislators' consideration is an example of a coalition.

Coalitions can develop into more permanent partnerships or even lobbies. A *lobby* is a group of people who seek to influence government policymakers on a particular issue. The Health Action Lobby (HEAL) is one example (see http://www.healthactionlobby.ca). This lobby was formed in 1991 and represents 35 national health organizations (including the CNA) with a cross-section of stakeholder groups, including health care providers, health regions, institutions, and facilities. HEAL is particularly concerned with upholding the unique qualities of the Canada Health Act. The purpose of HEAL is to influence health care policy at the federal level (HEAL, 2017).

EXERCISING POWER AND INFLUENCE: POLICY AND POLITICS

Previous sections have provided examples of how nurses can use different power strategies or sources of power to influence change. The following section provides a more in-depth look at policy and political action.

The Policy Process and Politics

The policy process involves developing, implementing, and evaluating policy on the basis of the best evidence available. Within health care settings, policies enforce specific structures and processes that are associated with quality, safe outcomes. They are considered organizational standards that must be followed. Hand hygiene policy, for instance, is based on the best available evidence of how to prevent infection transmission. Employees, patients, and visitors in health care settings are expected to comply with this policy, and health care settings have quality and safety departments that monitor and document adherence rates. People may be at risk when policies are not followed. In health care organizations, nurses typically play a key role in reviewing best evidence and updating policies on a regular basis. Nurses' involvement in policy work may take place within unit-based or hospital-wide shared-governance councils.

A controversial nursing policy is mandatory nurse-to-patient ratios. Nurse-to-patient ratios are one way to define nurses' workloads. Ratio legislation is based on a large body of global research evidence that demonstrates that as nurses' workloads increase, patient morbidity and mortality rates increase, and nurses are at greater risk for injury and emotional burnout (Aiken et al., 2014). Mandatory nurse to patient ratio legislation currently exists in the US, Australia and Wales. In the US, California enacted mandatory ratios over a decade ago, and this legislation resulted in improved nurse staffing levels. Impact on patient outcomes are still being evaluated (Mark et al., 2013). Ratio policies must be enforced, but some policy experts believe that this approach to safe staffing limits hospital administrators' capacity to respond to patient population needs in a flexible, cost-effective fashion. In 2015, The RN Safe Staffing Act was passed as federal legislation. Every publicly funded health care organization in the US is accountable for having safe nurse staffing levels. Rather than mandated ratios, health care organizations have safe staffing plans that use a variety of strategies to ensure adequate staffing levels. This approach permits more flexible use of the nursing workforce (American Nurses' Association, 2015).

Public policy is intended to ensure effective, equitable service and resource distribution for the public. Public policy, however, is closely intertwined with **politics**. Politics is based on the use of power to control or manipulate policy decisions. Politicians typically represent different values-based approaches to making decisions that influence the distribution of public resources, such as those associated with the social determinants of health (e.g., housing, transit, education). The competitive values-based positions of politicians and the complexity of public health often result in policies that do not adequately address fundamental inequities in society (Fafard, 2008). In Canada, the federal government is accountable for raising funds for public health needs, but the provincial governments are primarily responsible for making health policy. The fact that two levels of government are involved in health resource management and decision making adds to the complexity of Canadian health policy (and politics). Take, for example, planning for the health human resources (HHR) supply in Canada. Although many actors are involved in this policy area, no pan-Canadian HHR policy exists to "smooth" the distribution of health care providers across the country. "Many have called for a health human resources process or table at which policy discussions encompassing all health professions could take place. We do not have such a process in Canada; instead, we have a variety of actors attempting to react to current and perceived future pressures" (Wilson, 2013, p. 30).

EXERCISE 12.5

1. Take a look at the websites of the Canadian Nurses Association (https://www.cna-aiic.ca/en) and the Canadian Federation of Nurses Unions (https://nursesunions.ca). What policy work is underway? What political activities are posted on the websites? You may consider getting involved around an issue of significance to you.

2. Another source of information about nurses' involvement in policy and politics is the website of your provincial or territorial nursing association or union. Use the "search" field to look up "policy" or "position statements" on the association website. As one example, the Registered Nurses' Association of Ontario website (http://rnao.cahttp://www.rnao.org/) contains many resources on political action along with health and nursing policy, toolkits, and position statements.

3. After viewing the websites of national and provincial or territorial nursing associations and unions, select a topic of interest to you. Within your own sphere of influence (e.g., your peers at work, friends, and family), what can you do to raise awareness about this topic?

4. One way to get involved in policy development within your organization is through committee work or shared governance councils. Political awareness begins with nurses' knowledge of opportunities to participate in policymaking within their own units, departments, and organizations. Scope out opportunities to engage in policymaking at different levels within your organization. This is the first step toward making a commitment to action.

A basic policymaking framework appears in Fig. 12.1. An assumption about public policy is that good data will lead to good policy. As depicted in Fig. 12.1, the process begins with the *synthesis* of best available evidence. A major problem is the separation that typically exists between researchers who generate evidence from decision makers who need the evidence when making policy decisions. One way that researchers have been able to gain policymaker attention is by aligning themselves with other stakeholder groups (e.g., working with coalitions) and creating a sense of urgency. Another important consideration is the packaging of evidence. Policymakers have multiple stakeholder interests to address, and they have limited time to distill and synthesize the best evidence on specific topics. A whole body of science, known as knowledge translation, focuses on the best ways to present evidence for different stakeholder groups, including government policymakers and the public (White et al., 2016). In Fig. 12.1, the *knowledge translation* box makes a critical difference in how evidence is transferred to policymakers and how it is weighted in relation to other policy inputs.

Does scientific evidence even appear on some policymaking agendas? According to Fafard (2008), "how a given issue is framed can also have an enormous impact on the place of evidence and what evidence is considered relevant" (p. 10).

The *policymaking* box represents a process of (1) setting an agenda, (2) formulating a policy, (3) adopting the policy, (4) implementing the policy, and (5) evaluating policy outcomes. Government agendas, which influence policymaking, typically consist of three distinct streams. The "problem" stream deals with issues that have immediacy and public attention (e.g., teen suicide and cyber-bullying). The "policy" stream deals with public ideals that are more abstract and more difficult to understand and to act upon; these agenda items may be outside public awareness or have limited public awareness (e.g., a comprehensive cancer care strategy). The "political" stream consists of priorities for re-election; these agenda items often overlap with those of problem streams because they have public appeal (e.g., an official Family Day). Government agenda items therefore depend on salient social, ethical, and political implications—that often supersede the evidence (Howlett & Ramesh, 2003).

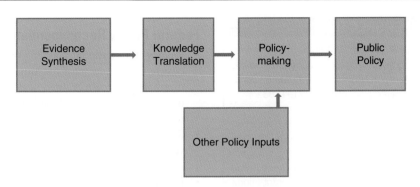

Fig. 12.1 A basic policymaking framework.

During the policy formulation phase, policymakers often consult with interest groups, academics, and other governments. A range of possible policy actions are drafted to address the agenda issue. Childhood obesity is an example of a problem stream issue. Policy actions depend on how this issue is framed. If obesity is considered an individual behaviour problem, for instance, policy actions might include policies aimed at changing individual behaviours, such as diet and exercise regimens. The government, for instance, might formulate policy to remove vending machines with junk food and high sugar drinks from schools. Another policy might be family tax breaks for children's recreational and sports program fees. Policy formulations are rarely clear or straightforward, and they are typically tempered by sociocultural and political forces that carry greater weight than the scientific evidence. When technical or knowledge experts are invited to participate in policy formulation, nurse experts have an opportunity to promote evidence-informed practices. Nurses often serve as experts on public health and health care services policies. One Canadian nurse policy expert is Dr. Gail Tomblin Murphy. Tomblin Murphy's area of expertise is health human resource (HHR) planning. Throughout the world, there are notable shortages of nurses and doctors. Evidence-informed HHR planning and policy development ensure that the number of health care providers is adequate to meet the burgeoning demands of aging populations. Tomblin Murphy is director of the World Health Organization/Pan American Health Organization (WHO/PAHO) Collaborating Centre on Health Workforce Planning and Research, Dalhousie University. She has served as a technical expert for WHO/PAHO policy

development, and she has advised Canadian policymakers at provincial and federal levels. According to Tomblin Murphy, HHR planning in Canada has been based on historical and political factors rather than the needs of populations. In many instances, HHR policies are reactive—based on perceived deficiencies—rather than systematic, proactive plans for the future (Tomblin Murphy & MacKenzie, 2013).

After assembling information from diverse groups on a range of possible actions, decisions have to be made about what action(s) to take. *Public policy* decision making may involve hundreds of people (e.g., Cabinet decision making) and decision-making rounds to "chunk" decisions on complex issues. Public policy rarely arises from one discrete decision. Some policy decisions include regulation, public expenditures, and tax measures. Policy research on the role of evidence in government decision making indicates that research evidence is not always used or sought out. The following Literature Perspective provides more insights into the drivers for policymaking.

Based on the research findings, the authors made policy recommendations for local, provincial, and national levels. A summary of these recommendations follows:

POLICY RECOMMENDATIONS

Local Policy Recommendations

- Involve community agencies in assisting immigrants with physician access:
  - Provide community centre transportation (e.g., a van).
  - Arrange for physicians to come to the community centre on specified dates.
  - Offer translation services through neighbourhood volunteers.

LITERATURE PERSPECTIVE

Resource: Asanin, J., & Wilson, K. (2008). "I spent nine years looking for a doctor": Exploring access to health care among immigrants in Mississauga, Ontario, Canada. *Social Science & Medicine*, 66(6): 1271–1283.

In Canada, approximately 20% of the total population consists of immigrants, and every year, about 250 000 new immigrants arrive in Canada, accounting for two-thirds of annual population growth. Although these immigrants make significant economic and social contributions to our society, research suggests that immigrants have difficulty getting social benefits and health care. This qualitative study explored access to health care among immigrants in one Canadian neighbourhood. This research approach was chosen because most research on access to care in Canada is done with national-level survey data that do not provide detailed insights into subpopulation groups like immigrants. In many instances, public policy decisions are based on these high-level data. Focus group interviews generated three categories of accessibility that were concerning for immigrant participants: geographical, sociocultural, and economic. In this immigrant neighbourhood, access to primary care was rarely obtainable. Several participants said that they were not comfortable leaving their neighbourhood to seek out medical care (geographical accessibility). Participants reported language difficulties with expressing their health concerns in English and interpreting medical directions in English. For many cultural and religious reasons, the Canadian biomedical model of care was deemed inappropriate by the majority of participants. There were notable differences in conceptions of health and healing between immigrants and the Canadian health care system (sociocultural accessibility). Cost was a barrier for immigrants requiring prescription medications, and in some instances, the medicare 3-month waiting period was an issue for recent immigrants, particularly immigrants with young children (economic accessibility). Some participants felt that foreign-trained physicians and nurses might aid their situation.

Provincial Policy Recommendations

- Re-assess the 3-month waiting period in provinces that require it (e.g., British Columbia). This waiting period appears to legally contradict the "accessibility" principle of the *Canada Health Act.*
- Speed up the process by regulatory bodies to access the qualifications of foreign-born doctors and nurses.

Federal Policy Recommendations

- Review the national Skilled Worker Program to ensure its adequacy for meeting public needs. Large numbers of foreign-trained health care providers are unemployed or in unskilled jobs, highlighting the ineffectiveness of the current program.
- Re-evaluate the *Canada Health Act* principles (25 years old) to determine whether they accurately reflect the needs of current immigrants.
- Include immigrants ("local experts") in commissioned studies on public health policy (this point is important at every level).

IMPLICATIONS FOR PRACTICE

Although this was a formal study, it portrayed a way that health care providers can make better connections with priority and vulnerable populations such as immigrant populations, Indigenous peoples, individuals with mental health and addiction issues, and people with chronic health conditions. One-on-one conversations and informal focus groups can be organized at community centres and not-for-profit agencies in neighbourhoods where these populations are located. Making genuine inquiries about subpopulation needs is an important way for health care providers to build a trusting relationship with the community. Accurate portrayals of population needs come from the "local experts." Individuals or focus group participants can also be engaged to offer possible solutions for existing problems and influence policy.

The actual implementation of policy may involve a complex series of additional decisions, often related to funding. Imagine that a provincial Minister of Health, in response to the issue of childhood obesity, declares a policy that physical activity will be increased in public schools. This broad policy may even include the transfer of funds to school boards. Although the policy must be implemented, the specifics on how to do so will rest with school boards, schools, teachers, and families. Clearly, a high-level decision can initiate a domino effect of subsequent decisions. The implementation phase may be the policy phase most in need of research evidence to operationalize actions at the local level. It is particularly critical at the local level during this phase for nurses to collaborate with other stakeholders in designing and implementing an evidence-informed program that truly meets the needs of the affected community or population (Fafard, 2008). Depending on the complexity of the policy, implementation may take place over a prolonged period of time and go through multiple adaptations. What happens when factors, such as time constraints, are present? An example of public health policy complexity is the World Health Organization's pandemic alert about an impending H1N1 influenza epidemic. Canadian policy analysts evaluated policies that arose at the federal, provincial, and local public health levels (Rosella et al., 2013). The analysts interviewed policymakers from five provinces (British Columbia, Alberta, Ontario, Quebec, and Nova Scotia), and they reviewed public documents with detailed accounts of H1N1 policies and recommendations. Policies were organized into four major categories: vaccine priority, use of adjuvanted vaccine for pregnant women, use of school closures as a containment approach, and use of the N95 respirator as personal protective equipment. The analysts uncovered three competing ideologies that influenced policymakers. Evidence-based ideology characterized policymakers who made decisions based on the best research evidence. Policy-based ideology represented policymakers who believed that science was a minor component of policymaking. For them, "evidence is meant to inform policy rather than drive policy" (p. 3). Pragmatist or hybrid ideology were policymakers who only accepted traditional research forms of evidence, specifically epidemiological evidence. The analysts discovered that a significant barrier to timely, effective policymaking was different ideological beliefs or interpretations of evidence and how to use it in policymaking. When time pressures exist, policymakers often rely on their previous belief systems or ideologies. Existing belief systems can cloud or override new, emerging evidence. Another barrier to effective policymaking for the H1N1 epidemic was competing interests. In this instance, there were unions who were interested in protecting their members; professional societies (e.g., for children, pregnant women) advocating for their specialty interests; and community interest groups (e.g., vulnerable populations). "At different jurisdictional levels in Canada, provincial and local level decision-makers needed to balance science with the overall needs and contextual factors of their community" (p. 6).

The analysts uncovered numerous tensions that challenged emergency public health policy actions. They recommended that whenever possible, proactive, pre-planned approaches should be in place, ready to enact. They cautioned, however, that pre-planned strategies, based on best evidence, must be flexible enough to accommodate local contexts.

Sources of evidence used by researchers and policy makers include the Cochrane Collaboration (health policy) and the Campbell Collaboration (social policy and education). These are international examples of not-for-profit organizations that critically evaluate the evidence available to inform policy decisions. The Cochrane Library has over 5 000 systematic reviews on health-related topics. Most universities have subscriptions to the Cochrane Library. Cochrane Library publications are considered a gold standard for making policy decisions related to health care.

EXERCISE 12.6 Visit the Cochrane Collaboration website at http://www.cochrane.org. Check out the website's features. Go to the "About us" page and click on "Newcomer's guide" to find out more about the organization. Go to the Cochrane Summaries website at http://summaries.cochrane.org.

1. Search a health term of interest to you and locate a summary to share with your class or your peers. You may also choose to share what you have learned by listening to a podcast under Cochrane Summaries.
2. Consider the public policy implications of your topic. Recommend one broad policy action based on Cochrane Summaries information.

POLICY ADVOCACY AND NURSING

Policy advocacy refers to nurses' capacity as individuals or members of professional associations and coalitions to influence policymakers. As discussed above, other policy inputs from key stakeholder groups can significantly impact the policymaking process, and an understanding of the formal government process of policy development helps nurses know when and how to present evidence, voice their concerns, and recommend potential policy actions.

Policy advocacy often begins with raising public awareness of the issue(s). An example is the social determinants of health and the inequities that exist within certain populations. Nurses provide care to at-risk populations in different settings (e.g., acute care, home care, public health clinics), and they are ideally placed to collect and share stories of people's lives that can raise awareness about health inequities. This practice is common in the United Kingdom where public health nurses are assigned to monitor and report on unsafe or unhealthy living conditions of their patients. Advocacy roles harness nurses' expert power to obtain access to needed health and social services for patients.

Professional associations and unions often offer campaign toolkits to assist nurses' advocacy work (see Chapter 21 on collective nursing advocacy). The Royal College of Nurses in the UK created a healthy workplace toolkit to support nurses' campaigns within their organizations to ensure quality practice environments for staff and patients and families. See https://www.rcn.org.uk/healthy-workplace/healthy-workplaces. The toolkit consists of five domains, such as work–life balance and dignity at work. Each section provides a brief overview of supporting research evidence with a checklist of indicators that nurses should look for within their workplaces. Each section includes resources, such as position statements, and website addresses to relevant national workforce policies, including bullying and harassment policies. Of importance is a "pledge page" in the toolkit where individuals or groups of nurses can design their own actions plans to address workplace concerns. What types of nurse campaigns can you join within your province, territory or nationally? To find out, visit the websites of your nurse associations and unions.

Nurses often become political through a quest to know more, to build expert power. The impetus to learn more and to do more is often driven by an inequity trigger. When there are power inequities, nurses can decide to use their power or to remain powerless. Nurses possess a great deal of expert power based on formal education and professional experiences. Although the impetus to make a difference begins with individual choice, political knowledge is synergized through collective action, such as networking, campaigning, joining coalitions, and lobbying.

EXERCISE 12.7 A model of political activism proposed by Leavitt et al. (2007) can be applied to the political development and activism of individual nurses in both professional and legislative political arenas. Assess yourself to see where you fit within this model—from apathy to leading the way. Based on where you fall within this model of political activism, consider two things you can do right now in your health care organization to move yourself further along this model's continuum.

1. *Apathy:* no membership of professional organizations; little or no interest in legislative politics as they relate to nursing and health care.
2. *Buy-in:* recognition of the importance of activism within professional organizations (without active participation) and legislative politics related to critical nursing issues.
3. *Self-interest:* involvement in professional organizations to further one's own career; the development and use of political expertise to further the profession's self-interests.
4. *Political sophistication:* high level of professional organization activism (e.g., holding office at the municipal or provincial level) moving beyond self-interests; recognition of the need for activism on behalf of the public and the profession.
5. *Leading the way:* serving in elected or appointed positions in professional organizations at the provincial or federal level; providing true leadership on broad health care interests in legislative politics, including seeking appointment to policymaking bodies and election to political positions.

? A SOLUTION

Carol was taken aback by what her friend said, but then she reflected on the types of shows that are on TV—and most do not portray nurses as intelligent, autonomous practitioners. So she decided to change her friend's view of nursing. Carol started by telling her friend about the life-changing experience she had during labour in which the nurse's help led to the safe delivery of her daughter. Having a professional there to coach and reassure them was essential to Carol's partner as well. Carol told her friend about a few of the expert nurses she knows from clinical experiences. She gave her friend examples of how nurses use their knowledge and skills to make a difference in the quality and safety of care delivery every day. Telling stories makes a difference. Carol's experiences had a powerful effect on her friend. She apologized for not knowing more about nursing and for making assumptions. Perhaps a number of people have the same ideas. Carol was glad for the apology but decided to go further. She went online to The Truth About Nursing Web site (http://www.truthaboutnursing.org) to learn more about how she could help improve nursing's image. The founder and executive director of The Truth About Nursing, Sandy Summers, discovered the hard truth about the public's perceptions of nursing when she was a graduate student at Johns Hopkins School of Nursing. Sandy and

her fellow graduate students banded together to create a not-for-profit organization to support a positive professional image of nurses. Their work has included campaigns to change the image of nurses on shows such as *Grey's Anatomy*. The Truth About Nursing has given TV shows that positively portray nurses, such as *Call the Midwife*, its award of excellence for showing the full range of what nurses do. The Web site gave Carol additional ways to take collective action to change how others think about nursing. Carol is proud to be entering the nursing profession and plans to speak to everyone she knows about the value of nursing. She will also keep a log of all those occasions when her care has made a positive difference for someone—and hopes to have a very large log! Carol and a group of nursing students at her school have contacted their provincial professional association to offer help in scanning the media for negative portrayals of nurses—so that they can collectively mount campaigns against media that undervalue or disrespect nursing. This situation led Carol to think about ways that she can use the power she has to make a difference for her new profession.

What approach might work for you in a similar situation? Have a look at Chapter 26 does it offer any information that might help with this kind of situation?

THE EVIDENCE

Eggertson (2011) examined the impact of emotional abuse and bullying in the workplace on nurses. The statistics in this article are staggering. A 2005 National Survey of the Work and Health of Nurses showed that 44% of female nurses and 50% of male nurses in Canada reported being exposed to hostility or conflict by people they work with. (Conflict management and workplace violence are discussed in Chapters 24–26.) The article also discusses the findings of a 2010 study by Mallette and colleagues on horizontal violence at the University Health Network in Toronto. This study found even higher levels of horizontal violence: 95% of nurses had observed horizontal violence and 71% identified themselves as targets. As part of

their research, Mallette and colleagues created an online curriculum that included a role-playing scenario where nurses could choose avatars to represent them in a virtual world. This allowed the nurses to safely role play different responses to bullying scenarios.

Eggertson concludes: "A genuine investment in coaching and mentoring nurses on how to value and respect one another will pay off, not only for nurses, but also for the patients they serve" (p. 20). Moreover, she states that "changing the workplace culture also requires managers and their supervisors to act immediately if nurses report bullying to them, and to back up nurses who have been hurt" (p. 20).

❋ NEED TO KNOW NOW

- Select positive and powerful role models.
- Form alliances with other new nurses: create your own support network.
- Join committees in your institution and/or professional nursing organizations.

- Contribute your talents to a topic of importance to you.
- Stay informed. What are current nursing policies in your organization? What are health policies at local, provincial or territorial, and national levels? Are they evidence-informed?

CHAPTER CHECKLIST

- Power is not finite: it expands by sharing it with others.
- Leaders can empower nurses and others by providing access to organizational empowerment structures (opportunities, information, supports, resources).
- Access to these empowerment structures (also called "power tools") is a catalyst for psychological empowerment—how nurses feel about themselves in their workplace.
- Psychological empowerment has four main dimensions: (1) meaning, (2) impact, (3) self-determination, and (4) competence.
- Nurses who are structurally and psychologically empowered are more satisfied and less likely to burn out or leave the organization.
- Another way to catalyze nurses' belief in themselves is through leader-empowering behaviours.
- Empowering leaders express confidence in their staff; they publicly value nursing; they involve nurses in making important decisions about health care delivery; and they support nurses in reaching their professional goals.

- Empowering work environments are known for strong nurse leadership at all levels, positive nurse–physician relationships, safe staffing, professional development opportunities, and giving nurses more control over practice. Some theorists and scholars consider nursing an oppressed group because of socialization practices that treat nurses as inferior. Horizontal violence, incivility, and bullying are associated with oppressed cultures.
- Nurses can build powerful professional identities by accentuating why they are irreplaceable. For instance, nurses make a positive difference in better, safer patient outcomes.
- Power strategies include networking and coalition building.
- The policy process should be based on best evidence, but other policy inputs, such as lobbying by special interest groups, can diminish the use of evidence during policymaking. However, evidence is important in every phase of the policy process.
- Policy engagement and political activism begin with nurses' desire to make a difference.

TIPS FOR USING INFLUENCE

- Make nursing your career, not just a job.
- Develop a powerful professional identity.
- Invest in your nursing career by continuing your education.
- Develop networking skills.

- Engage in policy advocacy by finding out what you can do through your provincial or territorial and national professional nursing associations and unions.

Visit the Evolve website for Suggested Readings, Internet Resources, and additional resources related to the content in this chapter: http://evolve.elsevier.com/Canada/Yoder-Wise/leading/.

REFERENCES

Aiken, L., Sloane, D., Bruyneel, L., Van den Heede, K., Griffiths, P., & Sermeus, W. (2014). Nurse staffing and education and hospital mortality in nine European countries: A retrospective observational study. *The Lancet, 383*(9931), 1824–1830.

American Nurses' Association. (2015). *ANA commends introduction of the Registered Nurse Safe Staffing Act (4/29/15)*. Retrieved from: http://www.nursingworld.org/Functional-MenuCategories/MediaResources/PressReleases/2015-NR/ANA-Commends-Introduction-of-the-Registered-Nurse-Safe-Staffing-Act.html.

Asanin, J., & Wilson, K. (2008). "I spent nine years looking for a doctor": Exploring access to health care among immigrants in Mississauga, Ontario, Canada. *Social Science & Medicine, 66*(6), 1271–1283. https://doi.org/10.1016/j.socscinied.2007.11.043.

Benner, P. (2001). *From Novice to Expert: Excellence and Power in Clinical Nursing Practice*. Upper Saddle River, NJ: Prentice Hall Health. commemorative ed. Retrieved from:

http://nursesunions.ca/sites/default/files/cfnu_workload_paper_pdf.pdf.

Bradbury-Jones, C., Sambrook, S., & Irvine, F. (2011). Nursing students and the issue of voice: A qualitative study. *Nurse Education Today, 31*, 628–632.

Bryant, T. (2009). *An introduction to health policy*. Toronto, ON: Canadian Scholars' Press.

Canadian Nurses' Association-Canadian Federation of Nurses' Unions. (2014). *Joint Position Statement: Workplace Violence and Bullying*. Retrieved from: https://cna-aiic.ca/~/media/cna/page-content/pdf-en/Workplace-Violence-and-Bullying_joint-position-statement.pdf.

Canadian Nurses' Association-Canadian Medical Association. (2013). *Principles to Guide Health Care Transformation in Canada*. Retrieved from: https://www.cna-aiic.ca/~/media/cna/files/en/guiding_principles_hc_e.pdf.

Cicolini, G., Comparcini, D., & Simonetti, V. (2014). Workplace empowerment and nurse's job satisfaction: A systematic literature review. *Journal of Nursing Management, 22*, 855–871.

Cziraki, K., & Laschinger, H. (2015). Leader empowering behaviours and work engagement: The mediating role of structural empowerment. *Nursing Leadership, 28*(3), 10–22. https://doi.org/10.12927/cjnl.2016.24455.

Dahinten, V. S., Lee, S. E., & MacPhee, M. (2016). Disentangling the relationships between staff nurses' workplace empowerment and job satisfaction. *Journal of Nursing Management, 24*, 1060–1070.

Dahinten, S., MacPhee, M., Hejazi, S., et al. (2013). Testing the effects of an empowerment-based leadership development programme: Part 2—staff outcomes. *Journal of Nursing Management, 22*(1), 16–28. https://doi.org/10.1111/jonm.12059.

Daveluy, M.-C. (2018). Jeanne Mance. In *Dictionary of Canadian Biography* (Vol. 1). University of Toronto/Université Laval. Retrieved from: http://www.biographi.ca/en/bio/mance_jeanne_1E.html.

DiNapoli, J. M., O'Flaherty, D., Musli, C., Clavelle, J., & Fitzpatrick, J. (2016). The relationship of clinical nurses' perceptions of structural and psychological empowerment and engagement on their unit. *Journal of Nursing Administration, 46*(2), 95–100.

Dong, W., Fung, K., & Chan, K. (2010). Community mobilisation and empowerment for combating a pandemic. *Journal of Epidemiology and Community Health, 64*, 182–183. https://doi.org/10.1136/jech.2008.082206.

Duchscher, J. E. (2009). Transition shock: The initial stage of role adaptation for newly graduated registered nurses. *Journal of Advanced Nursing, 65*(5), 1103–1113. https://doi.org/10.1111/j.1365-2648.2008.04898.x.

Eggertson, L. (2011). Targeted: The impact of bullying, and what needs to be done to eliminate it. *Canadian Nurse, 107*(6), 16–20.

Fafard, P. (2008). *Evidence and Healthy Public Policy: Insights from Health and Political Sciences*. Ottawa, ON: National Collaborating Centre for Healthy Public Policy/Canadian Policy Research Networks. Retrieved from: http://www.ncchpp.ca.

Goedhart, N., Van Oosten, C., & Vermeulen, H. (2017). The effect of structural empowerment of nurses on quality outcomes in hospitals: A scoping review. *Journal of Nursing Management, 25*, 194–206.

Green, J., Wyllie, A., & Jackson, D. (2014). Social networking for nurse education: Possibilities, perils and pitfalls. *Journal of Contemporary Nurse, 47*(1-2), 180–189. https://doi.org/10.1080/10376178.2014.11081919.

HEAL. (2017). Retrieved from: http://www.healthactionlobby.ca/about-us.html.

Health Canada. (2009). *Office of Nursing Policy*. Retrieved from: http://www.hc-sc.gc.ca/ahc-asc/branch-dirgen/spb-dgps/onp-bpsi/index-eng.php.

Hersey, P., Blanchard, K., & Natemeyer, W. (1979). Situational leadership, perception and impact of power. *Group and Organizational Studies, 4*, 418–428.

Howlett, M., & Ramesh, M. (Eds.). (2003). *Studying public policy: policy cycles and policy subsystems* (2nd ed.) Don Mills, ON: Oxford University Press.

International Council of Nurses. (2017). *Position Statement: Prevention and Management of Workplace Violence*. Retrieved from: http://www.icn.ch/images/stories/documents/publications/position_statements/ICN_PS_Prevention_and_management_of_workplace_violence.pdf.

Kanter, R. M. (1993). *Men and women of the corporation* (2nd ed.). New York, NY: Basic Books.

Kramer, M. (1974). *Reality shock: why nurses leave nursing*. St. Louis, MO: Mosby.

Laschinger, H., Finegan, J., & Wilk, P. (2009). Context matters: The impact of unit leadership and empowerment on nurses' organizational commitment. *The Journal of Nursing Administration, 39*(5), 228–235.

Laschinger, H., Gilbert, S., Smith, L., et al. (2010). Towards a comprehensive theory of nurse/patient empowerment: Applying Kanter's empowerment theory to patient care. *Journal of Nursing Management, 18*, 4–13. https://doi.org/10.111/j.1365-2834.2009.01046.x.

Leavitt, J. K., Chaffee, M. W., & Vance, C. (2007). Learning the ropes of policy and politics. In D. J. Mason, J. K. Leavitt, & M. W. Chaffee (Eds.), *Policy & politics in nursing and health care* (5th ed., pp. 34–46). St. Louis, MO: Saunders.

MacPhee, M., Jackson, C., & Suryaprakash, N. (2009). Online knowledge networking: What leaders need to know. *Journal of Nursing Administration, 39*(10), 415–422 doi:0.1097/NNA.0b013e3181b9221f.

Mark, B., Harless, D., Spetz, J., Reiter, K., & Pink, G. (2013). California's minimum nurse staffing legislation: Results from a natural experiment. *Health Services Research*, 48(2), 435–454. https://doi.org/10.1111/j.1475-6773.2012.01465.x.

McGillis Hall, L., MacDonald-Rencz, S., Peterson, J., et al. (2013). *Moving to action: Evidence-Based Retention and Recruitment Policy Initiatives for Nursing*. Ottawa, ON: Canadian Foundation for Healthcare Improvement and Office of Nursing Policy. Retrieved from: http://www.cfhi-fcass.ca/sf-docs/default-source/reports/Moving-to-Action-McGillis-Hall-E.pdf?sfvrsn=0.

McIntyre, M., & McDonald, C. (2010). *Realities of canadian nursing: professional, practice, and power issues*. Philadelphia, PA: Wolters Kluwer Health.

Purpora, C., Blegen, M., & Stotts, N. (2012). Horizontal violence among hospital staff nurses related to oppressed self or oppressed group. *Journal of Professional Nursing*, 28(5), 306–314.

Regan, S., Wong, C., Laschinger, H., Cummings, G., Leiter, M., & Read, E. (2017). Starting out: Qualitative perspectives of new graduate nurses and nurse leaders on transition to practice. *Journal of Nursing Management*, 25(4), 246–255. https://doi.org/10.1111/jonm.12456.

Rosella, L., Wilson, K., Crowcroft, N., Chu, A., Upshur, R., & Goel, V. (2013). Pandemilc H1N1 in Canada and the use of evidence in developing public health policies—a policy analysis. *Social Science and Medicine*, 83, 1–9.

Rush, K., Adamack, M., Gordon, J., Meredith, L., & Janke, R. (2013). Best practices of formal new graduate nurse transition programs: An integrative review. *International Journal of Nursing Studies*, 50(3), 345–356. https://doi.org/10.1016/j.ijnurstu.2012.06.009.

Sauer, P. (2012). Do nurses eat their young? Truth and consequences. *Journal of Emergency Nursing*, 38(1), 43–46.

Smith, B. (2012). Social networking and professional pitfalls. *International Journal of Orthopaedic and Trauma Nursing*, 16, 63–64. https://doi.org/10.1016/j.ijotn.2012.03.001.

Spreitzer, G. (2007). Taking stock: A review of more than twenty years of research on empowerment at work. In J. Barling, & C. Cooper (Eds.), *The Sage handbook of organizational behavior vol. 1*. (pp. 54–73). Los Angeles, CA: Sage.

St-Pierre, I., & Holmes, D. (2008). Managing nurses through disciplinary power: A Foucauldian analysis of workplace violence. *Journal of Nursing Management*, 16, 352–359. https://doi.org/10.1111/j.1365-2834.2007.00812.x.

Stam, L., Laschinger, H., Regan, S., & Wong, C. (2015). The influence of personal and workplace resources on new graduate nurses' job satisfaction. *Journal of Nursing Management*, 23, 190–199.

Sullivan, E. J. (2013). *Becoming influential: A guide for nurses* (2nd ed.). Upper Saddle River, NJ: Pearson Education.

Summers, S. (2014, January). Changing how the world thinks about nursing. *Canadian Nurse*, 26–30.

Ten Hoeve, Y., Jansen, G., & Roodbol, P. (2014). The nursing profession: Public image, self-concept and professional identity. A discussion paper. *Journal of Advanced Nursing*, 70(2), 295–309. https://doi.org/10.1111/jan.12177.

Tomblin Murphy, G., & MacKenzie, A. (2013). Using evidence to meet population healthcare needs: Successes and challenges. *Healthcare Papers*, 13(2), 9–21.

Trus, M., Razbadauskas, A., & Doran, D. (2012). Work-related empowerment of nurse managers: A systematic review. *Nursing and Health Sciences*, 14(3), 412–420.

Udod, S. (2008). The power behind empowerment for staff nurses: Using Foucault's concepts. *The Canadian Journal of Nursing Leadership*, 21(2), 77–92.

Udod, S., & Racine, L. (2014). A critical perspective on relations between staff nurses and their nurse manager: Advancing nurse empowerment theory. *Canadian Journal of Nursing Research*, 46(4), 83–100.

Uhlrich, B., Krozek, C., Early, S., Ashlock, C., Africa, L., & Carman, M. (2010). Improving retention, confidence, and competence of new graduate nurses: Results from a 10-year longitudinal database. *Nursing Economics*, 28, 448–462.

Upton, J., Fletcher, M., Mado-Sutton, H., et al. (2011). Shared decision making or paternalism in nursing consultations? A qualitative study of primary care asthma nurses' views on sharing decisions with patients regarding inhaler device selection. *Health Expectations*, 14(4), 374–382. https://doi.org/10.1111/j.1369-7625.2010.00653.x.

White, K., Dudley-Brown, S., & Terhaar, M. (Eds.). (2016). *Translation of evidence into nursing and health care* (2nd ed.). New York, NY: Springer.

Wilson, R. (2013). Policy and evidence in Canadian health human resources planning. *Healthcare Papers*, 13(2), 28–31.

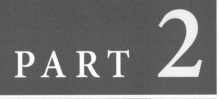

PART 2

Managing Resources

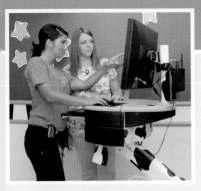

13

Caring and Communicating in Nursing With Technology

Gillian Strudwick, Richard Booth

This chapter describes how nurses can best work with technology to deliver clinical care. Nurses work in a variety of settings where technology is currently present, and where new technology is being introduced on a regular basis. Nurses need to know how to incorporate these technologies into their workflow, as well as be able to appropriately use these technologies during the clinical encounter. This chapter includes sections on the types of technologies that many nurses use in their practice, future technologies that may soon enter the clinical environment, how nurses can integrate technology into clinical care, standards and terminologies adopted by nursing associations, and special topics related to caring, communicating, and managing with technology. In the future, clinical environments where nurses work will become more advanced with regard to the types and ways in which technologies are used to deliver care. Nurses need to obtain the appropriate level of competencies to be able to use these technologies in clinically meaningful ways. As well, nurses should be equipped with the knowledge and skill to be able to influence decisions regarding technology acquisition by health care organizations.

OBJECTIVES

- Describe trends in the adoption and use of health information technology.
- Define nursing informatics.
- Discuss the types of technologies used in various clinical practice environments.
- Identify technologies that may enter clinical practice environments in the future.
- Analyze the influence of technology on clinical care.
- Learn techniques to support the use of technology in the clinical encounter.
- Describe how compassionate care can be delivered in the presence of technology.
- Discuss strategies to support the successful implementation and adoption of health information technologies.

- Explore ways that technology can be used to support patient safety and deliver evidence-based care.
- Learn about how nursing schools in Canada incorporate nursing informatics into their entry-to-practice programs.
- Describe the role of the nurse leader as it relates to nursing informatics.
- Identify ways to engage consumers and patients in health information technology selection, adoption, and use.
- Learn about nursing standards and terminologies.

TERMS TO KNOW

artificial intelligence

barcode medication administration

care planning tools

clinical decision support systems

clinical information system

compassionate care

computerized provider order entry

electronic health record

electronic medical record

electronic medication administration record

hardware

health information technologies

hospital information system

medication administration technology

monitoring technologies

nursing informatics

nursing informatics competencies

nursing leadership

patient engagement

patient portals

patient safety

robotics

software

standards

technology adoption

telehealth

terminology

workflow

❓ A CHALLENGE

Dana is an early career registered nurse in a small, rural hospital who is interested in technology and how it can enhance client care. The nursing leadership in their hospital is collaborating with leadership from the information management department, medicine, and allied health to implement an integrated electronic health record with other small rural hospitals in the geographical area and have asked Dana to be a staff nurse representative on the team. This electronic health record system will include nursing documentation, computerized provider order entry, clinical decision support, barcode-enabled electronic medication administration, laboratory results reporting and viewing, electronic care planning, and a patient portal. Additionally, it is the intention of the collaborating hospitals to standardize as much of the electronic health record design content as possible. During the design phase of the project, Dana was asked to consult with her colleagues and offer input on the following questions:

- What nursing assessments and documentation fields should be included in the electronic health record system?

- How will the electronic health record be incorporated into nursing workflow?
- In what ways would you like to see clinical decision making supports present in the electronic health record?
- What types of hardware are most appropriate in your care setting?
- When is the best time to for nurses to engage in professional development specific to this new technology? What methods should be utilized to deliver this professional development?
- Are there nursing terminologies or standards that should be incorporated into the nursing assessments and documentation fields in the electronic health record?
- How can other nurses, patients, and families be engaged in the implementation of the electronic health record and patient portal?

Dana and her colleagues need to offer comprehensive and future-minded input.

How do you think Dana should gather this input with and from her nursing colleagues?

INTRODUCTION

Canadian health care organizations rely heavily on technologies to support care delivery in all clinical settings. Nurses use technologies, such as digital thermometers, electronic health records, electronic vitals devices, smart intravenous pumps, computers on wheels, and glucometers, in many health settings to support the completion of nursing assessments and provision of nursing care. Many of these technologies have been introduced into

settings where nurses have worked for a number of years, and have been incorporated into the routines and working patterns of nurses in a variety of different environments, such as primary care clinics, hospital medical units, mental health inpatient settings, community care, and public health contexts. For nurses, technology is often critical for the completion of necessary assessments and to provide care. It can therefore be difficult to function when a device is broken, the power is turned off, the system is "down," or there is a lack of availability of equipment. Thus, nurses' use of technology has become an essential component in providing adequate nursing care. In the future, as technology becomes more pervasive in clinical environments, nurses will be required to incorporate technology into their practice in new ways.

In many Canadian hospital and clinic environments, patient records (or parts of them) are kept electronically in systems called electronic health records (EHRs) (Auditor General of Canada, 2010; Chang & Gupta, 2015). These computerized patient records provide nurses and other health professionals with an electronic way of documenting clinical care and obtaining relevant health information to support clinical decision making. In recent years, there have been some modifications to these EHR systems that allow some patients in Canada to have access to parts or all of their health record (Gheorghiu & Hagens, 2017). Providing patients with electronic access to their health record is often referred to as Open Notes (Delbanco et al., 2015), and can often be accessed through a patient portal (HealthIT.gov, 2015). This is not to be confused with a personal health record, which is a health record owned and maintained by individual patients themselves, without health professional access. Across the country, there is significant work going on to implement new EHR systems, update current EHR systems, or add certain functions and features to enhance the various technologies' ability to support the delivery of high-quality and safe patient care. According to the Healthcare Information Management Systems Society, the adoption of more sophisticated functions and features of EHR systems is much lower in Canada then it is in the United States (Healthcare Information and Management Systems Society, 2014). Therefore in the coming years, there is likely to be a number of implementations, updates, and modifications of EHR systems across the country.

To be able to work effectively in environments with numerous technologies and the presence of EHR systems, nurses need to have the appropriate level and types of competencies to be able to use these technologies in ways that best support their work. Canadian nurses must understand how to incorporate these technologies into their workflow, as well as how they can be used during clinical encounters in ways that do not detract from the relationship between the nurse and the patient. This chapter provides an overview of several

technologies that nurses may encounter and use in their clinical practice, as well as review some of the practice considerations with regard to how they can be meaningfully integrated into work patterns to support the delivery of safe and effective nursing care.

NURSING INFORMATICS

When considering nurses' use of technology in clinical settings, the term nursing informatics is often used. The Canadian Nursing Informatics Association (CNIA) and the Canadian Nurses Association (CNA) have endorsed the definition of nursing informatics in the following way: "Nursing informatics science and practice integrates nursing, its information and knowledge and their management with information and communication technologies to promote the health of people, families and communities worldwide" (International Medical Informatics Association, 2009). Nursing informatics can improve nurses' decision-making capabilities through the "collection, extraction, aggregation analysis and interpretation of standardized data, using the emerging principles and methods of data science" (Canadian Nurses Association, 2017).

Electronic health records are one technology that can support nurses in collecting relevant nursing data in standardized ways that can then be extracted and analyzed to support decision making. The data collected through these systems can support decision making at a number of levels, including the direct care level, the unit level, and the organizational level. Because nurses are required to document their assessments and clinical care, this information can be collected through EHR systems. Automated ways of extracting data can be used where the information is pulled from specific fields where nurses document within the EHR. This information can be combined with other data from the EHR and analyzed to identify trends and relationships. Insights gleaned from this data can then be used to support nurses in making clinical decisions. This, however, can only be done if data is captured within the EHR in a standardized way. Nurses with informatics knowledge and skills can support organizations implementing or modifying their systems to ensure that nursing documentation is captured in standardized ways that support the principles of nursing informatics.

Nursing informatics is a thriving subspecialty of nursing that combines nursing science, information science, and computer science. Like any knowledge-intensive profession, nursing is greatly affected by the growth of both scientific advances and technology. Thus, a group was formed in 2002 to support nursing informatics in Canada called the Canadian Nursing Informatics Association (CNIA) (Canadian Nursing Informatics Association, n.d.). The goals of this group are shown in Box 13.1. The organization hosts an annual conference, has a website, provides updates and news on nursing informatics topics through a regular newsletter, and collaborates with a number of organizations, such as the Canadian Nurses Association and Canada Health Infoway, to operationalize its goals. Across Canada, many provinces and territories also have jurisdictional nursing informatics groups, such as the Ontario Nursing Informatics Group.

Data, information, knowledge (CNA, 2001), and wisdom are the foundation of nursing informatics and all nursing communication (Englebardt & Nelson, 2002; Matney et al., 2011; Mastrian & McGonigle, 2009; Staggers & Nelson, 2009). The core of this model is the transformation of data into information and then into knowledge for use at the point of care, or what has been called *practice-based evidence*. It requires access to real-time clinical data housed in comprehensive repositories, such as EHR systems with robust analytical tools (Remus & Kennedy, 2012). Having actionable data available at the point of care enhances the credibility of information used to direct and coordinate patient-centric care. *Data* are discrete entities that describe or measure something

---

BOX 13.1   Goals of the Canadian Nursing Informatics Association

Goals

1 "To strategically seek out partnerships and networking opportunities to provide leadership and expertise for Nursing Informatics in Canada"
2 "To foster innovation by expanding and disseminating knowledge about nursing and health informatics for nurses and the health care community"
3 "To engage in national and international nursing and health informatics initiatives"
4 "To create awareness about the value of standardized data in health care to facilitate knowledge driven care and health system use"

Canadian Nursing Informatics Association. (n.d.). History. Paragraph 4. Retrieved from https://cnia.ca/history/

---

without interpretation. Numbers are data; for example, the number 30, without interpretation, means nothing. *Information* consists of defined, interpreted, organized, or structured data. The number 30 defined as millilitres, minutes, or hours has meaning. *Knowledge* refers to information that is combined or synthesized so that interrelationships are identified. For example, the number 30, when included in the statement "All patients who had indwelling bladder catheters for longer than 30 days developed infections," becomes knowledge, something that is known. *Wisdom*, the appropriate use of knowledge to manage and solve human problems (American Nurses Association, 2008; Englebardt & Nelson, 2002; Matney et al., 2011; Mastrian & McGonigle, 2009; Staggers & Nelson, 2009), occurs when a nurse chooses a specific, tailored means of preventing urinary tract infections in patients with long-term catheter use. The transformation of data into knowledge facilitates decision making, new discoveries, and the creation of designs. Wisdom allows for the application of designs in addressing clinical problems.

In practice, skilled clinicians synthesize data and information quickly, interpreting and comparing new data with previous information about the patient to reach knowledgeable conclusions. Much of the data's potential value is lost, however, if not stored where others can retrieve and use them in a timely manner to synthesize new information and knowledge.

Data from many patients analyzed and synthesized in scientific studies are combined to provide evidence for best practices in patient care. Evidence-informed practice either reassures us that our approach to patient care is correct or the evidence redirects our thinking. Technology has influenced both the availability and the applicability of evidence for practice.

TECHNOLOGIES

In its broadest definition, technology is defined as an application of knowledge, often in the form of equipment or machinery. Within Canadian health care settings, the term *technology* is often used broadly as well. For example, the term *technology* in health care could describe equipment used to conduct scans such as MRIs and CT, medical devices such as infusion pumps, monitors such as those used for ECGs, information systems such as EHRs, and communication systems such as telehealth. It has also been argued that more basic but essential equipment and devices, such as bedpans, are also a form of technology. Within this chapter, technologies in health care that are electronically based are discussed and described. Thus, the definition of technology used within this chapter is that of the application of knowledge in the form of electronic devices and/or systems in clinical environments.

Nurses in Canada work in environments with many technologies present. Nurses rely upon these technologies every day for completing nursing assessments, such as taking a blood pressure; and providing nursing care, such as delivering intravenous fluids via an infusion pump. For more than a decade, many nurses in Canada have been documenting either all or part of their assessments and nursing care in EHR systems. These systems often have other features and functions that support clinical decision making, provide access to timely information, automate processes, and support specific nursing processes such as administering medication. Despite the potential benefits of using these technologies, nurses need to continue to think critically with regards to their practice. If a result obtained from an assessment using a medical device does not seem congruent with a clinical assessment, nurses should consider redoing the assessment, performing the assessment manually, or gaining information from another source. Technology is not without fault. It needs to be maintained and replaced over time. On occasion it may malfunction. As well, nurses need to use information obtained from technology to inform their own thinking and decision making. Additionally, nurses may feel a sense of fatigue with the amount of technology used in a clinical setting, particularly when many new technologies are implemented in a setting in a short period of time.

The following section describes some of the common types of technologies currently present in Canadian clinical practice environments where nurses work, as well as some of the technologies that nurses may use in the future. Although there are many technologies present in these settings, this section of the chapter will focus on the following:

- Medical devices and monitoring technologies
- Electronic health record systems
- Patient portals
- Telehealth
- Future technology

The list and types of technologies described in this section of the chapter are not meant to be exhaustive, but rather represent an overview of the various technologies that nurses may use in different clinical settings within Canada.

MEDICAL DEVICES AND MONITORING TECHNOLOGIES

Electronically based medical devices are used in just about every clinical environment where nurses work in Canada. In mental health clinical care settings, nurses may use glucometers to assess blood glucose levels. On medical and surgical units, infusion pumps may be used to deliver intravenous fluids. In primary care clinics, nurses may use vital signs devices to assess blood pressure, heart rate, oxygen saturation, and temperature. These electronic medical devices are primarily used by nurses to perform a specific purpose. In the above examples, this purpose may be to assess a blood glucose level, deliver intravenous therapy, or obtain vital sign measurements. In each of these cases, nurses need to have knowledge of how the device works and how to best use it with the individual patient, often taking into consideration patient differences: for example, the size of the blood pressure cuff to be used. Thus nurses should have the appropriate level of knowledge and professional development to use these medical devices in their practice setting. In many cases, medical device professional development is learned "on the job"; however, more complex medical devices typically require more intensive and perhaps formal professional development. For example, given the complexity of using smart infusion pumps, Accreditation Canada has established a required organization practice specific to this device that specifies professional development expectations (Accreditation Canada, 2017). Therefore health care organizations that deliver care using smart infusion pumps typically deliver formal infusion pump education to nurses on a yearly basis.

EXERCISE 13.1 Select a health care setting in which you have completed or are currently completing your practice placement. What medical devices are used? Make a list of these devices and their functions. If the medical device was not working properly or was not available, could you still perform the assessment or care that the device was created to support? What professional development were you provided with regard to how to use the medical device? Are there other clinical settings where this medical device could be used?

Medical devices that support both patients and health professionals have been developed for and are used in a number of clinical settings. Several of these devices use speech recognition (SR) software. SR refers to electronic devices and programs that permit data entry by human speech (also known as *computer speech recognition*). The term *voice recognition* is also used to refer to speech recognition. SR converts spoken words to machine-readable input. SR applications in everyday life include voice dialling (e.g., "Call home"), call routing (e.g., "I would like to make a collect call"), and simple data entry (e.g., stating a credit card or account number). In health care, SR can be used to prepare structured documents, such as radiology reports (Ringler et al., 2015), order tests, or dictate notes, such as mental status exams (Derman et al., 2010). In all of these examples, the computer gathers, processes, interprets, and executes audible signals by comparing the spoken words with a template in the system. If the patterns match, recognition occurs and a command is executed by the computer. Voice technology allows untrained personnel or those whose hands are busy to enter data in an SR environment without touching the computer. Voice technology also allows people with physical challenges to function more efficiently when using a computer. SR systems recognize a large number of words but are still in their infancy. The speaker must use staccato-like speech, pausing between each clearly spoken word, and an SR system must be programmed for each user so that it recognizes a specific user's voice patterns.

Monitoring technologies are commonly used in Canada. These technologies were initially used primarily in intensive care and cardiac care units for physiological monitoring, however there have been more recent uses of some of these systems in other settings, including home and community care settings. Opportunities for data generated from monitoring technologies to populate specific fields within EHR systems have been implemented in some Canadian clinical settings. In these settings, nurses need to pay particular attention to the data generated from these monitoring devices, because the act of transcribing them into the clinical record is not a cue for assessing the outputs of the monitors. Common physiological monitoring systems measure heart rate, blood pressure, and other vital signs. They also monitor cardiac rhythm; measure and record central venous, pulmonary wedge, intracranial, and intra-abdominal pressures; and analyze oxygen and carbon dioxide levels in the blood. Intracranial pressure (ICP)-monitoring systems monitor the cranial pressure in critically ill patients with closed head injuries, or postoperative craniotomy patients. The ICP, along with the mean arterial blood pressure, can be used to calculate perfusion pressure. This allows assessment and early therapy as changes occur. When the ICP exceeds a set pressure, some systems allow ventricular drainage. Similarly, monitoring pressure within the bladder has recently been demonstrated to accurately detect intra-abdominal hypertension as measures of maximal and mean intra-abdominal pressures and abdominal perfusion pressure are made. Intra-abdominal hypertension occurs with abdominal compartment syndrome and other acute abdominal illnesses. Routine intra-abdominal pressure (IAP) monitoring has been recommended for those critically ill patients subjected to shock and subsequent resuscitation (Kirkpatrick et al., 2007).

Continuous dysrhythmia monitors and electrocardiograms (ECGs) provide visual representation of electrical activity in the heart and can be used for surveillance and detection of dysrhythmias and for interpretation and diagnosis of the abnormal rhythm. Although they are not new technology, these systems have grown increasingly sophisticated. More important, integration with wireless communication technology permits new approaches to triaging alerts to nurses about cardiac rhythm abnormalities. The need for wireless approaches to decrease response time to dysrhythmia alarms was demonstrated in a study of remote cardiac telemetry nurses who detected a valid rhythm disturbance an average of 72% of the time but required physically checking alarms every 2.1 to 6.2 minutes while simultaneously carrying their patient load (Billinghurst et al., 2003).

Monitoring technologies can sometimes be programmed to alert when the monitor reading falls outside of a predetermined parameter. Nurses should be involved in determining the appropriate parameters in which alerts and sounds can be generated so that alert fatigue is avoided. Alert fatigue occurs when there are so many alerts and noises that nurses become desensitized to these alerts. Ensuring that these alerts are only fired when clinically appropriate is one way to manage the possibility of alert fatigue.

EXERCISE 13.2 Identify a health care setting with a monitoring technology present that alerts when patient parameters fall outside defined limits. Can you think of the parameters that may have been used to determine when the monitor would alert? Who would make this decision? Where would the evidence or clinical guideline be obtained from? You notice that nurses in the area seem to have alert fatigue. What might have caused this? Are there any patient safety issues as a result of alert fatigue?

Other technologies used in clinical settings where nurses work include patient surveillance systems. Patient surveillance systems are designed to provide early warning of a possible impending adverse event. One example is a system that provides wireless monitoring of heart rate, respiratory rate, and attempts by a patient at risk of falling to get out of bed unassisted; this monitoring is via a mattress coverlet and bedside monitor.

ELECTRONIC HEALTH RECORD SYSTEMS

Electronic health record systems are secure computerized patient record systems where nurses and other health professionals can obtain and document clinical information for their patients. Multiple terms are used to describe these systems by health professionals. Commonly used terms include hospital information system (HIS), clinical information system (CIS), electronic medical record (EMR), and electronic health record (EHR). Both the terms EHR and EMR have gained widespread use, with some health informatics users assigning EHR to the global concept as well as their use in hospital settings, and EMR to more specific uses, like primary care settings. There are many different types of EHR system software, and many different vendors that sell these systems. In local hospitals, health authorities/regions, and primary care clinics, these EHR systems tend to have nicknames. For example, one Ontario mental health organization refers to their EHR system as *I-CARE*, and a nearby pediatric hospital refers to their EHR system as *Kid-Care*. These systems are not only present in hospital and primary care clinics but can also be used in community care settings and in public health contexts. EHR systems are most often accessed on a computer, often over a network. Among the many forms of data often included in EHR systems are patient demographics, health history, progress and procedure notes, health problems, medication and allergy lists (including immunization status), laboratory test results, radiology images and reports, and advanced directives.

EHR systems can have a variety of features and functions. Some organizations implement all of these features and functions at the same time. This is referred to as a "big-bang" implementation. Other organizations transition over a period of time from a paper-based system to an electronic system. This implementation may be called a "phased" approach. During this transition period, some processes are done electronically

and other processes are done on paper. When both electronic and paper is used, the term *hybrid environment* is used. Common features and functions of an EHR system include the following:

- Nursing documentation
- Computerized provider order entry (CPOE)
- Electronic medication administration record
- Barcode medication administration
- Care planning
- Clinical decision support systems

Nursing documentation completed in EHR systems is often done through the completion of electronic templates, forms, and flowsheets that capture discrete forms of data. For example, if a nurse wants to document a mental status examination of a recently assessed client, the nurse may have the option of selecting a mental status form in which aspects of the assessment are listed. The nurse would then identify the assessment findings through the selection of assessment values through drop-down menus, radio buttons, tick boxes, and other discrete selections. Additionally, nurses often have the ability to write narrative or free-text documentation to support discrete forms of data collection. Often nurses find it difficult to convey a complete overview of a patient through discrete methods, and therefore a narrative note is written to bring together and explain the discrete data already documented. In a study of acute care nurses' use of EHR systems, nurses appreciated having the ability to view trends in discrete data over time to support their decision-making process (Strudwick et al., 2018).

> **EXERCISE 13.3** Consider how you have documented, or observed your preceptor documenting, patient assessments and clinical care. Was this done on paper, a computer, or both? How did you or your preceptor document this information? Did you or your preceptor use discrete forms of documentation, narrative forms of documentation, or both? What are the benefits and drawbacks of the documentation methods that you have used or observed?

Computerized provider order entry (CPOE) is a function of the EHR system that allows physicians, nurse practitioners, dentists, and other health professionals to enter orders into the EHR system electronically (Niazkhani et al., 2009). Often, predetermined order sets, and parameters for orders that meet best practice guidelines, are available in these systems to give the ordering health professional the ability to ensure that orders reflect evidence-based practice. Additionally, there may be clinical decision support tools embedded into the CPOE function. For example, if a medication is ordered that the patient has an allergy to, an alert or pop-up may appear that provides the health professional with this information. The health professional can review the alert or pop-up and make a decision based on this information, as well as other information (e.g., patient preference, previous experience) that the health professional is aware of. One of the benefits of CPOE is that when new orders are entered, these systems often automatically alert those health professionals that need to know about the new order, and may also auto-populate areas of the record. For example, if a new medication is ordered, the order may be sent to pharmacy to be verified and the dispensing of the medication completed. This medication order may also automatically populate the medication administration record so that the nurse will know to give this medication. A systematic review by Charles et al. (2014) identified that CPOE systems in hospitals can support the reduction of medication errors, especially when used in combination with other technologies that support patient safety.

Electronic medication administration records are a function of an EHR system that allow nurses the ability to view and document medication administration for their patients. Often electronic medication administration records are auto-populated by new orders entered through the CPOE function. Similar to paper-based medication administration records, this electronic function allows nurses to complete and document the rights of medication administration and to document that medication has been given. In many cases, nurses use the electronic medication administration record function in combination with medication administration technology.

In **barcode medication administration**, a nurse is required to scan a patient identifier, such as a wrist band with a barcode present. The nurse then scans a medication package with a barcode also present. If these scans match the medication that was ordered in the electronic medication administration record, the medication can be safely administered. A recent literature review identifying the impact of barcode medication administration technology on medication administration safety showed that medication error rates typically decrease when this

technology is used (Strudwick et al., 2018). In a study by Poon et al. (2010), the use of barcode medication administration may have contributed to a reduction in medication errors by approximately 50%.

RESEARCH PERSPECTIVE

Resource: Strudwick, G., Clark, C., McBride, B., Sakal, M., & Kalia, K. (2017). Thank you for asking: Exploring patient perceptions of barcode medication administration practices in inpatient mental health settings. *International al Journal of Medical Informatics*, 105: 31–37.

Medication errors can be reduced with the use of barcode medication administration only if the technology is used during the majority of times medications are administered. The use of this technology is challenging in mental health inpatient settings where patients are mobile and not necessarily spending large amounts of time in a single location, such as a hospital bed. In an effort to identify how to improve barcode scanning rates in an inpatient mental health setting to improve patient safety, 52 patients were interviewed by a peer support worker using a semi-structured interview guide. The purpose of these interviews was to identify patient perceptions of the technology and to gather insights from patients on how to improve scanning rates. Results of the thematic analysis of the interview transcriptions identified the following six themes: (1) management of information; (2) privacy and security; (3) stigma; (4) relationships; (5) safety and comfort; and (6) negative associations with technology. Findings of this study led to changes at the organization with regard to how patients could be identified during the medication administration process. Patients now have the option to wear a barcoded wristband, have a photo taken with an affiliated barcode, or have a photo identification, such as a passport, scanned and affiliated with a barcode.

EXERCISE 13.4 Reflect on a time when you administered medications to a patient. Where did you find the medication administration record? Was it available on a computer or was it printed on paper? How did you verify all of the *rights* of medication administration? Was technology used to support any of these processes?

Care planning tools are sometimes present as a function of an EHR system that allows health professionals to document patient and health professionals' goals, their plan of care, and progress toward achieving these goals. As this tool can often be accessed by any member of the health professional team, all health professionals typically have the ability to document that certain care planning elements were followed or completed, and their efficacy.

The EHR system and its various feature and functions can be accessed through a variety of different hardware options. Placing computers or handheld devices *patient-side* permits nurses to enter data once, at the point of care, rather than on a paper *cheat sheet* that is transcribed into the EHR system at a later time. Documentation of patient assessments and care that is provided patient-side saves time, gives others more timely access to the data, and decreases the likelihood of forgetting to document vital information. Point-of-care devices and systems that fit with nurses' workflow, personalize patient assessments, and simplify care planning are available. Patient-care areas with point-of-care computers have improved the quality of patient care by decreasing errors of omission, providing greater accuracy and completeness of documentation, reducing medication errors, providing more timely responses to patient needs, and improving discharge planning and teaching. These systems can eliminate redundant charting and facilitate patient hand-offs from shift to shift or between care areas.

> **EXERCISE 13.5** Think about the data you gather as you care for a patient through the day. How do you communicate information and knowledge about your patient to others? Does the EHR system support the way you need this information organized, stored, retrieved, and presented to other health care providers? How easy is it for you to find information in the EHR system that you need to use to make clinical decisions?

Clinical decision support systems (CDSSs) are interactive functions of the EHR system designed to assist health care providers with decision-making tasks by mimicking the inductive or deductive reasoning of a human expert. The basic components of a CDSS include a knowledge base and an *inferencing mechanism* (usually a set of rules derived from the experts and evidence-informed practice). The knowledge base contains the knowledge that an expert nurse would apply to data entered about a patient and information to solve a problem. The inference engine controls the application of the knowledge by providing the logic and rules for its use with data from a specific patient.

Exercise 13.6 illustrates the use of an expert system for determining the maximum dose of pain medication that can safely be given to a patient after an invasive procedure. The knowledge base contains eight items that are to be considered when giving the maximum dose. The inference engine controls the use of the knowledge base by applying logic that an expert nurse would use in making the decision to give the maximum dose. This decision frame states that if pain is severe (A) or a painful procedure is planned (B), and there is an order for pain medication (C), and the time since surgery is less than 48 hours (H), and the time since the last dose is greater than 3 hours (G), and there are no contraindications to the medication (D) or history of allergy (E) or contraindication to the maximum dose (F), then the "decision" would be to give the dose of pain medication. The rules are those that expert nurses would apply in making the decision to give pain medication.

> **EXERCISE 13.6** Mr. Chugh's heart rate is 54 beats per minute. Colin is about to give Mr. Chugh his scheduled atenolol (Tenormin) dose. When Colin scans Mr. Chugh's armband and the medication barcodes, the computer warns them that atenolol should not be given to a patient with a heart rate less than 60 beats per minute. What should Colin do?

One of the advantages of CDSSs is that they permit the novice nurse to benefit from the decision-making expertise and judgement of experts. Nurse leaders must be aware of the usefulness of decision support systems for nursing and that the development of CDSSs applicable to nursing practices is just beginning. Clinical experts are needed to develop both the knowledge in the database and the logic used to develop the rules for its application to a particular patient in a particular circumstance. Advanced critical-thinking skills are needed to develop logic and rules. When these are in place, patient-care quality can be standardized and improved.

HARDWARE AND DEVICES FOR ELECTRONIC HEALTH RECORDS SYSTEMS

Placing the power of computers for both entering and retrieving data at the point of patient care is a major thrust in the move toward increased adoption of EHR systems. Many hospitals and clinics are using a number of computing devices in the clinical setting—desktop, laptop, tablets, and smart phones—as we learn about both the possibilities and limitations of different hardware solutions. Theoretically, nurses may work best with robust mobile technology. Installing computers on mobile carts, also known as *Workstations on Wheels*, or *WOWs*, may create work efficiency and time savings. However, if the cart is cumbersome to move around or if concern about infection risk is associated with moving the cart from one room to another, some organizations favour keeping one cart stationed in each patient-care room. Nurses who work in community and homecare settings may bring a laptop, tablet, or smart phone into a patient's home so that they can access and document information in the presence of a patient. Therefore ensuring that hardware is durable, can be easily cleaned, and has a long battery life is important.

New hardware for patient information systems has advantages and disadvantages. Purchasing a few portable devices, such as tablet computers, may be less expensive than placing a stationary computer in each patient room. In addition, each caregiver on a shift can be equipped with a portable device. Portable devices allow access to information at the point of care, both for retrieval of information and entry of patient data. The disadvantages of handheld technology stem from their size and portability. They have a small display screen, which limits the amount of data that can be viewed on the screen and the size of the font. They can be put down, forgotten, dropped and broken, and are a target for theft. Portable devices must also be stored in a convenient and safe location when they are not in use and have their batteries recharged as needed. Moreover, wireless technology may not always operate with the speed required by busy health care workers in fast-paced environments. For nurses who work in community and homecare environments, especially in rural and remote parts of Canada, there may be challenges with regard to finding wireless Internet or being outside of an area with cell phone coverage.

Management of the hardware designed to host clinical information system software is important. Nurse leaders must make knowledgeable decisions about the type of hardware to use, the education needed to use it effectively, and the proper care and maintenance of the equipment. Important questions to ask include the following: What data and information do we need to gather? When and where should it be gathered? How difficult is the equipment to use? Has the hardware been tested sufficiently to ensure the purchase of a dependable product? Nursing leaders should advocate for direct care nurses to be involved in the selection of the hardware used in their care settings.

Patient Portals

As an extension of a traditional EHR system, **patient portals** are technologies that provide patients with electronic access to all or part of their health record, along with other functions, such as booking appointments or communicating with a health professional (Irizarry et al., 2015). Some patient portals may allow patients to also contribute information to their record through structured questionnaires and other means of providing information electronically. Health professionals may suggest to their patients to complete certain questionnaires before arriving at their appointment so that they have some preliminary information to begin their more focused assessment.

In the United States, the movement to make health professional notes more readily available and accessible to patients through an electronic means began in Boston in the 1990s. The movement is now called OpenNotes (Open Notes, 2018). Over the last several years, the OpenNotes movement has expanded to various parts of the world and to different clinical areas. To date, there are more than 10 organizations in the world that provide mental health patients with access to their health professional notes, with 2 of these organizations being in Canada (Open Notes, 2017). One study of the use of OpenNotes indicated that providing mental patients with access to their health professional notes may support their journey toward recovery (Kipping et al., 2016). Although patients generally like having access to patient portals, a literature review on the efficacy of this technology for improving clinical outcomes and health service utilization has shown that there have been mixed results (Goldzweig et al., 2014). Box 13.1 describes potential benefits of providing patients with access to their clinical record through Open Notes in the patient portal. Box 13.2 provides some suggestions for documenting when patients are able to easily read the clinical record through Open Notes in the patient portal.

EXERCISE 13.7 Consider the last time you document-ed a nursing assessment. How would you feel if the patient you assessed read that documentation? Would they understand this documentation? If not, how might you be able to help them do so? Consider whether the language you used conveyed compassion for the individual. Was the language used patient or provider centric?

BOX 13.2   Potential Benefits of Open Notes in Patient Portals

1 Demonstrating respect and reducing stigma
2 Empowering patients
3 Organizing care and tracking progress
4 Providing a tool for behaviour change
5 Enhancing trust and the therapeutic relationship
6 Make care safer
5 Potential for reducing workload

Open Notes. (2017). Open Notes Mental Health. Retrieved November 8, 2017, from https://www.opennotes.org/tools-resources/for-health-care-providers/mental-health

Telehealth

Telehealth is the use of telecommunications and information technologies for the provision of health care to individuals at a distance and the transmission of information to provide that care (Coach, 2015). Telehealth employs two-way interactive videoconferencing and high-speed telephone lines, fibre optic cables, and satellite transmissions. Patients sitting in front of the teleconferencing camera can be diagnosed, treated, monitored, and educated by nurses and physicians. ECGs and radiographs can be viewed and transmitted. Sophisticated electronic stethoscopes and dermascopes allow nurses and physicians to hear heart, lung, and bowel sounds and to look closely at wounds, eyes, ears, and skin. Ready access to expert advice and patient information is available no matter where the patient or information is located. Patients in rural areas and prisons especially benefit from this technology. In 2010, Canada had 5710 telehealth systems in place in at least 1175 communities, servicing the 21% of the Canadian population who live in rural or remote areas (Praxia Information Intelligence and Gartner Incorporated, 2011). Not only did patients experience significant savings in terms of travel time and costs as a result of these services, but more than 80% reported satisfaction, better capability to manage their care, and measurable improvements in clinical outcomes and hospitalizations. A telepsychiatry project in southern Ontario that delivered mental health crisis interventions to patients at multiple locations in the province yielded positive outcomes, but leadership, team dynamics, and the involvement of front-line staff were critical to the success of the project (Bhandari et al., 2011).

Although not a formal part of telehealth, telecommunication technologies can support distance learning with enhanced opportunities to engage students in online classrooms. In Saskatchewan, nursing students in rural and northern communities are able to attend lectures with nursing professors at campuses in Prince Albert, Saskatoon, and Regina. With online or "virtual" classrooms, students from anywhere in the world with computer access can log into a university's online learning system via the Internet. In providing health education and other health information, the Internet fosters communication, collaboration, resource sharing, and information access.

FUTURE TECHNOLOGY

With the rapid evolution of technology in all areas of society, there is a range of emergent forms of technological innovation that will likely become more present within health care settings in the coming decades. From artificial intelligence (AI), robotics, and the Internet of Things (IoT), the future role of the nurse in relationship with these evolving types of future technologies has yet to be fully conceptualized. In this section, an overview of these evolving types of technologies in health care and their connection to a future nursing role will be examined.

Artificial intelligence is defined as "the ability of a digital computer or computer controlled robot to perform tasks commonly associated with intelligent beings" (Britannica.com, 2018, para 1). Over the last decade, there have been sizable increases in the use of this type of technology in a range of health-related activities. One of the most well-known examples of AI in health care is the use of IBM Watson in oncology care (Doyle-Lindrud, 2015). IBM Watson is a supercomputer that uses AI and cognitive computing capabilities to assist clinicians in making decisions regarding oncology diagnoses and treatment. IBM Watson's ability to understand natural language and analyze unstructured data provides the system with the ability to generate hypotheses related to specific oncology care–related questions posed by clinicians. IBM Watson is also able to draw from published literature and other large data repositories of genetic data to further refine these hypotheses for clinician inspection to support decision making. Although the capabilities of IBM Watson are still evolving, the development of clinical decision support tools featuring AI is a growing area in health care that will likely expand significantly in the future. Another area of technology development that has been highly dependent on AI is that of robotics.

Robotic technology, which has seen increasing use in many areas of society, also brings a range of promising functionalities and capabilities to health care. For instance, the use of robotics in surgery has become a well-established area of practice over the last decade (Estes et al., 2017). Similarly, other aspects of health care have also begun to witness the use of autonomous or semi-autonomous types of robots. For instance, AI personal service robots, social robots, and other types of personal assistive robots have begun to find uses within a range of home, community, and institutional health care settings (Bemelmans et al., 2012; Moyle et al., 2018). One of the most developed social robots currently in existence is the *Pepper robot*, which has begun to see use in a variety of social and health care settings over the last few years (Aaltonen et al., 2017; Niemelä et al., 2017). Pepper is a humanoid robot that speaks a variety of languages and can verbally socialize with people (Purvis, 2017). Although still in development and testing, the potential of robotic technology to support health care practices, tasks, and other psychosocial elements of nursing care are all emergent areas of development that will likely continue to grow in the coming decades (Booth, 2016).

Internet and mobile technology will also likely continue to grow in power and capability, especially within health care settings. Although use of the Internet is well established in most modern Western health care settings, a range of newer types of processes and relationships with this form of technology will continue to evolve in the future. The *Internet of Things* (IoT) is used to describe a network of both physical and digital devices that are interlinked and can communicate with each other. To date, a range of IoT devices currently exists, including smart home devices (e.g., smart

thermostats, robot vacuum cleaners) and, increasingly, various types of wearable devices (e.g., Fitbits, smart watches). Because IoT generates a seamless functionality between a range of physical and digital devices (i.e., a Google Home can be used to command a smart home thermometer or activate an online music player), a wide variety of health care applications, such as remote monitoring, assistive device use, and personalized medicine processes, can be made possible. Although the use of IoT technology has significant potential within health care, there are also many ethical and privacy implications of this type of connectivity between devices that have yet to be fully explored or researched (Kim, 2014).

EXERCISE 13.8 Think about the kinds of technology that you use in your everyday life but have not used in a clinical setting. Consider also technologies that you have heard about but have not had a chance to use. Are there any applications of these technologies to health settings and for nurses? What benefit might there be to patients and health professionals if these technologies were used in health settings? What drawbacks are there from using this technology?

IMPACT OF TECHNOLOGY ON CLINICAL CARE

Technology use in clinical care settings has led to improvements in care quality and the safety of care delivery. For example, patient information in an electronic clinical information system is organized and legible. Nurses may be able to see all of the medications prescribed for a patient in one location; doses are written clearly, and medication names are spelled correctly. The patient problem list shows acute and chronic health conditions and complete allergy information. Abnormal findings are highlighted or identified in some way and can be graphed and compared with interventions. Alerts signal nurses that critical information has been entered in the electronic record. For example, critical test results signal the need for provider notification and intervention. An alert that a patient is at risk for falling signals the need for additional monitoring and interventions to ensure safety.

When standards for care are not being followed, some EHR systems can generate alerts, reminders, or suggestions. Rules remind health care providers to perform required care. When documentation is not recorded for medication administration—IV tubing change, or wound care, for example—the system might generate a reminder based on rules that have been agreed to by providers. Evidence-informed practices are integrated in the process of care as providers are guided to select the most appropriate course of action. Nurses need to remember to use their critical-thinking skills when assessing the alerts and suggestions generated via technology.

Errors are avoided by eliminating the problem of illegible handwriting. Computerized order entry also eliminates the nursing time required for clarification of illegible and incomplete orders. Transcription is no longer required, orders are sent directly to the performing department, and patient-care needs are communicated more clearly and quickly to all clinicians. Computerized decision-making support has been shown to significantly reduce the rate of initiation of inappropriate prescriptions involving drug–disease contraindications, drug–age contraindications, excessive duration of therapy, and therapeutic duplication prescriptions (Tamblyn et al., 2003).

Nurses spend much time documenting patient-care activities. Clinical documentation in an EHR system improves access to patient information and increases documentation efficiency and organization (Canada Health Infoway, 2005). This should allow nurses to spend more time in direct patient care, but no clear link has been made between electronic nursing documentation systems and the resulting time spent in direct patient-care activities (Detwiller, 2006). In a study in which electronic documentation was introduced in a small rural hospital, 75% of respondents agreed that nurses have less time to give hands-on care with the use of the electronic system (Detwiller, 2006). Detwiller (2006) noted that many variables can affect time, including the design of the system, policies and procedures, and the experience of the staff. In a critical care unit setting, automatic downloads of patient vital signs, ventilator settings, and IV intakes remove the need to record these items by hand and provide time savings for nurses. An integrated EHR system eliminates the need to collect certain patient information (such as chronic conditions, allergies, or previous medical history) more than once because it is readily accessible in the system. As a result, nursing time is not spent searching for this information or asking the patient the same questions multiple times.

A Canadian study reported that 7.5% of patients who were admitted to hospital experienced one or more adverse events, with medications and injectable solutions found to be the second most common causes of adverse events (Baker et al., 2004). Technologies that are used to automate medication dispensing and administration may decrease this source of error, improve quality of care, and reduce associated costs. These technologies include automated medication-dispensing devices, barcode medication administration, and electronic medication administration records (Strudwick et al., 2018).

Automated medication administration systems can ensure that the right patient gets the right medication, in the correct dose, by the appropriate route, and at the specified time. These systems may even support the reduction of medication theft in some settings. However, it is imperative that this new information technology does not impede nurses' care of patients. Wulff et al. (2011) conducted a mixed-methods systematic review of research evidence evaluating relationships between medication administration technologies (MATs) use and incidence of medication administration incidents (MAIs) and preventable adverse drug events (ADEs). They concluded from their review of 12 studies, including one from Canada, that findings were generally positive about MATs and MAIs on patient safety but noted that the level of evidence overall was equivocal. A concern raised in the review was the development of problematic workarounds when introducing MATs that could compromise patient safety (Koppel et al., 2008). Workarounds are ways of completing tasks in unintended ways, or ways other than those officially designed. During the introduction of an automatic medication-dispensing system in a larger Canadian tertiary care centre, workarounds emerged to fill the gap between prescribed and actual work practices, activities, and processes (Balka et al., 2007). Workarounds develop when new technologies hinder workflow (Perras et al., 2009). Further, the technologies carry the potential for introducing different types of medication errors, such as completing tasks with minimal reflection and less checking because of overreliance on a machine.

Closed-loop electronic prescribing, dispensing, and barcode patient identification systems reduce prescribing errors and adverse drug events and increase confirmation of patient identity before administration. A clinical and economic impact study of technologies for medication dispensing and administration in Canadian hospitals found inconsistent results in the time spent on medication-related tasks by pharmacists and nurses (Perras et al., 2009).

The introduction of technology has the potential to increase nurses' productivity. MacDonald (2008) describes technology as a way to support knowing the patient; professional development in state-of-the-art technology can save time that nurses consistently report as a barrier to knowing the patient. Home health care nurses who perceived the usefulness of wireless PDAs incorporated for 1 month in their daily activities were more likely to adopt the technology (Zhang et al., 2010).

Although there are many benefits to implementing technology, including EHR systems in clinical practice, there have been some documented unintended consequences (Gephart et al., 2015). Challenges related to fitting the technology into nursing workflow may result in the use of workarounds (Koppel et al., 2008). Current EHR systems are often challenging to navigate, which may provide a risk of nurses missing important pieces of clinical information to inform their decision making (Strudwick et al., 2018). These factors may influence nurses' acceptance of the technology and, if not properly addressed, could lead to resistance. Ensuring that nurses are engaged in the selection of technology, as well as implementation and evaluation activities, may support the mitigation of these challenges.

BOX 13.3 Documentation Considerations When Using Open Notes in Patient Portals

1 Invite patients to read their notes.
2 Promote transparency to patients and their family members by discussing what they have read in their notes with them.
3 Avoid or define medical jargon.
4 Use plain language.
5 Engage patients in the documentation.
6 Develop options if a patient's access to notes may carry more risks than benefit.
7 Discuss the diagnosis.
8 Create a plan if your patients are unsure about what they are reading, or if they become upset reading their notes.

Open Notes. (2017). Open Notes Mental Health. Retrieved November 8, 2017, from https://www.opennotes.org/tools-resources/for-health-care-providers/mental-health

---

TECHNOLOGY, THERAPEUTIC COMMUNICATION, AND COMPASSIONATE CARE

A cornerstone of providing compassionate nursing care in any care setting is therapeutic communication between the nurse and patient. As described in previous sections of this chapter, health care settings where nurses work have become permeated with technology in recent years. Nurses now use computers, smart phones, tablets, and a number of other electronic devices when interacting with patients. Outside of health care settings, there have been concerns regarding how these various forms of technologies influence communication during face-to-face interactions; however, there has been less discussion within the nursing profession with regard to how these technologies may influence therapeutic communication, and thus how these technologies can be most effectively used in the clinical encounter to deliver compassionate care. To date, there have been articles written on this topic with physician populations (Duffy et al., 2016; Lanier et al., 2017; Mickan et al., 2014; Street et al., 2017). This section provides an overview of a few of these papers, and their potential implications for nurses.

In a study by Street and colleagues, physicians were observed interacting with patients while also using an electronic health record (Street et al., 2017). Patients became less participative when their physicians were typing more during the interaction. Similarly, when physicians were looking at the computer more often, there was more silence during the interaction. These findings suggest that nurses should be mindful of how much typing they are doing and where they are looking during the encounter. Nurses need to demonstrate that they are engaged in the conversation with the patient, and that the electronic health record is used as a tool to support care.

A study by Fleischmann and colleagues was conducted to determine if the introduction of tablets during ward rounds would decrease the amount of time physicians spent completing necessary tasks required of the medical record, in comparison to a computer-based record system (Fleischmann et al., 2015). Findings suggested that the tablet better supported this particular workflow of the physician, and thus allowed physicians to spend more time at the bedside with patients and less time completing tasks associated with the medical record. Although tablets may be a viable option for some nurses, an analysis of whether a tablet could feasibly be used and incorporated into nursing workflow would be required. As nurses value spending time with their patients, identifying ways that technology can be leveraged to support providing additional time, would be of value.

A paper written by Voran describes ways that physicians can effectively use technology during patient interactions (Voran, 2017). Suggestions from this paper applicable to nurses include: (1) pointing to the screen and showing patients what you are typing; (2) actively looking at the patient and not the technology; (3) beginning the interaction by talking to the patient and then bringing in the technology; and (4) telling patients why you are using the technology.

In summary, technology use within nursing practice has brought about many improvements to care; however, careful attention must be paid to how nurses use the technology during clinical encounters with patients to ensure that therapeutic communication is maintained. Box 13.4 provides an overview of some strategies that can be used when incorporating technology into the clinical encounter.

> **BOX 13.4 Strategies for Incorporating Technology Into the Clinical Encounter**
>
> 1 Explain to the patient what you are using the technology to accomplish. It can be helpful for a patient to know what value the technology brings, and why it is beneficial to be used in the particular context.
> 2 Position the technology in a way that the patient can see what you are doing. If using a computer screen, do not position it between you and the patient. Feel free to point to the screen and show the patient what you are doing.
> 3 Pay attention to the patient. Focus on the patient. Try to focus on the technology secondary to focusing on the patient.
> 4 If the patient looks uncomfortable with your use of technology, ask them about it. If you are using a technology that can be used after the interaction is over, e.g., EHR system, consider waiting until the person has left to initiate use.

Strudwick, G., & Xie, L. (2018). Incorporating technology meaningfully into the clinical encounter: A nursing perspective. *Nursing Informatics Bulletin*, 11(7), 9.

IMPLEMENTING TECHNOLOGY IN CLINICAL SETTINGS

Considerable thought and work is put into the implementation of technologies in clinical settings. Many people are usually involved in this work, ranging from those in finance, procurement, housekeeping, operations, leadership and information technology to infection control, patient safety and quality, health professional groups, nurses, and nursing leadership. Selection of an EHR system may be one of the most important decisions of a chief nursing officer and the nursing leadership team (Hannah, 2005). Nursing leaders play an extremely important role in EHR (and other technology) decision making within Canada. However, nursing leaders need to have the appropriate level of informatics competencies to be able to effectively do so (Kennedy & Moen, 2017). Whereas nursing informatics competencies of relevance to nurse leaders have been identified in the United States, work is currently being completed to identify those of relevance to Canadian nursing leaders (Kassam et al., 2017).

Making a decision on an EHR system may require that leaders take their direction from direct care health professionals that will ultimately ensure the success and sustainability of the technology. Nurse leaders and direct care nurses must be members of the selection team, participate actively, and have a voice in the selection decision. Remember, nurses are knowledge workers who require data, information, and knowledge to deliver effective patient care. The EHR system must make sense to the people who use it and fit effectively with the processes for providing patient care. The involvement of a team of professionals in care provision should advocate that the EHR system has the capacity for interprofessional care planning. It may be useful to make site visits at organizations already using the software being considered for selection. Discussions at site visits include both the utility and performance of the software and the customer service and responsiveness of the vendor.

Successful development and implementation of nursing information technology depends on nurses working in partnership with organizational leadership, information systems vendors, and systems analysts to create tools that truly benefit nurses. Patient safety and care may be affected when nurses are not involved in decisions related to the development and implementation of new technology or fail to receive adequate pre-implementation professional development. The technologically savvy nurse has the potential to contribute know-hows and experiential insights to decisions about technology that earlier generations of nurses may lack. Nurses need to have the systems and tools to provide patient care effectively, efficiently, and safely. Direct care nurses must work with informatics nurses and information system developers and programmers in systems development, implementation, and ongoing improvement. Nurses should be key partners in every phase of the clinical information life cycle (Benham-Hutchins, 2009). By combining computer and information science with nursing science, the goals of supporting nursing practice and the delivery of high-quality nursing care can be achieved (Delaney, 2007).

Once a system is selected, the successful implementation of an EHR system is related to a combination of individual, group, and organizational factors (Nagle & Catford, 2008). If any one of the people, processes, or technology is not adequately addressed, an EHR system implementation has a high risk of failure. Leadership, engagement, communication, process redesign, and support must be considered in the acquisition and implementation of information systems.

The Literature Perspective identifies areas of success and lack of success in Canada's implementation of electronic health information technology (HIT).

PATIENT SAFETY AND TECHNOLOGY

The patient-care environment is complex and associated with adverse events (Baker et al., 2004). Approximately 8% of patients admitted to Canadian acute care hospitals were found to experience one or more adverse events. Of these patients, 36.9% were judged to have highly preventable adverse events (Baker et al., 2004). As the largest health care provider group, nurses understand the risks to patient safety and are in a position to implement preventive measures (Nicklin & McVeety, 2002). In addition to physical challenges, resource challenges, and interruptions characteristic of nursing work, nurses are challenged by inconsistencies and breakdowns in care communication. Communication and information difficulties are among the most common nursing workplace challenges and are frustrating and potentially dangerous for patients. Mistakes in the nurse–patient process, a failure to know the patient, and a lack of patient involvement in decision making threaten patient safety (Bournes & Flint, 2003; MacDonald, 2008; O'Hagan et al., 2009). For example, O'Hagan et al. (2009) found twice as many self-reported medical errors

---

LITERATURE PERSPECTIVE

Resource: Rozenblum, R., Jang, Y., Zimlichman, E., et al., (2011). A qualitative study of Canada's experience with the implementation of electronic health information technology. *Canadian Medical Association Journal*, 183(5): E281–E288.

Although many Canadian provinces have made some progress toward the implementation of information technologies, and Canada Health Infoway has invested almost $1.6 billion in e-health initiatives over the past decade, Canada has lagged behind other Western countries in its uptake of EHRs. To address this situation, Canadian researchers conducted a case study to assess areas of achievement/success and lack of success/effectiveness in adoption of EHRs. The study involved a review of Canada Health Infoway documents and the completion of interviews with national and provincial stakeholder groups. Successful aspects of the e-strategy included its com-

prehensive national approach to the standards for health information technology, which allowed for interoperability across jurisdictions and a framework for collaboration and idea sharing; successful lobbying for health information technology, and the acquisition of political and financial support; and successful health information technology applications, namely digital imaging technology and provincial patient registries. Less successful aspects included the absence of an e-health policy that would foster effective adoption strategies by clinicians; a lack of meaningful engagement of clinicians; a lack of alignment of the e-health plan with needs of clinicians; a lack of flexibility in incorporating change; and a focus on national rather than regional interoperability. Thus, this article suggests that health organizations must work together to achieve appropriate e-health technologies across the country, and ensure that strategies to engage clinicians in the process are used.

among Canadian adults who perceived lack of involvement in decision making about their care compared with those who perceived involvement. Followers have the opportunity to upwardly influence a culture of safety by actively advocating for listening to and knowing patients and involving patients in decisions about their own care.

Information technology is an essential tool for advancing patient safety (Canada Health Infoway, 2005). Nurses rely increasingly on information technology to improve patient safety by reducing medical errors, enhancing clinical decision making, and promoting patient-centric care. In a national Canadian study of nurses and senior nurse managers across health care delivery sectors, researchers studied the factors that affected nurses' adoption of technologies and their perceptions of confidence and efficiency in using technologies (Wang et al., 2004). Technologies were grouped into the following categories: communication tools, information systems, diagnostic devices, and therapeutic devices. Researchers found that nurses in direct care used communication tools and information systems less than nondirect care nurses, and older nurses were less confident in the use of these tools and systems. Confidence in using technology was associated with the adequacy of professional development, regardless of age, education level, or area of practice. EHR systems and automated medication-dispensing systems were perceived as efficient or useful by about 60% of practical nurses and registered nurses and less than half of psychiatric nurses (Wang et al., 2004).

A critical use of information has been in the area of the medication management process. This process involves high-risk and high-volume activities (Saginur et al., 2008). Although new applications have been developed to provide support for all aspects of the process, uptake of the various technologies has been shown to vary significantly (Saginur et al., 2008). Saginur et al. (2008) conducted a cross-sectional survey of the uptake of medication safety technologies by 100 of Canada's largest acute-care hospitals. The survey studied the major technologies from a Canadian Agency for Drugs and Technology in Health (CADTH) systematic review. The most commonly used technologies were clinical pharmacy services (97%), followed in descending order by pharmacy-based intravenous admixture services (81%), computerized decision support modules for pharmacy order entry systems (77%), unit-dose medication distribution systems (75%), computerized medication administration records (MARs) (67%), and automated dispensing (56%). Computerized physician order entry (CPOE), computerized decision support systems (CDSS) for CPOE, and barcoding for medication dispensing and medication administration were used in less than 10% of hospitals. Although hospitals used fewer of the technologies with less evidence of effectiveness, these technologies were high priorities for uptake.

TECHNOLOGY AND INFORMATICS IN NURSING EDUCATION

The informatics educational needs of nursing students and faculty across Canada have been a priority for CNIA for almost two decades, beginning with a national study of informatics opportunities, preparedness, and information and communications technology (ICT) infrastructure and support (Canadian Nursing Informatics Association, 2003). For the past two decades, Canadian nursing informatics leaders have been envisioning a nationwide nursing informatics strategy, which culminated in an e-nursing strategy commissioned by CNA (2006). The CNA's (2006) e-nursing strategy identified the need for integrating technology competencies into undergraduate, graduate, and continuing nursing education as one of its top goals. In May 2011, the Canadian Association of Schools of Nursing (CASN) announced a three-year funded initiative in partnership with Canada Health Infoway to integrate technology into the curriculum of 91 nursing degree-granting colleges and universities across Canada. This work resulted in the identification of entry-to-practice nursing informatics competencies that are in the process of being integrated into undergraduate nursing education programs (Canadian Association of Schools of Nursing, 2012). Some schools of nursing have chosen to implement a stand-alone nursing informatics course, whereas other schools have decided to integrate nursing informatics education into the various other courses already being taught. Additionally, some schools have decided to incorporate technologies such as electronic medication administration records into both theoretical aspects of content delivery, as well as in more practical ways, such as simulation (Booth et al., 2017). One of the challenges of delivering nursing informatics education at the entry-to-practice level is the comfort and knowledge of nursing faculty. There are currently several initiatives targeted at better understanding and improving the capacity of nursing educators to be able to deliver this necessary informatics education.

NURSE LEADERS AND NURSING INFORMATICS

Despite the fundamental value and impact of informatics in advancing evidence-informed, patient-centred health care, many Canadian nurse leaders do not have the requisite informatics knowledge and skill to be able to adequately advocate for nurses with regard to this topic (Remus & Kennedy, 2012). Nurse executives need to supplement traditional roles with nursing informatics competencies if they are to provide leadership that transforms health care (Kennedy & Moen, 2017). Nurse leaders must be aware of how technologies fit into the delivery of patient care and the strategic plan of the organization in which they work. They must have a vision for the future and be ready to suggest solutions that will assist nurses across specialties and settings to improve patient-care safety and quality. Informatics competencies for nurse leaders have been identified in the United States (Yen et al., 2017), and work is currently underway to identify these competencies of relevance in the Canadian setting (Kassam et al., 2017). Once this work is completed, it is hoped that efforts to support the development of these competencies among both current and future nursing leaders can be identified and worked toward.

Although nurses in formal nursing roles play a critical role in advancing the use of technology in clinical practice settings, every nurse can embrace technology to improve nursing practice. Some strategies to accomplish this objective include the following:

1. Having clinicians partner with their information technology staff so that they drive EHR system initiatives.
2. Involving nurses in decisions about the process, design, and workflow in system integration initiatives.
3. Investing in EHR system professional development for nurses.
4. Leveraging opportunities to use information technology to enable quality improvement (Nagle & Catford, 2008).

Nurses at all levels should advocate for patients and family members to be engaged in the selection, implementation, use, and evaluation of technologies that are used with or for them (Strudwick & Strauss, 2017). Patients and family can be engaged through committees, advisory councils, and by interviewing them about their perceptions and ideas about a particular technology.

PROFESSIONAL, ETHICAL NURSING PRACTICE AND NEW TECHNOLOGIES

Technology has and will continue to transform the health care environment and the practice of nursing. Nurses are professionally obligated to maintain competency with a vast array of technological devices and systems. Baseline informatics competencies are required for all nurses to function in the 21 century.

Because of the increasing ability to preserve human life with technology, questions about living and dying have become conceptually and ethically complex. Conceptually, it becomes more difficult to define extraordinary treatment and human life because technology has changed our concepts of living and dying. A source of ethical dilemmas is the use of invasive technological treatment to treat patients with extraordinary means and to prolong life for patients with limited or no decision-making capabilities. Nurses are concerned with individual patient welfare and the effects of technological intervention on the immediate and long-term quality of life for patients and their families. Patient advocacy remains an important function of the professional nurse.

Safeguarding patients' welfare, privacy, and confidentiality is another obligation of nurses. Security measures are available with computerized information systems, but it is the integrity and ethical principles of system end users that provide the final safeguard for patient privacy. System users must never share the passwords that allow them access to information in computerized clinical information systems. Each password uniquely identifies a user to the system by name and title, gives approval to carry out certain functions, and provides access to data appropriate to the user. When a nurse signs on to a computer, all data and information that are entered or reviewed can be traced to that password. Every nurse is accountable for all actions taken using their password. All nurses must be aware of their responsibilities for the confidentiality and security of the data they gather and for the security of their passwords. Nurses should be aware of the privacy legislation that applies to them and their work setting.

Nurse leaders must promote ethical practice in the use of technology. One way is to make use of an ethics committee in their institutions and to assign knowledgeable nurses to serve on these committees. Nurse managers must ensure that policies and procedures for collecting and entering data and the use of security measures (e.g., passwords) are established to maintain the confidentiality of patient data and information. Nurse managers must also be knowledgeable patient advocates in the use of technology for patient care by referring ethical questions to the organization's ethics committee.

Nursing Data Standards

Data from within and across patient populations are needed to build evidence from practice and to use evidence in practice. These data are also needed to quantify and describe nursing practice and its impact on the quality of care provided and on patient outcomes. Collecting a set of basic data from every patient at every health care encounter through an EHR system makes sense because comparisons can be made among many patients, institutions, or countries, in almost any combination imaginable, as well as for individual patients and patient groups across time. However, to do so, nurses need to collect this basic set of data from all patients during these encounters using a consistent way of defining each data element. This information should be collected through electronic systems and should not add a documentation burden to nurses. Thus a set of nursing data standards to identify what data elements comprise the basic data set, and what standardized terminology to use, is required.

In the 1980s, Canadian nursing leaders became concerned about the absence of nursing information available in national databases, such as the Canadian Institute for Health Information's (CIHI) management information system (MIS) and Discharge Abstract Database (DAD), seemingly making invisible nursing's contribution to patient, organizational, and system outcomes (Doran et al., 2011; Kleibet et al., 2011). To address this information gap, the CNA convened the first nursing minimum data set (NMDS) conference in the early 1990s to promote the entry, accessibility, and retrievability of nursing data (Canadian Nurses Association, 2000; Haines, 1993).

More recently, there has been a reinvigoration of this work by nursing informaticians Dr. Lynn Nagle and Peggy White through a national approach culminating each year in a National Nursing Data Symposium (NNDS) (Nagle & White, 2016). Through the NNDS working groups made up of nurses in the domains of clinical practice, clinical administration, policy, research, and education, work is being led across the country to advance nursing data standards. The Canadian Nurses Association and the Canadian Nursing Informatics Association recently published a joint position statement advocating for the use of the Systematized Nomenclature of Medicine-Clinical Terms (SNOMED-CT), and the International Classification of Nursing Practice (ICNP), to represent nursing documentation in Canada (Canadian Nurses Association, 2017). Additionally, this joint position statement identified the Canadian Health Outcomes for Better Information and Care (C-HOBIC) and the Logical Observation Identifiers Names and Codes (LOINC) Nursing Physiologic Assessment Panel as the possible minimum data sets (Canadian Nurses Association, 2017). As organizations go forward in their implementation of EHR systems, it will be imperative that forms and screens be developed that provide nurses with the ability to document on the minimum data set elements through the documentation that they would complete on their patients, as well as using the terminology of SNOMED CT and ICNP. Nursing leaders play a critical role in advocating for this during the selection and implementation of EHR systems.

CONCLUSION

Technology is and will continue to become increasingly connected in the future, linking people and information together in the rapidly changing world of health care. With new technology comes the need for a new set of competencies. By participating in designing this exciting future, nurses will ensure that their unique contributions to patient and family health and illness care are clearly and formally represented.

? A SOLUTION

The leadership in Dana's organization understands that technology by itself does not improve quality and safety; a project that introduces technology must also consider the people and processes impacted. The new **electronic health records** system must support clinical processes, and nurses are integral to ensuring this outcome. Without nurses' involvement, the new system would not be aligned with patient-care processes, would not deliver the anticipated benefits, and would not be successful.

To ensure nurses are involved in the decision-making process, Dana requested that a nurse specialist from the hospital be brought onto the project full time. This nurse engaged clinicians through all the stages of the project. Initially, nursing staff created a storyboard that outlined their perspective on how a clinical information system could support their practice to deliver safe, quality care. Nursing staff were involved in reviewing and providing feedback for the system build, device selection, process and workflow redesign impacted by the system, and professional development and implementation.

Dana requested that nursing staff trial the hardware and recommended the type, number, and location of the devices required to support an efficient workflow. As nurses used the clinical information system to plan and document care, as well as administer medications, they noted that a variety of devices and carts were required. Nursing staff provided ongoing feedback for improvements to the software and hardware.

THE EVIDENCE

The field of nursing informatics and the body of research on the topic of technology use among nurses is constantly growing and evolving. The pace of technology development and rapid entry of everyday technologies to consumer markets makes it difficult for researchers to keep up with the ever-changing landscape. Fortunately, nurses in both leadership and clinical practice roles can obtain the necessary knowledge and skills related to informatics and the principles of technology use that can be applied both now and in the future. Thus, knowledge and skills learned today won't become obsolete as advanced technologies enter the field. Nurses can ensure that they are prepared to work with new technologies and can support the facilitation of new technologies into clinical practice settings. To do this, however, we need nurse researchers with a focus on nursing informatics and technology use among this profession. The evidence for using technology to support nurses in being able to provide better patient care and make more informed clinical decisions will need to continue to grow as we work with new technologies and learn to work with technology differently.

✳ NEED TO KNOW NOW

- Nurses need to be engaged in decision making regarding the selection, implementation, use, and evaluation of new technology in any clinical care setting.
- Nursing documentation should be captured in a standardized way in any electronic health record systems as per the position statement from the Canadian Nurses Association and the Canadian Nursing Informatics Association.
- Nurse leaders need to have the appropriate type and level of informatics competencies to be effective in their roles.
- Nurses need to understand how they can effectively use technology as a tool to support their work as a nurse.

CHAPTER CHECKLIST

Nurses are the key personnel in the health care system to mediate the interaction between science, technology, and the patient because of their unique holistic viewpoint and the 24/7 role of vigilant health care providers who preserve the patients' humanity and optimal functioning and promote health. The challenge for the profession is to continue to provide patient-centred care in a technological society that strives for efficiency and cost effectiveness. Nurse administrators, managers, and staff must provide leadership in managing information and technology to meet the challenge.

- Nurses will continue to encounter new health information technologies in their work environments regardless of the clinical context in which they practice.
- Nursing informatics is the convergence of nursing science, computer science, and information science.
- Nurses in all areas of practice should have the appropriate informatics competencies to perform their roles.
- A variety of health information technologies is available in clinical practice environments where nurses work, including medical devices, monitoring devices, EHR systems and patient portals, and telehealth.
- In the future, numerous new technologies will be incorporated into nursing clinical care and environments where nurses work.
- Nurses need to consider the influence of the use of technologies on the care they deliver.
- Technology should be thoughtfully incorporated into clinical encounters to not jeopardize the delivery of compassionate care.

- Nurses should be aware of strategies to support the implementation and adoption of technology in clinical settings where they work.
- Nurses should have a basic understanding of the nursing standards and terminologies used in Canada, and their importance to nurses and the nursing profession.
- Consideration should be given to the ways that technology can be applied to patient safety and delivery of evidenced-based care.
- Nurses should learn about the use of technology during their entry-to-practice education.
- Nursing leaders should have the appropriate informatics knowledge and skill to advocate for the appropriate selection, adoption, and use of technologies in practice.
- Nurses should identify ways to engage consumers and patients in health information technology selection, adoption, and use.

Visit the Evolve website for Suggested Readings, Internet Resources, and additional resources related to the content in this chapter: http://evolve.elsevier.com/Canada/Yoder-Wise/leading/.

REFERENCES

Aaltonen, I., Arvola, A., Heikkilä, P., & Lammi, H. (2017). Hello Pepper, May I Tickle You? In *Proceedings of the companion of the 2017 ACM/IEEE international conference on human-robot interaction—HRI '17* (pp. 53–54). New York, NY: ACM Press.

Accreditation Canada. (2017). *Accreditation Canada*. Retrieved from: https://accreditation.ca/standards.

American Nurses Association. (2008). *Nursing informatics: Scope and standards of practice.* Silver Spring, MD: Nursesbooks.org.

Auditor General of Canada. (2010). *Electronic health records in Canada—an overview of federal and provincial audit reports.* Retrieved from: http://www.oag-bvg.gc.ca/internet/English/parl_oag_201004_07_e_33720.html.

Baker, G. R., Norton, P. G., Flintoff, V., et al. (2004). The Canadian Adverse Events Study: The incidence of adverse events among hospital patients in Canada. *Canadian Medical Association Journal, 170*(11), 1678–1686.

Balka, E., Kahnamoui, N., & Nutland, K. (2007). *Who is in charge of patient safety? Work practice, work processes, and utopian views of automatic drug dispensing systems.* https://doi.org/10.1016/j.ijmedinf.2006.05.038.

Bemelmans, R., Gelderblom, G. J., Jonker, P., & de Witte, L. (2012). Socially assistive robots in elderly care: a systematic review into effects and effectiveness. *Journal of the American Medical Directors Association, 13*(2), 114–120. e1.

Benham-Hutchins, M. (2009). Frustrated with HIT? Get involved! *Nursing Management, 40*(1), 17–19.

Bhandari, G., Tiessen, B., & Snowdon, A. (2011). Meeting community needs through leadership and innovation: A case of virtual psychiatric emergency department. *Behaviour & Information Technology, 30*(4), 517–523.

Billinghurst, F., Morgan, B., & Arthur, H. M. (2003). Patient and nurse-related implications of remote cardiac telemetry. *Clinical Nursing Research, 12*(4), 356–370.

Booth, R. G. (2016). Informatics and nursing in a post-nursing informatics world: future directions for nurses in an automated, artificially intelligent, social-networked healthcare environment. *Canadian Journal of Nursing Leadership, 28*(4), 61–69.

Booth, R. G., Sinclair, B., Strudwick, G., Brennan, L., Morgan, L., Collings, S., et al. (2017). Deconstructing clinical workflow: Identifying teaching-learning principles for barcode electronic medication administration with nursing students. *Nurse Educator, 42*(5), 267–271.

Bournes, D. A., & Flint, F. (2003). Mis-takes: Mistakes in the nurse-person process. *Nursing Science Quarterly, 16*(2), 127–130.

Britannica. (2018). *Artificial Intelligence.*

Canada Health Infoway. (2005). Pan-Canadian electronic health record: Quantitative and qualitative benefits. Retrieved from: https://www2.infoway-inforoute.ca/Admin/Upload/Dev/Document/VOL1_CHI%20Quantitative%20&%20Qualitative%20Benefits.pdf.

Canadian Association of Schools of Nursing. (2012). Nursing Informatics Entry-to-Practice Competencies for Registered Nurses. *CASN*, 1–15.

Canadian Association of Schools of Nursing. (2011, May 19). *Re: Education of next generation of nurses to include effective clinical use of information and communication technologies [web log message].* Retrieved from: http://www.casn.ca/en/Whats_new_at_CASN_108/items/104.html.

Canadian Nurses Association. (2017). *Nursing informatics. Joint position statement,* 1–7. Retrieved from: https://www.cna-aiic.ca/en/~/media/cna/page-content/pdf-fr/nursing-informatics-joint-position-statement.

Canadian Nursing Informatics Association. (2012). *History.* Retrieved from: https://cnia.ca/history/.

Canadian Nurses Association. (2001). What is nursing informatics and why is it so important? *Nursing Now: Issues and Trends in Canadian Nursing, 11,* 1–4.

Canadian Nurses Association. (2000). *Collecting data to reflect nursing impact: A discussion paper.* Ottawa, ON: Author. Retrieved from: http://www.cna-aiic.ca/CNA/documents/pdf/publications/collct_data_e.pdf.

Canadian Nurses Association. (2006). *E-Nursing strategy for Canada.* Ottawa, ON: Author.

Canadian Nursing Informatics Association. (2003). *Assessing the informatics education needs of Canadian nurses educational institution component: Educating tomorrow's nurses where's nursing informatics?* http://www.cnia.ca/documents/OHIHfinal.pdf.

Chang, F., & Gupta, N. (2015). Progress in electronic medical record adoption in Canada. *Canadian Family Physician, 61*(12), 1076–1084.

Charles, K., Cannon, M., Hall, R., & Coustasse, A. (2014). Can utilizing a computerized provider order entry (CPOE) system prevent hospital medical errors and adverse drug events? *Perspectives in Health Information Management, 11,* 1b (fall).

Coach: Canada's Health Informatics Association. (2015). *Canadian telehealth report.* Toronto, ON: Author, 2015.

Delaney, C. (2007). Nursing and informatics for the 21st century. *Creative Nursing, 12*(2), 4–6.

Delbanco, T., Walker, J., Darer, J. D., Elmore, J. G., & Feldman, H. J. (2015). Open notes: Doctors and patients signing on. *Annals of Internal Medicine, 153*(2), 121–126.

Derman, Y. D., Arenovich, T., & Strauss, J. (2010). Speech recognition software and electronic psychiatric progress notes: Physicians' ratings and preferences. *BMC Medical Informatics and Decision Making, 5*(3), 1–7.

Detwiller, M. (2006). *Enhancing the quality of health care delivery through the use of electronic clinical documentation (unpublished master's thesis).* Victoria, BC: Royal Roads University.

Doran, D., Mildon, B., & Clarke, S. (2011). *Toward a National Report card in nursing: A knowledge synthesis.* Toronto, ON: Nursing Health Services Research Unit (Toronto site) and Lawrence S. Bloomberg Faculty of Nursing, University of Toronto.

Doyle-Lindrud, S. (2015). Watson will see you now: A supercomputer to help clinicians make informed treatment decisions. *Clinical Journal of Oncology Nursing, 19*(1), 31–32.

Duffy, F. F., Fochtmann, L. J., Clarke, D. E., Barber, K., Hong, S. H., Yager, J., et al. (2016). Psychiatrists' comfort using computers and other electronic devices in clinical practice. *Psychiatric Quarterly, 87*(3), 571–584.

Englebardt, S. P., & Nelson, R. (2002). *Health care informatics: An interdisciplinary approach.* St. Louis, MO: Mosby.

Estes, S. J., Goldenberg, D., Winder, J. S., Juza, R. M., & Lyn-Sue, J. R. (2017). Best practices for robotic surgery programs. *JSLS: Journal of the Society of Laparoendoscopic Surgeons, 21*(2), e2016 00102.

Fleischmann, R., Duhm, J., Hupperts, H., & Brandt, S. A. (2015). Tablet computers with mobile electronic medical records enhance clinical routine and promote bedside time: a controlled prospective crossover study. *Journal of Neurology, 262*(3), 532–540.

Gephart, S., Carrington, J. M., & Finley, B. (2015). A systematic review of nurses' experiences qith unintended consequences when using the electronic health record. *Nursing Administration Quarterly, 39*(4), 345–356.

Gheorghiu, B., & Hagens, S. (2017). Use and maturity of electronic patient portals. *Studies in Health Technology and Informatics, 234,* 136–141. https://doi.org/10.3233/978-1-61499-742-9-136.

Goldzweig, C., Orshansky, G., Paige, N. M., Towfigh, A. A., Haggstrom, D. A., Miake-Lye, et al. (2014). Electronic patient portals: Evidence on health outcomes, satisfaction, efficiency, and attitudes. *Annals of Internal Medicine, 159*(10), 677–687.

Haines, J. (1993). *Leading in a time of change: The challenge for the nursing profession.* Ottawa, ON: Canadian Nurses Association. A discussion paper Retrieved from: http://trove.nla.gov.au/version/36478507.

Hannah, K. J. (2005). Health informatics and nursing in Canada. *Health Care Information Management and Communications in Canada, 19*(3), 45–51.

Healthcare Information and Management Systems Society. (2014). *Canada EMR adoption model.* Retrieved from: https://app.himssanalytics.org/emram/scoreTrends .aspx.

HealthIT.gov. (2015). *What is a patient portal?* Retrieved from: https://www.healthit.gov/providers-professionals/ faqs/what-patient-portal.

International Medical Informatics Association. (2009). *IMIA-NI definition of nursing informatics updated.* Retrieved from: https://imianews.wordpress.com/2009/08/24/ imia-ni-definition-of-nursing-informatics-updated.

Irizarry, T., De Vito Dabbs, A., & Curran, C. R. (2015). Patient portals and patient engagement: A state of the science review. *Journal of Medical Internet Research, 17*(6), 1–15.

Kassam, I., Nagle, L., & Strudwick, G. (2017). Informatics competencies for nurse leaders: Protocol for a scoping review. *BMJ Open, 7*(12), e018855.

Kennedy, M., & Moen, A. (2017). In J. Murphy (Ed.), *Nurse leadership and informatics competencies: Shaping transformation of professional practice in forecasting informatics competencies for nurses in the future of connected health.* 2017 IMIA and IOS Press. https://doi.org/10.3233/978-1-61499-738-2-197.

Kim, J. T. (2014). Privacy and security issues for healthcare system with embedded rfid system on internet of things. *Advanced Science and Technology Letters, 72,* 109–112.

Kipping, S., Stuckey, M. I., Hernandez, A., Nguyen, T., & Riahi, S. (2016). A web-based patient portal for mental health care: Benefits evaluation. *Journal of Medical Internet Research, 18*(11), 1–9. https://doi.org/10.2196/jmir.6483.

Kirkpatrick, A. W., DeWaele, J. J., Ball, C. G., et al. (2007). The secondary and recurrent abdominal compartment syndrome. *Acta Clinica Belgica, 62*(Suppl), 60–65.

Kleib, M., Sales, A., Doran, D. M., C., et al. (2011). Nursing minimum data sets. In D. M. Doran (Ed.), *Nursing outcomes: State of the science* (2nd ed., pp. 487–512). Sudbury, MA: Jones and Bartlett.

Koppel, R., Wetterneck, T., & Telles, J. L. (2008). Workarounds to barcode medication administration systems: Their occurence, cause and threat to patient safety. *Journal of the American Medical Informatic Association, 15,* 408–423.

Lanier, C., Dominicé Dao, M., Hudelson, P., Cerutti, B., & Junod Perron, N. (2017). Learning to use electronic health records: Can we stay patient-centered? A pre-post intervention study with family medicine residents. *BMC Family Practice, 18*(1), 1–11.

MacDonald, M. (2008). Technology and its effect on knowing the patient: A clinical issue analysis. *Clinical Nurse Specialist, 22*(3), 149–155.

Mastrian, K., & McGonigle, D. (2009). *Nursing informatics and the foundation of knowledge.* Toronto, ON: Jones and Bartlett Publishers.

Matney, S., Brewster, P. J., Sward, K. A., Cloyes, K. G., & Staggers, N. (2011). Philosophical approaches to the nursing informatics data-information-knowledge-wisdom framework. *Advances in Nursing Science, 34*(1), 6–18.

Mickan, S., Atherton, H., Roberts, N. W., Heneghan, C., & Tilson, J. K. (2014). Use of handheld computers in clinical practice: a systematic review. *BMC Medical Informatics and Decision Making, 14*(1). https://doi.org/10.1186/1472-6947-13-56.

Moyle, W., Bramble, M., Jones, C., & Murfield, J. (2018). Care staff perceptions of a social robot called Paro and a look-alike Plush Toy: A descriptive qualitative approach. *Aging & Mental Health, 22*(3), 330–335.

Nagle, L. M., & Catford, P. (2008). Toward a model of successful electronic health record adoption. *Healthcare Quarterly, 11*(3), 84–91.

Nagle, L. M., & White, P. (2016). *Collected once—multiple uses national nursing data standards symposium proceedings list of acronyms.* Retrieved from: https://cnia.ca/wp-content/ uploads/2017/05/Proceedings-from-National-Nursing-Data-Standards-Symposium-2016.pdf.

Niazkhani, Z., Pirnejad, H., Berg, M., & Aarts, J. (2009). The impact of computerized provider order entry systems on inpatient clinical workflow: A literature review. *Journal of the American Medical Informatics Association, 16*(4), 539–549. https://doi.org/10.1197/jamia.M2419.

Nicklin, W., & McVeety, J. E. (2002). Canadian nurses' perceptions of patient safety in hospitals. *Canadian Journal of Nursing Leadership, 15*(3), 11–21.

Niemelä, M., Arvola, A., & Aaltonen, L. (2017). Monitoring the acceptance of a social service robot in a shopping mall. In *Proceedings of the companion of the 2017 ACM/IEEE international conference on human-robot interaction - HRI '17* (pp. 225–226). New York, NY: ACM Press. https://doi. org/10.1145/3029798.3038333.

O'Hagan, J., MacKinnon, N. J., Persaud, D., et al. (2009). Self-reported medical errors in seven countries: Implications for Canada. *Healthcare Quarterly, 12,* 55–61.

Open Notes. (2017). *Open notes mental health.* Retrieved from: https://www.opennotes.org/tools-resources/for-health-care-providers/mental-health.

Open Notes. (2018). *Open Notes.* Retrieved from: https:// www.opennotes.org.

Perras, C., Jacobs, P., Boucher, M., et al. (2009). *Technologies to reduce errors in dispensing and administration of medication in hospitals: Clinical and economic analyses (Technology report no. 121).* Ottawa, ON: Canadian Agency for Drugs and Technologies in Health.

Poon, E., Keohane, C., Yoon, C., Ditmore, M., Bane, A., Levtzion-Korach, O., et al. (2010, May 6). Effect of barcode technology on the safety of medication administration. *The New England Journal of Medicine, 362*(18), 1698–1707.

Praxia Information Intelligence and Gartner Incorporated. (2011). *Telehealth benefits and adoption: Connecting people and providers across Canada: A Study Commissioned by Canada Health Infoway*. Retrieved from: https://www2 .infoway-inforoute.ca/Documents/telehealth_report_ summary_2010_en.pdf.

Purvis, K. (2017, October). *Meet Pepper the robot—Southend's newest social care recruit*. The Guardian.

Remus, S., & Kennedy, M. A. (2012). Innovation in transformative nursing leadership: Nursing informatics competencies and roles. *Nursing Leadership, 25*(4), 14–26.

Rozenblum, R., Jang, Y., Zimlichman, E., et al. (2011). A qualitative study of Canada's experience with the implementation of electronic health information technology. *Canadian Medical Association Journal, 183*(5), E281–E288.

Ringler, M. D., Goss, B. C., & Bartholmai, B. J. (2015). Syntactic and semantic errors in radiology reports associated with speech recognition software. In *Studies in Health Technology and Informatics*. 922. https://doi.org/ 10.3233/978-1-61499-564-7-922.

Saginur, M., Graham, I. D., Foster, A. J., et al. (2008). The uptake of technologies designed to influence medication safety in Canadian hospitals. *Journal of Evaluation in Clinical Practice, 14*(1), 27–35.

Staggers, N., & Nelson, R. (2009). Overview of nursing informatics. In K. Mastrian, & D. McGonigle (Eds.), *Nursing informatics and the foundation of knowledge* (pp. 83–96). Toronto: Jones and Bartlett Publishers.

Street, R. L., Liu, L., Farber, N. J., Chen, Y., Calvitti, A., Weibel, N., et al. (2017). Keystrokes, mouse clicks, and gazing at the computer: How physician interaction with the EHR affects patient participation. *Journal of General Internal Medicine*, 1–6. https://doi.org/10.1007/s11606-017-4228-2.

Strudwick, G., Clark, C., McBride, B., Sakal, M., & Kalia, K. (2017). Thank you for asking: Exploring patient perceptions of barcode medication administration practices in inpatient mental health settings. *International Journal of Medical Informatics, 105*, 31–37. https://doi.org/10.1016/ j.ijmedinf.2017.05.019.

Strudwick, G., McGillis Hall, L., Nagle, L., & Trbovich, P. (2018). *Acute care nurses' perceptions of electronic health record use: A mixed method study (April)*, 1–10. https:// doi.org/10.1002/nop2.157.

Strudwick, G., Reisdorfer, E., Warnock, C., Kalia, K., Sulkers, H., Clark, C., et al. (2018). Factors associated with barcode medication administration technology that contribute to patient safety: An integrative review. *Journal of Nursing Care Quality, 33*(1), 79–85.

Strudwick, G., & Strauss, J. (2017). *Methods for engaging patients and family members in mental health contexts in digital health researchtechnology in psychiatry summit at Harvard Medical School and McLean Hospital.*

Strudwick, G., & Xie, L. (2018). Incorporating technology meaningfully into the clinical encounter: A nursing perspective. *Nursing Informatics Bulletin, 11*(7), 9.

Tamblyn, R., Huang, A., Perreault, R., et al. (2003). The medical office of the 21st century (MOXXI): Effectiveness of computerized decision-making support in reducing inappropriate prescribing in primary care. *Canadian Medical Association Journal, 169*(6), 549–556.

Voran, D. (2017). Using technology to enhance patient-physician interactions. *Pm&R, 9*(5), S26–S33.

Wang, S., Nagle, L., Li, X., et al. (2004). *Building the future: An integrated strategy for nursing human resources in Canada: Technological change*. Ottawa, ON: The Nursing Sector Study Corporation. Retrieved from: https:// www.cna-aiic.ca/~/media/cna/page%20content/pdf%20 fr/2013/09/05/19/20/technological_change_e.pdf.

Wulff, K., Cummings, G. G., Marck, P., et al. (2011). Medication administration technologies and patient safety: A mixed-method systematic review. *Journal of Advanced Nursing, 697*(10), 2080–2095.

Yen, P.-Y., Kennedy, M. K., Phillips, A., & Collins, S. (2017). Nursing informatics competency assessment for the nurse leader. *Journal Nursing Administration, 47*(5), 271–277.

Zhang, H., Cocosila, M., & Archer, N. (2010). Factors of adoption of mobile information technology by homecare nurses. *CIN: Computers, Informatics, Nursing, 28*(1), 49–56.

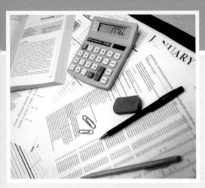

14

Managing Costs and Budgets

Karen Spalding, James Tiessen

This chapter focuses on methods of financing health care and specific strategies for managing costs and budgets in patient-care settings. As well, it explores factors that escalate health care costs, sources of health care financing, cost containment and health care reform strategies, and their implications for nursing practice. Various budgets and the budgeting process are explained. In addition to clinical competency and caring practices, nurses must understand the cost issues in health care delivery and the ethical implications of financial decisions to contribute fully to the health and healing of patients and populations.

OBJECTIVES

- Explain the major factors that are escalating the costs of health care.
- Evaluate different approaches to health care funding and their implications.
- Differentiate between variable and fixed costs, revenue, and expenditures in relation to a specified unit of service, such as a hospital visit, a hospital stay, or a procedure.
- Provide examples of cost considerations for nurses working in clinical environments.

- Discuss the purpose of and relationship between the operating and capital budgets.
- Explain the budgeting process.
- Identify variances on monthly expense reports and what they indicate.
- Understand how to develop a basic full-time equivalent (FTE) labour budget.

TERMS TO KNOW

budget
budgeting process
capital budget
case mix groups (CMGs)
cost centre
costs
expenditures

fixed costs
full-time equivalent (FTE)
nonproductive hours
operating budget
opportunity cost
price
productive hours

productivity
revenue
unit of service
utilization
variable costs
variance
variance analysis

❓ A CHALLENGE

Fraser Health is one of the fastest-growing health authorities in Canada, comprising over one-third of the entire population of British Columbia. Its emergency department visits are growing despite a provincial and regional focus on preventive strategies and community alternatives to acute care. One of its largest sites is the Surrey Memorial Hospital, which sees 100 000 emergency department visits annually. Rajesh works at Surrey Memorial Hospital as a nurse manager in the emergency department. Although Rajesh has made some progress in filling vacancies and reducing overtime in the department, he continues to struggle with vacancy rates in the 8% range. Provincial revenues are not growing fast enough to keep pace with the demand for health care services. Consequently, Rajesh needs to find ways to improve efficiency in his department, reduce less value-added expenditures (such as overtime), and meet the demand for emergency services while still staying on budget.

What would you do to work toward these improvements if you were Rajesh?

INTRODUCTION

Health care costs in Canada continue to rise at a rate greater than general inflation (Canadian Institute for Health Information [CIHI], 2017). In 2017, total health expenditure in Canada was 11.5% of the gross domestic product (GDP), an increase of over 2% since 2000 (CIHI, 2017, p. 44). Drug expenditures have almost doubled during that same period and account for approximately 16.5% of total spending (CIHI, 2017). In 2017, Canada spent $242 billion on health care, or an average of $6604 per capita (CIHI, 2017, p. 4). Approximately 70% of total health expenditure is financed by the public sector, and the rest is financed by the private sector. By comparison, health care spending in the United States reached $3.3 trillion in 2016, or $10 348 per capita (Centers for Medicare & Medicaid Services, 2018).

The significant portion of the GDP spent on health care can pose problems to the economy. Public-sector funds may need to be diverted from needed social programs, such as child care, housing, education, transportation, and the environment, to support health care. Nurse managers, of course, cannot directly affect health care spending at provincial or national levels. However, in their units and organizations they must be financially aware as they make decisions so that resources are used as both efficiently and equitably. This approach is captured in the Canadian Nurses Association's Code of Ethics, which states directly that nurses make fair decisions about the allocation of resources under their control based on the needs of persons receiving care. They advocate for fair treatment and fair distribution of resources (Canadian Nurses Association, 2017).

WHAT ESCALATES HEALTH CARE COSTS?

Total health care costs are a function of the price and the utilization rates of health care services (Costs = Price × Utilization) (Table 14.1). Price is the rate that health care providers set for the services they deliver, such as the hospital rate or physician fee as well as the unit prices of medications and supplies. Utilization refers to the quantity or volume of services provided, such as the number of diagnostic tests undertaken or the number of patient visits.

Price inflation in medications and supplies, as well as growing labour costs, are leading contributors to increasing prices for health care services. In recent decades, the rise in health care prices has dramatically outpaced general inflation. Examples of factors that stimulate price inflation are provider incomes that rise faster than average worker earnings and the high prices and utilization of prescription medications.

Many provinces are moving to group purchasing of medications and supplies as a method to control costs. Group purchasing organizations (GPOs), which purchase goods in high volumes to obtain discounts, are able to deliver lower unit prices and savings to their members. To achieve the best economies of scale, health care organizations who are members of GPOs must

TABLE 14.1 Relationship of Price and Utilization Rates to Total Health Care Costs

Price	×	Utilization Rate	=	Total Cost	% Change
$1.00		100		$100.00	0
$1.08[a]		100		$108.00	+8.0%
$1.08		105[b]		$113.40	+13.4%
$1.08		110[c]		$118.80	+18.8%

[a]8% increase for inflation.
[b]5% more procedures done.
[c]10% more procedures done.

standardize supplies and drug formularies as much as possible. HealthPRO is Canada's national group procurement group, comprising more than 800 health care facilities (HealthPRO, n.d.).

Several interrelated factors contribute to an increased utilization of medical services. These include a lack of appropriateness or effectiveness of some types of care, consumer beliefs and attitudes, health care financing, pharmaceutical usage, and changing population demographics and disease patterns. For example, a review of trends in health care utilization in British Columbia indicated that only 5% of the population had high-complexity chronic conditions or were frail in residential care. However, these groups together represented over 42% of total provincial health care expenditure (British Columbia Ministry of Health, 2010). Identifying inappropriate or ineffective medical procedures has led to national initiatives to demonstrate the efficacy of interventions and to decrease variations in physician practice. The Canadian Agency for Drugs and Technologies in Health (CADTH), for example, reviews the effectiveness of medical devices and medications annually and provides health care decision makers with evidence-based information on those that provide the best value.

Our attitudes and behaviours as consumers of health care also contribute to rising costs. In general, we prefer to "be fixed" when something goes wrong rather than practice prevention. When we need "fixing," expensive high-tech services typically are perceived as the best care. Many of us still believe that the physician knows best, so we do not seek much information related to costs and effectiveness of different health care options. When we do seek information, it may not be readily available, accurate, or understandable. Also, we are not accustomed to using other, less costly health care providers, such as nurse practitioners, if they are accessible.

The way health care is financed in Canada also contributes to rising costs. Because a large portion of health care spending is financed through taxation and not directly by consumers, users of the system are less aware of the direct costs involved with even something as simple as a visit to the emergency department. Effectively, no direct financial disincentive exists for overutilization.

Most physicians are not connected to the health care system as full employees. Rather, they tend to be independent contractors who drive the utilization of services such as diagnostic tests, procedures, and in-hospital bed days. As contractors, they are largely paid through models that include fee-for-service elements that can provide incentive for a physician to do, and bill for, more, rather than less, work. Physicians, however, are not directly accountable for the costs borne by a health region, hospital network, or a community care environment.

Changing population demographics are increasing the volume of health services needed as well. For example, chronic health problems increase with age, and the number of older adults in Canada is rising. In 2016, almost 6 million Canadians were 65 or older, a number that is expected to double in the next 25 years as the share of the population in that age group grows from 17% to 25% (United Nations Population Division, 2017).

HOW IS HEALTH CARE FINANCED?

Health care in Canada is financed through a mix of public and private funding. Approximately 70% of health care services are publicly financed, and another 30% are financed by third-party insurance plans and/or privately. Private health care delivery is regulated and tends to apply to less acute or noncore, rather than basic, health care services (Makarenko, 2010). Although each province and territory determines the services its public plan provides, those plans must comply with the principles of the *Canada Health Act* (Government of Canada, n.d.), which are as follows:

- **Public administration.** Government insurance plans pay for insured services. (Note that delivery can be private).
- **Comprehensiveness.** Necessary physician and hospital services are covered.
- **Universality.** All insured citizens are covered.
- **Portability.** Provisions exist so citizens travelling or moving between provinces and territories remain covered.
- **Accessibility.** Citizens have reasonable access to services, including no barriers associated with ability to pay. This prohibits extra billing.

Examples of publicly funded services include hospital admissions, emergency department visits, general practitioner visits, and most home health and public health services, such as immunizations and vaccines. Private health insurance is the second major source of health care funding in Canada. Most Canadians have some form of private health insurance to complement their publicly funded basic insurance. Examples of third-party or private financing include those services reimbursed through extended health and private corporate insurance plans. These typically help cover dental care, eyewear, and physiotherapy and massage therapy services not included under public health insurance. Individuals who are nonresidents of the province or territory in which they are treated pay directly for health care services when they do not have insurance. Costs paid by individuals—*out-of-pocket expenses*—include deductibles, additional fees, and co-insurance typically related to services such as dental care and prescription medications.

EXERCISE 14.1 As a student or recently qualified nurse, how aware are you of the costs and financing of health care in Canada? What kinds of strategies could be employed to increase the awareness of consumers and health care providers about the subject? As a health care provider, what can you contribute to ensuring a cost efficient and effective system?

APPROACHES TO HEALTH CARE FINANCING

In Canada, the primary source of funding for hospitals and health regions is a fixed, global budget transfer from the provincial or territorial government. The annual amount is typically based on historical spending, inflation, and politics rather than a zero-based assessment (e.g., where previous expenditures are not considered and budgets are based on starting from zero) of the type and volume of services provided (Sutherland, 2011). The advantages of this approach to funding include predictability and autonomy to move resources from one priority to another based on demand. A major disadvantage is that global budgets often do not grow at the same rate as demand, and this can make wait times for services longer and create other gaps in services.

Activity-based funding (ABF), although commonly used internationally, has recently gained prominence in the Canadian health care context. ABF funds health care organizations based on the type and quantity of services provided, paid at a set unit price. Although provincial or territorial governments still provide money, this mechanism in some settings creates a powerful incentive to find efficiencies because organizations are able to retain the difference in funding between the payment and the actual cost of delivering the service (Sutherland, 2011). Many provinces have adopted a mixed funding approach that combines global funding and ABF to reduce wait times yet still control health care spending. Since 2011, Ontario began to replace some global funding with a type of ABF, referred to as "Quality-based Procedures," that pays for treating several diagnoses (e.g., pneumonia, congestive heart failure) and interventions (e.g., knee/hip replacement, cancer surgery), and recommends care pathways and associated quality indicators (Ontario Ministry of Health and Long Term Care, n.d.).

Most health care organizations do not pay their physicians directly, with some exceptions. The shares of physician payments that are "alternative" (not fee-for-service) range broadly across Canada and across medical specialties. In eastern Canada, for example, more than 45% of total specialists' payments are alternative; the ratio in Quebec is 18%. In BC, for 17% of family medicine, payments are alternative, and in Ontario, the share is 55% (Mattison & Wilson, 2017, p. 13). Pay-for-performance (P4P) is another funding method that is becoming more common in Canada. As opposed to ABF, which funds organizations based on the volume of procedures, P4P provides funding incentives based on a predetermined set of quality outcomes (e.g., wait times) and outcome measures (e.g., hemoglobin A1C testing) (Sutherland, 2011). In British Columbia, the Emergency Department Decongestion P4P program is reported to have decreased emergency department wait times (Ministry of Health Services, Fraser Health, and Vancouver Coastal Health, 2009). This approach to funding can lead to innovation in care delivery, if the incentives are large enough to fund improvements on a cost-neutral basis.

Direct billing to the consumer is a form of financing that is less common in the public health sector in Canada. Most direct billing occurs if nonresidents of a province or territory are underinsured or not insured. As an example, new immigrants are often not granted public health insurance without a required waiting period, usually three months. Refugees and refugee claimants however can access some coverage through the Interim Federal Health Program (Association of Ontario Health Centres, n.d.). Should a health care facility need to provide services that require direct billing, collecting payment can be challenging.

BOX 14.1 **Health Care Financing Approaches**

Method	Key Points
Global funding	A set amount of funding distributed to a health care organization annually, not directly tied to volume or types of services.
Activity-based funding (ABF)	Funding that is based on a set price for a specific service and distributed based on volume.
Fee-for-service	Funding for every service provided based on a set fee.
Pay-for-performance (P4P)	Funding incentives provided for a specific quality outcome, such as reduced waiting time.
Direct billing	Direct billing of patients for the services provided.

Major health care financing approaches are summarized in Box 14.1. Researchers do not agree on the exact effects of these approaches on cost and quality (Sutherland, 2011; Mattison & Wilson, 2017). However, consideration of these effects is important because changes in payment systems have implications for how organizations provide care.

USING ACTIVITY TO INFORM THE BUDGET

Case mix groups (CMGs) represent a patient classification system used to group the types of inpatients a hospital treats. The CMG system is modelled after American Diagnosis Groups (DRGs) and developed by the Canadian Institute for Health Information (CIHI) (Manitoba Centre for Health Policy, 2010a). CMGs are assigned after a person is discharged from hospital, at which time the patient chart is reviewed and coded. The abstract produced from the review is sent to CIHI, which uses a computer algorithm to sort cases into CMGs. CMGs can either be categorized as typical or atypical, such as long-stay outliers. Most provinces and territories have been sending data to CIHI for inclusion in the discharge abstract database (DAD) since at least the mid-1990s.

CMGs can be a useful source of data for nurse managers to use in determining the types of services and resources required to care for patients within their portfolio. For example, a general medical unit may appear to care for a large range of medical problems, but after evaluating the CMGs, it may become evident that as few as three or four CMGs actually make up the majority of the patient population. This information allows nurse managers to plan resources more accurately to meet the specific needs of patients.

Although CMGs can help categorize patients' health problems more precisely, the need to understand the level of resources required for those patients is important. As a result, CIHI established resource intensity weights (RIWs). Each CMG is assigned a weight representing the relative value of resources that cases within that CMG are expected to consume, as well as an expected length of stay. Generally, it is reasonable to assume that the more acute the patient, the higher the RIW (such as a critical care unit patient). However, the RIW is not always a good proxy for acuity, especially when we consider a rehabilitation patient. In this case, the patient is no longer acutely ill but requires high levels of resources and so would be assigned a relatively high RIW (Manitoba Centre for Health Policy, 2010b). Age and other co-morbidities also play a factor in RIW calculation, as these factors can have a major effect on the resources required to care for different patients with the same diagnosis.

There are also case mix methods for classifying patients in acute ambulatory, continuing, long-term and home care, rehabilitation, and in-patient psychiatry. The groups defined by these methodologies are, like the CMGs, associated with expected resource usage (Canadian Institute for Health Information, n.d.).

THE CHANGING HEALTH CARE ECONOMIC ENVIRONMENT

Health care is a major public concern, and rapid changes are occurring in an attempt to restrain costs and improve the health and wellness of Canadians. As shown in Box 14.2, strategies shaping the evolving health care delivery system include primary health care reform, patient-focused funding (PFF) or activity-based funding (ABF), and regionalization. These strategies affect both the cost and utilization of health care services.

BOX 14.2   Health Care Delivery Reform Strategies

Strategies	Key Features
Primary health care reform	Focus on nonhospital, early treatment of health problems, with an emphasis on prevention to reduce overall costs.
Patient-focused funding or activity-based funding	A system whereby an organization is reimbursed at a set price per case based on agreed-upon outcomes, such as wait time targets.
Regionalization	An operating model where several health entities are merged into one organizational structure with the intent of reducing overhead and creating efficiencies.

EXERCISE 14.2 Work with two–three student colleagues for this exercise. For each strategy listed in Box 14.2, think about the incentives for health care providers (individuals and organizations) to change their practice patterns. Are there incentives to change the quantity of services used per patient or the number or types of patients served? Are there incentives to be efficient? List the incentives. How might each strategy affect overall health care costs? (Think in terms of the effect on utilization and price.) What effect on quality of care might each of the strategies have?

BENDING THE COST CURVE

With health care spending accounting for about 40% of provincial and territorial budgets in Canada (CIHI, 2017), the concept of "bending the cost curve" has never been more prevalent. Therefore most jurisdictions in Canada are exploring new ways of providing services to maximize efficiencies and, most important, to reduce demand. The emphasis on primary health and community care is an attempt to reduce the burden of hospitalization, particularly for people with multiple chronic illnesses. By reducing demand at the front door, the need to expand services and build new capital infrastructure is reduced, avoiding costs that otherwise would be borne by taxpayers. Primary health care clinics and providers can treat many people for the same cost as a single overnight hospital stay.

PFF and ABF, mentioned earlier, are gaining some acceptance in many provinces and territories. However, their impact on efficiency has elicited mixed reviews (Sutherland, 2011; Mattison & Wilson, 2017). It is assumed that by paying per case or unit of service, hospitals and health care providers will strive for efficiencies that increase outputs (e.g., inpatient services) and reduce waste (and garner more payments). Another related hypothesis is that health care organizations will work hard to be more efficient and provide services at less than the unit cost allocated, allowing the provider organization to retain the residual amount. In both cases, the drive for greater efficiency is the primary motivator for jurisdictions to experiment with this approach.

Regionalization is an organizational structure many provinces have gone to in an effort to reduce overhead and administrative costs, drive standardization, and create clinical efficiencies. When several hospitals and community care services operate under one umbrella, the need for separate support services, such as human resources, finance, and procurement of goods and services, is reduced, theoretically lowering system costs (Church & Barker, 1998). As funders of health care demand more value for money, the push to further consolidate back office or overhead functions continues to grow. It is suggested that the goals of regionalization in Canada have not been realized as fully as possible, mostly because physicians and primary care settings are usually not part of these structures (Marchildon, 2015).

WHAT DOES THE HEALTH CARE ECONOMIC ENVIRONMENT MEAN FOR NURSING PRACTICE?

Although the health care economic environment is ever changing, nurses must value themselves as health care providers and think of their practice within a context of organizational viability and quality of care. To do this, they must add "financial thinking" to their repertoire of nursing skills and be mindful that the services they provide add value for patients. Services that add value are of high quality, affect health outcomes positively, and minimize costs. The following sections help develop financial thinking skills and ways to consider how nursing practice adds value for patients by minimizing costs.

COST-CONSCIOUS NURSING PRACTICES

Knowing and Controlling Costs

Understanding what is required for a department or employer to remain financially sound requires that nurses think about not only the costs associated with individual patients but also revenue and expenses more globally, while actively considering how to control costs to the system as a whole.

It may not be obvious that revenues and costs should be concerns of nurses, who, after all, focus first on patient care. However, applying a fundamental economic concept, "opportunity cost," shows that this matters at department, organizational, and system levels. Opportunity costs arise because resources, including time, are scarce with respect to needs, so using them implies trade-offs. For example, a bed used for a patient who does not have to be in hospital is one not used for someone who needs acute care. This principle is also used when evaluating new health care technologies or programs, as the benefits of innovations, such as drugs or other interventions, are measured in terms of dollars or other outcomes (e.g., gains in Quality Adjusted Life Years, QALYs) and compared with existing practices (Palmer & Raftery, 1999).

As direct caregivers and case managers, nurses are constantly involved in determining the type and quantity of resources used for patients. Resources include supplies, personnel, and time. Nurses need to know what costs they generate by their decisions and actions. They also need to know what items cost and how they are paid for so they can make cost-effective decisions. For example, nurses need to know per-item costs for supplies so that they can appropriately evaluate lower-cost substitutes.

Although nurses must develop and implement their plans of care with full knowledge of the cost implications, cost alone does not drive care. They must continue to advocate for patients while working within cost and contractual constraints. Moreover, when nurses understand the funding practices of their organization, they can help patients maximize the resources available to them.

Using Time Efficiently

The adage that "time is money" is fitting in health care and refers to both the nurse's time and the patient's time. When nurses are organized and efficient in their care delivery and in scheduling and coordinating patients' care, the organization will save money. Doing as much as possible during each episode of care is particularly important to decrease repeat visits and unnecessary service utilization. Because length of stay (LOS) is the most important predictor of hospital costs (Finkler et al., 2007), patients who stay extra days cost the hospital a considerable amount and increase congestion. Decreasing LOS also makes room for other patients, thereby potentially increasing patient volume and reducing wait times. Nurses can become more efficient and effective by evaluating their major work processes and eliminating areas of redundancy and rework. Clinical information systems that support integrated practice at the point of care will also increase efficiency and improve patient outcomes.

Another important element of efficiently managing nursing resources is appropriate scheduling. Staffing decisions can be categorized into three general types: strategic, logistical, and tactical (College and Association of Registered Nurses of Alberta, 2008). Strategic decisions are judgements that establish overall approaches to nursing care (such as skill mix) and models of care delivery (see also Chapter 15). Logistical decisions are overall staffing directions, at unit and team levels, relative to baseline staffing, made to achieve appropriate patient care and management objectives. These include replacement staffing methods (e.g., float pools, relief lines, developing algorithms) and scheduling approaches (e.g., self-scheduling and 7.5-hour shifts). Tactical decisions are those made on a shift-to-shift basis that change schedules to safely meet patient needs in light of patient acuity or staffing availability (College and Association of Registered Nurses of Alberta, 2008). Appropriate staffing decisions of course must be made in accordance with any collective agreements and organizational policies, such as overtime policy.

Many public health care institutions also use managerial tools, such as Lean and Six Sigma, to reduce inefficiencies. Lean is a process redesign method used to reduce waste through process improvement tools, such as value stream mapping and 5S (Liker, 2003). Six Sigma focuses on improving the quality of processes and reducing errors (Keller & Pyzdek, 2009). Many provinces have begun using techniques such as Lean. Saskatchewan was the first province to introduce Lean across its entire health system (Government of Saskatchewan, 2013), and subsequently other provinces have embraced these techniques (Milne et al., 2014).

Evaluating the Cost-Effectiveness of New Technologies

The adoption of new technologies can present dilemmas in managing costs. In the past, if a new piece of equipment was easier to use or benefitted the patient in any way, providers were apt to want to use it for everyone, no matter how much more it cost. Now they may be forced to decide which patients really need the new equipment and which ones will have satisfactory outcomes with the current equipment. Essentially, these nurses analyze the cost effectiveness of the new equipment with regard to different types of patients to allocate limited resources. This new and sometimes difficult way of thinking about patient care may not always feel like a caring way of nursing. However, such decisions conserve resources without jeopardizing patients' health and thus create the possibility of using saved resources to provide other health care services, to the same patient or others. This is another example of applying the idea of "opportunity cost."

EXERCISE 14.3 Last year, a new positive-pressure, needleless system for administering IV antibiotics was introduced. Because the system was so easy to use and convenient for patients, the nurses in the contracted home IV therapy agency ordered it for everyone. Typically, patients get their IV antibiotics four times each day. The minibags and tubing for the regular procedure cost the agency $22 a day. The new system costs $24 per medication administration, or $96 a day. The agency receives the same per-diem (daily) payment for each patient. Discuss the financial implications for the agency if this practice is continued. Generate some optional courses of action for the nurses to consider. How should these options be evaluated? What secondary costs (e.g., the cost of treating fewer needle-stick injuries) should be included?

Predicting and Using Nursing Resources Efficiently

Because health care organizations are service institutions, the largest part of their operating budget is labour. For hospitals, nurses are the largest group of employees and account for most of the labour budget. Staffing, as mentioned, is the major area nurse managers can influence in managing costs. Supply management is the secondary area. To understand why this is so, it is helpful to understand the concepts of fixed and variable costs.

The total fixed costs in a unit are those costs that do not change as the volume of patients changes. In other words, with either a high or a low patient census, expenses related to facilities costs such as heat and light, support costs, administrative salaries, and salaries of the minimum number of staff to keep a unit open must be paid. Variable costs are costs that vary in direct proportion to patient volume or acuity. Examples include nursing and direct care staff, supplies, and medications.

In hospitals and community health care agencies, patient classification systems are often used to help managers predict nursing care requirements (see also Chapter 15). These systems differentiate patients according to acuity of illness, functional status, and resource needs. Some nurses do not like these systems because they believe they do not properly capture the essence of nursing. Although this may be true to a degree, these systems nonetheless can be good predictors. Misguided efforts to sabotage classification systems by incorrectly or inaccurately coding patient care with the hope for better staffing work primarily to prevent the development of tools to better manage practice. Used appropriately, patient classification systems can help evaluate and manage changing practice patterns and patient acuity levels as well as provide information for budgeting processes.

EXERCISE 14.4 Given the definitions for fixed and variable costs, which type do nurse managers have the greatest influence over?

Using Research to Evaluate Standard Nursing Practices

Nurses use research to restructure their work to ensure they add value for patients. For example, Koellinget al. (2005) studied the effect of patient education by a nurse educator on the clinical outcomes of patients with heart failure. In this randomized, controlled trial, one group of patients received standard discharge information whereas the other group received standard discharge information plus 1 hour of one-on-one education from a nurse educator. These patients were contacted by telephone after discharge to collect data concerning posthospitalization clinical events, symptoms, and self-care practices. Patients who received the additional 1-hour teaching session with the nurse educator showed improved clinical outcomes, increased adherence to self-care management, and reduced costs of care because of a reduction in readmissions. The costs of care, including the costs associated with the additional education session, resulted in average savings of $2823 per patient in the education group as compared with the control group. The findings from this economic evaluation support the implementation of nursing education programs for patients with chronic heart failure as evidenced by improved patient outcomes and reduced costs. Box 14.3 summarizes some cost-conscious strategies for nursing practice.

BOX 14.3 Strategies for Cost-Conscious Nursing Practice

1. Knowing and controlling costs
2. Using time efficiently
3. Discussing the cost of care with patients
4. Meeting patient rather than provider needs
5. Evaluating the cost-effectiveness of new technologies
6. Predicting and using nursing resources efficiently
7. Using research to evaluate standard nursing practices

LITERATURE PERSPECTIVE

Resource: Jones, C. B., & Gates, M. (2007). The costs and benefits of nurse turnover: A business case for nurse retention. *Online Journal of Issues in Nursing*, 12(3).

Nurse turnover is a continual concern for nurse administrators and nurse managers, particularly in times of nursing shortages. The authors of this article present a review of the literature related to the costs and benefits associated with nurse turnover. They confirmed the widely held belief that the costs of nurse turnover tend to exceed the benefits of hiring new staff. However, they also note that the literature does not quantify the actual costs associated with nurse turnover as related to the economic benefits associated with nurse retention.

The authors determined that the cost of nurse turnover ranges from US$22 000 to over US$64 000 per nurse, or about 1.3 times the departing nurse's salary. Nurse turnover costs include those associated with advertising and recruitment, vacancy (i.e., agency nurses, overtime), hiring and orientation, and termination. Determining the true costs of nurse turnover is difficult because it is challenging to calculate indirect costs (such as productivity loss or loss of organizational knowledge) and those associated with retaining nurses (such as ongoing education or rewards and recognition events). Other costs that are hard to estimate are associated with potential increases in nurse errors, a poorer work environment and culture, organizational knowledge loss, and additional turnover. The authors note that there are benefits of nurse turnover, although these are not typically quantified. These benefits include the lower salaries of newly hired nurses, savings from bonuses, new ideas and innovations brought by new nurses, and the possible elimination of poor performers.

The authors call for a business case supporting nurse retention. A business case provides information about the value of a project or investment based on a cost-benefit analysis.

Implications for Practice

This literature review demonstrates the challenges of attempting to quantify the actual costs of nurse turnover. It highlights the value of developing a robust business case as a means of determining the associated costs and benefits. Such a business case has the potential to drive organizational human resource practices in the areas of nurse recruitment and nurse retention programs.

EXERCISE 14.5 A community nursing organization performs an average of 36 intermittent catheterizations each day. A prepackaged catheterization kit costs the organization $17, but not every component of the kit is used each time. The four items in the kit, purchased separately, cost $5 each. What factors should be considered in evaluating the cost effectiveness of the two sources of supply?

BUDGETS

The basic financial document used in most organizations is the budget—a detailed financial plan for carrying out the activities an organization wants to accomplish for a certain period. A budget is stated in terms of dollars and includes proposed revenues (money received for providing goods or services) and expenditures (money spent on goods and services). The budgeting process is an ongoing activity in which plans are made and revenues and expenditures are managed. The management functions of planning and control are tied together through the budgeting process.

A budget requires that managers establish explicit program goals and expectations. Changes in health care practices, payment methods, technology, demographics, and regulatory factors must be forecast to anticipate their effects on the organization. Planning encourages an evaluation of different options and helps achieve a more cost-effective use of resources.

Health care organizations use different types of interrelated budgets. The major budgets discussed in this section are the operating budget and the capital budget. Managers also use long-range notional budgets, which are incorporated in *strategic plans* (Finkler & McHugh, 2007). Table 14.2 provides summary descriptions of budget types and indicates the degrees of nurse manager input into related decision making.

Operating Budget

The operating budget is the financial plan for the day-to-day activities of the organization. The expected revenues and expenditures generated from daily operations, given a specified volume of patients (the activity budget), are stated in it. Preparing and monitoring the operating budget, particularly the expenditure portion, can be a time-consuming job.

The expenditure part of the operating budget consists of a labour budget and a supply and expense budget for each cost centre. A cost centre is an organizational unit for which costs can be identified and managed. The labour budget is the largest part of the operating budget for most nursing units (see The Evidence).

Before the labour budget can be established, the volume of work predicted for the budget period must be calculated. A unit of service, which is a measure of the work being produced by the organization, is used. Units of service may be, for example, patient days, clinic or home visits, hours of service, admissions, deliveries, or treatments. Another factor needed to calculate the workload is the patient acuity mix. The formula for calculating the workload or the required patient-care hours for inpatient units is as follows:

Workload volume = Hours of care per patient day × Number of patient days (Table 14.3).

The workload is either established by the financial office and given to the nurse manager or calculated by nurse managers who forecast volumes. Forecasts usually start with a baseline of the last year's actual workload statistics and predict whether the volume in the upcoming year will be higher or lower. Nurse managers should inform administration about any factors that might affect the accuracy of the forecast, such as changes in physician practice patterns, new treatment modalities, or changes in inpatient versus outpatient treatment practices.

The next step in preparing the labour budget is to determine how many staff members will be needed to provide care. (This topic is also discussed in Chapter 16; which is available on Evolve.) Because some people work full time and others work part time, full-time equivalents (FTEs) are used in this step, rather

TABLE 14.2	**Characteristics of Budgets and the Role of Nurse Managers in Related Decisions**	
	BUDGET TYPE	
	Operating	Capital
Time frame	Fiscal year	One year or more
		Depreciation costs attributed yearly
Expenditure items	Labour, supplies, training, travel	Buildings, equipment, major renovations
Financing types	Global, activity based funding (ABF), Pay for performance	Yearly capital fund allocation; project-based applications to government; charitable fund-raising
Nurse manager input by role level		
Unit level	Significant	Moderate
Organizational level	Limited	Minimal

TABLE 14.3   **Workload Calculation (Total Required Patient-Care Hours)**

Patient Acuity Level[a]	Hours of Care Per Patient Day (HPPD)[b]	×	Patient Days[c]	=	Workload[d]
1	3.0		900		2700
2	5.2		3100		16 120
3	8.8		4000		35 200
4	13.0		1600		20 800
5	19.0		400		7600
Total			10 000		82 420

[a]1, low; 5, high.
[b]HPPD is the number of hours of care on average for a given acuity level.
[c]1 patient per 1 day = 1 patient day.
[d]Total number of hours of care needed based on acuity levels and numbers of patient days.

than positions. Generally, one FTE equates to working 37.5 hours per week, 52 weeks per year, for a total of 1950 hours of work paid per year. One-half of an FTE (0.5 FTE) equates to 18.75 hours per week. The 1950 hours paid to an FTE in a year consist of both productive hours and nonproductive hours. **Productive hours** are paid time that is worked. **Nonproductive hours** are paid time that is not worked, such as vacation, statutory holidays, orientation, education, and sick days. Before the number of FTEs needed for the workload can be calculated, the number of productive hours per FTE is determined by subtracting the total number of nonproductive hours per FTE from total paid hours. Alternatively, payroll reports can be reviewed to determine the percentage of paid hours that are productive for each FTE. Finally, the total number of FTEs needed to provide the care is calculated by dividing the total patient-care hours required by the number of productive hours per FTE (Box 14.4).

The total number of FTEs calculated by this method represents the number needed to provide care 24/7 each year (including relief). It does not reflect the number of positions or the number of people working each day. In fact, the number of positions, or head count, may be much higher, particularly if many nurses are part time. On any given day, some nurses may be scheduled for their regular day off or vacation and others may be off because of illness. Also, some positions that do not involve direct patient care, such as nurse managers or unit secretaries, may not be replaced

BOX 14.4   **Productive Hours Calculation**

Method 1: **Add all nonproductive hours/FTE and subtract from paid hours/FTE**

Example:

Vacation	20 days
Holiday	7 days
Average sick time	4 days
TOTAL	37 days

37 × 7.5 hours = 277.5 nonproductive hours/FTE
1950 − 277.5 = 1672.5 productive hours/FTE

Method 2: **Multiply paid hours/FTE by percentage of productive hours/FTE**

Example: Productive hours = 85.8%/FTE (1672.5 productive hours of total 1950 = 85.8%)
1950 × 0.858 = 1672.5 productive hours/FTE

Total FTE Calculation

Required Patient-Care Hours ÷ Productive Hours Per FTE = Total FTEs Needed
82 420 ÷ 1672.5 = approximately 49 FTEs

FTE, Full-time equivalent. Based on a 7.5-hour shift pattern or 37.5 hours/week.

during nonproductive time. Only one FTE is budgeted for any position that is not covered by other staff when the employee is off.

EXERCISE 14.6 Look at the number of patient hours per day at each acuity level listed in Table 14.3. Raise the hours linked to Acuity Level 2 by 35% (1.8 hours), and lower those associated with Acuity Level 4 by 23% (3 hours). Keep the total number of patient days the same and calculate the required total workload. Discuss how changes in patient acuity affect nursing resource requirements.

The next step is to prepare a daily staffing plan (ratios for day, evening, and night shifts) and to establish positions through the development of a rotation or annual schedule. Once this plan is established, the labour costs that comprise the labour budget can be calculated. Factors that must be addressed include straight-time hours, overtime hours, differentials and premiums, raises, and benefits (Finkler & McHugh, 2007). Differentials and premiums are extra pay for working specific times, such as evening shifts, night shifts, or holidays. Benefits usually include health and life insurance, Canada Pension Plan payments, and retirement plans. Benefits often cost an additional 23%–27% of a full-time employee's salary.

EXERCISE 14.7 If the percentage of productive hours per FTE is 80%, how many worked or productive hours are there per FTE? If total patient-care hours are 82 420, how many FTEs will be needed?

The supply and expense budget includes a variety of items used in daily unit activities, such as medical and office supplies, minor equipment, and books and journals; it also includes orientation, training, and travel. Each expense category generally has its own budget line and expense code. Although different methods are used to calculate the supply and expense budget, usually the previous year's expenses are used as a baseline. Ideally, this baseline is adjusted for projected patient volume and specific circumstances known to affect expenses, such as predictable staff turnover, which increases orientation and training expenses; a percentage factor would be added to adjust for inflation. However, the reality in many Canadian jurisdictions is that budgets rarely grow as quickly as actual expenses, and managers are expected to find efficiencies to arrive at a balanced budget.

The final component of the operating budget is the revenue budget which projects the revenue from a variety of sources that the organization will receive for providing patient care. Historically, nurses have not been directly involved in developing the revenue budget. The anticipated revenues are calculated according to the specifics of the nursing area or program. Data about the volume and types of patients and funding streams (i.e., global funding, ABF) are necessary to project revenues in any health care organization. Even when nurse managers do not participate in developing the revenue budget, learning about the organization's revenue base is essential for good decision making.

Capital Budget

The capital budget reflects expenses related to the purchase of major capital items, such as equipment and physical plant. A capital expenditure must have a useful life of more than 1 year and exceed a cost level specified by the provincial or territorial government. The minimum cost requirement for capital items in health care organizations is usually from $2000 to $5000, although some organizations have different levels. Anything below that minimum is considered a routine operating cost.

Accounting rules separate capital costs from operating expenses because to incur the former in the year they are made makes costs seem too high. Therefore these costs are spread out over time as capital items are depreciated. This means that each year, over the useful life of the equipment, a portion of its cost is allocated to the operating budget as an expense. This procedure is required as part of the generally accepted accounting principles governing each province, but it does not affect the bottom line of the manager's budget.

Organizations usually set aside a fixed amount of money for capital expenditures each year, and also rely on their own charitable foundations to raise money for much-needed equipment and facility upgrades. Complete well-documented justifications for new resources must be provided to the associated Ministry of Health because the competition for limited resources is stiff. Such justifications should include the projected amount of use; any services that will be duplicated or replaced; safety considerations; the need for space, personnel, or building renovations; the effect on operational revenues and expenses; and the resource's contribution to the strategic plan.

THE BUDGETING PROCESS

The phases in the budgeting process are similar in most health care organizations, although the budgeting period, budget timetable, and level of manager and employee participation vary. Budgeting is done annually and in relation to the organization's fiscal year. A fiscal year exists for financial purposes and can begin at any point on the calendar, but it is generally from April 1 to March 31. The major phases in the process include gathering information and planning, developing unit and departmental budgets, negotiating and revising, and later using feedback to evaluate budget results and improve plans (Finkler & McHugh, 2007). Each health care organization develops a timetable with specific dates for implementing the budgeting process. The timetable may be anywhere from 3 to 9 months. Box 14.5 outlines the budgeting process.

Gathering Information and Planning

The information-gathering and planning phase provides managers with data essential for developing their individual budgets. This phase begins with an environmental assessment that helps the organization understand its position in relation to the entire community. The assessment includes, for example, the changing health care needs of the population, influential economic factors, such as inflation and unemployment, differences in payment, and patient satisfaction.

BOX 14.5   Outline of the Budgeting Process

1. Gathering information and planning
   - Environmental assessment
   - Mission, goals, and objectives
   - Program priorities
   - Financial objectives
   - Assumptions (employee raises, inflation, volume projections)
2. Developing unit and departmental budgets
   - Operating budgets
   - Capital budgets
3. Negotiating and revising
4. Evaluating
   - Analysis of variance
   - Critical performance reports

Modified from Finkler, S. A., Kovner, C. T., & Jones, C. (2007). *Financial management for nurse managers and executives* (3rd ed.). St. Louis, MO: Saunders

---

Next, the organization's long-term goals and objectives are reassessed in light of the organization's mission and the environmental assessment. Doing so helps nurse managers situate the budgeting process for their individual units in relation to the whole organization. At this point, programs are prioritized so that resources can be allocated to programs that best help the organization achieve its long-term goals. It is important to know the organization-wide assumptions that underpin the budgeting process, such as salary increases, inflation factors, and volume projections for the next fiscal year.

Specific, measurable financial objectives are then established, and the budgets must meet these objectives. The financial objectives might include limiting expenditure increases or reducing labour costs by designated percentages. Nurse managers also set operational objectives for their units that are in concert with the rest of the organization. At this point, units or departments interpret what effect the changes in operational activities will have on them. For instance, how will using case managers and care maps for selected patients affect a particular unit? Establishing unit-level objectives is also a good way to involve staff nurses in setting the future direction of the unit.

Developing Unit and Departmental Budgets

Based on the information gathered, managers can develop operating and capital budgets for their units or departments with their financial managers. These budgets are often developed in tandem because each affects the other. For instance, purchasing a new monitoring system will have implications for the supplies used, staffing, and staff training.

Negotiating and Revising

The negotiating and revising phase is an important part of the budgeting process that may or may not take place at the nurse manager level. This phase is complex because changes in one budget usually require changes in others. Learning to defend and negotiate budgets is an important skill for nurse managers. Success depends upon knowing how costs are allocated and clearly communicating which resources are contained in each budget category. It is vital to clearly and specifically explain how insufficiently resourced care affects patient, nurse, and organizational outcomes.

Evaluating and Monitoring the Budget

Evaluating, the final and ongoing phase of the budgeting process, relates to the control function of management. Feedback is obtained regularly so that organizational activities can be monitored and adjusted to maintain efficient operations. Variance analysis, the major control process used, involves identifying differences between projected and actual costs. For expenses, a favourable, or positive, variance means that the budgeted amount was greater than the amount spent. An unfavourable, or negative, variance means that the budgeted amount was less than the amount spent.

Positive and negative variances cannot be interpreted as good or bad without further investigation. For example, if fewer supplies were used than were budgeted, this difference would appear as a positive variance, showing that the unit saved money. This variance would be good news if it meant that supplies were used more efficiently and patient outcomes remained the same or improved. However, this variance would suggest a problem if using fewer or less-expensive supplies led to poorer patient outcomes. This variance might also indicate that exactly the right amount of supplies was used but that the patient census (the average number of patients per day or other time period) was less than budgeted.

MANAGING THE UNIT-LEVEL BUDGET

At a minimum, nurse managers are responsible for meeting the fiscal goals related to the personnel and the supply and expense parts of the operations budget for their unit of operation. Typically, monthly expense reports of operations (see Table 14.4) are sent to nurse managers, who then investigate and explain the underlying cause

TABLE 14.4   Statement of Operations, Current Month

Description	Actual ($)	Budget ($)	Variance ($)	Variance (%)
REVENUES				
Contributions from the province/territory	167 615	163 635	3 980	2
Patients	206 865	194 624	12 241	6
Recoveries and other revenue	131 559	161 522	(29 963)	−19
Total	**506 039**	**519 781**	**(13 742)**	**−11**
EXPENSES				
Salaries and wages	8 179 882	8 105 135	(74 747)	−1
Benefit compensation	1 564 280	1 555 934	(8 346)	−1
Sick and severance pay	304 621	312 878	8 257	3
Purchasing services	121 327	15	(121 312)	−808 747
Physician fees	48 422	60 412	11 990	20
Medical supplies	535 945	543 799	7 854	1
Sundry and other expenses	330 694	302 152	(28 542)	−9
Health service provider	115 714	122 443	6 729	5
Total	**11 200 885**	**11 002 768**	**(198 117)**	**−2**
Excess/(deficiency) of revenue over expenses before amortization	(10 694 846)	(10 482 987)	(211 859)	—
AMORTIZATION				
Net invested in capital assets	126 348	123 689	−2 659	−2
Total	**126 348**	**123 689**	**−2 659**	**−2**
Excess/(deficiency) of revenue over expenses after amortization	(10 821 194)	(10 606 676)	(214 518)	—

RESEARCH PERSPECTIVE

Resource: Dahlberg, K., Philipsson, A., Hagberg, L., Jaensson, M., Hälleberg-Nyman, M., & Nilsson, U. (2017). Cost-effectiveness of a systematic e-assessed follow-up of postoperative recovery after day surgery: A multicentre randomized trial. *British Journal of Anaesthesia*, 119(5): 1039–1046.

A Swedish randomized control trial compared the health care costs generated by day-surgery patients who used a mobile phone application "Recovery Assessment by Phone Points" (RAPP) with patients who received standard care over a two-week period. The RAPP app, installed on the patients' phones, asked them to answer a few questions daily about their recovery. One question, for example, was, "Do you want to be contacted by a nurse?" Both groups were provided with the same information on who to contact if they had concerns, including Sweden's 24-hour helpline.

The researchers assessed all patients in terms of their quality of life both before their operations and after the two-week period. They also recorded the numbers of visits to providers, both RNs and physicians, and attributed costs to these. A total of 719 participants, roughly equally split between the two groups, participated.

The average cost of equipping patients with the RAPP was about € 19 (C$30), including the app cost and the time spent by RNs helping them download and learn it. The costs of phone calls and visits with RNs or physicians were also estimated.

Analysis of the findings showed that the differences in perceived quality of life after the surgery did not significantly differ between the patient groups. The mean cost for health care use in the 2 weeks postsurgery for the RAPP group was €37, compared with €61 for the control group who received standard care. Subtracting the cost of the RAPP gives a net saving of about €5 per patient. Although this seems a trivial amount, if used widely, the savings would be significant. Further, the cost of the RAPP would probably be lower if it were to more widely adopted.

Implications for Practice

Surgery patients can be anxious upon discharge to their homes. This anxiety can be heightened if they are not confident that they can maintain regular contact with providers who can advise them. Using an app like the RAPP can assure patients that their providers are ready to help them, if they need it. This makes them less likely to seek an in-person or even telephone contact when they feel unsafe.

Though the study was conducted in Sweden, the lesson is clear and applicable more widely. Hospitals can consider employing this type of app to reduce clinically unnecessary consultations by day-surgery patients. The time and money saved can be more efficiently allocated to other uses.

of variances greater than 5%. Many factors can cause budget variances, including unexpected changes in patient census or patient acuity, vacation or sick time, and staffing levels or mix. To accurately interpret budget variances, nurse managers need reliable data about these factors.

Nurse managers can control *some* but not all of the factors that cause variances. After the causes of variances are determined and if they are controllable by the nurse manager, steps are taken to prevent the variance from occurring in the future. However, even uncontrollable variances that increase expenses might require actions by nurse managers. For example, if supply costs rise drastically because a new technology is being used, the nurse manager might have to look for other areas where the budget can be cut.

> **EXERCISE 14.9** Examine Table 14.4 and identify major budget variances for the current month. Are the variances favourable or unfavourable? What additional information would help you explain the variances? What are some possible causes for each variance? Are the causes you identified controllable by the nurse manager? Why or why not? Is a favourable variance on expenses always desirable? Why or why not?

Productivity

Productivity is the ratio of outputs to inputs, which can be written as output/input. In nursing, outputs are nursing services as measured by hours of care, number of home visits, and so forth. The inputs are the resources used to provide the services, such as personnel hours and supplies. Productivity can be increased by decreasing the inputs or increasing the outputs.

Hospitals often use hours per patient day (HPPD) as a measure of productivity. For example, if the standard of care in a critical care unit is 12 HPPD, then 360 hours of care are required for 30 patients for 1 day. When 320 hours of care are provided, the productivity rating is 113% ($360 \div 320 = 1.13$), which means either productivity increased or needed care was not delivered. One must consider the quality component in any productivity model related to care.

In home care, the number of visits per day per registered nurse is one measure of productivity. If the standard is 5 visits per day but the weekly average was 4.8 visits per day, then productivity is lower than expected. Similar to the case of costs, variances in productivity are not inherently favourable or unfavourable, so they need investigation and explanation. For example, an explanation of the variance (4.8 visits per day) might include the fact that one visit took twice the amount of time normally spent on a home visit because of client needs, thus preventing the nurse from making the standard 5 visits per day. The extra time spent on one client was productive time but not adequately accounted for by the visits per day measure.

Staff Nurses and Budgets

Although they are not directly accountable for the budget, staff nurses play an important role in meeting budget expectations. Many nurse managers find that routinely sharing the unit's budget and budget-monitoring activities with staff nurses fosters an appreciation of the relationship between cost and the mission to deliver high-quality patient care. Having access to cost and utilization data allows staff nurses to identify patterns and participate in selecting appropriate, cost-effective practice options that work for both staff and patients. Nurse managers and staff nurses who work in partnership to understand that cost versus care is a dilemma to manage, rather than a problem to solve, will develop innovative, cost-conscious nursing practices that produce good outcomes for patients, nurses, and the organization.

💡 A SOLUTION

Rajesh started by reviewing his staffing clerks and frontline nurse leaders' processes in scheduling vacation and relief, and their decision making regarding overtime approval. He met with the patient care coordinators (PCCs) and staffing clerks and reinforced the approval processes and the policy on vacation scheduling. All overtime had to be approved by Rajesh, and he would review the overtime report on a monthly basis.

Rajesh calculated that he needed an additional four full-time equivalents (FTEs) for regular relief positions to fill short-term vacancies and vacation leave at straight time. They discovered that when the staffing clerk was stressed and busy, they sometimes went directly to the staff member they knew was available, even if doing so resulted in overtime. Thus Rajesh developed a casual clerk position to assist the staffing clerk on a periodic basis so that more time was available to go through casual call lists to find short-term replacements at straight time. They also cleaned up the casual call list to ensure that people who weren't actually available were taken off the list. This update made the staffing and casual clerks' jobs more efficient by dramatically reducing the calls required to find someone. Rajesh ensured that the vacation scheduling policy was adhered to, which meant that all vacations were scheduled by December of the preceding year so that relief workers could be prebooked well in advance. He worked with the PCCs and their manager on decision-making algorithms that could make better decisions regarding whether extra staff were required when patient volumes were high. All of these efforts appear to be reaping dividends; the emergency department's overtime rate has dropped by 30%, and Rajesh anticipates further reductions.

Would this be a suitable approach for you? Why or why not?

▌ THE EVIDENCE

Nursing services are a major cost component of health care delivery in Canada, so efficient staffing and scheduling are critical to maintaining effective health care services, while managing expenditures. A multi-site, collaborative study at four health care organizations (a pediatric hospital, a continuing care health centre, a pediatric rehabilitation hospital, and a community-based hospital) in Ontario explored innovative approaches to these activities.(Moreau et al., 2010).

This study focused on developing "evaluative strategies and tools for identifying and optimizing promising nurse staffing and scheduling practices" (p. 139). The nurses and those responsible for nurse staffing and scheduling were either interviewed or participated in focus groups for the study. Data from the interviews and focus groups were analyzed to create logic models and evaluation frameworks for each site's nurse staffing and scheduling model, as well as to answer five "evaluability" questions related to the design, implementation, and evaluation of each model (p. 139). The study provided the participating health care organizations with tools, resources, and knowledge to conduct effective evaluations of nursing staff and scheduling models.

The researchers found that evaluability assessments can be catalysts for change and improvements in nurse staffing and scheduling models; evaluability assessments can provide effective tools for stakeholder collaborations; and evaluation is an essential tool for improving nurse staffing and scheduling models.

✳ NEED TO KNOW NOW

- Determine the most commonly used equipment and how much it costs.
- Know the costs and charges (if applicable) of the 20 most frequently used supplies on your unit.
- Know how to retrieve literature related to best practice in staffing according to patient acuity and patient census.
- Know how to retrieve literature related to cost savings in nursing practice.

CHAPTER CHECKLIST

Financial-thinking skills are the cornerstone of cost-conscious nursing practice and are essential for all nurses. Nurses must also determine whether the services they provide add value for patients. Services that add value are of high quality, positively affect health outcomes, and minimize costs.

Understanding what constitutes costs and why organizations must remain cost conscious to provide sustainable services is basic to financial thinking in health care. Knowing what is included in operating and capital budgets, how they interrelate, and how they are developed, monitored, and controlled is also important. Considering the ethical implications of financial decisions and collectively managing the cost–care dilemma are imperative for cost-conscious nursing practice.

- Total health care costs are a function of the prices and the utilization rates of services.
- In Canada, the government is the major source of funding for health care services, followed by private insurance companies. Individuals are the third major payer.
- Health care is financed through a range of mechanisms, including a global budget transfer from the provincial and territorial governments, activity-based funding, fee-for-service, pay-for-performance, and direct billing.
- Because health care needs typically exceed available resources, it is important to focus on efficiency because money and/or time saved can be directed to help meet these excess demands. This is a use of the concept "opportunity cost".
- Nurses and nurse managers directly influence an organization's ability to remain on budget.
- Cost-conscious nursing practices include the following:
- Knowing and controlling costs.
- Using time efficiently.
- Discussing the cost of care with patients.
- Meeting patient rather than provider needs.
- Evaluating cost-effectiveness of new technologies.
- Predicting and using nursing resources efficiently.
- Using research to evaluate standard nursing practices.
- Nurse managers have the most influence on costs in relation to managing personnel and supplies.
- Variance analysis is the major control process in relation to budgeting.

■ TIPS FOR MANAGING COSTS AND BUDGETS

- Know the major changes in the organization and how they might affect the organization's budget.
- Analyze the supplies you use in providing care and what is commonly missing as one way to make recommendations about supply needs.
- Evaluate what each of your patients would find most helpful during the time you will be caring for them.

- Decide which of your actions create costs for the patient or the organization.
- Be aware of how changes in patient acuity and patient census affect staffing requirements and the unit budget.
- Examine the upsides and downsides of the cost–care dilemma thoughtfully.

Visit the Evolve website for Suggested Readings, Internet Resources, and additional resources related to the content in this chapter: http://evolve.elsevier.com/Canada/Yoder-Wise/leading/.

REFERENCES

Statutes
Canada Health Act, RSC 1985, c. C-6 (Canada).

Texts
Association of Ontario Health Centres. (n.d.). *Refugee and newcomer health.* Retrieved from: https://www.aohc.org/refugee-and-newcomer-health.

British Columbia Ministry of Health. (2010, October 8). *Presentation to the Health Operations Committee.*

Canadian Institute for Health Information. (n.d.). *Case mix.* Retrieved from: https://www.cihi.ca/en/submit-data-and-view-standards/methodologies-and-decision-support-tools/case-mix.

Canadian Institute for Health Information. (2017). *National Health Expenditure Trends, 1975 to 2017.* Toronto, ON: Author. Retrieved from: https://www.cihi.ca/sites/default/files/document/nhex2017-trends-report-en.pdf.

Canadian Nurses Association. (2017). *Code of Ethics for Registered Nurses.* Retrieved from: https://www.cna-aiic.ca/~/media/cna/page-content/pdf-en/code-of-ethics-2017-edition-secure-interactive.

Centers for Medicare and Medicaid Services. (2018). *National Health Expenditure, "NHE Fact Sheet".* Retrieved from: https://www.cms.gov/research-statistics-data-and-systems/statistics-trends-and-reports/nationalhealthexpenddata/nhe-fact-sheet.html.

Church, J., & Barker, P. (1998). Regionalization of health services in Canada: A critical perspective. *International Journal of Health Services: Planning, Administration, Evaluation, 28*(3), 467–486.

College and Association of Registered Nurses of Alberta. (2008). *Evidence-informed staffing for delivery of nursing care: Guidelines for registered nurses.* Retrieved from: http://www.nurses.ab.ca/Carna-Admin/Uploads/Evidence_Nursing_Care.pdf.

Finkler, S. A., Kovner, C. T., & Jones, C. (2007). *Financial management for nurse managers and executives* (3rd ed.). St. Louis, MO: Saunders.

Finkler, S. A., & McHugh, M. (2007). *Budgeting concepts for nurse managers* (4th ed.). St. Louis, MO: Saunders.

Government of Canada. (n.d.). (1985). Canada Health Act. R.S.C.. c. C-6. Retrieved from: http://laws-lois.justice.gc.ca/eng/acts/c-6/page-1.html#h-6.

Government of Saskatchewan. (2013). Saskatchewan Health Care Management System. Retrieved from: https://hqc.sk.ca/Portals/0/documents/lean-faq.pdf.

HealthPRO. n.d. "About". Retrieved from: https://portal.healthprocanada.com/web/healthpro-public/home.

Jones, C. B., & Gates, M. (2007). The costs and benefits of nurse turnover: A business case for nurse retention. *Online Journal of Issues in Nursing, 12*(3). Retrieved from: http://ojin.nursingworld.org/MainMenuCategories/ANA-Marketplace/ANAPeriodicals/OJIN/TableofContents/Volume122007/No3Sept07/NurseRetention.aspx.

Keller, P., & Pyzdek, T. (2009). *The Six Sigma handbook* (3rd ed.). McGraw-Hill Education.

Koelling, T. M., Johnson, M. L., Cody, R. J., et al. (2005). Discharge education improves clinical outcomes in patients with chronic heart failure. *Circulation, 111,* 179–185.

Liker, C. (2003). *The Toyota way: 14 management principles from the world's greatest manufacturer.* New York, NY: McGraw-Hill Professional.

Makarenko, J. (2010, October 22). *Canada's health care system: An overview of public and private participation.* Retrieved from: https://www.mapleleafweb.com/features/canada-s-health-care-system-overview-public-and-private-participation.html.

Manitoba Centre for Health Policy. (2010a). *Concept: Case Mix Groups (CMG™)—Overview*. Retrieved from: http://mchp-appserv.cpe.umanitoba.ca/viewConcept.php?conceptID=1094.

Manitoba Centre for Health Policy. (2010b). *Term: Resource Intensity Weights (RIW™)*. Retrieved from: http://mchp-appserv.cpe.umanitoba.ca/viewDefinition.php?definition-ID=103807.

Marchildon, G. P. (2015). The crisis of regionalization. *Healthcare Management Forum, 28*(6), 236–238.

Mattison, C. A., & Wilson, M. G. (2017). *Examining the Effects of Value-based Physician Payment Models*. McMaster *Health Forum*. Retrieved from: https://www.mcmasterforum.org/docs/default-source/product-documents/rapid-responses/examining-the-effects-of-value-based-physician-payment-models.pdf?sfvrsn=2.

Milne, V., Pendharkar, S., & Winkel, G. (2014). *From the factory floor to the emergency department: Hospitals explore lean method. Healthy debate*. (Sept. 11). Retrieved from: http://healthydebate.ca/2014/09/topic/lean.

Ministry of Health Services, *Fraser Health, and Vancouver Coastal Health*. (2009, March 2). *Innovation reduces ER congestion in lower mainland [Press release]*. Retrieved from: http://www2.news.gov.bc.ca/news_releases_2005-2009/2009HSERV0019-000256.htm.

Moreau, K., Maxwill, H., Sorfleet, C., et al. (2010). Innovative approaches to staffing and scheduling [Special Issue]. *Nursing Leadership, 23*, 138–139.

Ontario Ministry of Health and Long Term Care (n.d.). *Quality-based procedures, health system funding reform*. Retrieved from: http://www.health.gov.on.ca/en/pro/programs/ecfa/funding/hs_funding_qbp.aspx.

Palmer, S., & Raftery, J. (1999). Economics notes: Opportunity cost. *BMJ: British Medical Journal, 318*(7197), 1551.

Sutherland, J. M. (2011, March). *Hospital payment mechanisms: An overview and options for Canada*. Ottawa, ON: Canadian Health Services Research Foundation. Retrieved from: http://www.cfhi-fcass.ca/Libraries/Hospital_Funding_docs/CHSRF-Sutherland-HospitalFundingENG.sflb.ashx.

United Nations Population Division. (2017). *World population prospects*. Retrieved from: https://esa.un.org/unpd/wpp/DataQuery/.

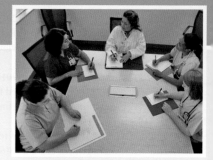

15

Care Delivery Strategies

Susan Sportsman
Adapted by Heather MacMillan

This chapter presents models of nursing care delivery used in health care organizations. It explores the historical development and structure of the case method; functional nursing; team nursing; primary nursing, including hybrid forms of this approach; and nursing case management. The chapter also summarizes the benefits and disadvantages of each model and describes the roles of nurse manager and staff nurse in each model. In addition, the chapter reviews care strategies that influence care delivery, such as disease management, differentiated practice, and "transforming care at the bedside."

OBJECTIVES

- Define the nursing care delivery models used in health care.
- Describe the role of the nurse manager and the staff nurse in each model.
- Describe disease management programs.
- Summarize the differentiated nursing practice model and related methods to determine competencies of nurses who deliver care.
- Consider the impact of Transforming Care at the Bedside (TCAB) on the delivery of care in a nursing unit.

TERMS TO KNOW

case management model
case manager
case method
charge nurse
clinical nurse leader (CNL)
clinical pathway
differentiated nursing practice
disease management
expected outcomes
functional nursing

nursing care delivery model
nursing case management
outcome criteria
partnership model
patient allocation
patient-focused care model
patient outcomes
primary nurse
primary nursing
staff mix

Synergy Model
team nursing
total patient care
Transforming Care at the Bedside (TCAB)
unregulated care providers (UCPs)
variance

The charge nurses in a newly built 50-bed long-term care facility, comprised of two different units, were finding it increasingly difficult to make patient assignments because of the layout and design of the 3000-square-metre facility. Furthermore, throughout the shift, the nursing staff were having problems remaining engaged with the activities on the units because of the distance between nursing stations. Also, the design of the units made it difficult for a nurse to ask for help when needed. After occupying the facility for several months and trying numerous methods to enhance teamwork and communication among the staff, it was apparent that a more formal process was needed to resolve these problems. As the patient care manager (PCM) and registered nurse, David was tasked with resolving the problems. What would you do if you were David?

INTRODUCTION

A **nursing care delivery model** is the method used to provide care to patients, that is, the way in which health care services are delivered (Agency for Clinical Innovation, 2013). Because nursing care is viewed by some as a cost rather than a method of cost savings, it is logical for organizations to evaluate their method of providing patient care for the purpose of saving money, while still providing quality care. In this chapter, various models of nursing care delivery are discussed, including **total patient care**, also known as **patient allocation** (King et al., 2014); **functional nursing**; **team nursing**; **primary nursing**, including hybrid forms; and **nursing case management**. In addition, the influence of **disease management** programs, **differentiated nursing practice**, and **Transforming Care at the Bedside (TCAB)** is discussed.

Each nursing care delivery model has advantages and disadvantages, and none is ideal. Some models are conducive to large institutions, whereas others work better in smaller settings. Managers in any organization must examine the organizational goals, the unit objectives, patient population, staff availability, and the budget when selecting a care delivery model. A historical overview of common care models is designed to convey the complexity of how care is delivered. Each of these models is still used within the broad range of health care organizations. In addition, these models often serve as the foundation for new and innovative care delivery models. Finally, it is important to consider that although no one model fits all settings, models of nursing care organization do need to strive to maximize positive outcomes for hospitalized patients and the broader health care system (Dubois et al., 2013).

TOTAL PATIENT CARE (PATIENT ALLOCATION)

The total patient care method, or patient allocation method, of nursing care delivery is the oldest model of providing care to patients. This model should not be confused with *nursing case management*, which is introduced later in the chapter.

The premise of the **case method** is that one nurse provides total care for one patient during the entire work period. This method was used in the era of Florence Nightingale (1820–1910), when patients received total care in the home. Today, total patient care is used in critical care settings—acute medical settings where one nurse provides total care to one or two critically ill patients, or to a group of patients, depending on the clinical setting, over the course of a shift (Duffield et al., 2010, p. 2243). Nurse educators often select this method of care when students are learning to provide care for patients. Variations of the case method exist, and it is possible to identify similarities among them after reviewing other models of care delivery described later in this chapter.

Model Analysis

In most hospital and inpatient settings, during an 8- or 12-hour shift, the patient or group of patients receives consistent care from one nurse. The nurse, patient, and family trust one another and work together toward specific goals. Total patient care remains popular with patients, as the care is seen as being consistent and high quality, provided by highly qualified nursing staff (Duffield, et al., 2010). The nurse may choose to deliver this care with a task orientation that can serve to negate the holistic perspective (Shirey, 2008). Because the nurse is with the patient during most of the shift, even subtle changes in the patient's status are easily noticed (Fig. 15.1).

In today's costly health care environment, total patient care provided by one nurse, typically a registered nurse (RN), is very expensive. Is it realistic to use a highly skilled and extremely knowledgeable professional nurse to provide all the care required in a unit that may have 20 to 30 patients? In a time of a global

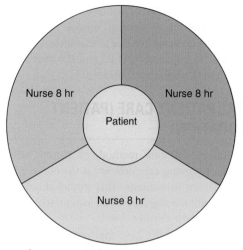

Fig. 15.1 Case method of nursing care delivery for an 8-hour shift.

nursing shortage, there may not be enough nurses to use this model or funding to provide for this model of care.

Nurse Manager's Role

When using the total patient care model, the nurse manager must consider the expense of the system. The nurse manager is obligated to weigh the expense of a registered nurse (RN) or registered psychiatric nurse (RPN) versus the expense of licensed or registered practical nurses and unregulated care providers (UCPs) in the context of the outcomes required. See Chapter 7 for the differences between regulated and unregulated health care workers. UCPs, as the name connotes, are caregivers who are not licensed as health care providers and are known by many titles, including *home support workers*, *personal support workers*, *resident aides*, and *health care aides* (Harris & McGillis Hall, 2012). When a patient requires 24-hour care, a nurse manager must decide the type of nurse to be deployed to best meet the needs of the patient and whether supervised UCPs might be used.

The Role of the Staff Nurse

In the total patient care model, the staff nurse provides holistic care to a group of patients during a defined work time. The physical, emotional, and technical aspects of care are the responsibility of the assigned nurse. This model is especially useful in the care of very complex patients who need active symptom management provided by an RN or specially educated nurse—for example, a patient in an acute pain management setting or a

critical care unit. The staff nurse who is assigned to total patient care must complete the complex functions of care, such as assessment and teaching the patient and family, as well as the less complex functions of care, such as personal hygiene. Nurses have been found to like this model, as there is a greater degree of autonomy and control over the care provided to their patients (Duffield et al., 2010).

> **EXERCISE 15.1** You have recently accepted a position at a home health care agency that provides 24-hour care to patients. You are assigned a patient who has care provided by an RN during the day, a licensed practical nurse in the evening, and a home support worker at night. You are the day RN. You are concerned that the patient is not progressing well and that you are not getting adequate information from the other care providers indicating whether the patient's status is changing or improvements need to be made to the patient's care plan.
>
>   What specific assessments should you make to validate your concerns? How would you assess and justify any change in staffing? What recommendations would you make to the nurse manager, and why?

FUNCTIONAL NURSING

Functional nursing became popular in the 1940s during World War II, when there was a war-related shortage of nurses (Duffield et al., 2010). At the time, many nurses joined the armed forces to care for the soldiers. To provide care to patients at home, hospitals began to increase the number of practical nurses and UCPs.

Functional nursing is a model for providing patient care in which each regulated and unregulated member of the care team performs specific tasks for a large group of patients. These tasks are in part determined by the scope of practice defined for each type of caregiver and the complexity of care required. For example, an RN may be responsible for all assessments, and practical nurses and UCPs may be responsible for collecting data that can be used in assessments. Regarding treatments, one RN may administer all intravenous (IV) medications, a licensed practical nurse may provide oral medications, and two special care aides may do all hygiene tasks, check supplies, and take all vital signs (Fig. 15.2).

Regulated nurses (RNs, licensed practical nurses, registered practical nurses) have specialized nursing skills and advanced nursing skills, which means that the process of functionally dividing the nursing work among qualified personnel can become complicated. In

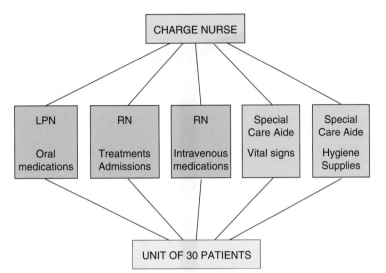

Fig. 15.2 Functional model of nursing care delivery. *LPN*, Licensed practical nurse; *RN*, registered nurse.

this model, the division of nursing work is similar to the division of work used in assembly-line systems in manufacturing. Just as an auto worker becomes an expert in attaching fenders to a new vehicle, the staff nurse becomes an expert in the specific tasks associated with their role in functional nursing. A charge nurse is an RN responsible for delegating and coordinating patient care and staff on a specific unit. In some cases, the charge nurse may ultimately be the only person familiar with all the needs of any individual patient.

Model Analysis

Functional nursing has several advantages. First, each nurse becomes efficient at specific tasks, and much work can be done in a short time. Another advantage is that UCPs can be trained and supported to perform a limited number of specific tasks very well. The organization benefits financially from this model because care can be delivered to a large number of patients by mixing a small number of regulated nurses and a larger number of UCPs.

Although financial savings may be the impetus for organizations to choose the functional nursing model, the disadvantages may outweigh the savings (Fig. 15.3). A major disadvantage is the fragmentation of care. The physical and technical aspects of care may be met, but the psychological and emotional needs of patients and families may be overlooked. Patients and families can become confused about who they should consult because many different health care providers are involved in their care per shift. Moreover, the different staff members may be so busy with their assigned tasks that they may not have time to communicate with one another about the patient's progress. Because no one care provider oversees patient care from beginning to end, the patient's response to care may be difficult to assess. Critical changes in patient status may go unnoticed. Fragmented care and ineffective communication can lead to patient and family dissatisfaction and frustration. Exercise 15.2 provides an opportunity to imagine how a patient would react to the functional method and also to imagine how the nurse may feel.

EXERCISE 15.2 Imagine that your mother is a patient at a hospital that uses the functional model of patient-care delivery. She just had her knee replaced, and when you ask the practical nurse for pain medication, the practical nurse responds, saying, "I'll tell the medication nurse." The medication nurse comes to the room and says that your mother's medication is to be administered intravenously and that the IV nurse will need to administer it. The IV nurse is busy starting an IV on another patient and cannot give your mother the medication for at least 10 minutes. This whole communication process has taken 40 minutes, and your mother is still in pain.

Discuss your perception of the effectiveness of the functional method of patient care in this situation. How effective do you think communication among staff is when a patient has a problem? What could be done to improve this situation?

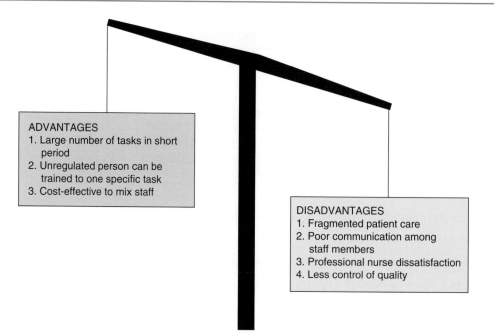

Fig. 15.3 Advantages and disadvantages of functional nursing.

The Role of the Nurse Manager

In the functional model, the nurse manager must be sensitive to the quality of patient care delivered and the institution's budgetary constraints. Because staff members are responsible only for their specific tasks, the role of achieving patient outcomes (the result of patient goals that are achieved through a combination of medical and nursing interventions with patient participation) becomes the nurse manager's responsibility.

Staff members can view this system as autocratic and may become discontented with the lack of opportunity for input. By using effective management and leadership skills, the nurse manager can improve the staff's perception that they lack independence. The manager can rotate assignments among staff within the legal limits of their role and as appropriate to each person's skill set to alleviate boredom with repetition. Staff meetings should be conducted frequently. They give staff the opportunity to express concerns and communicate about patient care and unit functions.

The Role of the Staff Nurse

The staff nurse becomes skilled at the tasks that are assigned to them, usually by the charge nurse. Clearly defined policies and procedures are used to complete

the physical aspects of care in a safe, efficient, and economical manner. However, the functional model of nursing may leave the professional nurse feeling frustrated because of the task-oriented role. Nurses are educated to care for the patient holistically and providing only a fragment of care to a patient may result in unmet personal and professional expectations of nurses.

> **EXERCISE 15.3** After 6 months of working on a unit that accommodates patients who have had general surgery, you realize that you are bored and frustrated with the functional model of delivering care. You have been administering all the IV medications and pain medications for your assigned patients. You have minimal opportunity to interact with the patients and learn about them, and you cannot be innovative in your care.
>
> What are some strategies you could use to resolve this dissatisfaction with the functional model of nursing care delivery?

The functional model of nursing care delivery works well in emergency and disaster situations. Each health care provider knows the expectations of the assigned role and completes the tasks quickly and efficiently.

Subacute care units, extended care facilities, and ambulatory clinics often use the functional model to deliver care efficiently.

TEAM NURSING

After World War II, the nursing shortage continued. Many female nurses who were in the military came home to start families instead of returning to the workforce. Because of criticisms of the functional model (discussed earlier), a new system of team nursing (a modification of functional nursing) was devised to improve nurse and patient satisfaction (Harris & McGillis Hall, 2012). "Care through others" is the hallmark of team nursing. This type of nursing care delivery remains in use, particularly when nursing shortages have resulted in organizations changing the staff mix (the proportion of regulated nurses and UCPs in a specific setting) and increasing the ratio of unregulated to regulated care providers.

In team nursing, a nurse team leader is typically responsible for coordinating a group of regulated and unregulated personnel to provide patient care to a group of patients. The team leader should ideally be a highly skilled leader, manager, and practitioner who assigns each member specific responsibilities according to role, licensure, education, ability, and the complexity of the care required. The members of the team report directly to the team leader, who then reports to the charge nurse or unit manager. Each unit has several teams, and patient assignments are made by each team leader. Fig. 15.4 provides an illustration of this model.

Model Analysis

Some advantages of team nursing, particularly when compared with the functional model, are improved patient satisfaction, decision making by staff nurses, which enhances their satisfaction, cost-effectiveness for the employer, and maximized team collaboration (Spruill & Heaton, 2014). Team nursing is seen by some nurses as the ideal approach to providing quality care (Rheaumeet al., 2015) and has been shown to lead to better system- and patient-level outcomes (Al Sayahet al., 2014). Many institutions and community health agencies currently use the team nursing method. Inpatient facilities may view team nursing as a cost-effective system because it works with a higher ratio of unregulated to regulated personnel. Thus, the organization has greater numbers of personnel for a designated amount of money.

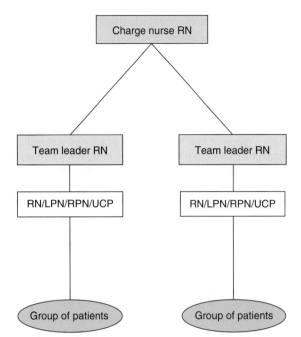

Fig. 15.4 Team nursing model. *LPN,* Licensed practical nurse; *RPN,* registered practical nurse; *RN,* registered nurse; *UCP,* unregulated care provider.

Team nursing has one major disadvantage, which can arise if the team leader does not have strong leadership skills. The team leader ideally should have excellent communication skills, delegation and conflict management abilities, strong clinical skills, and effective decision-making abilities to provide an optimal "team" environment for the members. The team leader must be sensitive to the needs of patients and, at the same time, be responsive to the needs of the staff providing direct care (Fairbrother et al., 2010; Shirey, 2008). The importance of communication in this model of care cannot be underestimated (Zimbudzi, 2013). When the team leader is not well prepared for this role, the team nursing method becomes a miniature version of the functional model, and the potential for fragmentation of care is high. For more details on developing leadership skills, see Chapter 2.

A recent systematic review of models of care in nursing (Fernandez et al., 2012) highlighted the predominance of team nursing models in the literature, suggestive of its popularity and longevity. In addition to the advantages of this model presented earlier, Fernandez and colleagues suggested that team nursing may present a better model for inexperienced staff to develop, especially in units where skill mix or experience is particularly diverse. In another systematic review designed to compare effectiveness of team nursing with total patient care, team nursing was also found to be more effective in achieving a number of outcomes (King et al., 2014).

EXERCISE 15.4 Think of a time when you worked with a group of four to six people to achieve a specific goal or accomplish a task. Perhaps in school you were grouped together to complete a project. Reflect on both the experience and the ability of the group to meet the set goal. Was one person the organizer or leader? If so, how was the leader selected? Think about your own role in the group. Do you see yourself as a leader or as a follower?

Now reflect on the membership of the whole group. Who assigned each member a component, or did you each determine what skills you possessed that would most benefit the group? Did you experience any conflict while working on this project? How did the concepts of group dynamics and leadership skills affect how your group achieved its goal? Are there any similarities between any of the models presented here and the function of your group?

The Role of the Nurse Manager

The nurse manager, charge nurse, and team leader must have management skills to effectively implement the team nursing method of nursing care delivery. In addition, the nurse manager must determine which nurses are particularly skilled and especially interested in becoming a charge nurse or team leader. Because the basic education of baccalaureate-prepared RNs emphasizes critical thinking and leadership concepts, they are likely candidates for such roles. The nurse manager should also provide an adequate staff mix and orient team members to the team nursing system by providing continuing education about leadership, management techniques, delegation, and team interaction. By addressing these factors, the nurse manager can help the teams function optimally.

The charge nurse functions as a liaison between the team leaders and other health care providers, because nurse managers are often responsible for more than one unit and may have other managerial responsibilities that take them away from the work of the unit. The charge nurse provides support to the teams on a shift-by-shift basis. Appropriate support from the charge nurse may

also include encouraging each team to solve its problems independently.

The team leader plans the care, delegates the work, and follows up with members to evaluate the quality of care for the patients assigned to their team. Ideally, the team leader updates the nursing care plans and facilitates patient-care conferences. Time constraints during the shift may prevent scheduling daily patient-care conferences or prevent some team members from attending those that are held.

The team leader must also face the challenge of changing team membership on a daily basis. Diverse work schedules and nursing staff shortages may result in daily changes in the staff mix of a team and a daily assignment change for team members. The team leader assigns the regulated and unregulated care providers to the type of patient care they are best prepared to deliver. Therefore the team leader must be knowledgeable about the legal limits of their scope of practice and associated skill sets of each role.

The Role of the Staff Nurse

Team nursing uses the strengths of each caregiver. Staff nurses, as members of the team, develop expertise in care delivery. Some members become known for their expertise in the psychomotor aspects of care. If one nurse is skilled in starting IVs, this nurse can then start all IVs for her team of patients. If another nurse is skilled in motivating postoperative patients to use the incentive spirometer and ambulate, this nurse would be assigned to the surgical patients. Under the guidance and supervision of the team leader, the collective efforts of the team become greater than the functions of the individual caregivers.

PRIMARY NURSING

A cultural revolution occurred in Canada and the United States during the 1960s. The revolution emphasized individual rights and independence from existing societal restrictions. This revolution influenced the nursing profession because nurses, as a group, were becoming dissatisfied with their lack of autonomy and began to focus more on professionalism and accountability (Shirey, 2008). In addition, the hierarchical nature of communication in team nursing caused further frustration. There was an awareness, at institutional levels, of declining quality of patient care. The search for increased autonomy and quality care led to the primary nursing model, which increases and emphasizes nurse accountability for patient outcomes.

Primary nursing, an adaptation of the total patient care model, was developed by Marie Manthey and introduced into hospital wards in 1968 as a model for organizing patient-care delivery that optimizes relationship-based care, in which one nurse functions autonomously as the patient's primary nurse throughout the hospital stay (Manthey, 2009; Nadeau et al., 2017). Primary nursing brought the nurse back to direct patient care. The primary nurse is a registered nurse who is accountable for managing all care aspects of specific patients throughout the hospital stay, even when the primary nurse is off duty (Carabetta et al., 2013; Nadeau et al., 2017). Care is organized using the nursing process (e.g., assess, diagnose, plan, implement, and evaluate). Advocacy and assertiveness are desirable leadership attributes for this care delivery model.

The primary nurse, preferably at least baccalaureate-prepared, is accountable for meeting outcome criteria – criteria that are the result of patient goals and that are expected to be achieved, and for communicating with all other health care providers about the patient (Fig. 15.5). Outcome criteria are the result of patient goals that are expected to be achieved through a combination of nursing and medical interventions. Consider the example of a patient with pulmonary edema who is admitted to a medical unit. His primary nurse admits him and then provides a written plan of care. When his primary nurse is not working, an associate nurse implements the plan. The associate nurse is a member of the primary nursing team and provides care to the patient according to the plan of care. If the patient develops additional complications, the associate nurse notifies the primary nurse, who has 24-hour accountability and responsibility. The associate nurse provides input to the patient's plan of care, and the primary nurse makes the appropriate alterations.

Model Analysis

Nadeau et al. (2017) cite numerous studies that identify the high quality of care, positive patient outcomes, and patient satisfaction all associated with primary care. Some studies found that primary care resulted in increased quality of care and patient satisfaction, whereas others found that the model made no difference to these parameters when compared with team nursing. Some findings suggest that although the use of primary care is favoured, and that there are some improvements in staff outcomes and patient well-being, more research is needed (Butler et al., 2011; Fernandez et al., 2012; Hodgkinson et al., 2011). Nurses practising primary nursing must possess a broad knowledge base and have highly developed nursing skills. Professionalism is promoted in this system of care delivery. Nurses experience increased job satisfaction because they can use their education to provide holistic and autonomous care

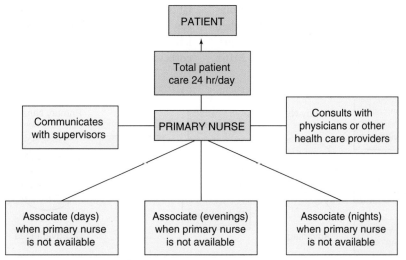

Fig. 15.5 Primary nursing model.

to patients. The high level of accountability for patient outcomes encourages nurses to further their knowledge and refine their skills to provide optimal patient care. However, if the primary nurse is not motivated or feels unqualified to provide holistic care, job satisfaction may decrease.

In primary nursing, patients and families are typically satisfied with the care they receive because they establish a relationship with the primary nurse and identify the caregiver as "their nurse." Because the patient's primary nurse communicates the plan of care, the patient can more easily move away from the sick role and begin to participate in their own recovery. By considering the sociocultural, psychological, and physical needs of the patient and family, the primary nurse can plan the most appropriate care with and for the patient and family.

A professional advantage of the primary nursing model is a decrease in the number of unregulated personnel. The ideal primary nursing system requires an all-nurse staff. The nurse can provide total care to the patient, from bed baths to complex patient and family education, even both at the same time. Unregulated personnel are not qualified to provide this level of inclusive care (Fig. 15.6).

A disadvantage of the primary nursing method is that the nurse may not have the experience or educational background to provide total care. Nurse leaders and managers are obligated to educate and support staff for a smooth transition from previous roles to the primary role. In addition, one has to ask whether the primary nurse is ready, willing, and capable of taking on this type of responsibility for patient care. In addition, communication gaps in relation to patient care may arise when another nurse is assigned to the patient when the primary nurse is away, or on days off (Klaasen et al., 2016).

> **EXERCISE 15.5** Mr. Faulkner is admitted to the medical unit with exacerbated congestive heart failure. Mohamed, RN, BSN, is Mr. Faulkner's primary nurse and will provide total care to Mr. Faulkner. Mohamed notes that this is Mr. Faulkner's third admission in six months for congestive heart failure–related symptoms. This is the first admission for which Mr. Faulkner has had a primary nurse.
>
> What do you think might be different about this hospital stay, with Mohamed providing primary nursing to Mr. Faulkner? Do you think any difference will occur in the continuity of care?

In times of nursing shortages, primary nursing may not be the model of choice. This model will not be effective if a unit has a large number of part-time nurses who are not available to assume the primary nurse role (which assumes responsibility for patients across shifts, over 24 hours). In addition, with the arrival of managed care in the 1990s, hospital stays were shorter than in the 1970s, when primary nursing became popular. Expedited stays make it challenging for primary nurses to adequately provide the depth of care required by primary nursing. If the patient is admitted on Monday and discharged on Wednesday, the primary nurse may have a difficult time meeting all patient needs before discharge if they are not working on Tuesday. The primary nurse must rely heavily on feedback from associate nurses, which can defeat the purpose of primary nursing. In addition, reductions in health care funding has caused administrators to consider ways to reduce the cost of care delivery. Because labour costs are the largest expense in health care delivery and nursing staff represent the largest portion of labour costs, attention has been given to reducing these costs with changes to the model of care delivery.

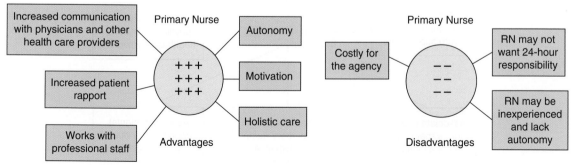

Fig. 15.6 Advantages and disadvantages of primary nursing. *RN*, Registered nurse.

The Role of the Nurse Manager

The primary nursing model can be modified to meet patient, nursing, and budgetary demands while maintaining the positive components that drove its conception. The nurse manager needs to determine the desire of staff to become primary nurses and then educate and support them accordingly. The associate nurses and all other health care providers need clearly defined roles. They also need to be aware of the primary nurse's role and the importance of communicating concerns directly to that nurse.

The nurse manager who implements this care delivery model experiences some benefits. Primary nursing provides the nurse manager an opportunity to demonstrate leadership capabilities, clinical competencies, and teaching abilities. In addition, the nurse manager roles of budget controller and unit quality manager remain in place. The traditional roles of delegation and decision making are typically relinquished to the autonomous primary nurse. The nurse manager functions as a role model, advocate, coach, and consultant.

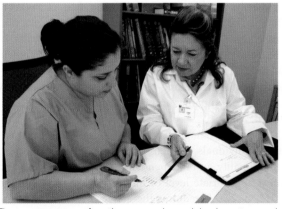

The nurse manager functions as a role model, advocate, coach, and consultant.

The Role of the Staff Nurse

The primary nurse utilizes many facets of the professional nursing role—caregiver, advocate, decision maker, teacher, collaborator, and manager. Because primary nurses cannot be physically present 24 hours a day, they must depend on associate nurses to provide care when they are not available. The associate nurse provides care using the plan of care developed by the primary nurse. Changes to the plan of care can be made by the associate nurse in collaboration with the primary nurse. This model provides consistency among nurses and shifts. To function effectively in this setting, staff nurses need experience and opportunities to be mentored in this role.

Because it usually is not financially possible for an employer to employ only highly qualified nurses, true primary nursing rarely exists. Some institutions have modified the primary nursing concept and implemented a partnership model to incorporate their current staff mix.

Primary Nursing Hybrid: Partnership Model

In the partnership model (or *co-primary nursing model*) of nursing care delivery, an RN is paired with another nurse (e.g., a technical assistant). The partner works with the RN consistently. When the partner is unregulated, the RN allows the assistant to perform basic nursing functions consistent with the provincial or territorial nursing regulatory body policy on delegation. Doing so frees the RN to provide "semi-primary care" to assigned patients. A partnership between an RN and a licensed practical nurse allows the latter to take more responsibility because the scope of practice for a licensed practical nurse is greater than that of a UCP. In some settings, the partnership is legitimized with an official contract to formalize the relationship. Rehabilitative care settings often use the partnership model to deliver care.

Primary Nursing Hybrid: Patient-Centred Care (PCC)/Patient-and Family-Centred Care (PFCC)

Another view of primary care is the care delivered in a patient-focused or patient-centred care model. Developed in the mid-1980s and 1990s, the patient-centred care model is a team-based approach to care incorporating principles of patient-centred care (PCC) (Hobbs, 2009; Mastro et al., 2014; Rathert et al. 2012) with the goals of (1) improving patient satisfaction and other patient outcomes, (2) improving worker job satisfaction, and (3) increasing efficiencies and decreasing costs. This model integrates principles from business and industry and features decentralized, efficient, coordinated, and integrated care (Pelzang, 2010). The interdisciplinary team formulates the plan of care after the primary nurse and the physician have assessed the patient.

Patient-focused care units require a change in the physical environment where care is delivered. Services such as laboratory tests and x-rays are decentralized to the bedside (Hobbs, 2009). Original models of a patient-focused care unit included an RN paired with a cross-trained technician who provided patient-side care including respiratory therapy, phlebotomy, and electrocardiographs. Modifications in this nurse-managed model include team members who provide direct care activities, such as recording vital signs, drawing blood, and bathing patients.

In a patient-focused care unit, the role and scope of the nurse manager expand. No longer is the individual just a manager of nurses. Now the nurse manager assumes the accountability and responsibility to manage nurses and staff from other, traditionally centralized departments. Because the care is focused on the needs of the patient and not the needs of the department, the role of the nurse manager becomes more sophisticated. The nurse manager orchestrates all the care activities required by the patient and family during the hospitalization. Implementing this philosophy and model of care requires building a culture of patient-centred care and developing a new understanding about one's beliefs,

attitudes, and practices toward providing care (Pelzang, 2010). A recent review of the literature suggests that although there is emerging evidentiary support for patient and family-centred care improving patient satisfaction, staff satisfaction, and enhanced staff–patient outcomes, there remain a limited number of studies that make up this evidence, and continuing work needs to be done in this area (Mastro et al., 2014).

NURSING CASE MANAGEMENT

Nursing case management, another nursing care delivery model, involves a complex set of expectations. Case management is the process of coordinating health care by planning, facilitating, and evaluating interventions across levels of care to achieve cost containment and quality outcomes.

The model first appeared in the 1920s when it was used by social workers and public health nurses working in community-based settings to identify and obtain resources for those most in need. In the 1970s, when a variety of factors forced health care costs upward, contemporary nursing case management began to be utilized in an effort to assure quality outcomes and cost containment (Fath, 2008; White & Hall, 2006).

In the United States during the mid-1980s, when acute care hospitals began to be reimbursed based on providing care for patient groups with particular diagnoses, nursing case management became a popular and effective method to manage shortened lengths of stay for patients and to prevent expensive hospital readmissions. In Canada, pieces of the case management model were adopted as length of stay and costs in health care settings were scrutinized; however, this change occurred primarily in community settings at first (Cawthorn, 2005). The nursing case management process can take place both "within the walls" and "beyond the walls" of the hospital. This model has been applied successfully in all health care settings, including acute, subacute, ambulatory settings, and long-term care facilities, as well as by insurance companies and in community settings (Cawthorn, 2005).

The case management model overall goal is to manage "individuals at their maximum level of comfort, functionality, and independence while at the lowest and most appropriate level of intensity of service" (Bower, 2012, p. 27). It requires the active involvement of the patient, the family, and diverse health care providers.

Health care organizations have tailored the case management system to meet their specific needs. Key elements of the case management model are the case manager and the clinical pathway.

Case Manager

Nurses, social workers, and other disciplines may work as case managers, bringing with them their discipline-specific skills and knowledge. Regardless of preparation, the National Case Management Network of Canada (2009) has identified the following six core standards to guide case manager practice.

1. *Client identification and eligibility for case management services:* Clients who meet the eligibility criteria for case management services are identified.
2. *Assessment:* In conjunction with the client, the case manager conducts and documents an individualized assessment using a structured process.
3. *Planning:* Client goals and priorities are documented and are reflected in the strategy for action agreed upon between the client and the case manager.
4. *Implementation:* Planned services, resources, and supports are initiated, coordinated, and adjusted as necessary.
5. *Evaluation:* A periodic reassessment is conducted to identify the client's current needs and to monitor progress within the client's individualized plan.
6. *Transition:* A process that supports disengagement or shift in the mechanisms for achieving client goals. (pp. 10–15)

Although there are inconsistencies among nursing professional associations about the education required for case managers, many prefer master's degree–prepared advanced practice nurses who have experience with the specific populations being served. Case managers are patient focused and outcome oriented. Their goal is to provide cost-effective care by integrating financial thinking into clinical services. In addition, case managers serve as advocates for the patient and the family. The National Case Management Network of Canada has developed the Canadian Core Competency Profile for Case Management Providers to guide case management. Case managers support client rights, are purposeful, are collaborative, support accountability, and strive for cultural competency (National Case Management Network of Canada, 2009).

Depending on the facility, several case managers may be engaged to coordinate care for all patients or one case manager may be assigned to a specific high-risk population (Fig. 15.7). It is essential for the case manager to have frequent interaction with patients and health care providers to achieve and evaluate expected outcomes.

Clinical Pathways

Many case managers use a clinical pathway to achieve patient outcomes. Also referred to as *multidisciplinary care pathways, integrated care pathways, critical pathways, care maps,* or *collaborative care pathways* (Kinsman et al., 2010), these patient-focused documents describe the clinical standards, necessary interventions, and expected outcomes for the patient at each stage of the treatment process or hospital stay. Clinical pathways are not appropriate for all patients and cannot replace professional clinical judgement; however, they

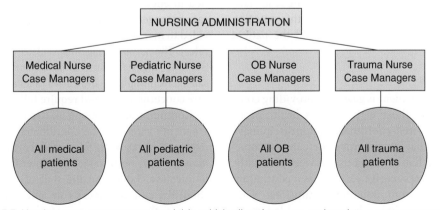

Fig. 15.7 Nursing case management model in which all patients are assigned to a case manager. *OB,* Obstetric.

do facilitate coordinated and well-organized care that links best available evidence to clinical practice (Rotter et al., 2010).

Clinical pathways are grids that outline the critical or key events expected to happen each day of a patient's hospitalization (D'Entremont, 2009). If a patient's progress deviates from the normal path, a variance is indicated. A variance alters the patient's progress through the normal clinical pathway. An analysis of variance is essential for effective utilization of a path. Circumstances that can cause a variance may be related to operations, the provider, patient, or clinical elements (De Bleser et al., 2006). Operational causes include broken equipment or interdepartmental delays. Changes in the practice pattern of the health care provider can affect the pathway and cause a variance. Complications in the patient's condition, such as a hemorrhage into the joint after total knee replacement, may increase total hospital days. A complication can inhibit the ability of the patient to meet a clinical indicator, and a patient's or family's refusal of a specific recommended component of care can create a variance.

Variances can be positive or negative. Negative variances occur when an action in care cannot take place. This may not have a major effect on patient's overall care; however, it can be a variance so extreme that the patient may need to come off the pathway altogether. A positive variance is an outcome that is achieved before it is expected (Kent & Chalmers, 2006). A patient undergoing a second hip replacement who attended preoperative classes and engaged in activities to "ready himself" for the surgery may actually leave the hospital sooner than predicted in a clinical path. The case manager on the orthopedic unit would view this outcome as a positive variance, as typically would the patient and family.

Model Analysis

Nursing case management is geared to providing comprehensive care for those with complex health problems. It delivers a well-coordinated multidisciplinary care experience that can improve the care outcome, decrease the length of stay, and use services efficiently. Families and patients receive care across a continuum of settings, often from different institutions. Case managers can often help break down invisible institutional barriers for the patient and family. Nurses often get a sense of satisfaction knowing that the patient and family received coordinated, quality care in a cost-effective manner across the spectrum of the illness or injury.

However, major obstacles exist in the implementation of case management services. Financial barriers, lack of administrative support, human resource inequities, turf battles, and a lack of information support systems have been identified as hurdles in the implementation of case management services (Powell & Tahan, 2010). Case management minimizes costs for those case types that have the potential of high resource consumption. Collaborative models of health care management that incorporate nurses, social workers, respiratory therapists, and physical or occupational therapists as case managers have demonstrated the ability to meet specific patient needs at significant cost savings (Powell & Tahan, 2010). Some health care institutions have developed departments of health care case management so that the professional background of each nurse case manager can be matched with the appropriate patient population and specific patient needs (Powell & Tahan, 2010).

The Role of the Nurse Manager

The nurse manager has increased demands when leading the case management system. The nurse manager must constantly assess whether resources are utilized appropriately, that care is delivered in the appropriate setting, and that case managers are adequately managing their caseloads—with particular attention to length of stay and cost (Cawthorn, 2005). Health care funding or institutional budgets for the care delivered can be tied to effective planning and care delivery within the case management process (e.g., incentives may be provided to meet specific targets, such as reducing infection rates). The nurse manager must also evaluate patient satisfaction, a key measure of quality of care. Low patient satisfaction might be indicative of a variety of service or care concerns and would require follow-up.

Communication among all departments involved in a patient's care must be coordinated. Because the case manager works with various departments, the nurse manager may need to facilitate interdepartmental communication. Educating the staff of other departments about the case manager's role and responsibilities will increase the effectiveness of the case management process.

The Role of the Staff Nurse

The staff nurse working with a patient who has a case manager as the coordinator of care provides patient care according to the case manager's specifications and must understand the extent of the case manager's role. Effective communication to facilitate care is the responsibility of both the case manager and the staff nurse.

CARE STRATEGIES THAT INFLUENCE CARE DELIVERY

Disease Management

Disease management has been in existence for many decades. However, in the late 1990s, disease management became a model of care that coordinates health care interventions and communication for those individuals whose self-care needs are significant (Lukewich et al., 2014). Those with chronic conditions who are viewed as higher consumers of health care dollars are the recipients of disease-managed care. Disease management programs for patients dealing with chronic illness build on the relationship with the health care team to prevent exacerbations and complications using evidence-informed guidelines and patient empowerment techniques to improve the overall health and well-being of the patient and family. The focus of this model of care is wellness, i.e., living well with a chronic disease. Determining the barriers to self-care is an essential element of successful disease-management programs.

Disease management programs consist of assessment to identify a specific population, comprehensive patient and family self-management education, use of evidence-informed practice guidelines, medical management based on treatment algorithms, and focused visits with the health care team in an ambulatory setting to assist with adherence to the treatment protocol (Powell & Tahan, 2010). Case managers often decide whether a patient meets the specific criteria for a disease-managed program.

Differentiated Nursing Practice (Staff Mix)

One factor that makes the development and implementation of any nursing care delivery model difficult is the variation in the level of education and experience of each nurse. Over the past 50 years, as multiple entry points to nursing (e.g., registered nurse, licensed practical nurse, bachelor of science in nursing) have grown and more is known about the length of time required for a nurse to move from novice to competent nurse (Benner, 2001), efforts have been made to document and validate differentiated nursing practice (Canadian Nurses Association [CNA], 2012b; Harris & McGillis Hall, 2012; Sharma et al., 2016; Suter et al., 2014).

Background of Differentiated Practice

Differentiated nursing practice, or staff mix, is a model of clinical nursing practice that combines different categories of health care personnel employed for the provision of direct client care (Harris & McGillis Hall, 2012) and therefore acknowledges the difference in each nurse's level of education, scope of employment and practice, professional standards, and organizational policies (CNA, 2012b).

In today's complex, fast-paced health care environment, nurses with a bachelor of science in nursing (BScN) practise at all points on the hospital pre-admission to post-discharge continuum, in the community, in long-term care facilities, and in various types of clinics. They develop and implement multi faceted plans for managing chronic disease, treating complex health conditions, and assisting in the transition from hospital to the community. They also collaborate with other disciplines, departments, and agencies and help design and facilitate a comprehensive, well-prepared discharge plan based on the unique needs of the patient and family. In Canada, all provinces except Quebec, require a bachelor's degree for nursing entry to practice or are in the process of moving to such a requirement.

Advanced nursing practice (ANP) (MacDonald et al., 2005) and advanced practice nurses (APN) (DiCenso et al., 2010) have been in existence in Canada for more than 40 years. In Canada, two advanced nursing practice roles are recognized: clinical nurse specialist (CNS) and the nurse practitioner (NP) (CNA, 2008). In most provinces and territories, a master's degree is required to achieve these designations. APNs function as clinical nurse specialists (CNS) or nurse practitioners (NP) (DiCenso et al., 2010). The CNS provides expert nursing care and plays a leading role in the development of clinical guidelines and protocols. They promote use of evidence, provide expert support and consultation, and facilitate system change. The NP provides direct care, focusing on health promotion and the treatment and management of health conditions. They have an expanded scope of practice that allows them to diagnose, order, and interpret diagnostic tests. They can also prescribe medications and perform certain procedures. Each province and territory has legislation in place that outlines the care and service permitted by an NP (CNA, 2018).

The varied educational backgrounds and philosophies of the nurses implementing a model of practice have a significant impact on the success of care delivery and the satisfaction of nurses and patients. This variation is further complicated by the experience of the nurse in the practice arena. Benner (2001), based on the Dreyfus model of skill acquisition, identified five stages of clinical competence for nurses: novice, advanced beginner, competent, proficient, and expert. Benner suggested that competence is typified by a nurse who has been on the job in the same or similar situations for 2 to 3 years. It follows that nurses who are either new graduates or in a new area of clinical practice may require more assistance than those with more experience. A group of nurses who are all at the novice or advanced beginner stage would be less likely than their more experienced counterparts to implement any type of delivery model effectively.

The competencies requirements entry-level nurses need to meet for safe and effective nursing practice are measured by national exams or entry to practice exams. For example, RN students across Canada take the National Council Licensure Examination (NCLEX) to assess their entry-level nursing practice competencies.

Differentiated Practice in the Clinical Setting

As the complexity of health care increases and the pressures of managed care rise, communication and critical thinking in nursing have become paramount. Differentiated practice in nursing can respond to changing health care systems, changing funding strategies, health human resource challenges, and rising acuities and complex health care needs in patients and their families.

However, despite a variety of efforts to differentiate the roles and competencies of nurses with various educational backgrounds and experience, the demands of the workplace, the chronic shortage of nurses, and the greater use of technology have made it difficult to differentiate nursing practice in many clinical settings, even among RNs with differing levels of education (Matthias, 2015). In addition, with the move away from more traditional models of nursing care delivery to models with emphasis on teamwork and interprofessional collaboration, the complexities

of determining staff or skill mix remain. Although the studies undertaken to look at staff mix and various outcomes have been criticized mainly because of strength of design, evidence from an increasing number of studies has shown an association between the level of in-hospital staffing by registered nurses (RNs) and patient mortality, adverse patient outcomes, and other quality measures (Needleman, 2017; Needleman et al., 2011; Sharma et al., 2016; Yang et al., 2015). As Sharma et al. (2016) have noted, finding the right staff mix is critically important in today's changing health care delivery landscape, workforce strategies, resource constraints, and changing patient needs across all care settings.

Clinical Nurse Leader

In response to a lack of differentiated practice in many health care settings and the increased emphasis on patient safety, the clinical nurse leader (CNL) role emerged in the early 2000s in Canada and is modelled on the American Association of Nursing description of the role. The CNL is a highly skilled master's degree–prepared nurse who has completed advanced studies in clinical care with a focus on the improvement of quality outcomes for specific patient populations at the point of care. The CNL coordinates and supervises the care provided by interdisciplinary team members. Like other leadership roles, the CNL role includes development of skills in preceptoring, mentoring, and coaching. The CNL may oversee the lateral integration of care for a distinct group of patients and may actively provide direct patient care in complex situations. The CNL uses evidence-informed practice to help ensure that patients benefit from the latest innovations in care delivery. The CNL collects and evaluates patient outcomes, assesses cohort risk, and has the decision-making authority to change care plans when necessary. This nurse functions as part of the interprofessional team by communicating, planning, and implementing care directly with other health care providers, including physicians, pharmacists, social workers, clinical nurse specialists, and nurse practitioners. The CNL is a leader in the health care delivery system in all settings in which health care is delivered, and implementation of the role may vary across settings (Schneider, 2014). Box 15.1 outlines the fundamental aspects of the CNL role, as defined by the AACN white paper on the clinical nurse leader (AACN, 2013).

BOX 15.1   Fundamental Aspects of the Clinical Nurse Leader

- Leadership in the care of the sick in and across all environments.
- Design and provision of health promotion and risk reduction services for diverse populations.
- Provision of evidence-based practice.
- Population-appropriate health care to individuals, clinical groups/units, and communities.
- Clinical decision making.
- Design and implementation of plans of care.
- Risk anticipation.
- Participation in identification and collection of care outcomes.
- Accountability for the evaluation and improvement of point-of-care outcomes.
- Mass customization of care.
- Patient and community advocacy.
- Education and information management.
- Delegation and oversight of care delivery and outcomes.
- Team management and collaboration with other health professional team members.
- Development and leverage of human, environmental, and material resources.
- Management and use of patient-care and information technology.
- Lateral integration for specified groups of patients.

American Association of Colleges of Nursing. (2013). Competencies and curricular expectations for clinical nurse leader education and practice. Retrieved from http://www.aacn.nche .edu/cnl/CNL-Competencies-October-2013.pdf.

The Synergy Model

Similar to the work of the AACN in developing the CNL, the American Association of Critical-Care Nurses adopted the Synergy Model as the framework for nursing practice as well as for the certification examination for the critical care nurse and the clinical nurse specialist. Some health care organizations have adopted this model as their model of care and it is being used in various health care settings (Ho et al., 2017). The Synergy Model identifies patient characteristics as "drivers" of the necessary competencies for nurses. Once patient priority needs are identified, the numbers and types of nurses are more accurately determined, creating a "synergy" between patient needs and nurse competencies. In settings with skill mix, staffing decisions are based on

legal scopes of practice and experience with the patient population.

The Synergy Model describes the following eight patient characteristics: resiliency, vulnerability, stability, complexity, resource availability, participation in care, participation in decision making, and predictability. The eight nursing competencies are clinical judgement, advocacy and moral employer, caring practices, facilitation of learning, collaboration, systems thinking, response to diversity, and clinical requirement (Kaplow & Reed, 2008). Each of the competencies is essential in providing holistic care to the patient. Depending on the acuity of the patient, some competencies emerge as priorities whereas others are used to a lesser extent (MacPhee et al., 2011). When there is synergy between the patient characteristics and the competency of the nurse, patient care is optimized (Brewer et al., 2007). The American Association of Critical-Care Nurses website provides information on the Synergy Model and its application in diverse care settings. Although the Synergy Model has been predominantly utilized in the United States, its use in Canada as a professional practice model has been explored in a pilot projects in British Columbia, Ontario, and Saskatchewan. Results of the pilot projects in British Columbia were positive, including enhanced communication among regulated and unregulated care providers and nursing leadership (British Columbia Nurses Union, 2010; Ho, et al. 2017; MacPhee et al., 2011).

Transforming Care at the Bedside

The variety of care delivery models and the complexity of patient needs, organizational structures, and technological advances require individual action to improve practice patterns in specific units. In 2003, the Robert Wood Johnson Foundation (https://www.rwjf.org) and the Institute of Healthcare Improvement (http://www .ihi.org) joined forces to create, test, and implement changes to dramatically improve care on medical and surgical units and enhance staff satisfaction (Osman & Nolan, 2013). The result was Transforming Care at the Bedside (TCAB), an initiative focused on empowering nurses and front-line staff in deciding on and implementing strategies that improve patient outcomes, facilitate collaborative team work, and support professional nursing practice.

The TCAB initiative is based on a set of five premises (Box 15.2) that serve as the underpinnings of four

BOX 15.2 Transforming Care at the Bedside Premises

- Patient-centred work redesign can create value-added care processes and result in better clinical outcomes and reduced costs.
- Effective care teams can have a positive impact on patient outcomes.
- Management practices and organizational culture have a significant impact on the work environment.
- Matching staff's knowledge and capabilities with work responsibilities enhances job satisfaction.
- Eliminating inefficiencies through work redesign enhances staff satisfaction and morale.

Viney, M., Batcheller, J., Houston, S., et al. (2006). Transforming Care at the Bedside: Designing new complex systems in an age of complexity. *Journal of Nursing Care Quality*, 21(2), 146.

BOX 15.3 Transforming Care at the Bedside Design Themes

- *Reliability:* The care for moderately sick patients who are hospitalized is safe, reliable, effective, and equitable.
- *Vitality:* Effective care teams continually strive for excellence within a joyful and supportive environment that nurtures professional formation and career development.
- *Patient-centredness:* Patient-centred care on medical/surgical units honors the whole person and family, respects individual values and choices, and ensures continuity of care.
- *Increased value:* All care processes are free of waste and promote continuous flow.

Modified from Viney, M., Batcheller, J., Houston, S., et al. (2006). Transforming Care at the Bedside: Designing new complex systems in an age of complexity. *Journal of Nursing Care Quality*, 21(2), 144, 146.

key design themes (Box 15.3). The four main categories serve as a framework for change and improving care on medical-surgical units.

The TCAB initiative was initially implemented at three pilot hospitals in the United States and was subsequently implemented in other hospitals across the United States and eventually Canada (Lavoie-Tremblay et al., 2013). The team members involved in implementation in each hospital began by asking "What do we know?" about each design theme. The group then was encouraged to tell stories about their work environment consistent with this theme. After the storytelling phase, the team members participated in a brainstorming session to come up with as many innovations as possible that could contribute to each theme. Innovations requiring minimal time and resources were then prioritized and selected for a rapid cycle trial. The CNA categorizes TCAB as an initiative for "improving work processes and optimizing the work of nurses" (CNA, n.d.).

Critical to practice changes, a rapid cycle trial is a process that encourages testing creative change on a small scale while determining potential impact (see Chapter 19 for more information on leading change). The process involves four stages—Plan-Do-Study-Act (PDSA). During the *plan phase*, the team defines the objectives and predicts how the identified change would contribute to design, how the change would occur, and what data collection methods would be needed. During the *do phase*, the team focuses on whether the change occurred as expected and, if not, what interfered with the plan. During the *study phase*, the team determines whether the innovation worked as predicted and what knowledge was gained. During the *act phase*, the team plans next actions.

The team and staff participating in the study rate the innovation in terms of adoption, adaptation, or discontinuation. The innovation is implemented for a short period (from a day to several weeks) at least twice during the prototype-testing phase and the pilot-testing phase. If the outcome of testing the innovation is positive, the new design can be easily spread to other participating sites.

CONCLUSION

Each nursing care delivery model identified in this chapter has strengths and weaknesses. There is no perfect method for delivering nursing care to all groups of patients and their families. Because of the variety of settings and organizational sizes, no one model addresses all needs. In addition, in times of local or national emergencies, the typical model of care may be replaced with one designed to best fit the urgency of the situation.

This chapter describes the traditional nursing care delivery models that have been used since the 20 century. The complexity of the current health care system, the shortage of health care providers, and the pressures to ensure patient safety and cost-effective care have led many organizations to explore alternative models to deliver patient care. The CNA (2011, p. 21) suggests that "nursing care delivery model design and staff-mix decision-making" is central to the future of health care and nursing in Canada. Furthermore, Ginette Rodger, past president of the CNA, stated that given the current state of interprofessional collaboration in health care settings, understanding the differences between "organizational" and "nursing care" delivery models is necessary and that specific, well-developed models of nursing care delivery need to exist (CNA, 2011, p. 4). Emerging nursing care delivery models, which are variations of traditional models of care, are being considered and tested in Canada, and efforts are being made to gain a better understanding of the principles needed to guide the development of nursing care delivery models as demonstrated by the Literature Perspective and the Research Perspective.

LITERATURE PERSPECTIVE

Resource: Wells, J., Manuel, M., & Cunning, G. (2011). Changing the model of care delivery: Nurses' perceptions of job satisfaction and care effectiveness. *Journal of Nursing Management*, 19: 777–785.

Wells, Manuel, and Cunning (2011) describe the implementation and evaluation of an adaptation of a total patient care (TPC) model in two acute care nursing units. Reports from nurses and administration that the traditional team nursing model of care contributed to inconsistent patient care and blurred lines of responsibility and accountability, and that patient confidentiality and privacy were at risk, prompted the exploration for alternative models of care. The authors used Lewin's change model (see Chapter 19) to support the implementation of the new TPC model of care. The authors initially asked the nursing staff what components they would like to see in the new model of care. Based on the suggestions from the nursing staff, TPC seemed to be the model most fitting. In the next phase, the physical environment of the nursing units was changed to facilitate the new model of care (e.g., centralized nursing station, separate medication room). Furthermore, educational sessions were offered to all nursing staff that provided an overview of the gaps between the old and new existing models of care, the potential benefits to nurses and patients of using TPC, and a review of the processes related to TPC (which included highlighting the nursing roles and scopes of practice of those working within the TPC, such as RNs, licensed practical nurses, or patient care coordinators). As the implementation proceeded, efforts were made to en-sure that those involved in the transition between models of care were part of the decision-making process regarding nursing practice issues.

This model of care was implemented in two acute nursing units with 52 beds and 78 permanent full-time staff in a regional health care facility. Job satisfaction was measured using the Index of Work Satisfaction (IWS) scale, empowerment was measured using the two subscales of responsibility and participation from the Perception of Empowerment Instrument (PEI), and the Care Delivery Effectiveness (CDE) tool was used to measure nurses' perception of the effectiveness of the provision of care. Data were collected before the change and again at 3 and 6 months after the change from nurses who had been on the unit for at least 6 months. Although adding to the limited and somewhat conflicting body of literature on TPC, the results suggested that TPC, or a modification of it, was more effective than the team nursing model previously used in the units; however, job satisfaction levels remained the same.

Implications for Practice

Although the study was undertaken in only one hospital over a discrete period of time, the results suggest that TPC is perceived by nurses to be a more effective nursing care delivery model than team nursing. The results also suggest that when planned change in nursing practice is being considered, involving and engaging the nursing staff and having organizational support is key. This is congruent with the guiding principles for nursing care delivery models outlined by the CNA (2012a).

RESEARCH PERSPECTIVE

Resource: Canadian Nurses Association. (2012a). *Nursing care delivery models: Canadian consensus on guiding principles*. Ottawa, ON. Retrieved from https://www.cna-aiic.ca/-/media/cna/page-content/pdf-en/nursing_care_delivery_models_e.pdf

The aim of this project was to gain consensus on guiding principles for decision making regarding nursing care delivery models. The project built upon three previously completed initiatives by the CNA related to nursing care delivery models and **staff mix**. These initiatives included an invitational round table discussion (CNA, 2011), a comprehensive literature review (Harris & McGillis Hall, 2012), and newly developed core principles for staff mix decision making (CNA, 2012b), all of which endeavoured to improve the transfer of knowledge into the practice setting related to nursing care delivery models and staff mix.

The article describes research undertaken to obtain a pan-Canadian consensus on overarching principles that could guide decision making about nursing care delivery models. Expert nurses from across the country were asked to rate and comment on 18 guiding principles, based on the previously mentioned initiatives. The survey results provided a prioritized list of 10 guiding principles for which consensus had been achieved:

1. Responding to the health care needs of patients, families, and communities is integral to the nursing care delivery model.
2. Staff competencies (knowledge, skills, abilities, attitudes) are a part of the nursing care delivery model.
3. The nursing care delivery model reflects an organization's patient population, best practices, professional standards, and research evidence.
4. Front-line nursing staff and nursing management are engaged in decision making about the nursing care delivery model.
5. The nursing care delivery model promotes quality and safe care, which is cost-effective and sustains the system.
6. Systematically collected data about patient outcomes and nursing human resources inform decisions about the nursing care delivery model.
7. A formal plan for the nursing care delivery model, including communication and educational strategies, considers patient and staff needs as well as the organizational mission.
8. Organizational structure and leadership across all levels supports the nursing care delivery model.
9. Staff mix based on patient care needs is a component of the nursing care delivery model.
10. Technology is a required component for implementing the nursing care delivery model. (CNA, 2012b, p. 17)

In addition to the need to consider all 10 guiding principles in the design of nursing care delivery models, the project's researchers also identified key messages from their research, which included involving front-line staff in the development of nursing care delivery models, that nursing care delivery models cannot be designed in isolation and need to consider the interdisciplinary nature of health care, and that nursing care delivery models must be flexible to meet individual patient needs.

Implications for Practice

Although the CNA's report highlights the principles needed to underpin nursing care delivery models, in a number of provinces, new "blended" models of care are being implemented. The blended models have aspects of traditional nursing care models but include elements of collaborative and patient-centred care to address current trends (Harris & McGillis Hall, 2012) while also responding to changes in funding, technology, and characteristics of patients cared for in health care organizations.

In Canada, examples of innovative nursing care delivery models being developed, implemented, and tested include the following:

1. Collaborative Nursing Practice (CNP) Acute Model (Vancouver Coastal Health Authority).
2. Nursing Demonstration Project: Building Better Nursing Care Delivery Models (Sunnybrook Health Sciences Centre).
3. Model of Care Initiative in Nova Scotia (a joint initiative for acute inpatient care).
4. Community Health Nursing Practice Models (Community Health Nurses of Canada).
5. The Ottawa Hospital's *Inter-Professional Model of Patient Care* (IPMPC) (CNA, 2011).

❓ A SOLUTION

As a patient care coordinator (PCC), David is responsible for ensuring the delivery of excellent patient care to patients admitted to a medical unit. The nurses on the unit were committed to this approach but encountered communication challenges. Collaborating with other members of the leadership team, receiving input from the staff nurses, and seeking out best practices from colleagues in the health care community provided David with a solution. They initiated a sit-down report for all nurses called the "team huddle" and established a "nurse buddy" system. The "team huddle" occurs at the beginning of the shift after each nurse has obtained the report from the nurse on the previous shift and has had the opportunity to review each patient's plan of care. The nurses are paged and notified that the "team huddle" will occur. The charge nurse who surveys each nurse on their workload and the projected times they would need assistance with patient care facilitates the "team huddle."

The "nurse buddy" system was initiated to provide the patient-side nurse with an immediate resource—someone other than the charge nurse. These two nurses provide each other with support on an "as-needed" basis. The "buddy" is assigned at the time the patient assignments are created and is in close proximity.

The staff response has been very positive. The charge nurse has a better understanding of the status of the patients, families, and staff. Staff nurses state they are more engaged, and thus better able to be involved with the unit's operational needs for the day. Patient care is planned collaboratively so that each nurse is available to the "buddy" when needed. Overall, teamwork and communication have been enhanced.

Would this be a suitable approach for you? Why or why not?

▌THE EVIDENCE

Wolf and Greenhouse (2007) recognized the need for health care system change and the importance of a well-developed care delivery model in addressing these changes. They suggested that it is not necessary to "start from scratch" in developing a model; many valuable lessons, learned from experience and scientific evidence, can be incorporated into new models. They also suggested three factors beyond the experience of the past should be considered in developing a new model. First, major health care trends, such as changes in patients, health care providers, information technology, and financing, as well as medical advances, must be considered. Second, what patients want and need should be identified. Some patient needs identified by the authors were traditionally expected, such as wanting a competent provider to meet their physical, emotional, and spiritual needs. However, others were not, such as wanting a provider to help sort through available information to find a solution that would be effective for them. Third, Wolf and Greenhouse (2007) suggested that developers must make structural (Who will do what?), process (How will it get done?), and outcome (What difference will it make?) decisions to ensure that the new model is in strategic alignment with the organization, sustainable over time, and can be replicated. The authors provide specific questions that can be helpful in making these structural, process, and outcome decisions.

✴ NEED TO KNOW NOW

- Consider the model of nursing care delivery used by an organization when selecting a position for employment.
- Anticipate that a national or local emergency could alter normal care delivery.

- Determine whether there are experienced nurses who provide clinical leadership in specific settings.

CHAPTER CHECKLIST

The roles of the nurse manager and staff nurse vary with each nursing care delivery model. Regardless of the model, the nurse manager must have strong leadership and management skills for the model to be effective. Numerous issues must be considered when a care delivery model is implemented. Without a competent manager with strong leadership skills and organizational support, none of the discussed models would be effective.

- A nursing care delivery model is the method nurses use to provide care to patients.
- Five models of nursing care delivery were presented, along with their advantages and disadvantages:
  - The *patient allocation*, or *total patient care*, model focuses on total patient care for a specific time period.
    - The nurse manager must consider the expense of this system and identify the level of education and communication skills of all staff members.
  - *Functional nursing* emphasizes task-oriented care for a large group of patients.
    - The nurse manager is responsible for achieving patient outcomes, whereas staff members are responsible only for their specific tasks.
    - The functional model is most often used in subacute care facilities.
  - In the *team nursing model*, a small team provides care to a group of patients.
    - The nurse manager needs strong management, critical thinking, and leadership skills.
    - The nurse manager functions as role model, advocate, coach, consultant, budget controller, and unit quality manager.
    - The partnership model pairs an RN with a partner (e.g., a technical assistant).
    - The patient-focused care unit employs a primary nurse and multi-skilled team members.
  - In the *primary nursing model* a registered nurse working with a team is responsible for planning and delivering care for a consistent group of patients.
    - The primary nurse is accountable for the patients' care 24 hours a day, from admission through discharge.

- The primary nurse plans, collaborates, communicates, and coordinates all aspects of patient care with other nurses as well as other disciplines.
- When the primary nurse is not working, an associate nurse implements the plan to provide care to the patient according to the primary nurse's specifications.
- The ideal primary nursing system requires an all-nurse staff.
- The *nursing case management model* is outcome-focused and is facilitated by a case manager, who directs unit-based care using a clinical pathway.
  - The nurse manager faces increased demands to move the patient through the system as quickly as possible.
  - Managed care is a way of organizing patient-care delivery with cost savings as the main goal.
  - The case manager plays a vital role in the management of care.
- The nurse manager and charge nurse are responsible for directing patient care, regardless of the nursing care delivery system. They apply the following key leadership and management concepts when directing patient care:
  - Accountability
  - Delegation
  - Critical thinking
  - Communication
  - Promotion of autonomy
  - Collaboration
- The *disease management model* of care assists those with chronic illnesses to manage their self-care to achieve optimal health.
  - The concept of differentiated nursing practice emphasizes two levels of nursing practice: technical and professional.
  - Each type of nurse has a specific role and particular responsibilities based on the nurse's education, experience, and clinical expertise.
  - All the nursing roles complement one another.
- Emerging models of professional nursing practice continue to evolve.

▮ TIPS FOR SELECTING A CARE DELIVERY MODEL

- Look at the organization and the population being served when selecting a care delivery model.
- Consider the organizational structure and processes when selecting the care delivery model.
- Understand that all models have advantages and disadvantages, and none is ideal.

- Know that every model has specific expectations for both managers and staff.
- Determine whether there are experienced nurses who provide clinical leadership in specific settings.

Visit the Evolve website for Suggested Readings, Internet Resources, and additional resources related to the content in this chapter: http://evolve.elsevier.com/Canada/Yoder-Wise/leading/.

REFERENCES

Agency for Clinical Innovation. (2013). *Understanding the process to develop a model of care.* New South Wales, Australia: Author. Retrieved from: https://www.aci.health.nsw.gov.au/__data/assets/pdf_file/0009/181935/HS13-034_Framework-DevelopMoC_D7.pdf.

Al Sayah, F., Szafran, O., Robertson, S., Bell, N., & Williams, B. (2014). Nursing perspectives on factors influencing interdisciplinary teamwork in the Canadian primary care setting. *Journal of Clinical Nursing, 23,* 2968–2979. https://doi.org/10.1111/jocn.12547.

American Association of Colleges of Nursing (AACN). (2013). *Competencies and curricular expectations for clinical nurse leader education and practice.* Retrieved from: http://www.aacnnursing.org/Portals/42/Academic Nursing/CurriculumGuidelines/CNL-Competencies-October-2013.pdf.

Benner, P. (2001). *From novice to expert: Excellence and power in clinical nursing practice.* Upper Saddle River, NJ: Prentice Hall.

Bower, K. (2012). Managing care: The crucial nursing-case management partnership. *Nurse Leader, 10*(6), 26–29.

Brewer, B. B., Wojner-Alexandrov, A. W., Triola, N., Pacini, C., Rust, J. E., & Kerfoot, K. (2007). AACN Synergy Model's characteristics of patients: Psychometric analyses in a tertiary care health system. *American Journal of Critical Care, 16*(2), 158–167.

British Columbia Nurses Union. (2010). *Provincial nursing workload project: Final report.* Burnaby, BC: Author. Retrieved from: https://www.bcnu.org/Documents/pnwp_report.pdf.

Butler, M., Collins, R., Drennan, J., Halligan, P., O'Mathuna, D. P., Schultz, T. J., et al. (2011). Hospital nurse staffing models and patient and staff-related outcomes. *Cochrane Database of Systematic Reviews, 7*(6). https://doi.org/10.1002/14651858.CD007019.pub2.

Canadian Nurses Association. (2008). *Advanced nursing practice: A national framework.* Ottawa, ON: Author. Retrieved from: https://www.cna-aiic.ca/-/media/cna/page-content/pdf-en/anp_national_framework_e.pdf.

Canadian Nurses Association. (2011). *Invitational round table. Nursing care delivery models and staff mix: Using evidence in decision-making.* Ottawa, ON: Author. Retrieved from: https://www.cna-aiic.ca/~/media/cna/page-content/pdf-en/roundtable_report_evidence_decision_e.pdf?la=en.

Canadian Nurses Association. (2012a). *Nursing care delivery models: Canadian consensus on guiding principles.* Ottawa, ON: Author. Retrieved from: https://www.cna-aiic.ca/~/media/cna/page-content/pdf-en/nursing_care_delivery_models_e.pdf.

Canadian Nurses Association. (2012b). *Staff mix decision-making framework for quality nursing care.* Ottawa, ON: Author. Retrieved from: https://cna-aiic.ca/~/media/cna/page-content/pdf-en/staff_mix_framework_2012_e.pdf.

Canadian Nurses Association. (2018). *Nurse practitioners.* Retrieved from: https://www.cna-aiic.ca/en/nursing-practice/the-practice-of-nursing/advanced-nursing-practice/nurse-practitioners.

Canadian Nurses Association, (n.d.). RN and baccalaureate education. Retrieved from: https://www.cna-aiic.ca/en/nursing-practice/the-practice-of-nursing/education/rn-baccalaureate-education

Carabetta, M., Lombardo, K., & Kline, N. (2013). Implementing primary care in the perianesthesia setting using a relationship-based care model. *Journal of Perianesthesia Nursing, 28*(1), 16–20.

Cawthorn, L. (2005). Online exclusives: Discharge planning under the umbrella of advanced nursing practice case manager. *Nursing Leadership, 18*(4). https://doi.org/10.12927/cjnl.2005.19033. Retrieved from: http://www.longwoods.com/content/19033.

D'Entremont, B. (2009). Clinical pathways: The Ottawa Hospital experience. *Canadian Nurse, 105*(5), 8–9.

De Bleser, L., De Waele, K., Vanhaecht, K., Vlayen, J., & Sermeus, W. (2006). Defining pathways. *Journal of Nursing Management, 14*(7), 553–563.

DiCenso, A., Bryant-Lukosius, D., Martin-Misener, R., Donald, F., Abelson, J., Bourgeault, I., et al. (2010). Factors enabling advanced practice nursing role integration in Canada [Special issue]. *Nursing Leadership, 23*, 211–238.

Dubois, C.-A., D'amour, D., Tchouaket, E., Clarke, S., Rivard, M., & Blais, R. (2013). Associations of patient safety outcomes with models of nursing care organization at unit level in hospitals. *International Journal for Quality in Health Care, 25*(2), 110–117.

Duffield, C., Roche, M., Diers, D., Catling-Paull, C., & Blay, N. (2010). Staffing, skill mix, and the model of care. *Journal of Clinical Nursing, 19*, 2242–2251.

Fairbrother, G., Jones, A., & Rivas, K. (2010). Changing model of nursing care from individual patient allocation to team nursing in the acute inpatient environment. *Contemporary Nurse, 35*(2), 202–220.

Fath, L. (2008). A primer for nursing case management. *Paediatrics and Child Health, 18*(1), S84–S86.

Fernandez, R., Johnson, M., Tran, D., & Miranda, C. (2012). Models of care in nursing: A systematic review. *International Journal of Evidence-Based Healthcare, 10*, 324–337.

Harris, A., & McGillis Hall, L. (2012). *Evidence to inform staff mix decision-making: A focused literature review.* Ottawa, ON: Canadian Nurses Association. Retrieved from: https://www.cna-aiic.ca/~/media/cna/page-content/pdf-en/staff_mix_literature_review_e.pdf.

Ho, E., Principi, E., Cordon, C., Amenudzie, Y., Kotwa, K., Holt, S., et al. (2017). The synergy tool: Making important quality gains within one healthcare organization. *Administrative Sciences, 7*(32), 1–8.

Hobbs, J. L. (2009). A dimensional analysis of patient-centered care. *Nursing Research, 58*(1), 52–62.

Hodgkinson, B., Haesler, E. J., Nay, R., O'Donnell, M. H., & McAuliffe, L. P. (2011). Effectiveness of staffing models in residential, subacute, extended aged care settings on patient and staff outcomes. *Cochrane Database of Systematic Reviews, 6.* https://doi.org/10.1002/14651858.CD006563.pub2.

Kaplow, R., & Reed, K. (2008). The AACN Synergy Model for patient care: A nursing model as a force of magnetism. *Nursing Economics, 26*(1), 17–25.

Kent, P., & Chalmers, Y. (2006). A decade on: Has the use of integrated care pathways made a difference in Lanarkshire? *Journal of Nursing Management, 14*(7), 508–520.

King, A., Long, L., & Lisy, K. (2014). Effectiveness of team nursing compared with total patient care on staff well-being when organizing nursing work in acute care ward settings: A systematic review protocol. *JBL Library of Systematic Reviews & Implementation Reports, 12*(1), 59–73.

Kinsman, L., Rotter, T., James, E., Snow, P., & Willis, J. (2010). What is a clinical pathway? Development of a definition to inform the debate. *BMC Medicine, 8*(31), 1–3.

Klassen, K., Groenewegen, T., Mitchell, L., & Wilson, S. (2016). From primary nurse collaborative nursing care team: Early feedback on a new model. *Healthcare Management Forum, 29*(3), 121–125.

Lavoie-Tremblay, M., O'Conner, P., Harripaul, A., Biron, A., Ritchie, J., Lavigne, G., et al. (2013). The effect of Transforming Care at the Bedside initiative on healthcare teams' work environments. *Worldviews on Evidence-Based Nursing, 11*(1), 16–25.

Lukewich, J., Edge, D. S., Vandenkerkhof, E., et al. (2014). Nursing contributions to chronic disease management in primary care. *Journal of Nursing Administration, 44*(2), 103–110.

MacDonald, M., Schrieber, R., & Davis, L. (2005). *Exploring new roles for advanced nursing practice: A discussion paper.* Ottawa, ON: Canadian Nurses Association. Retrieved from: https://www.cna-aiic.ca/-/media/cna/page-content/pdf-fr/exploring_new_roles_anp-05_e.pdf.

MacPhee, M., Wardrop, A., Campbell, C., et al. (2011). The synergy professional practice model and its patient characteristics tool: A staff empowerment strategy. *Nursing Leadership, 24*(3), 42–56.

Mastro, K., Flynn, L., & Pruester, C. (2014). Patient-and-family-centered care: A call to action for new knowledge and innovation. *JONA, 44*(9), 446–451.

Manthey, M. (2009). The 40th anniversary of primary nursing: Setting the record straight. *Creative Nursing, 15*, 36–38.

Matthias, A. D. (2015). Making the case for differentiation of registered nurse practice: Historical perspectives meet contemporary efforts. *Journal of Nursing Education and Practice, 5*(4), 108–114.

Nadeau, K., Pinner, K., Murphy, K., & Belderson, K. (2017). Perceptions of a primary nursing care model in a pediatric hematology/oncology unit. *Journal of Pediatric Oncology Nursing, 34*(1), 28–34.

National Case Management Network of Canada. (2009). *Canadian standards of practice for case management.* Author. Retrieved from: http://www.ncmn.ca/Resources/Documents/standards_of_practices_english-2014.pdf.

Needleman, J. (2017). Nursing skill mix and patient outcomes. *BMJ Quality & Safety, 26*, 525–528.

Needleman, J., Buerhaus, P., Pankratz, S., Leibson, C., Stevens, S., & Harris, M. (2011). Nursing staffing and inpatient hospital mortality. *New England Journal of Medicine, 364*, 1037–1045.

Osman, A., & Nolan, B. (2013). Critical evaluation of transforming care at the bedside application in a multi-model nursing practice: A reflect review. *Journal of Nursing Education and Practice, 3*(8), 67–74.

Pelzang, R. (2010). Time to learn: Understanding patient-centered care. *British Journal of Nursing*, *19*(4), 912–917.

Powell, S. K., & Tahan, H. A. (2010). *Case management: A practical guide for education and practice* (3rd ed.). Philadelphia, PA: Wolters Kluwer.

Rathert, C., Wyrwich, M., & Boren, S. (2012). Patient-centered care and outcomes: A systematic review of the literature. *Medical Care Research and Review*, *70*(4), 351–379.

Rheaume, A., Dionne, S., Gaudet, D., Allain, M., Belliveau, E., Boudreau, L., et al. (2015). The changing boundaries of nursing: A qualitative study of the transition to a new nursing care delivery model. *Journal of Clinical Nursing*, *24*, 2529–2537.

Rotter, T., Kinsman, L., James, E. L., Machotta, A., Gothe, H., Willis, J., et al. (2010). Clinical pathways: Effects on professional practice, patient outcomes, length of stay and hospital costs (Review). *Cochrane Database of Systematic Reviews*, *7*.

Schneider, J. (2014). Clinical nurse leader. *Home Healthcare Nurse*, *32*(9), 563–564.

Sharma, K., Hastings, S., Suter, E., & Bloom, J. (2016). Variability of staffing and staff mix across acute care units in Alberta, Canada. *Human Resources for Health*, *14*(74), 1–8.

Shirey, M. R. (2008). Nursing practice models for acute and critical care: Overview of care delivery models. *Critical Care Nursing Clinics of North America*, *20*(4), 365–373.

Spruill, C., & Heaton, A. (2014). Designing an innovative nursing care delivery model to promote continuity of care. *Journal of Obstetric, Gynecologic & Neonatal Nursing*, *43*(Suppl. 1), S40-S40.

Suter, E., Deutschlander, S., Makwarimba, E., Wilhelm, A., Jackson, K., & Lyons, S. (2014). Workforce utilization in three continuing care facilities. *Health Sociology Review*, *23*(1), 65–76.

Viney, M., Batcheller, J., Houston, S., & Belcik, K. (2006). Transforming Care at the Bedside: Designing new care systems in an age of complexity. *Journal of Nursing Care Quality*, *21*(2), 143–150.

Wells, J., Manuel, M., & Cunning, G. (2011). Changing the model of care delivery: Nurses' perceptions of job satisfaction and care effectiveness. *Journal of Nursing Management*, *19*, 777–785.

White, P., & Hall, M. E. (2006). Mapping the literature of case management nursing. *Journal of the Medical Library Association*, *94*(Suppl. 2), E99–E106.

Wolf, G., & Greenhouse, P. (2007). Blueprint for design: Creating models that direct change. *Journal of Nursing Administration*, *37*(9), 381–387.

Yang, P.-H., Hung, C.-H., & Chen, Y.-C. (2015). The impact of three nursing staff models on nursing outcomes. *Journal of Advanced Nursing*, *71*(8), 1847–1856.

Zimbudzi, E. (2013). Discovering the untapped benefits of team nursing in an acute haemodialysis unit of a major teaching hospital. *Journal of Nursing Education and Practice*, *3*(8), 149–153.

16

Staffing and Scheduling

Susan Sportsman,
Adapted by Bhavik B. Patel

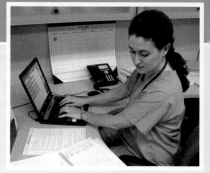

This chapter explores research regarding the relationship between staffing and various nurse and patient outcomes. It considers the interrelationship between the personnel budget and staffing plan. It also discusses measures for evaluating unit productivity and the impact of various staffing and scheduling strategies on overall staff satisfaction and continuity of patient care. These key points are critical to nurse managers' ability to deliver safe and effective care in their areas of responsibility while maintaining a high degree of employee satisfaction in the unit. Understanding the impact of nursing-sensitive indicators on patient outcomes helps managers control the unit's labour expenses. The ability to use this information and communicate about staffing to employees is critical to effectively managing productive services and being a valuable member of the leadership team.

OBJECTIVES

- Evaluate the impact of patient and hospital factors, nurse characteristics, nurse staffing, nurse outcomes, and other organizational factors that influence staff and patient outcomes.
- Relate how casual staff, float pools, overtime, mandatory overtime, and the use of supplemental agency staff affect nursing staff satisfaction and patient-care outcomes.

- Integrate current research into principles on effectively managing staff.
- Understand that scheduling seeks to meet patients' needs, nurses' personal scheduling needs, and budgetary needs in a balanced and fair manner.
- Understand and be able to evaluate activity reports on a unit's staffing and productivity.

TERMS TO KNOW

average daily census (ADC)
average length of stay (ALOS)
cost centre
direct care hours
factor evaluation system
fixed full-time equivalent (FTE)
forecast
full-time equivalent (FTE)
indirect care hours

labour cost per unit of service
mandatory overtime
nonproductive hours
nurse outcomes
nursing productivity
overtime
patient outcomes
percentage of occupancy
productive hours

prototype evaluation system
scheduling
staffing
staffing plan
unit of service
variable full-time equivalent (FTE)
variance report
workload

evolve *Go to Evolve http://evolve.elsevier.com/Canada/Yoder-Wise/leading/ to access the full chapter.*

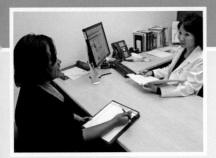

17

Selecting, Developing, and Evaluating Staff

Arden Krystal

Two of the most important functions of a nurse manager are interviewing and hiring employees for an organization. Once hired, it is essential that individuals understand the expectations associated with their role. Role clarity can improve performance, increase job satisfaction, and improve the quality of care delivered. Understanding role stress and ambiguity and how to avoid it is essential for the nurse manager and the employee to follow throughout the process of role development. This chapter also explores the process and tools of performance review as well as the role of the nurse manager as coach who empowers employees to grow as followers and develop their leadership skills in a learning environment.

OBJECTIVES

- Understand the concepts of role clarity, stress, and ambiguity.
- Define position description.
- Know how to approach the interview process when hiring a new employee.

- Describe the guidelines for performance reviews.
- Describe the various methods for reviewing performance
- Understand how collective agreements affect hiring decisions and performance reviews.

TERMS TO KNOW

coaching
empowerment
halo effect

performance review
position description
role ambiguity

role clarity
role conflict
role theory

evolve *Go to Evolve http://evolve.elsevier.com/Canada/Yoder-Wise/leading/ to access the full chapter.*

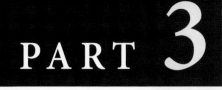

PART 3

Changing the Status Quo

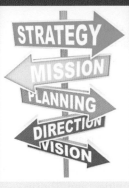

18

© Can Stock Photo Inc. / iqoncept

Strategic Planning and Goal Setting

Sandra Regan

This chapter discusses how organizations plan for the future, with a focus on the strategic planning process and goal setting. It also presents specific examples of strategic planning in health care organizations.

OBJECTIVES

- Understand the phases of the strategic planning process.
- Articulate the value and importance of conducting an assessment of external and internal environments.
- Review the purpose of an organization's mission statement, philosophy, goals, and objectives.
- Describe the four key steps in implementing a goal-setting program.
- Know the guidelines for developing SMART objectives.

TERMS TO KNOW

environmental assessment
goal setting

SMART objectives
strategic planning

SWOT analysis

💡 A CHALLENGE

In an effort to ensure patient safety, Ray, an early career registered nurse, and other staff nurses identified concerns with the interruptions they faced administering medications. Specifically, they were interrupted from medication administration to answer phone calls and random questions, redirect visitors, and check medications with nurses of other patients. Ray and the staff nurses wanted to bring their vision of patient safety to the process of medication administration on their unit. However, Ray and the staff nurses faced challenges in bringing this vision to reality because they lacked a clear plan. Ray agreed to take the lead on the matter and consider what he might do.

What do you think you would do if you were Ray?

INTRODUCTION

Given the rising costs of health care and our society's aging population, now, more than ever, health care organizations are under enormous pressure to deliver services while reducing expenses and containing costs. Major reforms are required, and the health care system has responded with the following initiatives:
- Empowering patients.
- Ensuring care across the continuum that is both coordinated and comprehensive.

- Ensuring appropriate utilization of resources, advanced technology, and the workforce.
- Focusing on health promotion and prevention.

Nurses are instrumental in developing, planning, and executing new strategies for the future, and thus are a major influence in the direction of health care. In the twenty-first century, technology has a strong influence on care delivery, nurse leaders, and organizations (Hirsch, 2014). Health technologies, defined as "the application of organized knowledge and skills in the form of devices, medicines, vaccines, procedures and systems developed to solve a health problem and improve quality of lives" (World Health Organization, 2007, p. 1), are rapidly advancing, and it is paramount for nurses to be at the forefront of influencing the implementation of new technologies. Doing so will require nurses to embrace the use of new technologies and evaluate their effectiveness. Across health care settings, new models of care will increasingly use and depend on new technologies. For example, mobile information technologies, such as handheld devices, are increasingly being used at the point-of-care by nurses to document patient care and improve safety and quality of care (Gregory & Buckner, 2014). By adopting and regularly using new technology, nurses will not only enhance their nursing expertise, but also earn the credibility to serve as advisors, directors, and influencers of technology. Nurses should be proactive and ensure that new technologies are used to meet nursing's information needs, to advance nursing practice, and to ensure nursing's continued viability.

The operational definition of *proactive* is simply "aggressive planning." It provides direction for one's efforts against which others must then react. Thus, greater control is possible so that one's vision becomes a probability, not just a possibility. The importance of proactive, thoughtful, and deliberate planning in the face of uncertainties cannot be overestimated. *Proactive* means that everyone in the organization manages their work and professional life and how they relate to the organization's goals and missions.

STRATEGIC PLANNING

Strategic planning is a process by which the guiding members of the organization envision their future and develop the necessary and appropriate procedures and operations to actualize that future. Planning is designed to encompass the organization's emphasis on mission

statements, strategic action plans, changes in policies and procedures, environmental factors affecting the organization, and the development and execution of new services.

The strategic planning process shown in Fig. 18.1 consists of the following key phases:

1. Assess the internal and external environments to determine those forces or changes that may affect the work of the organization or that may be crucial to its survival. These assessments entail analyzing the Strengths, Weaknesses, Opportunities, and Threats (SWOT analysis) facing the organization and the organization's ability to deal with change (SWOT analysis is also discussed in Chapter 8).

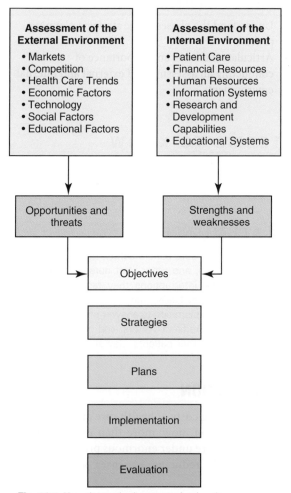

Fig. 18.1 Key phases in the strategic planning process.

2. Review the organization's mission, philosophy, goals, and objectives.
3. Determine major strategies, establish goals, and develop a plan of action to respond to the identified opportunities and threats. The best strategic option balances the organization's potential with the challenges of changing conditions, taking into account the values of its management and its social responsibilities.
4. Implement the plan of action.
5. Evaluate the strategic plan on a regular basis to determine its effectiveness and whether adjustments need to be made.

Reasons for Strategic Planning

In today's health care environment, which is marked by turbulence and complexity, strategic planning is imperative for health care organizations, from hospitals to home care, to remain responsive to internal and external forces. Therefore to survive the ongoing change and restructuring of the health care system, the strategic plan becomes the fundamental tool for creating and sustaining the organizational vision for the future. The strategic planning process leads to the achievement of goals and objectives, gives meaning to work life, and provides direction and improvement for the operational activities of the organization. Furthermore, a strong and dynamic strategic plan, if used, results in the efficient and effective use of resources and reflects the organizational culture and patient focus. Strategic planning occurs in large and small health care organizations and across sectors from hospitals to long-term care facilities to home health care agencies. Nurse leaders plan in a proactive, systematic manner because firstly, knowledge regarding philosophy, goals, and external and internal operations of the organization is necessary to lead change, and secondly, an understanding of the planning process is paramount to managing decisions.

Phases of the Strategic Planning Process

The strategic planning process is proactive, vision-directed, action-oriented, creative, innovative, and oriented toward positive change. For a strategic plan to succeed, a system must be developed that creates a plan for each approved initiative; this plan is integrated with a financial plan so that resources can be allocated and the time for implementation and the required capital resources can be determined (Ruder & O'Connor, 2007).

The strategic planning process involves developing a plan of action that covers 3 to 5 years. The initial phase—assessing the external and internal environments—is the most difficult. An environmental assessment is carried out to understand the specific internal and external forces that influence the health care setting (e.g., a hospital or community agency). Fig. 18.1 presents some of the key forces in an external and internal environmental assessment.

Visionary leaders ensure that those around them understand the direction the organization is taking (Ibarra & Obodaru, 2009). These visionaries search for a new path through a vigorous dialogue with various constituents, both internally and externally, because great visions will not actualize from solitary analysis (Ibarra & Obodaru, 2009). It is also important that visionaries test their ideas practically, based on current resources, from the following perspectives: financial, human resources, and overall organizational capabilities (Ibarra & Obodaru, 2009). True strategists provide an organization with more than a vision statement; "they articulate a clear point of view about what will transpire and position their organizations to respond to it" (Ibarra & Obodaru, 2009, p. 66). Although strategic planning often takes place at the executive level of an organization, nurse managers and staff nurses can provide a valuable perspective through established processes, such as committees. In addition, nurse managers and staff nurses often engage in clinical strategic planning processes at the unit level.

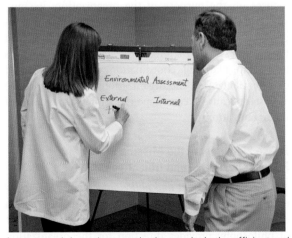

A strong and dynamic strategic plan results in the efficient and effective use of resources.

Phase 1: Assessment of the External and Internal Environments

External environmental assessment. An external environmental assessment takes place first in the strategic-planning process. The legal–political forces, economic forces, sociocultural forces, accreditation, technology, professional associations and unions, and regulatory bodies are assessed according to a SWOT analysis. By assessing and monitoring external forces, nurse leaders can make effective plans for their organization and develop creative and visionary programs that respond to external changes within the framework of their institutional mission and goals. An example of an external environmental assessment appears in Box 18.1.

> **EXERCISE 18.1** Research the demographics of the city you work or study in. Specifically, find information on age, socioeconomic factors (income, education, employment, and housing), and the ethnic origin of the population. What is the gap between the actual health care needs of the population and the services provided to patients in your particular placement setting?

Internal environmental assessment. Internal environmental assessment involves a SWOT analysis of the health care organization's structure, size, programs, financial resources, human resources, information systems, and research and development capabilities. It also includes a review of the education and training needs of staff and patient demands or needs. The management team involves all levels of staff in this assessment and focuses on the purpose of the organization; its mission and goals; the capabilities, skills, and relationships of various health care providers and related staff; and the weaknesses and strengths of staff in areas such as leadership, planning, coordination, research, and staff development. Also, the organizational climate must be assessed because it can shape the strategic direction of the organization.

Phase 2: Review of the Mission Statement, Philosophy, Goals, and Objectives

Mission statement and philosophy. A mission statement reflects the purpose and direction of the health care organization or a department within it. A statement of philosophy provides direction for the organization

---

BOX 18.1   An Example of an External Environmental Assessment

A community-based acute care hospital is undertaking a study to examine accessibility, availability, quality, and effectiveness of developing an orthopedic centre of excellence. One of the initial steps is to conduct an environmental scan. The hospital considered the following external forces:

- Legal–political forces, such as health care legislation, and provincial and territorial government health policy priorities, such as addressing wait lists, health promotion, and disease prevention.
- Economic forces, such as escalating health care costs and shifts in provincial and territorial funding as well as the cost of orthopedic care from admission to discharge.
- Sociocultural forces, such as the community organizations with volunteer groups supporting older adults.
- Accreditation Canada standards and accreditation processes.
- The diagnostic services available, including magnetic resonance imaging (MRI) and nuclear diagnostic imaging, along with the availability of rehabilitative and home health care services.
- The numbers and types of health care providers, including certified orthopedic physicians specialized in innovative joint replacement, operating room (OR) orthopedic nurses, orthopedic staff nurses (specialty certified), case managers, social workers, physiotherapists, occupational therapists, and pain management specialists and their respective unions and regulatory bodies.

Patient Trends

- Demographic and population trends (e.g., age, size, and distribution of the population, employment, socioeconomic indicators, education, ethnicity, and lifestyle issues, with particular emphasis on priority populations).
- Trends in health care (increased emphasis on wellness programs and enhanced technologies).
- Prospective users' input about current and future services.

---

and/or department. The content usually specifies organizational beliefs regarding the patient, health and nursing, the expectations of practitioners, and the commitment of the organization to professionalism, education, evaluation, and research. The importance of the mission statement cannot be overstated, yet it is questionable how many individuals in an organization, when asked, can articulate their organization's mission statement or its philosophy.

Covey (1990) considered that the mission statement is vital to the success of an organization and believed that everyone should participate in its development: "The involvement process is as important as the written product and is the key to its use" (p. 139). "An organizational mission statement, one that truly reflects the deep shared vision and values of everyone within that organization, creates a unity and tremendous commitment" (p. 143). Chapter 10 further discusses organizational mission statements.

> **EXERCISE 18.2** Form a small group of two to four students; you will work in this small group on several exercises in this chapter. Select a health care organization you are all familiar with. This could be a hospital, long-term care facility, public health unit, or home care agency. How effective is the organizational structure (i.e., is the organization operating effectively and efficiently?) in terms of the organization's mission, goals, and objectives? What human resources are present (refer to the organizational chart, note the various titles, and find out the number of employees)? Where are nurse leaders identified in the organizational chart? What information systems (give an example) are used in the organization?

Building on the example in Box 18.1, an example of a mission statement for a newly developed total joint replacement program within the orthopedic centre might be as follows: To provide quality care, to be integrated with the community, and to support a patient-centred approach to care.

Goal setting. Goal setting is the process of developing, negotiating, and formalizing the targets of an organization. If goals are not appropriate to the organization, frustration and poor performance could result (Hader, 2008).

The new joint replacement program might have five goals:

1. Provide comprehensive patient and family education across the continuum of care.
2. Develop protocols for standardized patient-care programs in terms of activities of daily living,

physiotherapy, occupational therapy, recreational exercise, and pain management.
3. Incorporate an interprofessional approach to patient care through a team consisting of physicians, nurse practitioners, nurses, case managers, social workers, physiotherapists, occupational therapists, nutritionists/dietitians, home support workers, and clergy or other spiritual support roles.
4. Enhance community support programs for arthritis patients.
5. Ensure that the website is current, with information and services available to patients.

> **EXERCISE 18.3** Continuing with the small group you created for Exercise 18.2, obtain and review the health care organization's mission statement. Based on what it says and means to you, create a goal statement that fits.

Specific goals are more likely to lead to higher performance than are vague or very general goals, such as "try to do your best." Feedback, or knowledge of results, is more likely to motivate individuals toward higher performance levels and commitment to goal achievements. For example, as organizations have become more focused on patient outcomes, they have been able to focus on specific goals and behaviours that result in better care.

Four key steps in the goal-setting process are as follows:

1. Set goals that are specific and adhere to a deadline.
2. Promote goal commitment by providing instructions and support to employees and managers.
3. Support the achievement of goals with appropriate feedback as soon as possible.
4. Monitor performance at appropriate intervals.

Objectives. Objectives are an important way to set out specific actions for goal achievement. Objectives tend to be short- or medium-term statements that support people's efforts to attain stated goals. The ability to write clear and concise objectives is an important aspect of nursing leadership. Effective objectives are known as SMART objectives. The acronym *SMART* refers to key attributes of effective objectives: namely, that objectives are *S*pecific, *M*easurable, *A*greed on (or some use the word *A*chievable), *R*ealistic, and *T*ime bound. Consider the following guidelines when developing SMART objectives:

Specific The objective statement must be properly constructed and describe exactly what is to be accomplished.

- It begins with the word *to*, followed by an action verb.
- It specifies a single result to be achieved.
- It specifies a target date for its attainment.

Measurable The objectives must be measurable.

- They provide the level of accomplishment of the end result.
- They leave no question as to what is expected.

Agreed On The objectives must be agreed on by all parties.

- There is mutual agreement by all parties on who will be responsible for execution and monitoring.

Realistic The objectives must be created within the realm of possibility and a challenge.

- They should not be unrealistic or unattainable.
- They must be written in the span of control for the specific team working toward the goals.
- The team has to be accountable for follow-through.

Time Bound The objectives should establish a time frame for which the activity or improvement must be achieved.

- The timeline and deadlines are adhered to.
- The timeline must be well-defined, avoiding statements such as "in the future."

Examples of SMART objectives appear in Box 18.2.

Phase 3: Identification of Strategies

The third phase of the strategic planning process involves identifying major issues, establishing goals,

and developing strategies to meet the goals. The term *strategy* can be defined as an organized and innovative plan that assists an organization to achieve its objectives. All departmental managers are involved in this process and are responsible for preparing a detailed plan of action, which may include the following: development of short-term and long-term objectives, formulation of annual department objectives, allocation of resources, and preparation of the budget. Table 18.1 identifies a plan of action for developing, implementing, and evaluating an orthopedic centre of excellence based on the internal and external environmental assessment in Box 18.1.

BOX 18.2   Examples of SMART Objectives

1. To provide training for 20 registered nurses in the use of the new electronic health record by June 1, of the current year.
2. To increase by 4 the number of medical–surgical units in the ABC hospital to implement electronic health records by August 31, of the current year.
3. To deliver 10 additional smoking cessation clinics per month in the local public health unit starting January 1, of the current year.

EXERCISE 18.4 Your group is working in home care within your region. The chair of the Professional Practice Council has assigned you to work on a planning committee with staff nurses and nurse managers from across the region in acute care, community, long-term care, and home care. The purpose of the committee is to devise long-term and short-term goals for nursing within the region.

The population of the community served by a local hospital is 55 000 and the population is aging. The older adult population will increase over the next 5 years. Many patients in the community are seeking assistance for arthritis complications such as building better bones and exercise programs, physiotherapy opportunities, and access to education.

The hospital has both an inpatient and an outpatient rehabilitation program with a specialized orthopedic unit; the inpatient orthopedic unit is staffed with nurses who are Canadian Nurses Association–certified in orthopedics and world-renowned Royal College of Physician and Surgeons of Canada–certified orthopedic surgeons. The hospital has implemented an early discharge program for patients who have had knee or hip replacement surgery. Nurses in home care are increasingly providing postoperative orthopedic care to these patients.

Considering the parameters of this strategic planning situation, in what direction should nursing in the hospital consider moving during the next 5 years to meet the needs of the community? How will you determine short-term and long-term plans? What additional information will your committee need to plan, realistically, for the next 5 months and the next 5 years?

TABLE 18.1 **Strategic Plan of Action for the Development, Implementation, and Evaluation of an Orthopedic Centre of Excellence**

Goal	Activities	Responsible Council	Time Frame
1. To develop an orthopedic centre of excellence	1.1 To conduct an internal and external environmental assessment • Primary and secondary service area • Demographic review • Out migration	Director of nursing Orthopedic manager Strategic planning director	January 2020
	1.2 To conduct a literature review related to each of these topics: • Orthopedic product lines • Innovative orthopedic joint replacement procedures • Programs related to orthopedics evidenced-informed practices for sjoint replacement	Orthopedic manager Operating room (OR) director Vice-president of medical affairs Director of rehabilitative services Nurse practitioner Staff nurse	January 2020
	1.3 To form an advisory committee comprising community representatives to oversee the development and implementation of the centre	Quality assurance director Physician champion Vice-president of patient-care services Orthopedic staff across the continuum of care Director of rehabilitation services Vice-president of medical affairs	February 2020
	1.4 To develop the organizational structure, mission statement, philosophy, and objectives, and revise accordingly	All parties	March 2020
	1.5 To develop policy and procedure manuals for staff in all areas	Orthopedic staff across the continuum of care Medical staff Standards staff Nurse practitioners Director of education Staff nurses	Ongoing
	1.6 To determine the business structure of the organization (i.e., legalities regarding partnerships, corporations, and proprietorship)	Nurse practitioners Medical staff Vice-president of medical affairs Orthopedic manager Vice-president of patient-care services Assistant vice-president of patient-care services Office of general counsel	Ongoing
	1.7 To develop a budget	Assistant vice-president of patient-care services Orthopedic manager/nurse manager	March 2020 Ongoing
	1.8 To develop a business site for the organization: • All renovations • Equipment • Supplies	Consultants and orthopedic manager	April 2020

Continued

TABLE 18.1 **Strategic Plan of Action for the Development, Implementation, and Evaluation of an Orthopedic Centre of Excellence—cont'd**

Goal	Activities	Responsible Council	Time Frame
	1.9 To develop a communications program (internal and external communications)	Communications office Patient engagement office Nurse practitioners Orthopedic manager Director of strategic planning Medical staff Staff nurses	February 2020 Ongoing
2. To implement and evaluate the effectiveness and efficiency of these programs	2.1 To develop patient questionnaires related to satisfaction regarding care provided	Nurse practitioners Orthopedic managers Quality assurance director Orthopedic front-line staff across the continuum Staff nurses	April 2020
	2.2 To develop cost-effective analysis studies to evaluate each of the programs being provided	Orthopedic manager	Ongoing
	2.3 To collect and collate data related to utilization of services by orthopedic patients	Nurse practitioners Staff across the continuum of care Pharmacists Medical staff Orthopedic manager Quality and patient safety director	Ongoing

Phase 4: Implementation

In the fourth phase of the strategic planning process, the specific plan of action is executed in order of priority. Implementation requires open communication with staff (this is paramount) regarding the priorities for the next year and subsequent periods; the development of revised policies and procedures regarding the changes; and the creation of area and individual objectives related to the plan. The specific plan needs to be focused on communications, programs, operations, a budget, and human resources.

Phase 5: Evaluation

The strategic plan is reviewed on a regular basis at all levels to determine whether the goals, objectives, and activities are on target. It is important to keep in mind that objectives may need to change in response to legislation, government funding, organizational budget constraints, restructuring, and other environmental factors. Therefore alternative activities may need to be used to adapt to respond to new situations. For example, imagine that an employer is informed that the budget must be decreased by $250 000 over the next 3 months. Management involves the staff in developing creative alternative methods for ensuring that the necessary changes will occur. Three months later, savings have been realized through restructuring, reducing expenses, and, when appropriate, using oral rather than intravenous medication administration.

The strategic planning process is similar in nature to the nursing process, as Fig. 18.2 shows.

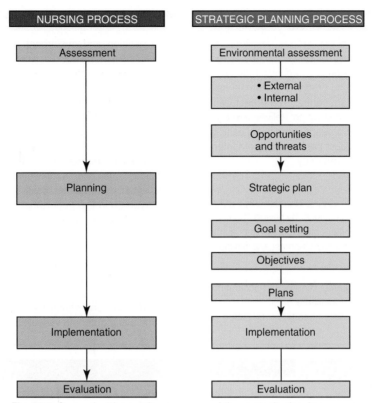

Fig. 18.2 Comparing the nursing process and the strategic planning process.

EXERCISE 18.5 With your small group, obtain a copy of the health care organization's strategic plan. You can often go to the website for a particular health care organization, hospital, long-term care facility, primary health care centre, home health agency, public health unit, or other health care related organization and type in "strategic plan" in the search box. Keep in mind that not all organizations will have their strategic plan on their website. If this is the case, you might contact a nurse leader in the organization and request a copy of the strategic plan. How does the strategic plan you obtained compare with what you have learned in this chapter about the key phases in the strategic planning process? Can you find information that illustrates most of the phases of the planning process?

The strategic planning process can also be useful to develop programs within organizations. The Literature Perspective below illustrates how one Canadian hospital applied the strategic planning process to develop a nursing strategic plan. Box 18.3 outlines key elements of a strategic plan to reduce breast cancer deaths in the workplace. Notice the goal setting and use of SMART objectives.

During the strategic planning process, an organization may identify significant gaps in health care services or the health care needs of specific populations. The Research Perspective below illustrates how an association used their strategic planning process to advocate for improvements in primary care delivery in one community in Ontario.

BOX 18.3   Mission Statement, Goals, and Objectives of a Breast Cancer Screening Program

Mission Statement

To reduce the leading cause of cancer deaths in women by delivering a comprehensive, organized, and evaluated breast cancer screening program for female health care workers in an acute care setting. The Breast Cancer Screening Program is committed to deliver a program that is sensitive to women's needs, builds on health-promoting behaviours, and fosters partnerships with interest groups in the health care community.

Overall Goals

To integrate health promotion strategies and medical practice to reduce mortality from breast cancer by having 100% of eligible female health care workers participate in annual mammography screening and conduct self-breast examinations.

Objectives

- To detect breast cancer earlier than would occur if organized screening were not available.
- To develop and implement a hospital mobilization plan for the program.

- To develop and implement a social marketing plan, including a health education component for the program.
- To articulate protocols and standards for health care providers associated with the program.
- To establish protocols for the interaction of the target population with the program.
- To develop and implement training and technical assistance for those associated with the delivery of the program.
- To develop a partnership with health care providers that will facilitate program delivery.
- To establish a regional breast screening service so that all women in the target population have equal access to breast screening.
- To document the follow-up of all women in whom an abnormality has been detected.
- To provide screening that is sensitive and acceptable to the target population.
- To evaluate the program on a continual basis, including needs assessment and measurement of process, economic, and outcome variables.

LITERATURE PERSPECTIVE

Resource: Jeffs, L., Merkley, J., Jeffrey, J., et al. (2006). Case study: Reconciling the quality and safety gap through strategic planning. *Canadian Journal of Nursing Leadership*, 19(2): 32–40.

A strategic planning process was applied to enhance the nursing professional practice environment at St. Michael's Hospital, Toronto, Ontario. The authors reported on the steps of the strategic planning process used to develop a nursing strategic plan (NSP). They concluded with several key lessons learned in the process, including the importance of linking a change agenda, such as enhancing the nursing professional practice environment, to an external strategic direction, such as patient safety.

Implications for Practice

The key lessons learned from the strategic planning process can help nurse leaders undertaking similar processes achieve success and avoid challenges commonly encountered in strategic planning processes.

RESEARCH PERSPECTIVE

Resource: Doey, T., Hines, P., Myslik, B., et al. (2008). Creating primary care access for mental health care clients in a community mental health setting. *Canadian Journal of Community Mental Health*, 27(2): 129–138.

The authors described how a strategic planning exercise conducted by the Canadian Mental Health Association was used as a point of advocacy to address the unique primary care needs of people with mental illness in Windsor-Essex County in Ontario. A Primary Care Working Group was established to explore options to provide mental health care within a primary care model. The working group reports on the process that led to the establishment of City Centre Health Centre, an interdisciplinary mental and primary care facility, and the patient-focused evaluation of the services provided.

In 2018, 10 years after publishing this research paper, the City Centre Health Centre continues to provide services in the community. They have updated their Strategic Plan—Vision 2020—as a means of planning future directions and ensuring they meet their mandate. See https://windsor-essex.cmha.ca/about-cmha/strategic-plan.

Implications for Practice

Strategic planning processes can be used to identify gaps in service delivery and to advocate for patient-focused strategies.

❓ A SOLUTION

The first step in addressing any problem is to define the problem and identify its root causes. Ray talked to the staff nurses on his floor. Their concerns about the disruptions during medication administration were also shared by nurses on other units. Given that the hospital had recently implemented a Professional Practice Council (PPC), Ray proposed, and the staff nurses agreed, that bringing their concerns forward to the PPC would be a first step in addressing the problem. Most hospitals and other health care settings have implemented PPCs or something similar as a forum for nurses, other staff, and nurse managers to discuss issues arising in practice, identify evidence-informed solutions, and make decisions. At the PPC, it was agreed that the goals of supporting nurses to meet medication administration standards and ensuring patient safety were shared among the staff nurses and nurse managers. To address these concerns, the PPC undertook the following:

1. It conducted an assessment of the internal environment, gathered information about medication errors, and interviewed staff nurses and nurse managers to gain their perspectives on the problem. The PPC also consulted with key people responsible for patient safety in the organization.

2. It obtained and reviewed provincial nursing regulatory body's standards for medication administration. It also reviewed and summarized research on medication administration and patient safety, identifying solutions that had been implemented in other health care settings to address similar concerns.

3. It established the following goal: to ensure that staff nurses were able to meet medication administration standards, minimize disruptions during medication administration, and ensure patient safety. To understand the resources required to support staff nurses, the PPC conducted an assessment of the process of "typical" medication administration on a unit, which included shadowing some staff nurses to identify the full nature of the problem.

4. It involved nursing staff and nurse managers in all aspects of planning to address the problem. During this process, the nursing staff felt a strong sense of ownership of the issue and the potential solutions. Nurse managers communicated the concerns to other key executives in the hospital, including the patient safety officer and the director of nursing.

5. After examining the standards, reviewing the research, and understanding the work processes that nurses enact to administer medication, the PPC identified solutions that could be implemented to minimize interruptions during medication administration. It reported its recommendations to the vice-president, Patient Care Services.

PPCs provide staff nurses with a strong professional voice within their organization. They are also an avenue for bringing professional and patient safety issues to the attention of managers, identifying a shared vision or goal, reviewing evidence, working on solutions, developing actions, and evaluating how the actions can make a difference for nursing practice and address patient safety issues.

Would this be a suitable approach for you? Why or why not?

▮ THE EVIDENCE

Connelly (2005) explored how six departmental nursing leaders dealt with high nurse turnover rates in their organization. The goal of the nursing leaders was to not have any new nurses leave the organization unless they were asked to leave.

The nursing leaders conducted a SWOT analysis through a focus group of staff nurses who had recently resigned from the organization. Based on feedback from the former staff nurses, a new strategic plan for nurse retention was developed, and the resulting new Welcoming Process transformed the nursing department as a whole.

The Welcoming Process incorporated six elements: establishing connections, greeting new staff, individualizing orientation, acceptance into the workgroup, checking in periodically, and supporting new staff. In addition to decreasing the nurse turnover rate, the organization realized significant cost savings by retaining the new nursing staff and improved nurse satisfaction of both the new nursing staff and the nursing leaders.

✳ NEED TO KNOW NOW

- Consider how a health care organization's vision and mission statement would affect your practice.
- Know the strengths, weaknesses, opportunities, and threats facing your health care organization.
- Listen for ideas about needs from your patients.

CHAPTER CHECKLIST

The operational effectiveness of any organization depends on its strategic planning. Nurse managers and leaders must be knowledgeable of the critical elements to facilitate the process.

- The strategic planning process leads to attainment of goals and objectives and provides meaning to work life and direction for the organizational activities.
- Strategic planning is similar in nature to the nursing process and involves the following:
- Assessment of the environment (internal and external) based on SWOT analysis

- Review of the organization's mission statement, philosophy, goals, and objectives
- Identification and development of strategies to respond to opportunities and threats
- Implementation of the plan of action
- Evaluation of the strategic plan.
- Nurses across the career continuum can play a pivotal leadership role in the development of visionary programs and services that meet the needs of patients by participating in planning processes at all levels of the organization and across all sectors of health care.

TIPS FOR PLANNING AND GOAL SETTING

- Be clear about the organization's mission and vision, ensuring that they meet the needs of those you serve, and stay true to them.
- Read and listen to a wide range of sources of information to determine what is happening and what

trends could affect you and your organization, and be flexible if changes are imminent.
- Be clear about your role in the organization and its success. Actively participate in the process.

Visit the Evolve website for Suggested Readings, Internet Resources, and additional resources related to the content in this chapter: http://evolve.elsevier.com/Canada/Yoder-Wise/leading/.

REFERENCES

Connelly, L. (2005). Welcoming new employees. *Journal of Nursing Scholarship, 37,* 163–164.

Covey, S. (1990). *The seven habits of highly effective people.* Toronto, ON: Simon & Schuster.

Doey, T., Hines, P., Myslik, B., et al. (2008). Creating primary care access for mental health care clients in a community mental health setting. *Canadian Journal of Community Mental Health, 27*(2), 129–138.

Gregory, D., & Buckner, M. (2014). Point-of-care technology: Integration for improved delivery of care. *Critical Care Nurse Quarterly, 37*(3), 268–272.

Hader, R. (2008). Know your targets, then align your goals. *Nursing Management, 39*(1), 6.

Hirsch, A. (2014). Technology management strategies for nurse leaders. *Nursing Management, 45*(2), 41–43.

Ibarra, H., & Obodaru, O. (2009). Women and the vision thing. *Harvard Business Review, 87*(1), 62–70.

Jeffs, L., Merkley, J., Jeffrey, J., et al. (2006). Case study: Reconciling the quality and safety gap through strategic planning. *Canadian Journal of Nursing Leadership, 19*(2), 32–40.

Ruder, S. M., & O'Connor, D. J. (2007). Strategic planning: What's your role? *Nursing Management, 38*(12), 54–56.

World Health Organization. (2007). *Health technologies: Report by the secretariat.* Geneva, Switzerland: Author. Retrieved from: http://apps.who.int/gb/ebwha/pdf_files/EB121/B121_11-en.pdf.

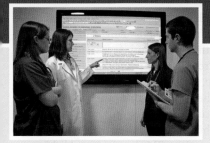

19

Nurses Leading Change: A Relational Emancipatory Framework for Health and Social Action

Marcia D. Hills, Nancy Clark, Simon Carroll

The purpose of this chapter is to introduce a change framework for nursing that proposes three processes necessary and sufficient to bring about change. It suggests that nurses leading change engage in the change process with people rather than imposing it on or around them. Leading change in this manner has the potential to engage nurses in an empowering transformational and relational experience. The proposed framework is emancipatory because it honours each individual's freedom of choice, multiple forms of knowledge, and it calls attention to health inequities and injustices. Therefore working with others within a context of freedom of choice and inclusivity makes this framework relational and emancipatory. Further, the chapter highlights the importance of a sociopolitical stance that calls attention to health inequities and social injustices. This stance suggests that leading change must address root causes of injustice through social action. Leading change from this perspective is dramatically different from most other change theories or frameworks. The framework is described according to three processes: creating collaborative relationships, engaging in critical dialogue, and reflection-in-action. This framework implements change through a series of iterative cycles that are explored with examples.

OBJECTIVES

- Describe a relational emancipatory framework for health and social change.
- Understand the components and elements of a relational emancipatory change framework.
- Describe how to apply the framework to nursing leadership in practice, project, or policy change.
- Develop a plan to bring about health and social change in practice.

TERMS TO KNOW

change theory
collaboration
emancipatory

leadership
participatory
power

relational
social justice

🔔 A CHALLENGE

A student group is taking an undergraduate course on Health and Healing Promoting Community and Societal Health. Of interest to the group is the health inequities experienced by immigrant and refugee groups in their local community. The group wants to develop a health promotion initiative aimed at increasing health care access. Amy, one of the students, had done some research in this area and found out that social determinants of health, for example, health literacy, gender, local geography, and social support networks, are playing an increasing role in primary health care accessibility. Amy asks: "How could the local primary health care team increase accessibility to health services for refugees?" and "What needs to be in place for newcomer families to utilize a primary health clinic?" Amy is also wondering about how they could develop an initiative that promotes accessible primary health care for newcomers.

If you were Amy, what community engagement strategies could you initiate to promote change?

INTRODUCTION

Baccalaureate-prepared registered nurses are being called upon to lead change in the workplace and in everyday practice. The move towards evidence-informed practice demands that all registered nurses be prepared to lead the change process, whether of a new practice, procedure, project, or program.

However, facilitating change requires an understanding that practice is linked to metacognitive competencies, such as critical thinking and self-reflexivity, which are not necessarily evidence based. Therefore a strict reliance on evidence-based competencies will be insufficient to bring about change (Josephsen, 2014). Traditionally, nursing leadership is connected to a formal role that nurses might take up, such as a team leader or nurse manager. Increasingly, these traditional formal leadership roles are important in nursing administration and management, but more contextual and relational approaches to leading change are required for addressing the complexities of the everyday practice of nursing. However, it is important to note that these more informal types of leadership role are often ambiguous and intimidating for novice practitioners.

Even within the more traditional roles of leadership, there is an important distinction to be made between managers and leaders. Pate (2013) explains, "Managers bring stability to complex workplaces by actions such as planning, staffing, controlling, organizing, and problem solving. Leaders, on the other hand, focus on creating a vision for the future, aligning people, and motivating and inspiring" (p. 186). The authors endorse this distinction and further suggest that nursing leadership needs to be conceptualized not only within traditional formal leadership but also in relation to leading change in everyday practices. This involves establishing a shared vision and forming a synergistic alliance with all stakeholders, inspiring them to move toward an unknown future that is transformational. Furthermore, when the authors use the word "change," this refers to a particular type of change—transformational change. Transformational change is distinctly different from the incremental change that is so often the focus of "quality improvement" projects in nursing. Drawing on relational emancipatory educational theory (Freire, 1972; Hills & Watson, 2011) and participatory approaches to knowledge development (Freire, 1972; Heron & Reason, 1997), the authors recommend using a relational emancipatory framework for leading change, whether nurses leading change are in formal or informal roles.

CRITIQUING CURRENT PERSPECTIVES/ THEORIES OF CHANGE

Most change theories or frameworks focus on planned change. These theories can be helpful in stable situations in which one is trying to make an incremental change, for example, making adjustments with quality improvement frameworks and models (Mills et al., 2018). Nursing students are typically introduced to planned change theories such as Lewin (1951), Reinkemeyer (1970), and Havelock (1973). The trans-theoretical model of change, which has remained popular since it was introduced in the 1990s, is linear and mostly draws on individualistic theories of behavioural change. Moreover, May (2002) and Freeman & Dolan (2001) critique change theory advanced by Prochaska et al., 1995, generally questioning its practical utility and the inherent limitations of an experience-centred focus. Using planned linear change theories was useful to their application in nursing leadership when cycles in society and health care were somewhat stable (low-complexity change) (Johnston, 2015). However, the highly complex, accelerated, and unpredictable change situations of contemporary everyday nursing require a contextualized approach.

Health care in Canada is in the midst of unprecedented change. Shrinking health care dollars, the increasing demand for services, human resources shortages, health care reform, increased complex health care needs of individuals and groups, and a growing body of research on the need for innovation mean that the health care system is unpredictable and chaotic. To address this complexity, nurses leading change can no longer rely on the typical planned change theories or frameworks. Chaos theory (sometimes referred to as complexity theory) and learning organizations theory have gained recognition as being useful in such unpredictable situations (Johnston, 2015). However, nursing needs to be thoughtful about how to adapt these theories to align with the relational and emancipatory values of nursing.

Some complex organizations, often referred to as *learning organizations*, are responsive to internal and external influences and try to survive and thrive in unpredictable environments, such as health care. They best respond and adapt when members of the organization work with others using the results of learning to achieve better results (Johnston, 2015). Senge (1990) identified five interrelated disciplines (or components) that converge to support innovation in learning organizations and that function effectively only when all are present, linked, and interacting. Senge's five disciplines of learning organizations are: systems thinking, personal mastery, mental models, shared vision, and team learning. These five concepts are congruent with the relational aspect of our framework but fall short of recognizing the impact of an emancipatory perspective.

More recently, Doane & Varcoe (2016) have recommended a relational view of leadership. As they state, "from a relational perspective, leadership is understood to be a relational process that occurs and is enacted among people and within contexts . . . it is understood that the influence of both formal and informal leaders is shaped by the specific contexts within which they are working, the people with whom they work, and the relationships among them" (p. 426). This relational view acknowledges that formal leaders may have more influence because of their position, but it also recognizes that "each person can have influence and be a leader regardless of that person's position within the organizational hierarchy position" (p. 426). Although Doane and Varcoe (2016) do not address change specifically, their relational view is congruent with the authors' relational emancipatory perspective. The authors expand the relational concept to include emancipation and draw attention to the sociopolitical factors that influence health and health care practice. From a relational emancipatory perspective, the authors argue that contemporary nursing leaders ought to act with communities to mitigate the increasing social inequities and injustices in health care.

Deficit approaches remain the dominant perspective in health care and are supported by most health professionals, including nurses. A recent development that influences nurses leading change is the focus on assets-based approaches, or what are sometimes referred to as strength-based approaches, with communities (Kretzmann & Mcknight, 1993), globally (Morgan et al., 2010), and, more recently, in nursing (Gottlieb, 2013). After many years of focusing on deficits and trying to fix problems, the results are limited and, in many cases, disheartening (Gottlieb, 2013). As Gottlieb (2013) further explains, "The deficit approach has yielded short term solutions that often have been proven to be unsustainable in the long term. People have difficulty maintaining change when motivated by fear and when reminded of their weaknesses, what they are missing, what is malfunctioning or dysfunctional" (p. xxii). Like others, Gottlieb (2013) calls for a profound shift in our thinking that moves from a narrow focus on a problem or deficit to a wider perspective. She argues, "The person, family, and community are situated in their context and history of their lives with their many facets, layers and complexities" (p. xxiii). Similarly, leading change draws on multiple forms of knowledge without privileging a leadership position or status.

Finally, in another area of research that reviewed "Large System Transformation" combining a realist review with a complex adaptive systems framework, Best et al. (2012) found that a key *simple rule* of successful systemic organizational change was that leadership needed to be *distributed*. The authors argued that *distributed leadership* "means focusing on the practices and relationships involved in leadership as well as developing shared and evolving leadership through purposeful mentoring strategies" (p. 433). Best et al. (2012) found that this approach activated key mechanisms that initiated and sustained successful change in large-scale health systems. It is clear that, although leadership does require formal, designated leadership roles, the actual functions of leadership need to be shared across organizations. This finding is congruent with a relational and emancipatory approach to leadership in nursing, as it presupposes actively engaging nurses at all levels in a participatory process of developing leadership skills through mentoring and allowing these capacities to be distributed across large health systems.

THE FRAMEWORK: PRESENTING AN ALTERNATIVE

The following section outlines the *what* of the change process. It answers the question: "What are the conditions that must be present for change to occur?"

The authors propose a change framework comprised of three interrelated components that are necessary and sufficient and that act in synergy to bring about change: creating collaborative relationships, engaging in critical dialogue, and reflection-in-action.

Defining Collaboration

Before detailing the first component, creating collaborative relationships, it is important to consider what we mean by *collaboration*. The process of nurses leading change should arguably always be collaborative, involving the change leader working together with stakeholders who are interested in bringing about the desired change and vice versa. We call this concept *leading from beside* (Hills, 2016). Others have described this process as *shared governance* (Porter-O'Grady, 2001; Finklemann, 2006; Anthony, 2004).

LITERATURE PERSPECTIVE

Resource: Hills, M. (2016). Emancipatory and collaborative: Leading from bedside. In William Rosa (ed). *Nurses as Leaders: Evolutionary Visions of Leadership* (pp. 293–309). Springer: New York.

Hills describes how nursing curriculum development and research focused on change were achieved through collaboration and emancipatory processes. She describes a major collaborative nursing program involving five postsecondary educational institutes who were successful in changing these five traditional nursing programs into a single visionary collaborative nursing program based on caring science. The essence of this approach to change requires learners to do research with people rather than on, to, or about them.

Implications for Practice

This change process is based on emancipatory and collaborative processes similar to those described in this chapter.

The following definition best captures the collaboration that is needed to lead the change process in this way. *Collaboration* is the creation of a synergistic alliance that honours and utilizes each person's contribution to create collective wisdom and collective action. Collaboration is not synonymous with cooperation, partnership, participation, or compromise. Those words do not convey the fundamental importance of being a relationship or the depth of caring and commitment needed to create the kind of reciprocity that is collaboration. Collaborators are committed to, care about, and trust in each other. They recognize that, despite their differences, each has a unique and valuable knowledge, perspectives, and experiences to contribute to the collaboration (Hills & Watson, 2011).

In creating collaborative relationships as part of a change process, all participants are viewed as contributing partners. The leader and the participants share responsibility and joint decision making. This type of collaboration demands that leaders relate person to person with all team members. It is not possible to develop a collaborative relationship with someone who assumes all responsibility and power, as with some traditional styles of team leadership, or who in some way is not truly present. Leading change requires a facilitation process that supports equitable power relations and community building of these relationships. All participants fully engage in the process to build their capacity and feel a sense of ownership that moves the change process forward.

Creating Collaborative Relationships

The first framework component is creating collaborative relationships. Three elements, when taken together, lead to collaborative relationships: partnership vs. individual action, sharing power vs. wielding power, and committed participation vs. mere involvement (Hills & Watson, 2011; Hills & Carroll, 2017a).

Developing Partnerships

How often have you encountered someone's decision to change things up by engaging the boss, choosing a charismatic leader, or securing the money without any consideration of who they will need to work *with* to get things changed?

The first element in creating collaborative relationships is to identify allies across and within groups who may have an interest in the proposed change, and to engage them as partners in the change process. This performed at the beginning of health promotion initiatives, and it is important to ask the questions: *Is there anyone else that should be at the table with us? Whose voices matter and need to be represented, and is anyone being excluded? How can we work through tensions and differences?*

> **EXERCISE 19.1** There are often various perspectives on health initiatives when working in multidisciplinary teams, and not everyone feels that they have a voice in the process of change. Think of a time when you were asked to lead a change initiative, and reflect upon what factors supported collaboration.
>
> What kinds of things do you feel needed to be present to ensure inclusion of diverse perspectives and voices? What strategies can be used to effectively promote meaningful engagement and inclusion?

Negotiating Power

The second element of creating collaborative relationships is negotiating power. It is not possible to talk about leading change without talking about power. The authors agree with Freire's (1972) contention that power dynamics exist in all relationships, organizations, and health and social structures. More recently Lather (2017) has deconstructed power relations through empirical research and argues that there needs to be a conscious empowerment that is built into research design. This critical praxis-oriented paradigm produces emancipatory knowledge that can also be applied to process of teaching and learning in communities. Lather draws on Cris Williamson, a feminist poet singer who claims "the changer and the changed" (p. 83). In a similar vein, nurses leading a change process need to be aware of power dynamics, understand how they operate, and know how to negotiate power effectively for inclusivity and positive social change to occur.

Power can be an inherent attribute in many leadership positions, such as being a team leader or a nurse manager or leader on a project. However, leaders always have a choice of how they negotiate power: they can choose to have power *over* others or to have power *with* others, and to use power for a social good. In the framework presented in this chapter, power is a relational process, negotiated through dialogue, reflexivity, and mutual interests. Negotiating power this way results in distributed leadership. Power lies at the centre of empowerment, and "[T]

he empowering act exists only as a relational act of power taken and given in the same instance" (Labonte, 1994, p. 49). Empowering behaviours of nurses leading change can be of paramount importance to the way that staff nurses react to their work environment and to the change (Greco, Laschinger & Wong, 2006). Many make the distinction between individual empowerment and community empowerment (Freire, 1972; Laverach & Labonte, 2000; Rendon, 2014; Wallerstein & Hammes, 1991). This distinction is important in that it serves different purposes; however, all empowering relationships are characterized by "power with" relationships that encourage full participation by all participants. This may challenge traditional approaches to leadership.

> **EXERCISE 19.2** Power is often correlated with a leadership role, as though leaders inherently have power and knowledge over health interventions and/or others. To some extent this is true, based on the social position and social constructions of leadership. However, power is a complex relational construct, which necessitates negotiation and reflexivity of environmental contexts in which nurses work. Leaders always have a choice about how to use power.
>
> What strategies could you use to operationalize power for the purpose of leading change?
>
> What strategies in working with people can mitigate power imbalances to promote meaningful social inclusion?

PARTICIPATION

The third element of creating collaborative relationships is participation. "Without participation there can be no partnerships, no negotiation of power or relationships" (Hills & Watson, 2011, p. 79). Participation requires a commitment that is not necessarily present when you are merely involved in or associated with an activity or project. Participation is a conscious choice to commit time, resources, and energy to a change project. Participation demands engagement. Chinn (2008) describes several strategies for creating full participation based on *power with* relationships, including giving every perspective full voice; demystifying all processes and structures; fully respecting different points of view; paying attention to the process itself so that how things are done is just as important and what is done; rotating and sharing leadership according to ability and willingness; valuing learning new skills so that opportunity is accessible to all; and sharing responsibility for the process of the group equally among everyone present. In every change project, it is critical to make the process for discussion and decision making transparent and participatory.

ENGAGING IN CRITICAL DIALOGUE

The second component of the relational emancipatory framework—engaging in critical dialogue—is the *backbone* of our relational emancipatory change framework. Critical dialogue encourages change agents to stay in a state of not knowing, to question taken-for-granted assumptions and habits, and to ask the unaskable. This approach is similar to the notion of transdisciplinarity, which uses reflexivity and critical consciousness to transcend disciplinary boundaries and enhance collaboration for social justice aims (Clark et al., 2015). To think critically does not mean to criticize, but rather to ask questions that examine both benefits and limitations of actions. In a relational emancipatory framework, this means that nursing knowledge is shared across different disciplines. Likewise, within the nursing discipline, nursing knowledge can be enhanced through interdisciplinary perspectives. This second component consists of operationalizing critical dialogue through interwoven elements: authentic listening and responding, critical questioning, and critical thinking.

AUTHENTIC LISTENING AND RESPONDING

Authentic listening and responding is the heart of critical dialogue. Being able to understand and to demonstrate that we understand another's issues, concerns, and interpretations is a precious gift that nurses leading change can develop. It means listening not only to the words of another but also to the meaning that is conveyed between the words, the feelings and experiences that are not expressed, and what remains to be known. When we are able to respond authentically in a way that the other feels understood, it allows change to occur. As Moustakas (1977) explains, "When we are listened to, it creates us, makes us unfold and expand. Ideas actually begin to grow in us and come to life . . . It makes us . . . feel free . . . there is an alternating current and that recharges us . . . we are constantly being re-created" (p. 82). Authentic listening and responding requires that

we suspend our judgements, assumptions, prejudices, and responses and hold space for the other's story and perspective.

> **EXERCISE 19.3** In discussing a change initiative, you find yourself disagreeing with your collaborator as you are trying to put forward your opinion. You realize that in this situation the collaborator does not share your point of view. You shift your stance and decide to fully listen and engage with your collaborator through authentic listening. In this case, how could you demonstrate understanding of the other collaborator's perspective?
>
> Provide one or two examples of a response that would effectively demonstrate authentic listening.

Critical Questioning (Problem Posing)

Freire (1972) suggests a three-phase methodology called problem posing. This process consists of listening as described above; participatory dialogue, which we discuss here; and action, which we discuss in the next section of this chapter. Nurses who are leading change can encourage critical dialogue by posing critical questions.

Freire differentiates problem posing from problem solving. With problem posing, you are not looking for immediate resolution but rather trying to discover "generative themes" that are inherent in the issue to be changed. Freire contends that by raising questions through dialogue, people become "masters of their thinking by discussing their thinking and views of the world explicitly and implicitly manifest in their own suggestions and those of their comrades" (p. 95). In other words, as leaders of change, nurses engage their colleagues in critical dialogue through posing questions that illuminate problematic conditions and challenges to be addressed. They begin to see a way forward by *hearing* each other's perspectives rather than by an outsider telling them what to do or giving them advice. Critical questioning "systematically invites colleagues to think critically . . . to construct peer relations instead of authority-dependent relations" (Freire, 1972, p. 41).

CRITICAL THINKING

Hills and Watson (2011) argue that "critical thinking is a process that requires that we consistently and critically question our assumptions that underlie our customary, habitual ways of being, thinking and acting in everyday life and work" (p. 100). Brookfield (1993) identifies four essential components of critical thinking: identifying and challenging assumptions, challenging the influence of context, imagining and exploring alternatives, and engaging in reflective scepticism.

Critical thinking requires the ability to identify and challenge assumptions as they are enacted in our daily lives. Questioning our assumptions or raising our awareness about the assumptions we are making can be challenging because it implies that our personal and/or political existence might rest upon faulty foundations. Asking questions such as *What constitutes a given reality? How do you know that?* or *Why must this be so?* begins to uncover our taken-for-granted ideas and assumptions about the world.

Critical thinkers are aware that practices, structures, and actions are contextual. They are tuned in to the nuances of a given situation and they understand the dynamics that occur because of the context. "Because they understand the complexity of context, they can respond instantaneously to a given situation even though they may have never previously been in such a situation" (Hills & Watson, 2011, p. 103). Critical thinkers can imagine and explore alternatives because they are aware that there are many possible ways to act other than the one that seems obvious. They are open and flexible and are willing to try different alternatives. Critical thinkers are wary of quick-fix solutions and have a healthy scepticism of situations that appear too easily remedied. Critical thinkers like to raise questions and are not intimidated, even when others' views may differ. Importantly, critical thinking is a developmental process that requires culturally safe strategies for leading change. Ways of thinking and acting may differ in multidisciplinary groups whose members have not been supported to develop critical reasoning (Josephsen, 2014).

> **EXERCISE 19.4** A clinical practice team is engaged in a cultural safety initiative for a community-based public health unit. You decide to have them identify five strategies they could use to develop critical thinking as a team-building exercise. What assumptions need to be addressed related to unexamined practices?

Reflection-in-Action (Praxis)

The third and final framework component is reflection-in-action. Put simply, reflection-in-action is the relationship between experience, theory, reflection, and action (Freire, 1972; Kemmis, 1985; Hills & Watson, 2011, Hills & Carroll, 2017b). To create transformational change, team members need to be provided with experiences so that they can discover reflecting and acting in the moment. We explore reflection-in-action here as a dialectic.

Theory is often talked about as something that belongs in the academy or in the classroom. We tend to think about theory as some form of abstraction that is separate from our practice and our lives. Kemmis (1985) challenges this thinking and suggests that reflection as dialectic looks inward at our thoughts and thought processes and outward at the situation in which we find ourselves. When we consider the interaction of the internal and the external, our reflection orients for further thought and action. Thus, reflection is meta-thinking—thinking about thinking—in which we consider the relationship between our thoughts and actions in a particular context (p. 140).

Kemmis argues that reflection is action-oriented, social, and political. There is a tendency to think of reflection as something that happens quietly within us; however, Kemmis suggests that to do so is "to ignore the very things that give reflection its character and significance: it splits thought from actions" (p. 141). Freire (1972) extends this thinking and describes reflection as praxis. Emancipatory action is informed by a dialectal movement from action to reflection to new action. "This dialectal way of viewing reflection-in-action reorients our consideration of this concept from one of searching for understanding or explanation to one of ethical action toward societal good (Hills & Watson, 2011, p. 121). This way of being in the world assists us as nurse leaders to develop *critical consciousness*, which can be defined as "a moral awareness which propels individuals to disembed from their cultural, social, and political environment and engage in a responsible critical moral dialogue with it, making active efforts to construct their own place in social reality and to develop internal consistency in their ways of being" (Mustakova-Possardt, 1998, p. 13). In this relational emancipatory framework, change agents (the team members) engage in moral questioning through critical self-reflexive practices required for building the literacy abilities required for self-evaluation and autonomous learning (Josephsen, 2014). Change agents require critical reflexivity to view situations from a variety of perspectives and to try out changes that have been agreed upon by the team.

EXERCISE 19.5 Action flows from practical and theoretical reflection. In considering the necessary conditions for change to occur, and as agents of change, nurse leaders need to be able to evaluate their actions for the promotion of ethics and social justice. What aspects of leading change are most important for transformative leadership to occur? In particular, what meaning does this have for changing socially unjust conditions of health.

THE CHANGE PROCESS: A RELATIONAL EMANCIPATORY FRAMEWORK

The previous section describes the *what* of the change process. In the following section, the *how* of leading effective change will be explored.

Nurses leading change using this relational emancipatory change framework create and implement change through iterative cycles of reflecting, planning, and acting that are based upon relational and emancipatory values. Through this process change is planned and operationalized. This process cycles through six phases: Initiation; Reflection and Planning; Action; Critiquing, Reflection and Planning; Follow-up Action; and Subsequent Cycles (Fig. 19.1).

It is important to note that this change process relies on an extended epistemology, consisting of four types of knowledge: experiential, representational, propositional, and practical. They will be introduced and described as they arise below.

Phase 1: Initiation

Nurses who lead change face two immediate tasks: to identify and engage key stakeholders and to gain clarity about the issue or problematic condition to be changed. In this context, a stakeholder is one who has a stake in the intended goal or aim of the change process. Critical questions related to stakeholder engagement include: *Who cares about this issue? Who has an interest in this issue?* and *Who has the capacity to influence this situation?*

With the team established and issue or condition to be changed identified, through team collaboration, the group turns its attention to establishing group processes and norms. They accept shared responsibility for the team process and shared decision making. In the context of continuing to build collaborative relationships, the group, acting as change agent, begins to create a shared vision,

a picture of where it is trying to go. What is the team's vision of what needs to be in place that is not there now? It asks such questions as: What do we want to see happen? What needs to be in place for us to feel/think that we have been successful? What will we take as evidence? In more traditional change frameworks, leaders are often identified and sought after as being visionary. As Pate (2013) describes, "[Nursing leaders] can create visions and influence others about quality care for patients and families, performance improvement, health care systems, and the profession, as they are always looking forward and thinking about the bigger picture" (p. 191). This quality is also important for nurses leading change in the proposed relational emancipatory change framework. However, in the proposed framework, power is always negotiated. In this way, nurses facilitate shared leadership to identify a shared vision to imagine what is possible.

Phase 2: Reflection and Planning

In this phase, the team develops and articulates the purpose and goals of the change process. It answers the question: What are we trying to achieve? The team reflects on what it knows about the situation and investigates what others have said about the issue. In other words, the team gathers what Heron & Reason (1997) identify as *experiential* and *propositional* knowledge: knowledge from our experiences and knowledge from the literature. This reflection is important because too often we jump into planning without first considering what we already know. The team then identifies goals to focus its change project. Once the purpose and goals are clear, the team articulates the activities that it will initiate to bring

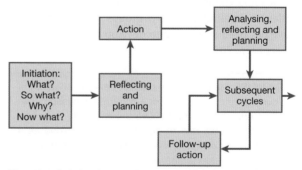

Fig. 19.1 Relational emancipatory change process. (Modified from Hills, M., & Carroll, S. (2017). Evaluating a community health program: Collaborative action evaluation. In Vollman, A. R., Anderson, E. T., & McFarlane, J. (Eds.), *Canadian community as partner: Theory & multidisciplinary practice* pp. (288–301). Philadelphia, PA: Wolters Kluwer.)

about the desired change. One common way to clarify the change that is required is to ask the question, *What would it look like if . . . ?* For example, when trying to lead a change project in nursing to change from a strictly biomedical perspective of nursing to a more humanistic and health promotion perspective of nursing, one could ask the question: *What would it look like if we practised from a nursing health promotion perspective?* From this question, the team could build a conceptual map or model that would identify the requisite key components to practise that way. At this time, the team also considers how it will evaluate what happens when change is initiated and new processes are implemented. Evaluation in a relational emancipatory framework moves beyond traditional forms of evaluation because it is underpinned by an emancipatory paradigm, participants are co-evaluators, evaluators are social activists, who focus on collective and systemic change, with the aim of transforming practice and structures (Hills & Carroll, 2017b).

Phase 3: Action

The action phase is critical in our relational emancipatory framework because it involves social action in the everyday practice of nursing. The team implements the identified components from the conceptual map or model and tries them out in practice. In this phase, the team is putting its propositional knowledge (gathered in Phase 1) up against its practical knowledge—knowing "how" to do something. Heron & Reason (1997) argue that the more that practical knowledge is grounded in experiential, presentational and propositional knowledge, the greater the evidence upon which to base change. During this phase, the team members collect evidence of the impact of the change in practice. Team members might learn of the impacts of change by observation or by discussing with others or in groups about their experiences. Note here that, despite its rigour, the proposed change process is a community development process, not community-based research. It is possible to actually utilize a rigorous research or evaluation process, such as Collaborative Action Research and Evaluation (CARE) (Hills et al., 2010; Hills & Carroll, 2017a; Hills & Carroll, 2017b), *but* it is not necessary to do so to bring about change.

Phase 4: Critiquing, Reflecting, and Planning

In this phase, by remaining critically conscious, the team critiques what it has learned from trying out planned change in practice. Team members reflect on what they learned in practice (practical knowledge) in relation to how they conceptualized the change (propositional knowledge). This reflection differs from that in Phase 1 because the initial reflection was based upon propositional and/or experiential knowledge but not upon practical knowledge. Heron and Reason (1997) suggest that, if propositional knowledge is not congruent with practical knowledge, then we need to change our theory not our practice.

Practical knowledge has primacy in a relational emancipatory change framework as it does in nursing generally. It is found in the action of nurses who are leading change. This type of knowledge synthesizes our conceptual knowledge (propositional) and our experiences (experiential) and our presentational knowledge in our actions, in our practice.

The team reflects on its experiences and plans for the next action phase. It considers questions such as: What do we need to know more about? What other changes do we need to try? What strategies can we use to understand and monitor these changes?

Phase 5: Follow-up Action

The team implements the agreed-upon activities to initiate further change in practice and continues to monitor the impact. Follow-up action is redistributed through participation and work of all stakeholders. The follow-up action integrates prior learning and critical reasoning and reflection.

Phase 6: Subsequent Cycles

A series of cycles are carried out following the same format. Heron and Reason (1997) recommend that 3–5 cycles are usually sufficient to bring about transformational change. As discussed by Hills and Carroll (2017b), "An advantage of this planning-acting-reflecting approach [is to] build capacity to continue an ongoing evaluation process as part of [initiating change]" (p. 298).

In summary, operationalizing a relational emancipatory framework for change requires that nurses leading change facilitate the process through cycles of action and reflection that build theory (propositional knowledge) from practice and collect evidence about what constitutes better practices. The team derives theory from practice and then tests theory in the real world of practice and reflects on their experiences in relation to propositional knowing. This relational participatory process articulates a way of knowing and acting that is both grounded in our experiential presence in the world and honours human capacity of sense-making and intentional action (Heron & Reason, 1997; Hills, 2016).

EXAMPLE OF STUDENT NURSES LEADING CHANGE USING A RELATIONAL EMANCIPATORY CHANGE FRAMEWORK

In this section, the authors describe how an undergraduate nursing student group applied the relational emancipatory framework for leading change in a community health course.[1] The authors also discuss some of the challenges and learnings that occurred during the process of integrating a relational emancipatory framework.

As previously mentioned, traditional approaches to leadership roles within nursing include assessments and evaluations that may not account for the lived realities of nurses and/or their clients. For the purpose of the student assignment, the student group applied a relational emancipatory framework to evaluate their health promotion initiative, which examines the relationship between social media and student mental health on a university campus. Their assignment was to theorize how a relational emancipatory framework could promote change for a social good and/or community development project. In part one of this student assignment, students collected data from observation, windshield surveys, publicly accessible information on the University of Victoria (UVic) website, and the lived experiences of student members of the impact of social media and their mental health and well-being. Although students did not interact directly with their chosen community of interest—students on the UVic campus—their project served as a critical pedagogical approach to teaching and learning. Simultaneously, students gained strategies for leading change and deeper understanding in critical consciousness and leading change (Jamel, 2017). In Phase 1: Initiation, students proposed to implement an interpersonal workshop to identify the community of interest and key stakeholders. Once students identified and discussed key stakeholders (e.g., members of the university residence, University of Victoria [UVic]

Residence Services, UVic Counselling Services, and the UVic faculty orientation team), they discussed how developing a plan of action (Phase 2) would start with establishing an inquiry group as a way to foster trust and promote equitable power relations and confidence within the group. Initiation and developing a plan of action included diverse faculty and student voices to examine how they would develop a health promotion initiative that would promote mental health and use of social media.

An excerpt from the student project highlights this process:

A workshop led by student mentors would be more relatable to the UVic residents than if it were led by instructors or community nurses. McGlynn-Stewart (2015) states that students were more receptive to their peers than the instructor in a discussion-based learning environment. As well, including students in leadership positions would foster community commitment and motivation to respond to community needs and desires. This would also give the volunteers an opportunity to gain experience in mentorship, as well as a way to build their resume (Barnes et al., 2018, pp. 6–7).

In Phase 3, students identified how they would act upon the model: in other words, how they would put a relational emancipatory model *into* action. In this phase, the students outlined the specific workshop activities that would be inclusive and sensitive to a variety of different learning styles and knowledges (experiential as well as propositional). This student group discussed how the process of the "Collaborative Action Evaluation" (CAE) (Hills & Carroll, 2017a) is not a step that is completed at the end of the program, but rather a process that is revisited at every step of the program to generate knowledge and change. Therefore students reflected that evaluation began with Phase 1 of the proposed project where stakeholders could evaluate what they would like to have addressed throughout the plan of action. Students noted that it is important to address values and link values throughout planning and evaluation. In this context, the use of social media may have either negative or positive impacts upon students' mental health. Through this process students described the cyclical nature of applying a relational emancipatory framework through "reflecting and planning", "action", "analysing, reflecting, and planning", and "follow-up action" (Hills & Carroll, 2017a). Building on community capacity

---

[1]The authors would like to acknowledge the valued participation of UVic BSN students for their contributions and for allowing us to use their example for this chapter.

and critical pedagogical approaches, this student group aimed to draw upon the knowledge and resilience of students within the university campus. In this way, the relational emancipatory framework served as a way to support empowerment of the community of interest.

In traditional approaches to leadership, evaluation usually comes after a change initiative has been implemented and may not include the experience of all participants in the process, including those impacted by the change. The student group described above applied a relational emancipatory framework to their evaluation process. Hills & Carroll (2017a) incorporate principles of such a framework throughout their Collaborative Action Evaluation Process (CAE). In a relational emancipatory process for leading change, this student group discussed that stakeholder collaboration includes and involves community-in-partnership in all phases of evaluation. Students argued that to have buy-in and action, program intervention must be continuous and collaborative, and that evaluation must also be participatory. That is, if a health promotion initiative on social media and student mental health were to occur, students would participate in evaluating what would be the impact of change. Finally, using the principles of a relational emancipatory framework, students suggested that an inquiry team would review and share evaluations with policy and decision makers. Evaluation results would be shared with key stakeholders and the team would continue to re-evaluate in subsequent cycles to ensure the continued relevance of the proposed program.

The authors found working with students who incorporated the relational emancipatory framework and its application to community health initiatives both rewarding and challenging. It was rewarding to see that students demonstrated increased consciousness about their position as nurses working with various participant groups and communities. This increased critical consciousness and enhanced students' capacity to critically engage with community health needs. Moreover, the assignment demonstrated that students could apply a model for leading change that was in partnership with people and that integrated diverse knowledge and perspectives. They demonstrated that values of social justice could be operationalized as a primary principle of ethical nursing (Canadian Nurses Association, 2017). Despite these advances, the authors also found that students struggled to work within an emancipatory paradigm because of abstract theoretical concepts and approaches that are rooted in traditional hierarchical leadership styles, traditional public health disease/deficit models. This finding may also be related to diverse metacognitive processes of those students who have not yet fully engaged with critical self-reflexive practices (Josephsen, 2014). To provide clarity and mitigate these tensions, the authors suggest that a relational emancipatory framework be applied as a heuristic approach at the beginning of courses in leadership as well as courses with a specific focus on health promotion. Additionally, more time could be made for nursing students to reflect on the process of leading change from a relational emancipatory framework. To engage in meaningful action, it will be important that experienced as well as novice nurse leaders integrate theory in action in real-world contexts to fully examine the usefulness of a relational emancipatory framework.

CONCLUSION

Now, more than ever, to make a positive impact in our discipline and across health care contexts, nurses have a moral responsibility to lead change that is both visionary and empowering. Given the complexity of the social world and its impact on everyday nursing work, it is argued that leadership must be transformative, attend to equitable power relations, be reflexive of theory and action, and engage in critical consciousness to uphold nursing's commitment toward social justice. The authors offer a relational emancipatory framework as an alternative approach to leadership for *nurses leading change*. This framework includes three general phases: Creating Collaborative Relationships; Engaging in Critical Dialogue; and Reflection in Action (Praxis). It is proposed that the change process is fluid and contextual and dependent upon collective engagement and integration of multiple ways of knowing, i.e., all voices. The BSN-student-led example demonstrates action and potential learnings from implementation of a relational emancipatory framework. Although this approach has its inherent challenges, it departs from traditional models by situating change in a context of *with*, *for*, and *by* nurses. You are invited to reflect upon a relational emancipatory framework for nurses leading change in the twenty-first century.

? A SOLUTION

Amy and the group decided to use a relational emancipatory framework and work through the six phases to bring about the desired change. In this context, to make change happen, they engaged not only key stakeholders, such as nurse practitioners, registered nurses, and physicians, but also settlement workers, child and youth workers, and local immigrant support workers. The student group realized that to support primary health care access and integration of Social Determinants of Health (SDOH) they would have to include wider community members. This team of stakeholders developed a conceptual model through a brainstorming activity by asking: *What it would look like if the access needs of newcomer families were met?* The team identified the need to have a greeter, translation services, patient navigator, linkages to settlement support, literacy resources, local social support networks, and resources available. The team decided to monitor the implementation of the change by collecting community stories from service users as well as service providers. This approach helped nurses evaluate the impact of the change initiative. They learned that having a greeter made them feel comfortable and welcomed. Consequently, the number of people accessing the primary health care clinic increased. Having a translations service also reduced language barriers. The families found that in-person translators worked more effectively than translators over the phone, whereas health care providers preferred phone interpretation because of its efficiency. In the next iteration of the planned change process, the team decided to adjust the conceptual model to provide in-person services for lower-literacy newcomers. Although several challenges remain, other primary health care centres have decided to integrate SDOH into their delivery of primary health care services for newcomers.

Would this process for leading change be a suitable approach in your workplace setting? Why or why not?

THE EVIDENCE

The benefits of participatory research have been explored and validated in systematic reviews of literature (Jagosh et al., 2012; Salimi et al., 2012; Greenhalgh et al., 2016). This broad approach has consistently been found to be particularly effective when used in highly complex settings, such as health systems and communities struggling with health inequities. The approach has been associated with the successful implementation and sustainability of health interventions that reflect the values of the communities affected by the health issues targeted. Nurses have often been participants in participatory and collaborative approaches aimed at developing positive change for patients, their families, and communities. These participatory research approaches see themselves as dedicated to relational and emancipatory processes with the goal of systemic transformational change.

※ NEED TO KNOW NOW

- Recognize when there is an opportunity for change.
- Engage stakeholders from the outset and in every phase of the change process.
- Understand group dynamics and processes and develop your group facilitation capacities.
- Be creative, use your imagination, and encourage others to do the same.
- Create a safe space for dialogue by exploring other perspectives and not knowing.
- Be an advocate for social justice in nursing by sharing nursing knowledge.

CHAPTER CHECKLIST

- Leading change
  - Nurses can uphold principles of social justice by operationalizing a relational emancipatory process for change.

- A relational emancipatory process is underpinned by emancipatory education theory and participatory approaches to knowledge development.

- Transformational change
  - Assets of team/group and community members are privileged to promote positive change.
  - Emancipation is fostered through collaborative action.
  - Reciprocity across and within stakeholder groups is necessary for collaborative action.
- Social contexts
  - Reflexivity of broader social contexts and relationships is required.

- Space is created for critical dialogue to occur.
- Social action is a reflexive process (reflection in action).
- Evaluation
  - Impact of social change must include the voice of those most impacted by the change initiative.
  - All participants co-evaluate.
  - Change must be systemic to transform practice and structures for the social good.

TIPS FOR LEADING CHANGE

- Be aware of your capacity to lead and develop your leadership strengths.
- Observe others leading change and note what they do and the impact it has.
- Keep a journal to track your experiences, goals, and learning about leading change.

- Be open to the unpredictability and chaos in the change process—go with the flow and process.
- Being rigid and inflexible will hinder your ability to lead change.
- Lead by engaging with others as a full participant in the process (leading from beside).

Visit the Evolve website for Suggested Readings, Internet Resources, and additional resources related to the content in this chapter: http://evolve.elsevier.com/Canada/Yoder-Wise/leading/.

REFERENCES

Anthony, K. (2004). "Shared governance models: the theory, practice, and evidence" online journal of issues in nursing. 9(1). Manuscript 4. Available: www.nursingworld.org/MainMenuCategories/ANAMarketplace/ANAPeriodicals/OJIN/TableofContents/Volume92004/No1Jan04/Shared-GovernanceModels.aspx.

Barnes, H., Bradshaw, E., Hubscher, R., Messelink, S., Morgan, J., & Young, Marissa. (2018). *Community health plan part II: Interpersonal workshops within the university of victoria.* Scholarly paper for Nursing 350, University of Victoria.

Best, A., Greenhalgh, T., Lewis, S., Saul, J. E., Carroll, S., & Bitz, J. (2012). Large-system transformation in health care: A realist review. *The Milbank Quarterly, 90*(3), 421–456.

Brookfield, S. (1993). On impostership, cultural suicide, and other dangers: How nurses learning critical thinking. *The Journal of Continuing Education in Nursing, 24*(5), 197–205.

Canadian Nurses Association. (2017). *Ethics for Registered Nurses.* Retrieved from: https://www.cna-aiic.ca/en/nursing-practice/nursing-ethics.

Chinn, P. (2008). *Peace and power.* London: Jones Bartlett.

Clark, N., Handlovsky, I., & Sinclair, D. (2015). Using reflexivity to achieve transdiciplinarity in nursing and social work. In L. Greaves, N. Poole, & E. Boyle (Eds.), *Transforming addiction: Gender, trauma, transdisciplinarity* (pp. 120–136). London: Routledge.

Doane, G., & Varcoe, C. (2016). *How to nurse: Relational inquiry with individuals and families in changing health and health care contexts.* Philadelphia: Wolters Kluwer/Lippincott Williams & Wilkins.

Finklemann, Ward, A. (2006). *Leadership and management in nursing.* New Jersey, US: Pearson Prentice Hall.

Freeman, A., & Dolan, M. (2001). Revisiting Prochaska and DiClemente's stages of change theory: An expansion and specification to aid in treatment planning and outcome evaluation. *Cognitive and Behavioral Practice, 8*(3), 224–234.

Freire, P. (1972). *Pedagogy of the oppressed.* London: Penguin Books.

Gottlieb, L. (2013). *Strengths-based nursing care: Health and healing for person and family.* New York: Springer.

Greco, P., Laschenger, H. K., & Wong, C. (2006). Leader empowering behaviours, staff nurse empowerment/burnout. *Nurse Leadership, 19*(4), 41–56.

Greenhalgh, T., Jackson, C., Shaw, S., & Janamian, T. (2016). Achieving research impact through co-creation in community-based health services: Literature review and case study. *The Milbank Quarterly, 94*(2), 392–429.

Havelock, R. G. (1973). *The change agent's guide to innovation in education.* Englewood Cliffs, NJ: Educational Technology.

Heron, J., & Reason, P. (1997). A participatory inquiry paradigm. *Qualitative Inquiry, 3*(3), 274–294.

Hills, M. (2016). Emancipation and collaboration: Leading from beside. In W. Rosa (Ed.), *Nurses as leaders.* New York: Springer, 293–310.

Hills, M., & Carroll (2017a). Collaborative action research and evaluation: Relational inquiry for promoting caring science literacy. In S. Lee, P. Palmer, & J. Watson (Eds.), *Global Advances in Human Caring Literacy.* New York: Springer, 115–130.

Hills, M., & Carroll (2017b). Evaluating a community health program: Collaborative action evaluation. In A. Vollman, E. Anderson, & J. McFarlane (Eds.), *Canadian Community as Partner.* Philadelphia: Wolters Kluwer.

Hills, M., Carroll, S., & Desjardins, S. (2010). Assets based interventions: Evaluating and synthesizing evidence of the effectiveness of the assets based approach to health promotion. In Health assets in a global context (pp. 77–98). New York, NY: Springer.

Hills, M., & Watson, J. (2011). *Creating a caring science curriculum: An emancipatory pedagogy for nursing.* New York: Springer, 346–372.

Jagosh, J., Macaulay, A., Pluye, P., et al. (2012). Uncovering the benefits of participatory research: Implications of a realist review for health research and practice. *Milbank Quarterly, 90*(2), 311–346.

Johnston, S. (2015). Leading change. In L. Grant (Ed.), *Leading and managing in canadian nursing.* Toronto: Yoder-Wise, 331–350.

Josephsen, J. (2014). (2014). Critically reflexive theory: A proposal for nursing education. *Advances in Nursing, Vol. 2014.* Article ID 594360, 7 pages.

Kemmis, S. (1985). Action research and the politics of reflection. In D. Boud, R. Keogh, & D. Walker (Eds.), *Reflection: Turning experience into learning (pp. 139–163).* London: Kogan Page.

Kretzmann, J. P., & Mcknight, J. L. (1993). *Building communities for the inside out: A path toward finding and mobilizing a community's assets.* Chicago: ACTA.

Labonte, R. (1994). Health promotion and empowerment: Reflections on professional practice. *Health Education Quarterly, 21*(2), 253–268.

Lather, P. (2017). Feminist perspectives on empowering research methodologies. In Patti Lather (Ed.), *(Post)Critical methodologies: The science possible after the critiques* (pp. 82–96). New York: Routledge.

Laverack, G., & Labonte, R. (2000). A planning framework for community empowerment goals within health promotion. *Health Policy and Planning, 15*(3), 255–262.

Lewin, K. (1951). *Field theory in social science.* London, UK: Tavistock.

May, C. (2002). Stages of change. A critique. *Behavior Modification, 26*(2), 223–273.

McGlynn-Stewart, E. M. (2015). Undergraduate student perspectives on the value of peer-led discussions. *The Canadian Journal for the Scholarship of Teaching and Learning, 6*(3). https://doi.org/10.5206/cjsotl-rcacea.2015.3.9.

Mills, L. W., Pimental, B. C., Palmer, A. J., et al. (2018). Applying a theory driven framework to guide quality improvement efforts in nursing homes: The lock model. *The Gerontologist, 58*(3), 598–605.

Morgan, A., Ziglio, E., & Davies, M. (2010). *Health assets in a global context: Theory, methods, action.* New York: Springer.

Moustakas, C. (1997). *Creative life.* New York: Van Nostrand Reinhold.

Mustakova-Possardt, E. (1998). Critical consciousness: An alternative pathway for positive personal and social development. *Journal of Adult Development, 5*(1), 13.

Pate, D. M. F. (2013). Nursing leadership from the bedside to the boardroom. *AACN Advanced Critical Care, 24*(2), 186–193.

Porter-O'Grady, T. (2001). Profound change: 21 century nursing. *Nursing Outlook, 4*(4), 182–186.

Prochaska, J., Norcross, J., & DiClemente, C. (1995). *Changing for good.* New York: Avon Books.

Reinkemeyer, A. M. (1970). Nursing's need: Commitment to an ideology of change. In *Nursing forum* (Vol. 9) (pp. 340–355). Oxford, UK: Blackwell Publishing Ltd. No. 4.

Rendon, L. (2014). *Sentipensante pedagogy: Educating for wholeness, social justice and liberation.* New York, NY.

Salimi, Y., Shahandeh, K., Malekafzali, H., Loori, N., Kheiltash, A., Jamshidi, E., et al. (2012). Is community-based participatory research (CBPR) useful? A systematic review on papers in a decade. *International Journal of Preventive Medicine, 3*(6), 386.

Senge, P. M. (1990). *The fifth discipline: The art and practice of the learning organization.* New York, NY: Doubleday.

Wallerstein, N., & Hammes, M. (1991). Problem-posing: A teaching strategy for improving the decision-making process. *Journal of Health Education, 22*, 250–253.

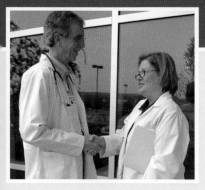

20

Building Teams Through Communication and Partnership

Colleen A. McKey,
with contributions by Mallory McKey, BScN Student

This chapter presents frameworks, concepts, and tools important for creating and maintaining effective teams. To ensure safety for patients and coworkers, health care providers must work together collaboratively and respectfully, communicate effectively, and develop dynamic partnerships. Research has demonstrated that teams are critical to patient safety and quality care because they encourage frequent and ongoing communication and interact with a system in which safeguards and supports are part of health care delivery. This chapter also provides an overview of the different types of teams, the qualities of team members, the importance of communication and conflict management in teams, the characteristics of effective teams, and the role of leadership in team success.

OBJECTIVES

- Describe the differences between a group and a team.
- Compare and contrast types of teams.
- Describe the qualities of a team member.
- Critique a team that functions synergistically, including the team's outcomes.
- Understand how generational differences can affect teams.
- Describe the value of team building.
- Explore the role of conflict in teams.
- Apply the guidelines for acknowledgement to a situation in your workplace.
- Explore the guidelines for effective communication.
- Explain why it is important for individuals to manage their emotions.
- Describe processes and importance of reflective practice, including mindfulness.
- Understand the concepts of interdisciplinary and interprofessional teams.
- Explain how leadership can contribute to team success.

TERMS TO KNOW

active listening
conflict
dualism

group
interdisciplinary team
interprofessional team

synergy
team

A large team provides care to medical patients and their families in an interprofessional Clinical Teaching Unit (CTU) in a large academic teaching hospital. The team members include physicians, registered nurses, licensed practical nurses, respiratory therapists, physiotherapists, occupational therapists, social workers, nurse practitioners, dietitians, pharmacists, discharge planners, and ancillary staff. Occasionally, specialists are consulted on specific cardiac, neurological, or gastrointestinal problems; they are intermittent team members who play a crucial role in medical care.

Recently, a new group of specialists joined the team. These specialists are known for their expertise and reputation. The existing team was excited to have the specialists join the CTU, particularly because they expected that there would be an increase in the number of referrals to the hospital. However, the integration of the new team members did not go smoothly. Clinical disagreements, communication breakdowns, and interpersonal conflicts arose. The experience evolved into a state of mutual distrust and perceived issues of control over clinical practice decisions.

As disagreements, insults, and complaints escalated on both sides, the situation came to a defining moment when one of the specialists said, "I'm never bringing any patients here. I'm sending them to another teaching hospital." The response from the CTU team was "Fine with us; we don't need you, your patients, or the hassle." It seemed unreasonable to continue to work "together" because, in fact, the two groups worked separately and sometimes against each other. This inability to work together was in direct conflict with the belief that the CTU team provided a valuable service and made a difference for both the patients and their families. This conflict posed a dilemma for the staff and everyone felt the situation was hopeless.

Team members felt that they could no longer function effectively and that further efforts to work together would be futile. All parties believed they had tried and failed. The new mantra was "Let's just cut our losses and move on." How does one create a team when no one believes it is possible and some believe that it is not even necessary?

If you were a CTU new graduate nurse, how would you feel working on this unit? What fears and anxiety would you have? What strengths do you feel you bring to the situation? What help/support would you need from your nurse manager? What actions would you take in your nursing role?

INTRODUCTION

Teamwork has become critical to safe quality care. We are in an era in which **teams** are accountable for patient outcomes. Health care organizations focus not only on safety and quality care but also on linkages with the public, consumer groups, other provider organizations, and government in the forms of accountability agreements and funding models. Team communication is the bedrock of safe quality care and will be increasingly important as teams negotiate with internal and external key stakeholders.

In our society, emphasis is often placed on individual achievement. However, we still need individuals to work together to achieve goals that one person alone would not be able to achieve. Teams often function with the yin and yang of cooperation and competition. They do so in many forums, from health care to sports. Sports teams are premier models of cooperation and competition. This model of teamwork represents the team member following the team coach with a focus on the team goal (Thelwell et al., 2017). To create and sustain teams that are able to function effectively in complex health care environments, it is important to understand what a team is, the different types of teams, when it is appropriate to create a team, and how to best utilize teams in the delivery of quality care.

GROUPS AND TEAMS

A **group** is a number of individuals assembled together or who have a unifying relationship. Groups could be all the parents in an elementary school, all the members of a specific church, or all the students in a school of nursing. The members of these various groups are related in some way to one another by definition of their involvement in a certain endeavour. A **team**, on the other hand, is a number of individuals who work closely together toward a common purpose and are accountable to one another. Not every group is a team, and not every team is effective.

A group of people does not constitute a team. A team is a group of interdependent individuals who seek out opportunities to combine their expertise to achieve common goals (Thompson, 2018). It has a high degree of interdependence geared toward the achievement of a goal or a task. Often, we can recognize intuitively when the so-called team is not functioning effectively. We say things such as, "We need to be more like a team" or "I'd like to see more team players around here." Consequently, in the process of defining *team*, effective versus ineffective teams should be considered. Teams have defined objectives, ongoing relationships, and a supportive environment and are focused on accomplishing specific goals. Teams are essential in providing cost-effective, high-quality care. As resources are expended more prudently, teams must develop clearly defined goals, use creative problem solving, and demonstrate mutual respect and support.

Types of Teams

A number of types of teams exist, each fulfilling a distinct purpose. As a first step, it is important to decide whether a team is required to reach a specific goal or address a specific issue. Often we create teams without a clear mandate, specific goals, or team roles. As a result, an effective team of individuals—no matter how knowledgeable, creative, and productive—can fail.

Understanding the different types of teams can be helpful in deciding which team approach is appropriate.

- *Manager-led team:* The manager is the team leader and controls the agenda, decisions, direction, and outputs of the team.
- *Self-managing team:* The manager sets the overall direction and defines the goal and outcome for the team. The members of the team determine the direction, strategies, and focus of the team to achieve the goal.
- *Self-directed team:* The manager identifies the outcome, and the team members determine the direction, strategies, methods, and focus to achieve the outcome. Often, these teams function in quality improvement initiatives to address quality challenges and opportunities.
- *Self-governing team:* This team is a collection of individuals who come together to create something new or address an opportunity or challenge. The team determines appropriate membership, sets its own direction, defines the outcomes, and then manages team performance and outcomes (Thompson, 2018).

The terms *management team* and *leadership team* are often used interchangeably in the literature and in organizations. There is, however, a distinct difference. Management teams typically focus on operational issues, such as described above, although leadership teams tend to focus on creating a strategic vision and working with teams to achieve this vision.

Each of these types of teams is appropriate for and often used in health care organizations. They assist in the achievement of organizational goals and address issues of competition (both internal and external) to the organization.

Interdisciplinary and Interprofessional Teams

Teams are essential to quality patient care. Nurses, physicians, dietitians, social workers, case managers, pharmacists, and physiotherapists, to name but a few, must work together to provide high quality cost-effective care for patients. This means that health care providers must understand the various roles and educational backgrounds of each discipline. Two types of teams, interdisciplinary teams and interprofessional teams, are common in health care settings.

An **interdisciplinary team** comprises members from different clinical disciplines who have specialized knowledge, skills, and abilities. They often work alongside one another and may or may not collaborate closely on patient care. Much of the care in hospitals is delivered through interdisciplinary teams. For example, nurses, surgeons, and physiotherapists work together to address the complex needs of a patient receiving postoperative care after orthopedic surgery. Each health care provider on the team has a specific role in patient care, often has their own approach to patient documentation, and may or may not meet together with other team members to discuss a patient's plan of care.

An **interprofessional team** comprises "different healthcare disciplines working together towards common goals to meet the needs of a patient population. Team members divide the work based on their scope of practice; they share information to support one another's work and coordinate processes and interventions to provide a number of services and programs" (Virani, 2012, p. 3). A body of literature has emerged highlighting the importance of interprofessional collaboration, which supports a deep degree of collaboration in both the academic and practice settings among team members. Studies of interprofessional teams have identified positive outcomes for clients (e.g., lower readmission rates, improved self-care), health care providers (e.g., higher rates of job satisfaction, retention in the workplace), and the health care system (e.g., cost savings associated with improved patient and health care provider outcomes) and the academic learning community (e.g., education and practice partnerships to support student learning) (Suter et al., 2012; Carter et al., 2016).

The Centre for Interprofessional Education, Toronto Academic Health Science Network (2017) developed the Interprofessional Care Competency Framework and Team Assessment Toolkit. This framework addresses six domains:

1. Patient/client/family/community centred care.
2. Communication.
3. Role clarity.
4. Conflict.
5. Team functioning.
6. Collaborative leadership.

In addition to focusing on collaborative teams in the health care setting, health professional educational programs, such as those in nursing and medicine, have included opportunities for interprofessional education. That is, students from different disciplines are encouraged to take courses or participate in educational initiatives together to learn about one another's role, share knowledge and skills, and learn how to collaborate (World Health Organization, 2013).

> **EXERCISE 20.1** Think of a team or group of which you were a part. How did the team function? Use the Team Assessment Exercise in Table 20.1 to assess aspects of the team more specifically. Address each of the identified areas and discover how well the team functioned. Think about roles, activities, relationships, and the general environment. Consider examples of shared decision making, shared leadership, shared accountability, and shared problem solving. These concepts can be used to evaluate the functioning of almost any team.

Key Concepts Related to Teams

In rare instances, a group of individuals may work as a team spontaneously, like kids in a schoolyard at recess. However, most teams learn about teamwork because they need and want to work together. Working together requires that individuals observe how they function in a group and that they unlearn self-limiting assumptions about the exclusive value of individual effort and authority that are contrary to cooperation and teamwork. Ineffective teams are often dominated by a few members, leaving others bored, resentful, or uninvolved. Leadership within an ineffective team may be autocratic and rigid, and the team's communication style, as a result, may be overly stiff, formal, and not focused on the team goal. Members tend to be uncomfortable with conflict or disagreement, avoiding and suppressing it rather than using it as a catalyst for change. When criticism is offered, it may be destructive, personal, and hurtful rather than constructive and problem-focused. Team members may begin to hide their feelings of resentment or disagreement, sensing that they

TABLE 20.1   Team Assessment Exercise

Are we a Team?

Directions: Select a team with which you work or in your educational program. Place a checkmark beside each item that is true of your team. If the statement is not true, place no mark beside the item.

1. The language we use focuses on "we" rather than "you" or "I".
2. When one of us is busy, others try to help.
3. I know I can ask for help from others.
4. Most of us on the team could say what we are trying to accomplish.
5. What we are trying to accomplish on any given work day relates to the mission and vision of nursing and the organization.
6. We treat each other fairly, not necessarily the same.
7. We capitalize on people's strengths to meet the goals of our work.
8. The process for changing policies, procedures, equipment is clear.
9. Meetings are focused on the goals we are focused on.
10. Our outcomes reflect our attention to goals and efforts.
11. Acknowledgement is individual and goal-oriented.
12. Innovation is supported by the team and management.
13. The group makes commitments to each other to ensure goal attainment.
14. Promises are kept.
15. Kindness in communication is evident, especially when bad news is delivered.
16. Individuals can describe their role in the overall work of the group.
17. Other members of the team are seen as trustworthy and valued.
18. The group is cost-effective and time-effective in attaining goals.
19. No member is excluded from the process of decision making.
20. Individuals can speak highly of their team members.

Tally the number of checkmarks and multiply that number by 5. The resultant number is an assessment of how well your team is functioning. The higher the score, the better the functioning.

©The Wise Group, 2007, Lubbock, Texas.

are inappropriate. Doing so creates the potential for later eruptions and discord. Similarly, the team avoids examining its own team dynamics. This can result in members waiting until after meetings to voice their thoughts and feelings about other team members, as well as what went wrong and why.

In contrast, an effective team is characterized by its clarity of purpose, commitment to goal achievement, and a high level of participation. It is also characterized by members' ability to listen respectfully to one another and communicate openly, which helps them handle disagreements in a professional manner and work through them rather than suppress them. Through goal-focused discussions of issues, the team reaches decisions by consensus or other predetermined ways. Roles and work assignments are clear. Members may share the leadership role and recognize that each person brings their own unique strengths to the work. This diversity of styles helps the team adapt to changes and challenges, as does the team's ability and willingness to assess its own strengths and weaknesses and respond to them appropriately. Signs that a team is functioning effectively include the following: discussions progress productively, team members have a good understanding of team-specific goals and tasks, team members listen to one another, the team manages disagreements, decisions are usually made by consensus, and feedback is given and received respectfully. MacGregor (1960), whose work is still relevant today, identified the characteristics of effective and ineffective teams (Table 20.2). This is supported by other authors including Thompson (2018) and Cahn & Abigail (2014). The Leader's Institute (2017) identified five characteristics of highly effective teams. Highly effective teams 1) have trust, 2) debate positively, 3) are mission oriented, 4) are results focused, and 5) work within and sustain a culture of

TABLE 20.2 Characteristics of Effective and Ineffective Teams

Characteristic	Effective Team	Ineffective Team
Working environment (Culture of leadership and have trust)	Informal, comfortable, relaxed	Indifferent, bored, tense, stiff
Discussion (Debate Positively)	Focused Shared by almost everyone	Frequently unfocused Dominated by a few
Objectives (Mission oriented)	Well understood and accepted	Unclear, or many personal agendas
Listening (Have trust)	Respectful—encourages participation	Judgemental—much interruption and "grandstanding"
Ability to handle conflict (Have trust and debate positively)	Comfortable with disagreement Open to discussion of conflicts	Uncomfortable with disagreement Disagreement usually suppressed, or one group aggressively dominates
Decision making (Results focused)	Usually reached by consensus Formal voting kept to a minimum General agreement is necessary for action; dissenters are free to voice opinions	Decisions often occur prematurely Formal voting occurs frequently Simple majority is sufficient for action; minority is expected to go along with opinion
Criticism (Have trust and debate positively)	Frequent, frank, relatively comfortable and constructive; directed at removing obstacle	Embarrassing, tension-producing, and destructive; directed personally at others
Leadership (Culture of Leadership)	Shared; shifts from time to time	Autocratic; remains clearly with committee chairperson
Assignments (Mission focused)	Clearly stated Accepted by all despite disagreements	Unclear Resented by dissenting members
Feelings (Have trust)	Freely expressed; open for discussion	Hidden; considered "explosive" and inappropriate for discussion
Self-regulation (Culture of leadership)	Frequent and ongoing; focused on solutions	Infrequent, or occurs outside meetings

Modified from MacGregor, D. (1960). *The human side of enterprise.* New York, NY: McGraw-Hill; The Leader's Institute. (2017). *Five characteristics of highly effective teams.* Retrieved from www.leadersinstitute.com.

leadership. The work of MacGregor and Leader's Institute is integrated in Table 20.2.

In today's health care system, complex patient safety, quality, and cost-effective care issues are at the forefront. Ongoing rounds of restructuring, realignment, budget cuts, declining patient days, ever-changing funding models and incentives, and staff adjustment abound. Effective teams will need to continue to engage in effective problem solving and increased creativity to improve health outcomes. The impact of effective teams on patient safety and quality care is critically important.

TEAM DEVELOPMENT

When individuals come together in a group, they spend considerable time in group processes or social dynamics, which allows the group to advance toward becoming an effective team and achieving set goals.

Moreover, when a team begins to develop, it is essential to establish ground rules for the team as well as build trust in the team, both of which are essential to collaboration, creativity, and achieving the desired goals.

Ingroups and Outgroups

Most of us want to be valued and recognized by others as a member of the team, one who knows or understands. Most people want to be at the core of decision making, power, and influence. In other words, they want to be part of the "in group," and researchers have demonstrated that those who feel a part of this group cooperate more, work harder, and are more enthusiastic and effective as a member of the team. The more people feel they are not a key member of the team, the more disenfranchised they feel and the more they may withdraw, work alone, and engage in self-defeating behaviours. Often, intergroup conflict results in a schism or a division that can prohibit the team from accomplishing its goals.

Team members need to get to know one another to feel part of the team. Therefore it is important to take the time at the formation of a new team to create group cohesion through clearly defined roles, group norms, ground rules, and team charters.

Power

Everyone wants to feel a sense of control over their work environments. A component of that control is power. Power is the ability to influence. Robbins et al. (2016) presented French and Raven's (1959) six key sources of power. The power sources are:

1. *Legitimate*: the power one holds by virtue of their role.
2. *Reward*: getting access to benefits.
3. *Coercive*: having the ability to punish.
4. *Expert*: based on competence and unique knowledge
5. *Referent*: based on a person's appealing qualities.
6. *Informational*: based on individual's extent of knowledge.

Thompson (2018) also speaks of *network power*. This type of power is reflected in the connections an individual has in their professional network. When faced with changes that individuals feel they cannot control, they experience a loss of that sense of power and influence. This can result from both overuse or abdication of power. Effective team members learn to use their power to bring about behaviours and strategies that support team goals.

EXERCISE 20.2 Think about a time when you were a member of a team in your workplace or observed a team during your clinical placement that was not able to successfully make a change in a patient-care practice. How did you, as a member or observer of the team, feel? What was the response from other members of the team towards you and each other? Did team members engage in dysfunctional interpersonal conflict to make others appear wrong? Using the content in this section of the chapter and reflecting on the preceding questions, answer the following:

- Do you believe that a perceived power differential was having an impact upon the team? If so, what was that? How did you reach this conclusion?
- What would be the warning signs that the team was becoming ineffective? What actions could you take to address the warning signs?

Using, Developing, and Being Appreciated for Skills and Resources

Each member of the team has unique skills and resources to bring to the team's goals and tasks. In its evaluation of the work environment, David Williams (2017) from Forbes says one of the most powerful indicators of a successful, supportive work environment is to remove fear of mistakes. When fear exists in the workplace it decreases the opportunities for innovation and change. This has significant consequences on employee performance and overall goal achievement. An effective and knowledgeable team leader is key to ensure that each team member feels recognized, encouraged, and utilized

---

BOX 20.1 Ground Rules

Vision
- One commonly understood goal to be jointly attained by the team.
- The desired future the team wants to achieve.

Values
- Respect and honesty in team interactions.
- Bringing the good news and bad news to the team.
- Living the values and competencies for each interprofessional member of the team.

Team Commitment & Norms and Team Accountability
- Only one person speaks at a time.
- Team meetings begin and end on time.
- An agenda is sent before the team meeting.
- Team decisions are made by consensus.
- If the team cannot make decisions by consensus, then majority plus one is employed.
- Team members complete assigned work between team meetings.

Modified from Leggat, S. (2007). Effective healthcare teams require effective team members: Defining teamwork competencies. *BMC Health Services Research, 7*, 17–27; Stuart, A. (2014). Ground rules for a high performing team. Paper presented at PMI Global Congress 2014, North America, Phoenix, AZ. Newtown Square, PA: Project Management Institute; Pilette, P. (2017). Team charters: Mapping clearer communication. *Nursing Management, 48*(5) 52–55.

---

to the fullest potential. When team members do not feel their skills are used, they are more prone to be in the outgroup, which can lead them to feel disengaged from the team and the workplace.

Ground Rules and Team Charters

One of the most helpful tools in team development is to have team members come to an agreement about the ground rules concerning their relationships with one another (Leggat, 2007; Stuart, 2014). Ground rules are the foundation "rules of the game" that focus on both team dynamics and processes. Multiple types of guidelines or rules can be used to set the context for how team members work together. An example of a set of guidelines is given in Box 20.1. A team's ground rules may go through multiple transitions and redesign over time, but the basic tenets essentially remain the same. People must agree on the goals and mission with which they are involved. They have to do so in an environment that is free of fear of retribution and allows freedom to express

ideas fully. They have to reach some understanding of how they will work together. Tenets or rules such as "We will speak respectfully" go a long way to avoid gossiping, backbiting, bickering, and misinterpreting others. An essential success factor for these team agreements is the willingness of members to be accountable for upholding the agreements and to give feedback when the agreements have been violated. Without rules, people have implicit permission to behave in any manner they choose, such as with anger, hostility, and unprofessionally. These ground rules are complemented with team charters. Pilette (2017) presents team charters as effective tools. The four elements of the team charter are: 1) vision, including aspirational goals; 2) values that drive behaviours; 3) team commitment and norms that reflect how team members treat each other; and 4) collaborative accountability to help ensure team effectiveness. Each of these four domains are affected by the values, beliefs, and behaviours reflected in the ground rules.

Trust

Trust can be a major concern among team members, and one of the first questions to come up often concerns what trust will look like in the team. In the early days of organizational development, MacGregor (1967) defined *trust* in the following way:

> Trust means: "I know that you will not—deliberately or accidentally, consciously or unconsciously—take unfair advantage of me." It means, "I can put my situation at the moment, my status and self-esteem in this group, relationship, my job, my career, even my life, in your hands with complete confidence." (p. 163)

The *Oxford English Dictionary* (2012) defines *trust* as "the belief in the loyalty, veracity, reliability, strength, etc., of a person or thing." Trust is fundamental to well-functioning teams. Leaders model trust through behaviours such as setting the ground rules and agreements by which the team will function and holding themselves and the team members accountable. Trust is probably the most delicate aspect within relationships and is influenced far more by actions than by words. What people do is often more powerful than what they say. Trust is a fragile thread that can be undone by one act. Once destroyed, trust is more difficult to re-establish than its initial creation. When speaking of trust, we often hear the adage "years to create and moments to destroy."

Trust is the basis on which each team member assumes a role in the activities and the progress of the team. Kouzes and Posner (2017) have focused their leadership work on personal best leadership practices that mobilize others to get extraordinary things done. They learned that leaders build high-performance teams through five key behaviours: modelling the way, inspiring a shared vision, challenging the process, enabling others to act, and encouraging the heart. Poorly performing teams show little evidence of these relational behaviours and, consequently, trust is low for the leader and among team members.

QUALITIES OF A TEAM MEMBER

Riggio (2013) identified seven qualities of a good team member. A good team member is:

1. Honest and straightforward. *The team member will tell others "what's what," regardless of whether it is good news or bad news.*
2. A person who shares the load. *The team member completes the work assigned and pitches in to help others.*
3. Reliable. *The team member can be trusted and looked upon as a valued and important member of the team.*
4. Fair. *The team member gives credit and takes credit as appropriate.*
5. Compliments others' skills. *The team member brings out and supports others' strengths and abilities.*
6. A person with good communication skills. *The team member utilizes a professional goal- oriented approach to all communication.*
7. A person with a positive attitude. *The team member looks at error as opportunity and keeps a realistic but positive attitude.*

EXERCISE 20.3 Think about the last team project in which you participated. What worked about the team? What did not work about the team? Was there a member who did not carry their share of the work? Was there a team member who was a "know it all"? How did you handle the situation? Was there a person on the team who took the lead? Now reflect on your own contribution as a team member in that same situation. Be honest—how many of the qualities of a good team member do you possess? In what areas could you improve? What are your strengths and where do you shine as a team member? Finally, what learning opportunities present themselves for improvement?

CREATING SYNERGY

Teams function with varying levels of effectiveness. The interesting part is that effectiveness can be created systematically. Effective teams are ones in which people work together to produce results and achieve a common goal that could not have been achieved by any one individual. This phenomenon is often described as synergy. In the physical sciences synergy is found in metal alloys. Bronze, the first alloy, was a combination of copper and tin and was found to be much harder and stronger than either copper or tin separately. This strength is not an additive strength (combining the strength of copper plus tin), but rather the strength comes from a unique combination of factors to create a unique strength that only applies to the end product, the bronze.

We see the same properties of synergy in human endeavours. Consider the silver-medal win of the Canadian women's hockey team in the 2018 Winter Olympics in PyeongChang, South Korea, for example. The success of the women's hockey team was the result of determination and hard work by all team members. Each member brought their own strengths and was focused on the goal and not self. The team as a whole knew how to best use the strengths of each individual team member. The women's ice hockey team won silver because its members knew how to work together to produce extraordinary results. Working cooperatively, an effective team produces results that no one team member could have achieved alone. Creating synergy requires a clear purpose. Each member of the team must understand the reason the team is together, determine what they each wish to accomplish (as delineated by defined goals and objectives), and express their belief in both the value and feasibility of the goals and tasks. Teams function best when the members can tell others about their purpose as well as define and operationalize succinctly the meaning and value of this purpose.

Synergy cannot occur when one team member becomes a self-proclaimed expert who has the "right" answer. Nor can synergy occur when people refuse to communicate. Each team member has good ideas, and these need to be shared. They are not shared, however, when someone does not feel valued. It can be difficult to speak up if you fear appearing wrong or inadequate.

The challenge each person faces is to push through discomfort and become a full participant in problem identification and resolution for the overall benefit of the team.

Our society tends to be dualistic in nature. Dualism means that most situations are viewed in terms of two opposing positions (right or wrong; yes or no), thus limiting the broad spectrum of possibilities that exists between. Exercising creativity and exploring numerous possibilities are important. Doing so allows the team to operate at its optimal level.

We have all known people who were self-proclaimed experts, to whom it was critically important that they be right and acknowledged as right and who become judgemental of others whose perspectives and opinions differ from theirs. Consequently, being able to tell the truth to one's team and to encourage team members to stretch and look at different ways of thinking and acting is vital. This ability requires strong skills in negotiation and conflict management; something for which few teams have been developed. If self-proclaimed experts think we are judging them, they will not hear the questions, the observations, or the veracity of the issue because the message seems to be suggesting they are wrong rather than originating from consideration of varied perspectives. The most valuable contribution employees can make to an organization is the creation of synergistic teams.

GENERATIONAL DIFFERENCES AMONG TEAM MEMBERS

Most workplaces have a mix of team members from different generations: Baby Boomers, Generation X, Generation Y, and Millennials. With each generation, the concept of work has been interpreted using the current and historical influences of the time. We live in a world of changing economic, geographic, and cultural environments as well as changing dominant discourses. To have effective teams, there is a need to understand the common and unique generational needs within the current and future workforces (Anderson & Morgan, 2017). For example, the perspectives of many Baby Boomers is influenced by having lived through post–World War II social change. Generation X-ers tend to be more accustomed to working independently, having grown up as part of the "latch key" generation where parents worked

outside the home. Once they entered the workforce, job stability was no longer guaranteed. Generation Y-ers tend to be characterized as more technology-savvy having grown up alongside the Internet and accustomed to accessing massive amounts of information. They are more aware of the values of cultural diversity and view education as one of the keys to success. Often within the nursing profession we hear the unfortunate phrase "eating our young." Nursing leaders must continue to focus on the value of nursing education, and engage nurses in goal-oriented discussion to collaboratively engage diverse teams in strategies to create effective work environments and teams.

Efforts to understand and bridge these generations can make the difference between a dysfunctional and an effective team. Chapter 2 discusses generational differences in more detail. Understanding and capitalizing on the unique attributes of a multigenerational team can help strengthen the team.

Understanding the diversity of team members is crucial at all stages of team development, but in particular during the formation of the team and when the team may encounter challenges and difficulties. Team building, discussed next, can help teams overcome challenges and achieve their goals. Team building can be the cornerstone to effective teams.

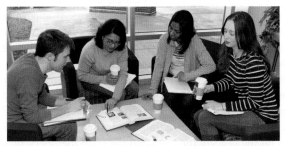

Teams can form strong relationships outside the work environment.

THE VALUE OF TEAM BUILDING

Team building can enhance functioning in any one or all of the following processes (Thorman & Mendonca, n.d.):

- *Living operating principles*: The establishment of goals, objectives, and decision-making approaches.
- *Packing up your troubles*: The relationships among the people doing the work.

BOX 20.2   Questions to Assess the Need for Team Building

1. What do you see as the issues currently facing your team?
2. What are the current strengths of your work group? What are you currently doing well?
3. Do other members of the team affect your ability to be as effective as you would like to be?
4. Does the leader of the team engage in activities or behaviours that prevent you from being as effective as you would like to be?
5. What would you like to accomplish at your upcoming team-building session? What changes would you be willing to make that would facilitate a more effective team and the accomplishment of the team goals?

• *Staff meeting check-ins*: Clearly defining performance expectations and team outcomes.

When organizations face challenges that require attention and resolution, team building is often one of the first interventions. Teams, in particular interprofessional teams, including learners, must function in a culture of learning (Carter et al., 2016). Difficulties can occur when organizations are under pressure and facing challenges. The team members feel tremendous pressure and struggle to function as a cohesive team. Team building can assist the team members to refocus and work in a more synergistic manner. A team-building exercise can teach a team how to set goals and priorities; help a team analyze the distribution of the workload using various team members' strengths; examine a team's process, norms, decision-making processes, and communication patterns; and promote the resolution of interpersonal conflicts or problems within the team. Often the focus is on the tasks of the team and the team members' processes, and interrelationships do not receive the education and support they require for team success.

Regardless of which areas are problematic, appropriate assessment of the team is essential. The difficulties may be in priority or goal setting, allocation of the work, team decision making, or interpersonal relationships among the members. Box 20.2 presents guidelines you can use to determine areas in which your team would benefit from team building.

The Research Perspective below examines the success of the team and the role team building plays.

RESEARCH PERSPECTIVE

Resource: McEwan, D., Ruissen, G., Eys, M., Jumbo, B., & Beauchamp, R. (2017). The effectiveness of team nursing on teamwork behaviors and teamwork performance. A systematic review and meta-analysis of controlled interventions. *PLOS One.* https://doc/10.1371/journalpone.0169604.

The authors undertook an extensive meta-analysis of team-building research that focused on four specific components of teams: goal setting, interpersonal relationships, problem solving, and role clarification. The meta-analysis included 103 articles published between 1950 and 2007 and expanded the original work conducted in 1999. The outcomes measured were cognitive, affective, process, and performance based. The results suggested that team-building activities have a moderately positive effect across all team outcomes, whereas the strongest effect existed for goal setting and role clarification. The size of the team can also be important, and teams of 10 or fewer members seem to have more success.

These findings indicated that most work teams need to be limited in size (with 10 or fewer members per group), and that the focus when forming the team is on clarifying the goals of the team and the role of each team member.

Implications for Practice

The implications of this meta-analysis are important for nursing practice. How often do we find ourselves in teams of more than 10 individuals? Is this really a team or a group of individuals who have come together to address or provide input on an issue? Often, when a team is formed, we look to people we like to work with, who think the same way we do, and who have a similar set of skills that we do. A team should be formed based on the knowledge and skills required to address the issue. When a team has varying skills and backgrounds, it is very helpful to take the time to clarify roles, set team goals, and use tools that help with problem solving. Try these strategies (or suggest the leader try these strategies) the next time you are asked to be part of a team.

CONFLICT AND TEAMS

Conflict Management

When thinking about conflict, it is helpful to realize that conflict is fundamental to the human experience and is an integral part of all human interaction (Porter-O'Grady & Malloch, 2014). **Conflict** is defined as two or more competing responses to a single event. It is a problem to be solved when differences exist between and among individuals or groups (Cahn & Abigail, 2014). Challenges arise when a breakdown in communication processes occurs that requires an appropriate response to preserve working relationships (Porter-O'Grady & Malloch, 2014). Conflicts are usually based on attempts to protect a person's self-esteem or to alter perceived inequities in power because most human beings believe that other people have more power. When a team leader recognizes conflict between two members of the team, they can follow a problem-solving approach. The following steps can be helpful:

- Identify the core concern for each team member.
- Discover the common ground to move forward.
- Work with each person, both separately and together, to establish mutually agreeable outcomes.
- Facilitate discussions and mutual goal-setting while setting clear expectations of outcome.

Assessing the state of the working relationship between the conflicted parties is essential, particularly if they work together on a regular basis.

Working together requires that team members understand how to conduct interpersonal relationships and communicate with their peers in respectful, supportive, and meaningful ways. It requires that team members be able to resolve conflicts among themselves and do so in ways that enhance, rather than inhibit, their working relationship. In addition, team members must be able to trust that they will receive what they need, while being able to count on one another to complete tasks related to team outcomes. To communicate effectively, people must be willing to confront issues and to openly express their ideas and feelings—to use interactive skills to accomplish tasks. In nursing, constructive confrontation has not been a well-used skill. Consequently, if communication patterns are to improve, the onus is on each individual to change communication patterns. In essence, for things to change, each of us must change. To create an environment that allows for conflict management, a number of contextual factors must be in place. These include a focus on the mission, a willingness to cooperate, a commitment to the team, and a commitment to address concerns that arise in the team.

Singleness of Mission

Every team must have a purpose—that is, a plan, an aim, or an intention. However, the most successful teams have a mission—some special work or service to which the team is 100% committed. The mission and purpose of the team must be clearly understood and agreed to by all (Thompson, 2018). The more powerful and visionary the mission, the more energizing it will be to the team. The more energy and excitement on the team, the more motivated all members will be to do the necessary work.

Willingness to Cooperate

Just because a group of people has a common reporting relationship within an organization does not mean that the members are a team. The boxes and arrows of an organizational chart are not in any way related to the technical and interpersonal coordination or the emotional investment required of a true team. In effective teams, members are required to work together in a respectful manner. Most of us have been involved in organizations in which people could accomplish assigned tasks but were not successful in their interpersonal relationships. Organizations can no longer afford to pay people who do not work collaboratively to achieve established organizational goals. Personal friendship or socialization is not required, but cooperation and civility are both necessities. Traditionally, interpersonal skills related to effective collaboration were considered to be soft skills, which are typically difficult to coach and to hold people accountable for. Contemporary organizations are now more inclined to hold accountable and discipline employees who demonstrate a lack of willingness to work cooperatively with team members.

Commitment to the Project

Commitment is a state of being compelled by one's passion for and dedication to a project or event—a mission. In other words, people go the extra mile because of their commitment. They do whatever it takes to accomplish the goal or see the project through to completion. Charles Garfield, an expert on team management, described what it was like to be a part of the team that created the lunar landing module for the first trip to the moon (Albrecht, 2003). People did all kinds of extraordinary things including working extended hours and shifts, calling in to see how the project was progressing, and sleeping over at their workstation so as not to be separated from the project—all because everybody knew that they were a part of something that was much bigger than themselves. They were all a part of sending a man to the moon, something that human beings had been dreaming about for many years. It was a historical moment, and people were intensely committed to making it happen.

Some people experience a gap between their commitment and the team or employer's mission and goals. Because we spend an extensive amount of time in the work setting, it is critically important to have both physical and mental well-being. If this is not the case, then trying a different project, position, or career move—one that might lead to passion—is important. Committing to yourself and your team to do your best at whatever you are now doing provides opportunities for you to grow and meet professional commitments as a team member. You will bring lessons learned to new teams and career opportunities. This approach honours patients as well as you and your co-workers.

Commitment to the Resolution

Being committed to a resolution means that team members are dedicated to finding a workable response to a problem. It means there is a willingness to hear and listen to others' perspectives, identify similarities and differences, and creatively seek solutions to resolve the areas of difference to reach a common ground. The parties need to then agree that they feel heard and agree to the resolution. This approach differs greatly from the compromise and majority vote that are part of the democratic process. When compromise exists, there is acquiescence or relinquishing of a significant portion of what was desired. Compromise generally leaves both parties feeling negative about themselves or the agreement. Consequently, most compromises must be reworked at some future date. Conflict can either be constructive or destructive (Table 20.3), but it is essential to effectively functioning teams (Cahn & Abigail, 2014).

Commitment to the resolution is integral to the needs of the team. One team member may disagree with another team member, but the successful work of the team could be at stake in this conflict. Without commitment to conflict management for the sake of the team's goals, individuals often have less impetus to seek common ground or to agree to disagree.

COMMUNICATION

The only thing humans do more often than communicate is breathe. Communication is the most important component of daily activities. It is essential to clinical practice,

TABLE 20.3   Aspects of Conflict

Destructive	Constructive
• Diverts energy from more important activities and issues	• Opens up dialogue regarding issues of importance, resulting in their clarification
• Destroys the morale of people or reinforces poor self-concepts	• Results in a focus on finding the solution to issues
• Creates differences in a group that cannot be addressed and leads to team paralysis	• Increases the involvement and commitment of individuals in issues
• Deepens differences in values	• Supports authentic communication with expression of individual needs
• Leads to actions and behaviours such as anger, anxiety, withdrawal, or combative communication	• Serves as an opportunity for mutual respect
	• Helps build cohesiveness among team members engaged in the conflict
	• Provides opportunities for professional growth

Modified from Cahn, D., & Abigail, R. (2014). *Managing conflict through communication* (5th ed.). New York, NY: Pearson.

to building teams, and to leadership. A person cannot be without communication. Cahn and Abigail (2014) define *communication* as the sending and receiving of messages that leads to a process of creating meaning in our interactions and relationships. It is the exchange of a message between two or more individuals. Communication can occur as a verbal or nonverbal exchange. Because communication consists of both verbal and nonverbal signals, individuals are continuously expressing thoughts, ideas, and opinions as well as emotions. Once the message is sent, it cannot be retracted; it can be amended, but the first impression of the communication is usually lasting. However, as important as this initial impression is, it is often an unconscious response or reaction.

Communication is learned from watching others. A host of poor examples can be seen in our everyday lives. Poor communication leads to relationship breakdowns, misunderstandings, high levels of emotion, judgement, and an excess of drama. Nursing programs teach students therapeutic communications to engage with patients and their families. However, there is less of a focus placed on effective communication in the workplace, even though communication is essential to building and maintaining effectively functioning teams.

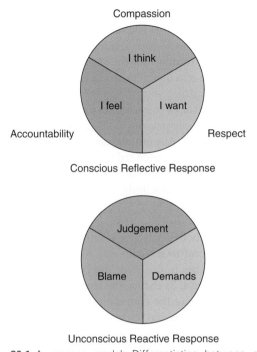

Conscious Reflective Response

Unconscious Reactive Response

Fig. 20.1 Awareness model: Differentiating between conscious and unconscious responses.

A basic model of communication patterns between the sender and the receiver appears in Fig. 20.1. Effective communication occurs when messages are transmitted between the sender and receiver in a respectful and goal-oriented manner (Robbins et al., 2016). Communication begins to break down as the rhythm of communication is disrupted. The sender–receiver pattern disintegrates into a nonrhythmic event, as described in Fig. 20.1. When non-rhythmic patterns develop, the participants may feel disrespected, upset, and even fearful.

Positive Communication Model

Whenever human beings are in distress, disengaged, or have an emotional reaction to a situation or the actions of another, a conditioned response is to move into one or all of the following: *blame, judgement,* or *demand.* These ideas are depicted in the awareness model that appears in Fig. 20.2. With effort and practice, it is possible to create a positive communication interaction that produces a significantly improved outcome.

When individuals are reacting at the feeling level, they tend to move unconsciously to blame. By taking accountability for these feelings, one can move out of blame and own one's feelings by stating: "I feel."

Communication Rhythm

Sender ——— Receiver

| Sender sends a message. | Receiver actively listens and receives. |

Communication Non-rhythm

Sender ——— Sender

Both parties send simultaneously. Neither party is receiving.

Sender ——— No Receiver

| Sender sends a message. | The receiver is preoccupied with another matter and is not attending. |

No Sender ——— Receiver

The receiver awaits a message or response. The sender "clams up," refusing to speak or send a message.

Receiver ——— Receiver

When both parties are striving to receive and neither party sends a message (e.g., teacher questions what students know and gets no response), silence reigns.

Fig. 20.2 Potential communication rhythms.

Likewise, when individuals are trapped in distress or reaction at the thinking level, they most often turn to judgement. By thinking compassionately, one can dismantle the judgement and state what one thinks in a compassionate way: "I think."

Finally, when in distress, we make demands that are often unreasonable. By calming oneself, one can find respect for the other human being and make a request: "I want."

Most broken relationships are stuck in blame, judgement, and demand. Being accountable, compassionate, and respectful helps clarify what goes on inside each of us. Everyone needs to feel as though their skills, tools, and contributions are needed and valued and that they are respected for what personal contributions they offer to the workplace, team, or group. A focus on strengths and contributions can be an effective means of establishing positive communication strategies.

Acknowledgement of peers, family, and significant others is viewed as recognizing and acknowledging others' strengths. We do not always give acknowledgement in a way that it can be received and valued. Box 20.3 provides guidelines for giving acknowledgement.

To deal with the three personal issues discussed in this section, team members must learn how to clearly and openly state their views and positions and be responsive and respectful as other members of the team do the same. In other words, team members must give and receive feedback constructively.

EXERCISE 20.4 During the next three days, find three opportunities to acknowledge a peer (e.g., a student) or acquaintance using the five guidelines for acknowledgement shown in Box 20.3. In addition, use the guidelines to accept at least one self-acknowledgement.

Communicating During Conflict

Cahn and Abigail (2014) proposed a framework to help guide effective communication during conflict called S-TLC. The S-TLC acronym stands for Stop, Think, Listen, Communicate.

Stop

As we communicate with others, we need to realize that the primary focus is not only the message we wish to deliver, but also the feelings and emotions we have related to the topic or discussion. In any communication, but especially in difficult situations, the ability to stop and take time out to consider the situation can prevent an interaction that you will regret. This strategy can be an effective way of de-escalating a situation by calling a time out and reconvening the meeting at a later time. It can also be an effective tactic to use when you need a few seconds to organize your thoughts. Stopping can mean withdrawing from a conversation for a few minutes or a few days or simply pausing to think about how you are going to respond. Any of these approaches can be effective. Stopping is not intended to be an act of avoidance but a way to take a time out to regroup so that you can re-engage more productively.

Think

Thinking is about analyzing a situation and how you want to respond to it. Cahn and Abigail (2014) noted three approaches to this step. You can try to 1) change the other person, 2) change the situation, or 3) change yourself. Knowing the communication goals you wish to reach is fundamental to this stage of the framework. Identifying those goals will help you choose which of the approaches to engage in.

Listen

This step is the most challenging. As another person begins to speak, we automatically begin to mentally prepare our response; in doing so, we miss vital pieces of the other person's message. True listening is a learned skill and provides a means for connecting with the other person. Giving your complete attention to the conversation and the other individual(s) engaged in the

---

BOX 20.3   Guidelines for Acknowledgement

1. Acknowledgement must be specific. The specific behaviour or action that is appreciated must be identified in the acknowledgement; for example, "Thank you for taking notes for me when I had to go to the dentist. You identified three key points that appeared on the test."

2. Acknowledgement must be "eye to eye" or personal. Look the person in the eye when you thank them. Do not run down the hall and say "Thanks" over your shoulder. Written appreciation also qualifies as "eye to eye."

3. Acknowledgement must be sincere, that is, from the heart. Each of us recognizes insincerity. If you do not truly appreciate a behaviour or an action, do not say anything. Insincerity often makes people angry or upset, thus defeating the goal.

4. Acknowledgement is more powerful when it is given in public. Most people receive pleasure from public acknowledgement and remember these occasions for a long time. For people who are shy and may prefer no public acknowledgement, this is an opportunity to work on a personal growth issue with them. Public acknowledgement is an opportunity to communicate what is valued.

5. Acknowledgement needs to be timely. The less time that elapses between the event and the acknowledgement, the more powerful and effective it is and the more the acknowledgement is appreciated by the recipient.

conversation is critical. Eye contact, positive nonverbal messages, and remaining open to understanding the other person's perspective are important activities that support listening.

Communicate

Cahn and Abigail (2014) offered two approaches to communication: linear and transactional. In the linear approach, the focus is on goals, purpose, and intention of the message. In the transactional approach, the focus is on the process of communication; that is, what and how we communicate with one another. The transactional approach can be very effective in resolving conflict because it considers that the conflict is not one-sided but a result of the behaviours of each person. Cahn and Abigail (2014) suggested that communication is like a dance; individuals need to engage and partner with each other to achieve a goal.

Factors That Hinder Effective Communication

Stress

In her classic work, Satir (1988) identified the connection between stress and self-worth that can evolve as a result of a breakdown in communication. Although much of her focus was in the area of family therapy, she was seen as a leader on the impact of stress upon communication. Satir's work has been further supported in the work of others, including Leslie (2016). Satir defined *stress* as a threat to positive self-worth. Individuals tend to feel stress or anxiety whenever there is an unconscious linking of feelings, behaviours, or comments from others to a lowering of self-esteem or an attack on self-worth. Leslie identifies behaviour and coping as the visible responses to stress while there is a need to widen our lens to the more invisible to understand our feelings, our aspirations, and our individual needs.

Stress Response Model. When a threat is identified, the receiver often reacts using one of these communication patterns: attribution of blame, placation, constrained cool-headedness, immaterial irrelevance, ineffective conflict management, or congruence (Thompson, 2018; Robbins et al., 2016; Bradley & Edinberg, 1990; Satir, 1988). The communication patterns, types of interaction, sources of the interaction, and related examples appear in Table 20.4. The pattern that produces effective communication—the one to strive for—is congruence. Congruent communication occurs when both the verbal and nonverbal actions fit the inner feelings of the sender and are appropriate to the context of the message. This communication pattern creates the kind of connection between the sender and the receiver that fosters respect, support, and the creation of relationship. Further discussion on stress appears in Chapter 29.

TABLE 20.4 Communication Patterns During Stress

Pattern	Interaction	Source	Example
Attribution of blame	Sender blames receiver	Fault-finder dictator acts superior as camouflage for fear and low self-esteem	Mostly "you" messages; for example, "You made a mistake."
Placation	Sender placates receiver	Sender's low self-worth; puts themself down	"I was wrong. I'm sorry. It's all my fault."
Constrained cool-headedness	Sender is correct and very reasonable without feeling or emotion	Feelings of vulnerability covered by cool analytical thinking	"I decided to use research data in coming to a solution."
Irrelevant	Sender is avoiding the issue, ignoring own feelings and feelings of the receiver	Fear, loneliness, and purpose-lessness	"Wait a minute. Let me tell you about . . ." (changes the subject)
Congruence	Sender's words and actions are congruent; inner feelings match the message	Any tension is decreased, and self-worth is at a high level	"For now, I feel concerned about the anger and hostility exhibited by Nurse X. I'm wondering what approach would de-escalate the situation."

Modified from Satir, V. (1988). *The new peoplemaking.* Mountain View, CA: Science & Behavior Books; and Bradley, J., & Edinberg, M. (1990). *Communication in the nursing context* (3rd ed.). Norwalk, CT: Appleton & Lange.

Communication Barriers

A number of communication barriers can interfere with clear, focused, and effective communication. Olen (1993) identified potential problems to allow both the sender and receiver to be prepared to minimize them.

- *Distractions:* Distractions most commonly come through sensory perceptions, such as poor lighting or background noise. Email and overly heavy workloads can also be distracting.
- *Inadequate knowledge:* The sender and receiver may have different levels of knowledge, particularly in this time of highly specialized and technical knowledge bases. For multiple reasons, one person may not seek clarity from the other.
- *Poor planning:* The process of organizing, planning, and clearly thinking through what needs to be communicated is very helpful. If the interaction is more spontaneous, it can more easily fall into a nonrhythmic pattern.
- *Differences in perception:* Both the sender and the receiver have their individual mental filters—the way in which they see the world. Because of this individuality, no two filters are the same. Thus, the same message is interpreted differently. Add to this, for example, sociocultural, ethnic, and educational differences, and it is easy to see how differences in perception can occur.
- *Emotions and personality:* Someone who is experiencing distress may not be able to receive another message or may have difficulty keeping their emotions out of an unrelated message. Most individuals, at some point, bring distress or problems from home to the workplace. If these remain unconscious, they can influence the work setting in a negative or nonproductive way.

Communication Pitfalls and Barriers

Effective communication suggests that the interaction is a rhythmic pattern that is respectful and clear, promotes trust, and encourages the expression of feelings and viewpoints. On the other hand, pitfalls in communication comprise actions, behaviours, and words that create distrust, are dishonouring, and decrease the feelings of self-worth in the receiver. Box 20.4 lists the major pitfalls of communication. Key barriers to communication include information overload, emotions, defensiveness, and manipulation of information (Robbins et al., 2016).

Guidelines for Effective Communication

A number of communication tools can help individuals communicate effectively. For example, Situation-Background-Assessment-Recommendation (SBAR) is a standardized approach to communication often used in health care settings to convey clinical information from one caregiver to another (Box 20.5). The purpose of communication tools is to create an environment in which the communicator can achieve the desired outcome. Box 20.6 lists some basic guidelines on how to communicate effectively and avoid misunderstandings. It is important to keep in mind that active listening, being compassionate, telling the truth, and being flexible are essential to the process of communicating effectively.

> **EXERCISE 20.5** In pairs or small groups, compare the guidelines for effective communication with the communication pitfalls. Give examples of each from your own recent personal experience. Hypothesize how you could have changed the pitfalls into a positive interaction.

Understanding Our Role on the Team

Use Active Listening

Active listening means being completely present with and focusing on the individual who is speaking. It means listening to the essence of the conversation, without judgement, so you can understand the speaker's intended message. Box 20.7 presents guidelines for active listening.

In active listening we avoid developing a defensive response or argument in our heads while the other person is still speaking. To listen actively, we must be absorbing words, posture, tone of voice, and all the verbal and nonverbal clues accompanying the message so that the intent of the communication can be received. Specific purposes used in active listening, including examples, appear in Table 20.5.

Be Compassionate

Being compassionate means showing concern for another's position and perspective. It means listening from a caring perspective—one that is focused on understanding the viewpoint of the other person rather than focusing on one's own point of view.

BOX 20.4 Communication Pitfalls

1. Giving advice

   It is so tempting to give advice when a coworker comes with an issue or problem. Do not! Most often what the person wants is to work through the issue by talking out loud. Just listen.

2. Making others wrong

   When telling others "our" story of distress, the adversary is always "wrong". The telling of the story to a third party only reinforces how right "I" am and how wrong, bad, or terrible the other person is. If you have an issue or problem, take the problem to the person with whom you have the issue.

3. Being defensive

   Defensiveness occurs when you do not listen, are hostile or aggressive, or respond as if attacked when there was no attack. Look for a physiological signal in your body so that you can identify your own distress. Stop. Breathe. Acknowledge that the message did not come out the way you intended, and begin again.

   Also, defensiveness can occur when met with hostile, aggressive behaviour from another. Rather than choose an emotional response or react to the attack, know that the other person's behaviour has nothing to do with you personally but is the response chosen by that person in a moment of stress. Any one of a dozen other responses could have been chosen. Understand that the person may be motivated by fear or hurt.

4. Judging the other person

   Evaluating another person as "good" or "bad", as someone you like or do not like, or judging the person's actions or behaviour as "stupid", "crazy", or "inappropriate" is a reflection of how you judge yourself. Who is the hardest person on you? Of course, you are. Know that you can have feelings about situations or behaviours without judging the other person in a negative way. Rather, you can feel compassion for their stress and fear, which often drives behaviour.

5. Being patronizing

   Speaking to others as if they are not equal to you as an individual fails to honour the person as a valued human being. To ensure that you understand their perspective, clarify what is of immediate concern to the person and endeavour to address that issue.

6. Giving false reassurance

   One of the great temptations is to "fix" things and make them better, to rescue the situation or the person involved. To accomplish this goal, sometimes we reassure inappropriately. Know that you do not have to fix every situation. You can support people to work through situations themselves.

7. Asking "why" questions

   When working in the team, refrain from asking "why" questions. These tend to create a defensive response in the other person. Instead, ask "What makes you think . . . ?"

8. Blaming others

   Saying things such as "You make me so angry" is blaming the other person for your feelings, which you choose at any given time. In nearly every situation, the responsibility for communication breakdown is a joint responsibility. You can always choose your response, even if that response is to say, "I can't discuss this with you now. I would like to talk about this later when I am calmer."

BOX 20.5 SBAR Communication

Miscommunication is the most commonly occurring cause of sentinel events and "near misses" in patient care. Situation-Background-Assessment-Recommendation (SBAR) is one of the most popular structured communication techniques used in health care and was created by health care providers at Kaiser Permanente of Colorado. It is used throughout North America and focuses on providing information to health care providers that can be easily applied to decision-making trees. SBAR honours the structured transfer of information.

Situation. The health care provider identifies the patient, the physician, the diagnosis, and the location of the patient. The health care provider describes the patient situation that has led to this SBAR communication.

Background. Next, the health care provider provides background information, which could include information relevant to the current situation, mental status, current vital signs (all of them), chief complaint, pain level, and physical assessment of the patient.

Assessment. The health care provider offers an assessment of the chief problem and describes the seriousness of the situation. Any specific changes in the patient's condition should be described.

Recommendation. The health care provider can make a request of the health team members.

Modified from NHS Institution for Innovation and Quality. (2014, February 20). SBAR. Retrieved from http://www.institute.nhs.uk.

BOX 20.6 Guidelines for Effective Communication

- Approach each interaction as though the other person has no knowledge of effective communication. Assume responsibility for creating the sender-receiver rhythm.
- Share your thoughts and feelings. Be self-revealing.
- Use casual conversation or "small talk": it can be important to relationships, particularly when it is light and humorous. It balances deep, meaningful talk.
- Acknowledge, praise, and encourage the other person; doing so is supportive and brings life and energy to the relationship.

- Present messages in a way that the other person can receive them.
- Take responsibility for any problem or issue you have with another and speak about it as your problem or issue also.
- Use language of equality even when position titles are not of the same level.

Modified from Olen, D. (1993). *Communicating: Speaking and listening to end misunderstanding and promote friendship.* Germantown, WI: JODA Communications.

BOX 20.7 Guidelines for Active Listening

1. Slow down your internal processes and seek data. Do not interrupt the speaker.
2. The more information you acquire through listening, the less interpretation you do (making up the missing pieces or motivations). The less information you have, the more interpretation you do.
3. Realize that the first words from the other person are not necessarily representative of inner thoughts and feelings. Be patient.
4. When listening, suspend your own beliefs, views, and judgements, at least temporarily. Attempt to understand the perspective of the other person, particularly if it is different from yours.
5. Realize that any judgements or "labels" strongly influence the manner in which you listen to the other person.
6. Appreciate the difference between understanding other people's perspective and agreeing with them. First strive to understand. Then you may agree or disagree.
7. Effective listening is based on an inner desire to learn about another's unique experience of the world.

Modified from Olen, D. (1993). *Communicating: Speaking and listening to end misunderstanding and promote friendship.* Germantown, WI: JODA Communications.

TABLE 20.5 Active Listening

Use of Active Listening	Examples
To convey interest in what the other person is saying	I see! I get it. I hear what you're saying.
To encourage the individual to expand further on his or her thinking	Yes, go on. Tell us more.
To help the individual clarify and understand the issue	Then the issue as you see it is . . .
To get the individual to hear what they have said in the way it sounded to others	This is your decision, then, and the reasons are . . .
	If I understand you correctly, you are saying that . . .
To pull out the key ideas from a long statement or discussion	Your major point is . . .
	You feel that . . .
To respond to a person's feelings more than to his or her words	I hear you say you feel strongly that . . .
	You don't believe that . . .
To summarize specific points of agreement and disagreement as a basis for further discussion	We seem to be agreed on the following points . . . But we seem to need further clarification on these points . . .
To express a consensus of group feeling	As a result of this discussion, we as a group have decided to . . .

Tell the Truth

Telling the truth is a strength of character that allows a person to express their position in an honest and fact-based manner. Telling the truth means speaking factually and consistently to express facts, feelings, and perspectives while acknowledging that they are those you hold to be true. One important component of telling the truth is respecting the perspectives of others while remaining true to your core values and beliefs. This is accomplished in an objective rather than subjective manner using neither a cynical nor a critical tone of voice. To be effective, we must be responsible for our integrity and our behaviour in our interactions with others.

Be Flexible

Being flexible reflects a willingness to hear another person's point of view rather than being solely committed to only one point of view. Flexibility is critical for a team to work well together. No single person has all the right answers. Therefore acknowledging that each person has something to contribute is important.

MANAGING EMOTIONS

Emotions within a team can be very positive or very challenging for the team members. Critical to team success is understanding the role emotions can play. Emotional intelligence is core to team success. Goleman & Boyatzis (2017) define emotional intelligence (EQ) as the ability to identify, assess, and control one's own emotions and the emotions of others. They present four domains of emotional intelligence. These are:

1. *Self Awareness:* the ability to recognize one's own strengths, weaknesses, values, and goals and their impact on others.
2. *Self-Management:* emotional self-control and adaptability to situations.
3. *Self-Awareness:* includes empathy and organizational awareness.
4. *Relationship Management:* includes the ability to work in a team and manage conflict as well as to coach and mentor.

Emotions are important components of organizational life. Most of us know of situations where a disagreement between two or more individuals has resulted in the dissolving of the relationship. The power of emotions and the inevitability of their presence influences interpersonal relationships, productivity, quality of work, and safety of patients. The impact of emotions should be a high priority when examining the functioning of the team. Research addresses the importance of emphasizing the "emotional intelligence" of individuals and team members (Cahn & Abigail, 2014). Those teams that address emotions are much more successful and create a positive work environment.

According to Bocialetti (1988) and Thompson (2018), people are sensitive to what happens when emotions are revealed. When goals, objectives, and tasks are disputed, employees see the following:

- Unprofessional behaviours including intimidation and bullying.
- A team member overstating or exaggerating points of view to appear right.
- Defensive and hostile responses by one or more members of the team.
- Concern for oneself to the point of self-absorption.
- Gossip.
- Attempts to stop or subvert the "real work" of the team.
- Conflict in the team that becomes unproductive and distracts the team from its purpose.

These behaviours can destroy the team. What are needed are behaviours that support team members in growing, learning, and achieving goals. On the other hand, the cost of suppressing emotions or "feelings" includes the following:

- Physical and psychological stress.
- Withdrawal from participation.
- Loss of energy and direction of the team.
- Lost opportunities for team learning.
- Hidden agendas.
- Prevention of others from being acknowledged.
- Decreased motivation.
- Weakening of the team members' ability to receive constructive feedback.
- The loss of one's influence.

These types of outcome indicate lack of emotional intelligence and are neither healthy nor constructive for team members. When emotions are managed appropriately, there are several positive outcomes for the team members, the team as a whole, and the organization.

Team effectiveness occurs when members of the team work together in a manner that is focused on a common goal and outcome. The frameworks and tools previously discussed are the basic foundations needed to be a productive and respected member of the team. Choosing to be a member of the team requires a conscious choice, one that requires the ability to engage in reflective practice.

REFLECTIVE PRACTICE

The process of reflective practice consists of the active, careful consideration of a belief or knowledge and can derive from "learning from experience." It is defined as a "learning and development process that includes the self-examination of one's professional practice, including experiences, thoughts, emotions, actions, and knowledge that enrich it" (Dube & Ducharme, 2015, p. 91). Using a reflective process allows the team member to see the world differently and, as a result of these new insights, see the work world differently, which can translate into acting differently. Thus, upon reflection of how an interaction progressed within the team, team members can examine how this event unfolded compared with how they might have wanted the event to occur. It is a time to look inward and examine beliefs, values, and behaviours. The opportunity for growth is when we identify specific behaviours to enact differently and make a commitment to actually enact them differently. Bringing issues to the conscious level is the first step in personal and professional growth.

MINDFULNESS AND COMPASSION

Jon Kabat-Zinn is a world-recognized expert on mindfulness. He defines mindfulness as an awareness that emerges by intentionally paying attention non-judgementally, in the present moment, and experiencing that moment to its fullest (Kabat-Zinn, 2013). Compassion, as described by Kabat-Zinn, is physical, mental, and emotional help for self and others. Compassion is a critical competence in nursing practice.

Brass (2016) presents the concepts of mindfulness and compassion in the context of nursing practice. These are linked and must be practised together in order for someone to be an effective member of a health care team. The author identifies challenges in enacting mindfulness and compassion within the nursing role. These challenges may include having personal

discomfort with looking inward or focusing on self in both our personal and professional lives. Often nurses' desires to provide compassion in care are challenged by factors such as tight schedules, a focus on outcomes at the exclusion of the individual patients, or individual nurses' experiences of emotional exhaustion or perceived vulnerability.

Brass (2016) promotes the concept of mindful compassion, believing it needs to begin with individual mindfulness and self-care before the nurse can provide compassionate care to patients. Through mindfulness and reflection nurses, and all members of the health care team, have an opportunity to create workplaces that support care of self and others to achieve patient care goals. Strategies can be incorporated into teams through self-assessment, team member feedback, and team development opportunities.

THE ROLE OF LEADERSHIP IN TEAM SUCCESS

The team leader plays a key role in the success of a team. Kouzes and Posner (2017) have identified five practices of exemplary leaders in their Leadership Practices Framework, presented in the Literature Perspective.

Teams usually have a formal leader as well as informal leaders (team members who by virtue of their knowledge and experience are seen by their peers as leaders). These leaders often have followers who learn from them, act on their behalf, and are inspired by them. In addition, teams function within large organizations that have leaders. Without the approval and the support of the leader, team building, which can be a costly endeavour in terms of consultation fees as well as work time and the resources of the team, is difficult to undertake and of questionable effectiveness. Although very strong teams may be able to educate themselves regarding some of the issues, such as establishing goals and priorities or clarifying their own team processes, addressing any kind of relationship issue among team members without a more objective party facilitating the process is exceedingly difficult.

Because leadership is such a pivotal part of smoothly functioning teams, it is illuminating to examine leaders more carefully. Effective leaders need to create opportunities for teams to be innovative and to be willing to give up the old way of doing things.

LITERATURE PERSPECTIVE

Resource: Kouzes, J. M., & Posner, B. Z. (2017). *The leadership challenge* (6th ed.). Hoboken, NJ: Jossey-Bass, John Wiley & Sons.

Kouzes and Posner's (2017) Leadership Practices Framework focuses on how leaders, either formal or informal, can mobilize people to get extraordinary things done. For example, informal leaders, such as novice nurses, can guide others along pioneering journeys to phenomenal accomplishments. The research and work that Kouzes and Posner have done establish relationships as the core of leading any change or initiative. Five key aspects of establishing and maintaining relationships constitute the heart of this leadership framework:

- **Model the way:** Credibility is the foundation of leadership. It is established by consistently *doing what you say you will do* or by *setting the example* for the other team members.
- **Inspire a shared vision:** Imagine exciting and enabling possibilities, and enlist others in these dreams through positive attitude, excitement, and hard work.
- **Challenge the process:** Seek innovative ways to change, grow, and improve—experiment and take risks.

- **Enable others to act:** Foster collaboration by promoting cooperation and building trust. Create a sense of reciprocity or give and take. Establish a sense of "we're all in this together".
- **Encourage the heart:** Novice leaders encourage their constituents to carry on. They keep hope and determination alive, recognize contributions, and celebrate victories.

When nurses use this framework to approach leadership, they can strengthen their skills. Each of the examples above provides a way for new, emerging, and established leaders to remain committed to the team in which they work.

Implications for Practice

Each of us has leadership qualities that we bring to every encounter. Think about using the strategies for each of the practices in dealing with patients, families, peers, co-workers, and the team. If each of us consciously engages in "doing what we say we will do" and "setting an example", imagine the positive impact this would have on ourselves and others. The five leadership practices speak to the core of the profession of nursing.

Contemporary leaders must do more than talk about innovation. They must behave in an inspirational way. Leaders must be willing to take risks and allow team members to take risks. Teams led by contemporary leaders make informed decisions and identify their successes and failures in ways that promote more innovation (Porter-O'Grady & Malloch, 2014). For the contemporary leader, team building is a natural process. This type of leader understands that the best in a person is tied intimately to the individual's deepest sense of themselves—to their spirit. Warren Bennis, a pioneer in the field of leadership, notes the importance of candour in leadership (Rosenbach et al., 2012). Candour manifests itself in improving team functioning. This may imply involving oneself in team building with the team. The risk in using candour is that the team leader is open to being vulnerable, to being judged by others, and to being wrong. However, if the leader has been a role model supporting the group norms and goals and has held team members to the group norm and goals, the team-building exercise will not degenerate into judging and placing blame.

If true leadership is about character development as much as anything, then character development is also beneficial for followers—that is, members of the team. An area of character development often addressed is

communication, particularly those aspects of speaking supportively that avoid placing blame and justifying and enhance understanding of the other person's message.

Leaders understand the multiple aspects of the issue of control. They take control of their lives rather than put themselves at the mercy of others. They have clarity regarding opportunities and areas for improvement. They focus time and energy primarily and almost exclusively on those situations, events, and behaviours over which they have control. Their activities are thus focused primarily on areas relating directly to them—not on world events or other external situations over which they have neither influence nor control.

Confidence, which loosely translates as faith or belief that one will act in a correct and effective way, is a key aspect of character. Thus, it follows that confidence in oneself can be closely tied to self-esteem, which is satisfaction with oneself. The greatest deterrent to self-esteem and self-confidence is fear. Fear is described by some as "false evidence appearing real". Kabot Zinn (2013) believes that a fear that rules our lives is our lack of self-belief in our own abilities. Issues related to self-esteem and fear can be addressed through the use of reflective practice and mindfulness and compassion.

？ A SOLUTION

The Challenge presented at the beginning of the chapter is a very complex one. It includes a number of issues: conflict that impacts individual nurses and other health care providers, patient and family outcomes, and the functioning of the Clinical Teaching Unit (CTU) as a whole. No easy responses to these issues exist. The common theme that affects each individual in the Challenge scenario is communication. Communication strategies for the CTU nurse and the nurse manager are explored here.

The CTU nurse must focus on recognizing the communication patterns that are occurring. Understanding the aspects of conflict and how these are impacting the nursing role is very important. As the nurse works with team members, it would be important not to use language that blames or judges others. Staying focused on the patient and family care issue and not the conflict can be difficult but achievable. Using the S-TLC framework would be especially helpful. Also, using SBAR principles can make

both verbal and written communication more effective. The nurse can also reflect on the communication pitfalls and identify areas for growth. The nurse can seek feedback from peers and the nurse manager on his or her communication strategies. Managing emotions and using the strategies identified in this chapter can help prevent an escalation of the conflict.

The nurse manager is in a challenging position. The manager must bring team members together to focus on the issues and not on individual team members. The nurse manager should also use the communication strategies identified in the preceding paragraph. The manager can draw on the organization's vision, mission, values, and goals to drive the work of the team. Support from the senior administration team would be essential to success. It is also important to ensure that the individuals who are on the team will help achieve a positive outcome.

■ THE EVIDENCE

The Canadian Interprofessional Health Collaborative (CIHC) is made up of health organizations, health educators, researchers, health care providers, and students from across Canada. The CIHC holds that interprofessional education and collaborative patient-centred practice are key to building effective health care teams. In 2008, the CIHC established its original working group to review the existing literature on competency frameworks in interprofessional education and interprofessional practice. From this work, the CIHC developed the National Interprofessional Competency Framework (2010). This framework provides an integrative approach to describing the competencies required for effective interprofessional collaboration. The framework comprises six competency domains that are essential for interprofessional collaborative practice. The six competency domains are as follows:

1. Interprofessional communication
2. Patient/family/community-centred care
3. Role clarification
4. Team functioning
5. Collaborative leadership
6. Interprofessional conflict resolution (Canadian Interprofessional Health Collaborative, 2010, p. 9)

One domain of this framework that has not been explored in this chapter is interprofessional

communication. Interprofessional communication occurs when members of the patient's health care team shares information, evidence, and recommendations to meet the patient's health care needs.

O'Daniel & Rosenstein (2008) and Foranda et al. (2016) describe the barriers to effective interprofessional communication and the strategies to enhance communication in the interprofessional teams. Common barriers to interprofessional communication include intergenerational issues, fears of loss of professional identify and lack of cultural sensitivity, ego, lack of confidence and structural hierarchies. The authors identify three key strategies to enhance interprofessional communication. These include engaging in open dialogue between the disciplines, engaging in collaborative interprofessional rounds, and using interprofessional committees to address patient care and practice concerns.

Many hospital and community health organizations design their models of patient care on models that promote interprofessional communication. Tools such as SBAR and interprofessional rounds can become important ways of supporting interprofessional communication.

The framework supported by interprofessional communication is used by health care educators, students, regulators, practitioners, employers, and accreditors. The framework is reproduced in Chapter 27.

✳ NEED TO KNOW NOW

- Remember that all team members are your colleagues.
- Learn to apply effective communication techniques, such as SBAR.
- View all members of the team as colleagues and team members who all share the outcomes of providing the best possible care for patients.

CHAPTER CHECKLIST

Nurse managers must help build teams. Although managers may not be the team leaders, they must ensure that the team can function effectively. The team members must be able to communicate with one another effectively, share a single mission, be willing to cooperate with one another, and be committed to achieving their objectives. Successful teamwork requires leadership, trust, and willingness to take risks.

- A team is an interdependent group of people that has the following characteristics:
  - Defined goals and objectives with a focus on accomplishing a task.
  - Members communicate effectively with one another.
  - Members have an ongoing relationship.
- An effective team is characterized by the following:
  - Clarity of purpose.
  - Informality.
  - Congeniality.
  - Commitment.
  - High level of participation.
  - Listening.
  - Effective communication.
  - Civilized disagreement.
  - Consensus decisions.
  - Clear roles and work assignments
  - Shared leadership.
  - Diversity of styles.
  - Self-assessment and self-regulation.
- Each team member will ask the following three questions:
  - Am I in or out?
  - Do I have any power or control?
  - Can I use, develop, and be appreciated for my skills and resources?
- One of the most helpful tools in team development is to have team members come to an agreement about the ground rules concerning their relationships with one another.
- Trust among team members is essential for successful teamwork.
- Characteristics of an effective team member include being adaptable, collaborative, committed, communicative, competent, dependable, disciplined, enlarging, enthusiastic, intentional, mission conscious, prepared, relational, self-improving, selfless, solution-oriented, and tenacious.
- Synergy allows a team to produce results that could not have been achieved by any one individual.
- Efforts to understand and bridge generational differences can contribute to the difference between a dysfunctional team and an effective team.
- Focusing on team members' strengths and acknowledging what they do well are key to team building.
- To be effective, acknowledgement must be specific, personal, sincere, timely, and public.
- Conflict can either be constructive or destructive, but conflict is essential to effectively functioning teams.
- When communicating during a conflict with another person, try the S-TLC approach to arrive at a productive outcome.
- Managing emotions is a key to successful team building.
- Leadership is a pivotal part of a well-functioning team.
  - Leaders rely on personal character development as much as on education.
  - Confidence is a key aspect of the leader's character. A "can-do" attitude is one of the most important confidence-building strategies a leader can adopt.
  - The leader must be willing to take risks and allow team members to take risks.

■ TIPS FOR TEAM BUILDING

- Commit to the purpose of the team.
- Develop team relationships of mutual respect.
- Communicate effectively and use active listening.

- Create and adhere to team agreements concerning function and process.
- Build trust.

Visit the Evolve website for Suggested Readings, Internet Resources, and additional resources related to the content in this chapter: http://evolve.elsevier.com/Canada/Yoder-Wise/leading/.

REFERENCES

Albrecht, K. (2003). *The power of minds at work: Organizational intelligence in action*. New York, NY: AMACOM.

Anderson, L., & Morgan, B. (2017). An examination of nurses' intergenerational communicative experiences in the workplace: Do nurses eat their young? *Communication Quarterly, 65*(4). https://doi.org/10.1080/01463373.2016.1259175.

Brass, E. (2016). How mindfulness can benefit nursing practice. *Nursing Times, 112*(18), 21–23.

Bocialetti, G. (1988). Teams and management of emotion. In W. B. Reddy, & K. Jamison (Eds.), *Team building blueprints for productivity and satisfaction* (pp. 62–71). Alexandria, VA: NTL Institute for Applied Behavioral Sciences.

Bradley, J., & Edinberg, M. (1990). *Communication in the nursing context* (3rd ed.). Norwalk, CT: Appleton & Lange.

Cahn, D., & Abigail, R. (2014). *Managing conflict through communication* (5th ed.). New York, NY: Pearson.

Carter, L., Beattie, B., Caswell, W., Fitzgerald, S., & Nowrouzi, B. (2016). An examination of interprofessional team functioning in a BScN blended learning program: Implications for accessible distance-based nursing education programs. *Canadian Journal of University Continuing Education, 41*(1). https://doi.org/10.21225/D5QW3Q.

Canadian Interprofessional Health Collaborative. (2010). A national interprofessional competency framework. Retrieved from: http://www.cihc.ca/files/CIHC_IPCompetencies_Feb2010.pdg.

Centre for Interprofessional Education, Toronto academic health science network. (2017). *Interprofessional care competency framework and team assessment toolkit*. Toronto: Centre for Interprofessional Education University of Toronto.

Dube, V., & Ducharme, F. (2015). Nursing reflective practice: An empirical literature review. *Journal of Nursing Education and Practice, 5*(7), 91–99.

French, J. R., & Raven, B. (1959). *The basis of social power*. Boston, MA: Cengage Learning.

Goleman, D., & Boyatzis, R. (2017). Emotional intelligence has 12 elements. What do you need to work on? *Harvard Business Review*. Retrieved from: https://hbr.org/2017/02/emotional-intelligence-has-12-elements-what-do-you-need-to-work-on.

Kabbat-Zinn, J. (2013). *Full catastrophe living: Using the wisdom of your body and mind to face stress, pain and illness* (2nd ed). New York, NY: Bantam Random House.

Kouzes, J. M., & Posner, B. Z. (2017). *The leadership challenge* (6th ed.). Hoboken, NJ: Jossey-Bass, John Wiley & Sons.

Leggat, S. (2007). Effective healthcare teams require effective team members: Defining teamwork competencies. *BMC Health Services Research, 7*, 17–27.

Leslie, M. (2016). Widening our lens, deepening our practice. *Satir International Journal, 4*(1), 5–20.

MacGregor, D. (1960). *The human side of enterprise*. New York, NY: McGraw-Hill.

MacGregor, D. (1967). *The professional manager*. New York, NY: McGraw-Hill.

McEwan, D., Ruissen, G., Eys, M., Jumbo, B., & Beauchamp, R. (2017). The effectiveness of team training on teamwork behaviors and teamwork performance: A systematic review and meta-analysis of controlled interventions. *PLOS One*. https://doc/10.1371/journalpone.0169604.

NHS Institution for Innovation and Quality. (2014, February 20). SBAR. Retrieved from: http://www.institute.nhs.uk.

O'Daniel, M., & Rosenstein, A. H. (2008). Professional communication and collaboration. In R. G. Hughes (Ed.), *Patient safety and quality: An evidenced based handbook for nurses*. Rockville, MD: Agency for Healthcare Research and Quality.

Olen, D. (1993). *Communicating: Speaking and listening to end misunderstanding and promote friendship*. Germantown, WI: JODA Communications.

Oxford English Dictionary. (2012). Oxford U.K: Oxford University Press.

Pilette, P. (2017). Team charters: Mapping clearer communication. *Nursing Management*, 52–55.

Porter-O'Grady, T., & Malloch, K. (2014). *Quantum leadership: Building better partnerships for sustainable health* (4th ed.). Sudbury, MA: Jones & Bartlett.

Riggio, R. (2013). Characteristics of good team members. *Psychology Today*. Retrieved from: www.psychologytoday.com.

Robbins, S., Coulter, M., Leach, E., & Kilfoil, M. (2016). *Management eleventh canadian edition*. Toronto, ON: Pearson.

Rosenbach, W., Taylor, W., & Youndt, M. (2012). *Contemporary issues in leadership* (7th ed). New York, NY: Taylor & Francis.

Satir, V. (1988). *The new peoplemaking*. Mountain View, CA: Science & Behavior Books.

Stuart, A. (2014). *Ground rules for a high performing team. Paper presented at PMI® Global Congress 2014—North America, Phoenix, AZ*. Newtown Square, PA: Project Management Institute.

Suter, E., Deutschlander, S., Mickelson, G., et al. (2012). Can interprofessional collaboration provide health human resources solutions? A knowledge synthesis. *Journal of Interprofessional Care, 26*(4), 261.

The Leader's Institute. (2017). *Five Characteristics of Highly Effective Teams*. The Leader's Institute. Retrieved from: www.leadersinstitute.com.

Thelwell, R., Harood, C., & Greenless, I. (2017). *The psychology of sports coaching: Research and practice*. New York, NY: Taylor & Francis Group.

Thompson, L. (2018). *Making the team: A guide for managers* (6h ed.). Upper Saddle River, NJ: Pearson Education.

Thorman, S., & Mendonca, K. (n.d.). *Team Building Toolkit*. University of California at Berkeley. Retrieved from: www.hr.berkeley.edu.

Virani, T. (2012). *Interprofessional Collaborative Teams*. Ottawa, ON: Canadian Health Services Research Foundation. Retrieved from: http://www.cfhi-fcass.ca/Libraries/Commissioned_Research_Reports/Virani-Interprofessional-EN.sflb.ashx.

Williams, D. (2017). *Six ways to Create a Supportive work Environment*. Forbes. Retrieved from: https://forbes.com/sites/davidkwilliams.

World Health Organization. (2013). *Interprofessional Collaborative Practice in Primary Health care: Nursing and Midwifery Perspectives*. Retrieved from: http:/www.int/hrh/resources/observer.

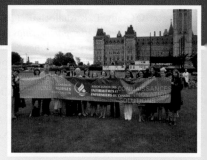

21

Collective Nursing Advocacy

Janice I. Waddell

In 2006, journalists Buresh and Gordon made a compelling case for ending the silence in nursing and challenged nurses to "envision how things would be if the voice and visibility of nursing were commensurate with the size and importance of the nursing profession" (p. 11). Today, nurses make critical contributions to nursing, health care, and public policy decisions. These decisions involve both the context and the content of their work. Education, knowledge, and experience empower nurses to actively participate in decision making that affects the workplace, health care delivery, and the social determinants of health. Professional nurses are expected to participate in decisions regarding practice. Collective action is one mechanism available to achieve that participation. Understanding collective action is critical if nurses' efforts to shape practice are to be successful.

OBJECTIVES

- Define what *collective action* means in nursing.
- Identify the three pillars, or program areas, that are essential to the improvement of nursing and health.
- Describe the role of nursing organizations in collective action (e.g., professional associations, labour unions, and regulatory bodies) and how nurses contribute to these organizations.
- Identify evidence on the need for and impact of nurses' collective action initiatives.
- Describe the three strategies nurses use most often to achieve collective action: shared governance, workplace advocacy, and collective bargaining.

- Understand the impact of organizational culture and leadership on nurses' abilities to engage in collective action.
- Evaluate how the participation of staff nurses in decision making has the potential to enhance job satisfaction and patient outcomes.
- Describe how new graduate and early career nurses can influence workplace, health care, and public policies.

TERMS TO KNOW

advocacy
collective action
collective bargaining
health equity
nursing governance

nursing professional practice
    council
organizational culture
professional association
professional governance

shared governance
subculture
union
whistle-blowing
workplace advocacy

❓ A CHALLENGE

Ann is an early-career registered nurse new to the role of patient care coordinator at Seaview Home Health Care. As a new graduate nurse Ann worked in a large urban hospital system in the role of staff nurse. She began her work at Seaview in a staff nurse position in home health care and soon thereafter assumed the role of patient care coordinator. They learned from their team that care provision was disjointed and ineffective, and client and nurse satisfaction levels were low. Moreover, issues were evident in the areas of delegation to and support for health care assistants, and family support and teaching were not consistently a part of nursing practice. After several months of assessing how nurses worked and learning which resources were available to support their practice, Ann determined that it would be beneficial to work with their team to redesign how care was delivered. Patient-centred care was a model of care that Ann was familiar with at the large city hospital where they had previously worked, but it was not a model that had been used at Seaview. Ann wondered if they could adapt the model used in the hospital to make positive differences in client outcomes and the delivery of care in home health care nursing.

If you were Ann how would you go about moving forward to adapt a patient-centred care model at Seaview Home Health Care? What factors would you need to consider? Who needs to be involved in the discussion of a shift to patient-centred care? How would you ensure their involvement?

INTRODUCTION

The excitement of beginning a career in nursing and assuming a leader's role and responsibilities is often balanced by events taking place in health care and society and the effect these events have on nursing, nurses, and the health care system. For instance, the impact of chronic illnesses such as HIV/AIDS and diabetes on families worldwide, public awareness of health inequities, and the promise of health equity are prominent influences on nursing in the twenty-first century. Health equity, or *equity in health*, is the absence of unfair or unjust differences in life circumstances and access to resources so that all persons have fair opportunities to achieve their full health potential (Reutter & Kushner, 2010, p. 271). Unfair or unjust differences most often relate to the social determinants of health, such as income, housing, access to essential services, and the environment. The knowledge gained in your nursing education provides a background for considering these issues and how you can work with others to make a difference in nursing practice, health care, and health equity.

Nurses are deeply involved in the complex clinical problems of individuals, families, and communities because nursing practice requires the acquisition, synthesis, and retrieval of knowledge to provide competent nursing care. Having the time and resources to engage in high-level preparation for good-quality, competent care can be achieved through the collective action and advocacy of nurses. Nurses make a difference in various ways and by using various means, which is the main focus of this chapter.

DEFINING COLLECTIVE ACTION AND ADVOCACY

Collective action is defined as activities that are undertaken by a group of people who have common interests or goals. Collective action is a benign phrase; it can be applied to many aspects of daily life. The concept of *advocacy* is normative and involves action to support a cause or an interest; it is often embedded in nursing codes of ethics. For example, the Canadian Nurses Association (CNA, 2017) *Code of Ethics for Registered Nurses* states, "Nurses endeavour, individually and collectively, to advocate for and work toward eliminating social inequities by supporting or recommending a cause or course of action, undertaken on behalf of persons or issues. It relates to the need to improve systems and societal structures to create greater equity and better health for all" (p. 4). The nature of advocacy has been widely discussed in the literature (Baldwin, 2003; MacDonald, 2007). Gadow's (1990) historic discussion of the manifestations of advocacy is relevant to a discussion of today's workplace advocacy. These manifestations include the following:

1. Ensuring that nurses have relevant information to support their practice.
2. Enabling nurses to learn about the organization in which they work.
3. Encouraging nurses to disclose their personal views on issues in the work environment.
4. Providing support to nurses to make and implement decisions.
5. Helping nurses clarify their personal values.

Collective action helps nurses advocate for patients, families, and communities in health care and the political arena. The purposes of collective action extend beyond the focus on patient care and practice environments to also focus on health equity and social justice (Spenceley et al., 2006).

Individually, nurses can find it challenging to advocate for changes to patient care, the health care system, and societal health. In the absence of collective action, the average individual has limited influence in achieving their purpose. Cultivating networks and developing a collective voice require strong leaders: that is, nurses with skill and knowledge in policy and political action. Traditionally, nurses have been able to exert a broad influence on health care by working together through their professional associations and unions. Working collectively requires that nurses understand the purposes and functions of the various nursing organizations, such as professional associations, unions, and regulatory bodies. It also requires that nurses who hold different positions and are at different points in their careers understand how they can participate in advocacy through collective action. Ultimately, it is well documented that to address systemic problems successfully, it is important for nurses to engage in collective action to create a strong, unified voice that speaks on behalf of the profession (Donovan et al., 2012; Mahlin, 2010; Mildon, 2013).

The history, purpose, and functions of key nursing organizations are described in this chapter. So too are examples of their influence. It is important that nursing students learn about each of these types of organizations and their functions and consider participation—as a student and registered nurse—as a professional responsibility in making a difference to nursing, health care, and public policy. Participation in the collective action of nursing organizations is an important aspect of career and leadership development, which begins with nursing students in the formative years of their nursing education (Mata et al., 2010).

EXERCISE 21.1 Joshua is a fourth-year nursing student who has just completed a practicum with a street outreach program. During the practicum, they learned that the growing lack of affordable housing in the community has led to serious health risks, including homelessness. Joshua also volunteers at the local shelter and sees that the number of people (including children) in the community who lack access to basic living resources such as shelter and food is growing. Joshua wonders how they can draw on his experiences and work toward positive change in the living conditions of people in his community. They are particularly motivated to engage in advocacy as a nurse after they graduate and has broached the subject with a few colleagues who have cautioned them that it is not really the nurse's role to take on this issue. If you were Joshua, how would you respond to those who do not consider advocacy to be part of nursing practice?

Doane and Varcoe (2015) assert that leadership "occur[s] in every moment of practice" provided by nurses in both formal and informal leadership roles (p. 421). Nurses who bring their voice and perspective to the policy arena are providing essential leadership within the profession. Often, registered and student nurses who work directly with patients or populations are in an excellent position to bring their care experiences, "stories," and knowledge to influence a nursing practice, the health care system, or a policy. For example, the Canadian Nursing Students' Association (CNSA) lobbied the president of MTV to end the production and airing of the TV show *Scrubbing In*, which presents stereotypes and inaccurate information on nurses. Then–CNSA president Carly Whitmore sent a letter and a petition signed by the membership to MTV to pull the show. After hearing from thousands of individual nurses and nursing students, and receiving letters and petitions from nursing associations including the CNSA and the CNA (Fig. 21.1), the network announced that "it would move the show from 10 pm to midnight, therefore cutting its viewership in half, review three of the remaining episodes to see if more clinical scenes featuring nursing skills could be added, and develop new online features to educate viewers about the real work and challenges that come with being a nurse" (Geller, 2014, p. 29). This collective action clearly made an important and real difference to the professional image of nursing.

EXERCISE 21.2 Identify two policy issues, in either the practice or academic setting, for which collective action by registered/student nurses has been taken. How did you come to know about these issues, and what was the registered/student nursing's role in addressing them? Is registered/student nursing's collective action in addressing these issues visible to the organization and the public? What difference did the advocates' collective action make on these issues?

NURSING ORGANIZATIONS AND COLLECTIVE ACTION

The International Council of Nurses (ICN, n.d.) identified three pillars, or program areas, that are essential to the improvement of nursing and health:

- Professional practice.
- Regulation.
- Socioeconomic welfare.

The national voice of registered nurses   Porte-parole national des infirmières et infirmiers

CANADIAN
NURSES
ASSOCIATION

ASSOCIATION DES
INFIRMIÈRES ET
INFIRMIERS DU CANADA

October 21, 2013

Stephen Friedman
President, MTV
Stephen.Friedman@mtvstaff.com

Dear Mr. Friedman,

Both as president of the Canadian Nurses Association, which represents more than 150,000 registered nurses (RNs), and as an RN of 36 years, I am truly saddened to learn of your network's new program, *Scrubbing In*. First hearing of this show from a young nurse, I am especially concerned about its impact on the new generation of nurses.

RNs provide expert care to their patients, helping them and their families through life's most difficult days. RNs work with people to help them heal and live healthier lives. Between birth and death, the number of interactions RNs have with their patients are among the highest of all health-care providers. *Scrubbing In*'s dramatized account of nurses' lives trivializes the critical work they perform. All of their hard work, from studying and gaining experience to answering nursing's call, will be overshadowed by typical 'reality' show fodder.

Moreover, both the American and Canadian nursing professions are facing real challenges — such as tighter health-care budgets, ever-evolving legislation that governs our practice and increasing demand from growing populations who are living longer lives (often with more complex, chronic illnesses). As we work to fight these real battles that affect our capacity to deliver the best care to patients, it's a shame that we have to add sexual objectification and negative stereotypes to the list because of *Scrubbing In.*

If you respect the nursing profession and the care we provide to millions of people every day, you will cancel *Scrubbing In.*

Regards,

Barbara Mildon

Barbara Mildon, RN, PhD, CHE, CCHN(C)
President

cc.   Jennifer Solari, Vice President of Communications — Jennifer.Solari@mtvstaff.com
      Shannon Fitzgerald and David Osper, executive producers for MTV — Shannon.Fitzgerald @mtvstaff.com and David.Osper@mtvstaff.com
      Janay Dutton and Nick Predescu, executives in charge of production for *Scrubbing In* —
      Janay.Dutton@mtvstaff.com and Nick.Predescu@mtvstaff.com
      Candice Ashton, senior publicist — Canadice.Ashton@mtvstaff.com

cna-aiic.ca

50 DRIVEWAY OTTAWA ONTARIO K2P 1E2 CANADA
TEL/TÉL 613-237-2133 ▪ 1-800-361-8404 ▪ FAX/TÉLÉC 613-237-3520

Fig. 21.1 Speaking out on behalf of all nurses: a Canadian Nurses Association letter advocating for the cancellation of *Scrubbing In.*

Most countries have nursing associations that advance the professional practice of nursing. These associations have regional or national collectives, and they are connected through the ICN, which serves as a unified, global voice for nursing. Regulatory bodies regulate the practice of nursing and license nurses. Nurses' unions advance the socioeconomic welfare of nurses. These three types of organizational functions (represented in the three circles shown in Fig. 21.2) appear in some form in most countries, and they may exist in three separate organizations or be combined in one or more organizations.

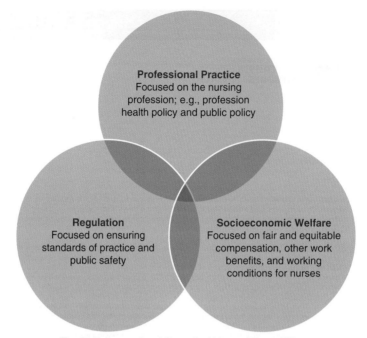

Professional Practice
Focused on the nursing
profession; e.g., profession
health policy and public policy

Regulation
Focused on ensuring
standards of practice and
public safety

Socioeconomic Welfare
Focused on fair and equitable
compensation, other work
benefits, and working
conditions for nurses

Fig. 21.2 International Council of Nurses' Three Pillars.

It is important to understand the mandates of the three pillars because specific types of advocacy and collective action flow from each one. The pillar of professional practice involves advocacy on behalf of the nursing profession to shape health care and public policy and inform decisions on behalf of the profession. Provincial and territorial professional nursing associations have generally held this mandate. Since 1924, registered nurse associations have had membership in the CNA, a national professional nursing association that connects nurses in Canada to the ICN (CNA, 2018).

The pillar of regulation involves regulatory bodies that ensure nurses provide safe, professional care. The nursing profession is self-regulating; it sets standards and monitors professional practice for quality and safety on behalf of the public. Self-regulation is a privilege of the profession: "through regulation there is the power to shape nursing. If we, as experts in our field, set our own universal standards of excellence in education and practice, then we can influence what nursing can contribute to health care across the globe" (Affara, 2005, p. 579). Regulatory bodies have been part of the nursing associations in almost every Canadian province, but recent legislation requires that this function be managed

separately to avoid perceived conflicts of interest. Nursing regulatory bodies and self-regulation are undergoing change in Canada as a result of new legislation for health care providers as well as greater government oversight. For example, many regulatory bodies are now required to establish mechanisms to ensure health professionals are maintaining their competence to practice. Students must learn about these changes and have in-depth knowledge of professional standards of practice as they relate to the changing landscape of self-regulation.

The pillar of socioeconomic welfare generally involves labour unions. **Unions** are organizations that undertake collective action on issues such as nurses' working conditions, salaries, and benefits (see also Chapter 7). Nursing unions exist in all Canadian provinces, each with membership of the Canadian Federation of Nurses Unions (CFNU). Nursing unions developed over the last quarter of the twentieth century with a mandate for **collective bargaining** on behalf of nurses. The first provincial nursing union was established in Saskatchewan in 1973, and others were established in the rest of the provinces over the next 14 years. Nursing unions have made significant gains in nursing salaries, working conditions, and policy for public health care and patient safety. *Collective bargaining* is a mechanism for negotiating a labour contract between the employer and representatives of the employees. It leads to "an agreement in writing entered into between an employer and a bargaining agent containing provisions respecting terms of conditions of employment and related matters" (*Canada Labour Code*, RSC, 1985, c. L-5, s. 3). Nursing unions enter into collective agreements with employers, such as health care organizations and government ministries. Collective agreements create the mutual obligation for employers and the representatives of the employees to meet at reasonable times to confer in good faith on wages, work hours, and other terms and conditions of employment (and any agreement or question arising from those terms and conditions). The purpose of unionization and collective bargaining by nurses is to secure fair and satisfactory conditions of employment, including the right to participate in decisions regarding nursing practice. As an example, Table 21.1 presents the registered nursing associations, regulatory bodies, and unions of registered nurses in the provinces and territories.

EXERCISE 21.3 Search your academic or practice placement setting websites to see if there is a collective agreement posted on the site. If so, examine the articles of the agreement. Are they related to practice issues or financial issues? What is the relationship between these two issue areas?

Professional Associations

A **professional association** is an alliance of practitioners within a profession that provides members with opportunities to meet leaders in the field, hone their own leadership skills, participate in policy formation, continue specialized education, and shape the future of the profession. They carry out a great deal of this work through collective action. The legacy of professional associations in nursing began with the formation of the ICN in 1899, an organization that was initially conceptualized and formed by a group of visionaries—including two Canadian nurses, Isabel Hampton Robb and Mary Adelaide Nutting, who were living in the United States at the time (Paul & Ross-Kerr, 2011). In 1908, representatives of 16 organized nursing bodies met in Ottawa to form the Canadian

National Association of Trained Nurses (CNATN). By 1924, each of the nine provinces had a professional nursing association with membership in the CNATN, and in that year, the national group changed its name to the Canadian Nurses Association (CNA) (http://www.cna-aiic.ca). Today, the CNA is a federation of provincial and territorial nursing associations and colleges representing over 150 000 registered nurses. The CNA's mission implies advocacy:

"CNA is the national professional voice of registered nurses, advancing the practice of nursing and the profession to improve health outcomes in a publicly funded, not-for-profit health system by:
- unifying the voices of registered nurses
- strengthening nursing leadership
- promoting nursing excellence and a vibrant profession
- advocating for healthy public policy and a quality health system
- serving the public interest" (CNA, n.d.).

The CNA realizes its mission through its ability to speak as the unified voice of Canadian nurses on matters of nursing, health, and public policy. Voice and presence are the essence of political power and influence; they are essential to the mission of professional associations as they advocate on a range of issues, including publicly funded health care, care delivery, nurse staffing models, evidence-informed practice, and the influence of poverty on health. As a nursing student, it is an important part of your education to remain current on the issues of the day and the mandates of your provincial or territorial, national, and international nursing associations. Professional association websites and social media make it easier to stay up-to-date on the latest issues and activities in the field.

Professional associations undertake collective action on a variety of topics, including changes to nursing practice, working conditions, care delivery models, public health care, and publicly funded health care. Nurses have been involved in creating healthy public policy in areas such as housing, poverty reduction, and the environment. Many strategies and tools are available to nurses who wish to engage in advocacy initiatives, and many of these have been developed and promoted by professional nursing associations.

Nurses contribute to the work of professional associations by identifying issues and submitting resolutions or

TABLE 21.1   Provincial and Territorial Registered Nursing Associations, Regulatory Bodies, and Unions

Province/ Territory	Professional Association	Regulatory Body	Professional Association AND Regulatory Body (Combined)	Union
British Columbia	Association of Registered Nurses of British Columbia (ARNBC) http://www.arnbc.ca	College of Registered Nurses of British Columbia (CRNBC) http://www.crnbc.ca		British Columbia Nurses' Union (BCNU) https://www.bcnu.org
Alberta			College and Association of Registered Nurses of Alberta (CARNA) http://www.nurses.ab.ca/Carna/index.aspx	United Nurses of Alberta (UNA) http://www.una.ab.ca
Saskatchewan			Saskatchewan Registered Nurses Association (SRNA) http://www.srna.org	Saskatchewan Union of Nurses (SUN) sun-nurses.sk.ca
Manitoba			College of Registered Nurses of Manitoba (CRNM) http://www.crnm.mb.ca	Manitoba Nurses Union (MNU) http://www.nursesunion.mb.ca
Ontario	Registered Nurses' Association of Ontario (RNAO) http://rnao.ca	College of Nurses of Ontario (CNO) http://www.cno.org		Ontario Nurses' Association (ONA) http://www.ona.org
Quebec			Ordre des infirmières et infirmiers du Québec (OIIQ) http://www.oiiq.org	Fédération interprofessionnelle de la santé du Québec (FIQ) http://www.fiqsante.qc.ca/fr/contents/pages/accueil.html
New Brunswick			Nurses Association of New Brunswick (NANB) http://www.nanb.nb.ca	New Brunswick Nurses Union (NBNU) http://www.nbnu.ca
Nova Scotia			College of Registered Nurses of Nova Scotia (CRNNS) http://www.crnns.ca	Nova Scotia Nurses' Union (NSNU) http://www.nsnu.ca
Prince Edward Island			Association of Registered Nurses of Prince Edward Island (ARNPEI) http://www.arnpei.ca	Prince Edward Island Nurses Union (PEINU) http://www.peinu.com
Newfoundland and Labrador			Association of Registered Nurses Newfoundland and Labrador (ARNNL) http://www.arnnl.ca	Newfoundland and Labrador Nurses' Union (NLNU) http://www.nlnu.ca
Yukon			Yukon Registered Nurses Association (YRNA) http://www.yrna.ca	
Northwest Territories and Nunavut			Registered Nurses Association of Northwest Territories and Nunavut (RNANT/NU) http://www.rnantnu.ca	

motions that can then be voted on by members. Resolutions or motions that are approved by the membership are shared with decision makers or governments on behalf of the nurse membership. It is important to review the kinds of resolutions that have been voted on by the membership of provincial or territorial associations and the CNA at annual general meetings and their outcomes.

Recently, the CNA formed a National Expert Commission on health to influence the government on nurse-led solutions for health care transformation (CNA, 2011). This initiative and others are clear examples of nurses working together to maximize nursing's voice and influence.

Canadian Nursing Students Association (CNSA) is the national professional voice of nursing students. Similar to other professional organizations, CNSA is guided by specific principles and objectives; specifically:

- to be the primary resource for Canadian nursing students
- to influence and advance innovation and social justice in the nursing curriculum
- to strengthen linkages and create new partnerships (http://cnsa.ca/about-us/objective-and-meetings/).

In relation to these overarching objectives, CNSA provides members with opportunities to meet leaders in the field, hone their own leadership skills, participate in policy formation, continue specialized education, and shape the future of the profession. The work and impact of CNSA leadership and members are accomplished through collective action.

Labour Unions

Today, 80% of nurses in Canada belong to unions, with nurses in managerial positions excluded from membership. Union stewards or regional representatives are elected to represent unionized nurses within regions, practice settings, or both. The CFNU is "the national voice of unionized nurses" with 156 000 nurses represented from unions in nine provinces (Canadian Federation of Nurses Unions, n.d.). Unions' collective bargaining agency is established under various provincial, territorial, and federal labour relations legislation. Although it is possible to bargain collectively without a union, the union model is commonly used.

Union activity in nursing and in health care has grown in the past 30 years and has been stimulated by health care reorganization, work redesign, and changes in patient care delivery models. Some of the major issues that have led to increased union activity in nursing are as follows:

- Lack of professional autonomy and professional practice models in nursing.
- Inadequate staffing and increased reliance on unregulated health care providers.
- The absence of procedures for the reporting of unsafe work environments and poor quality care.
- Mandatory overtime and work overload.
- Low wages and poor benefits.
- Workplace violence.
- The impetus to preserve publicly funded health care.
- Social justice issues.

As unions evolve to broader mandates of collective influence, they may work in concert with other associations and organizations. It is important that nonunionized nurse managers find ways to work with staff nurses who are union members and union representatives to advance the quality of work environments and patient care, as these interests are not mutually exclusive. In recent years, processes have evolved within unions to address issues of workload, safety, patient care, and other nursing practice issues through a joint problem-solving process between nursing staff and nurse managers.

Nurses who are nonunionized often have supervisory positions that include the authority to act in the interest of the employer in areas such as hiring, terminating, rewarding, and disciplining staff. Many supervisory nurses may think that they are unnecessarily placed in an adversarial relationship with unionized nurses in the hospital. However, supervisory nurses and nonsupervisory nurses both share concern for working conditions, practice standards, and the care delivery environment.

Regulatory Bodies

Self-regulation is a hard-won and essential component of nursing professionalism. Regulatory bodies have the important mandate of establishing professional standards of practice, educational requirements, and scopes of practice. Regulatory bodies exist in an environment of dynamic change and are affected by the evolution of legislation, the inclusion of models of interprofessional practice in health care, and the involvement of nurses in primary health care reform. Regulatory bodies also establish the required competencies for entry-level registered nurse practice, and these competencies are used to guide nursing education program recognition and development. Many provincial regulatory bodies have student representation programs that engage nursing students in learning about professional practice standards, scopes of practice, and ethical issues. Some regulatory bodies have workplace representatives to maintain connection with front-line nurses, and most have practice consultants available to assist registrants with practice questions or practice issues. The regulatory responsibilities of these organizations are discussed in more detail in Chapter 7, but their supportive roles to nurses and their ability to collectively educate and advocate on matters that are in the public interest should not be overlooked.

Inter-organizational Advocacy and Coalitions

At times, associations, regulatory bodies, and unions work together on common issues. For example, an association and a union may decide to work together on policies affecting workplace and care delivery systems. A regulatory body and an association might work together on the matter of expanded nursing practice roles. In addition, nursing associations join with other nonnursing associations to form partnerships in the interest of public policy. Examples include the Canadian Nurses Association, the Canadian Public Health Association, and the Canadian Medical Association, who work in partnership with national patient and consumer advocacy groups in the interests of safeguarding public health care.

Silas (2012) reported on a CFNU, CNA, Canadian Healthcare Association, and Dieticians of Canada initiative undertaken as a series of cross-national pilot projects designed to improve working conditions for nurses, that resulted in important lessons learned and recommendations (see Box 21.1).

EXERCISE 21.4 Visit the CNA website (http://www.cna-aiic.ca) for recent positions and publications on two key issues in nursing: (1) nurse fatigue and (2) nursing care delivery models and staff mix. Pay particular attention to the recommendations for each of these issues. From your perspective, are these recommendations followed in the health care organizations in areas where you have had clinical practice experience? What evidence is cited in making these recommendations? Based on your experience and what you have learned to date in your program, what recommendations for change would you make to your provincial or territorial and national nursing associations?

BOX 21.1 "Research to Action" Project Summary

In recognition of the need to support the practice of new graduates, the CFNU collaborated with the CNA, the Canadian Healthcare Association, and the Dieticians of Canada to initiate the "Research to Action: Applied Workplace Solutions for Nurses" project. Many initiatives across Canada were undertaken as part of Research to Action, all aimed at piloting and evaluating strategies that would improve the quality of working conditions for nurses (Silas, 2012). More details on this project, including lessons learned, can be found here: http://www.longwoods.com/content/22815. The project involved staff nurses in research and policy. Through the process of action research, nurses learned about the importance of supporting colleagues, the knowledge and skills required for professional development, mentorship models, and the partnerships and leadership needed to ensure that the initiatives continue to be valued as part of a quality work environment (Silas, 2012).

NURSING GOVERNANCE

The governance structure of an organization provides nurses with a framework for participating in decision making regarding their practice to ensure safe, quality care for their patients. The goal of governance structures is to establish an environment in which professional practice thrives (Clavelle et al., 2016). Professional nurses are expected to participate in decision making in their health care setting. Doing so provides nurses with greater autonomy and authority over practice decisions regarding care for patients and is a major component of job satisfaction (Kramer et al., 2008; Pittman, 2007). Nursing governance is the methodology or system by which a department of nursing controls and directs the formulation and administration of nursing policy. Organizational structure provides a framework for fulfilling the organization's mission. Organizational charts show the relationship among and between roles (see also Chapter 9). The structure of the organization and the relationship among the components of the structure are influenced by the individuals selected to interpret and implement the organization's philosophy. A particular form of governance evolves from the mission and values of the organization and the relationships among and between its components. Thus, nurse managers and leaders who enact their organization's mission and values on a daily basis support nursing more openly. To paraphrase an adage, behaviour speaks louder and has more clout than do organizational charts.

The three strategies nurses use most often to achieve collective action are professional governance, workplace advocacy, and collective bargaining. These strategies are not mutually exclusive. Moreover, as noted, governance is influenced by the context within which the organizational culture is embedded. *Organizational culture* is the implicit knowledge or values and beliefs within the organization that reflect the norms and traditions of the organization. Often, the culture itself dictates the avenue of collective action.

The culture of the geographical area influences the organizational culture, governance structure, and leadership approaches of a health care setting. Organizational culture comprises value systems and subcultures within organizations. Subcultures differ from the main culture with respect to core values, goals, and relationships, including approaches to issues and conflicts. For example, when a subculture is clearly rooted in the mission of the organization (e.g., delivery of quality care in a cost-effective environment), the possibility of genuine negotiation or problem solving is enhanced. A subculture has its own unique and distinctive features, even as other features overlap with those of the larger culture. Members may adhere to values that are specific to their group while espousing values of the larger society. The presence of congruent subcultures supports healthy relationships. Healthy relationships are an important variable in the development of a strong internal governance structure capable of supporting a professional practice environment that works well for everyone involved.

Too often, nurses and administrators are members of separate subcultures. Several factors may increase the distinct ideologies of the two groups, including the existence of a distant corporate structure and the presence of a union. Both factors may be considered external tensions. Administrators tend to take on greater decision making and be risk averse when faced with economic pressures and the need to maintain a healthy "bottom line." However, history shows that broader input, not less, from nurses at all stages

of their professional practice is important during these times.

> **EXERCISE 21.5** Identify four factors in your classroom and clinical practice experiences that have positively contributed to your sense of accomplishment and satisfaction and describe why these factors have had a positive impact. Compare your responses with those of three of your student colleagues. Are your experiences similar to the responses of others? Are you surprised by the responses?

Today, nurses expect a motivating, satisfying work environment that includes a role in decision making. Many nurses are and should be unwilling to remain outside the decision-making loop. Work redesign efforts to increase productivity and lower costs have placed a strain on the role of nursing and nurses in decision making. Supporting or creating a system that incorporates others in the decision-making process may be difficult for many in upper-management positions. However, high-performing organizations that provide quality health care have a climate that encourages participation by all stakeholders. Each stakeholder shares responsibility and risk, and that requires optimism and trust.

Professional Governance

Clavelle et al. (2016) identify accountability, professional obligation, collateral relationships, and effective decision making as the four key attributes of professional governance. *Professional governance* is further described as an extension and "maturation of the concept and practice of shared governance" (Clavelle et al., 2016, p. 308). Porter-O'Grady (2009) describes shared governance as a democratic, egalitarian, and dynamic process resulting from shared decision making and accountability. The shift from shared to professional governance reflects a response to the enhanced need for stronger interprofessional collaboration to offer integrated services that respond to the complex need of diverse clients across the age and care continuum (Clavelle et al., 2016). Professional governance must also focus on four essential elements of professional practice: accountability, partnership, ownership, and equity (Porter-O'Grady, 2009; Clavelle et al., 2016). The concepts, attributes, and characteristics of professional governance are presented in Table 21.2.

RESEARCH PERSPECTIVE

Resource: Clavelle, J. T., Porter-O'Grady, T., & Weston, M. J. (2016). Evolution of Structural Empowerment: Moving from shared to professional governance. *Journal of Nursing Administration*, 46(6): 308–312.

The authors of this study conducted a concept analysis of structural empowerment and shared governance with the goal of elucidating how each of these concepts has evolved and how each is currently used. References from 2006–2016 were selected from CINAHL, Medline, PupMed, and PsychInfo databases. The search was guided by the terms *shared governance, shared decision-making, Magnet/profession and professional, organization and relationship*, and *structural empowerment*. In addition, defining attributes, antecedents, and outcomes were reviewed individually and in relation to one another and to Kanter's structure theory of organizational power. The authors also reviewed the characteristics of collaboration, relationship, partnership/team work, nursing engagement, empowerment, change

management, professional practice, accountability, and decision making. Data analyses revealed specific shared governance attributes that have evolved over time that reflect professional governance. The aforementioned attributes include accountability, professional obligation, collateral relationships, and decision making (see Table 21.2).

Implications for Practice

Professional governance is determined to be an evidence-informed concept for implementation in health care organizations. Nurse leaders will need to determine to what extent the elements of professional governance currently exist in their institutions and to build an institutional culture in which these elements can be actualized through the provision of relevant supports and resources that foster the capacity of nurses and other health professionals to build strengths in collaboration, relationship, partnership/team work, nursing engagement, empowerment, change management, professional practice, accountability, and decision making.

TABLE 21.2   The Concept, Attributes, and Characteristics of Professional Governance

Concept	Definition	
Professional governance	The accountability, professional obligation, collateral relationships, and decision making of a professional, foundational to autonomous practice and achievement of exemplary empirical outcomes.	
Attribute	**Definition**	**Characteristics**
Accountability	The assurance that decisions and actions represent the standards of the profession and positively impact intended client, staff, and organizational outcomes	Intentionality Change management Speaking out Advocacy
Professional obligation	The professional, ethical, and legal responsibilities that influence practice within the profession, organization, or community	Legal Ethical Organizational engagement Professional involvement Knowledge seeking and growth Community engagement
Collateral relationships	The establishment, expression, and demonstration of equitable interprofessional relationships and interactions	Relational coordination Collective convergence
Decision making	The exercise of judgement grounded in the synthesis of evidence-based data to generate alternatives and make informed choices that drive actions and innovation within the profession and organization	Framework Identifying problems/opportunities Enacting the decision

From Clavelle, J. T., Porter-O'Grady, T., & Weston, M. J. (2016). Evolution of structural empowerment. Moving from Shard to professional governance. *Journal of Nursing Administration*, 46(6), p. 310.

Workplace Advocacy

Workplace advocacy is an umbrella term that encompasses advocacy activities within the practice setting. Workplace advocacy includes an array of activities undertaken to address the challenges faced by nurses in their

practice settings. These activities include career development, mentorship, participatory decision making, and the promotion of a quality work life for nurses and others with whom they work. The objective of workplace advocacy is to equip nurses to practice in a rapidly changing environment. Advocacy occurs within a context of evidence-informed and participatory decision making.

Participatory Decision Making and Collaboration

The Registered Nurses' Association of Ontario (RNAO, 2006) recommends that collaborative practice can be achieved by "incorporating nonhierarchal, democratic working practices to validate all contributions from team members" (p. 25). This is the essence of participatory decision making and can be achieved through a variety of means, including the establishment of professional practice councils. Where it is often difficult for individual nurses acting alone to effect change in nursing practice, a **nursing professional practice council** is a formal committee of nurses in a health care setting that identifies, reviews, and addresses issues that influence nursing professional practice (London Health Sciences, n.d.).

LITERATURE PERSPECTIVE

Resource: Porter-O'Grady, T. (2017). A response to the question of professional governance versus shared governance, *Journal of Nursing Administration*, 47(2): 69–71.

Porter-O'Grady highlights that the progressive growth and conceptualization of governance in nursing over the past three decades has been informed and influenced by both scholarship and practice. He describes governance as a means by which professions assume self-management and control over their unique practice and engage in partnerships with organizations toward responding to the needs of those they serve. Porter-O'Grady proposes that this partnership is an "agreement, not a hierarchy" (p. 70). This positioning of nursing as a partner with organizations is important, as it emphasizes that the profession of nursing is self-managed and hence nurses, both individually and collectively, have control over their practice. Porter-O'Grady describes that in the 1980s, when nursing governance was first being implemented into hospital systems, the term "professional governance" was considered by hospital administration to be akin to an "in-house union" (p. 69). The term "shared governance" was adopted by nurses as it was considered to be less contentious. Porter-O'Grady states that the more recent move to the term professional governance reflects the reality that nurses are self-governing, interdependent, and equitable—as well as accountable for nursing practice. Porter-O'Grady further contends that moving from shared to professional governance for nursing is a "transformation that requires continued expansion of structures and processes" (p. 70) for nursing to continue to grow in strength and equity.

Professional Values

"Professional values are beliefs and attitudes about what is good and right that generally are held in common by members of a profession and that are used to guide professional action" (Chinn & Kramer, 2011, p. 55). Professional values evolve through education in classroom settings, clinical assignments, and interactions with other nurses. Nurses have an opportunity to solidify their own values as skilled mentors, guide practice, and assist more novice nurses to engage in value clarification. Inherent in professional values are ethical codes, standards of practice, standards for protecting participants, and a willingness to challenge social traditions, cultural mores, and priorities for allocating resources (Chinn & Kramer, 2011).

Organizational patterns may segment the responsibility for the provision of care and the management of resources for that care. It is in the best interest of patients for nurses to participate in decisions regarding the provision of care and resources. The involvement of nurses can vary from none whatsoever to a high degree of input in virtually every decision affecting the conditions of employment and their practice. Nurses must be prepared and willing to participate.

> **EXERCISE 21.7** Identify three factors that you consider most empowering in a professional governance model. Would the presence of one or more of these factors influence you to practice in such an environment? If so, in what way would it influence your nursing practice?

Whistle-blowing

On occasion, individual nurses must act outside of their usual organizational channels of communication to advocate the interests of safety for themselves, colleagues, or patients. Sometimes, one nurse blows the whistle on unsafe actions, practices, and harms. Other times, a group of nurses supported by their professional associations or unions act together as whistle-blowers. **Whistle-blowing** within the scope of nursing is defined as "the action taken by a nurse who goes outside the organization for the public's best interest when it is unresponsive to reporting the danger through the organization's proper channels whereas reporting is the action taken by the nurse inside the channels of his or her organization to correct a dangerous situation" (Lachman, 2008, p. 126).

CONCLUSION

Nurses deploy a wide range of strategies to challenge the status quo and speak out against inequity and inequality. Nurses can advocate for change and influence public policy in a variety of ways, such as collective action, which will continue to benefit both the nursing profession and the outcomes of the diverse client populations that they serve.

❓ A SOLUTION

When planning any new change, and particularly a major change, it is important to include all of the stakeholders in the planning process. It is important that all Seaview Home Health Care staff, and particularly the nurses, bring their voice to the decision-making and planning processes for a change in the care delivery system that would affect each and every one of them, as well as the patients and families. Ann held numerous meetings with all involved staff on the units to discuss the idea of shifting to a patient-centred care delivery system and elicited input from all staff about their feelings, concerns, and thoughts regarding the proposed change. Ann then created a nursing professional practice council to review current evidence focused on the patient-centred care model and related patient outcomes. It was important to review best evidence-informed practices on a variety of topics, including staff mix and decision-making frameworks for quality nursing care. Locating evidence to support best practices was determined to be one of the activities of the nursing professional practice council. Ann was aware that some nurses would need additional support and education to support these efforts and arranged for a health region librarian to attend a staff meeting to discuss and outline the library support she could offer nurses in their research work. Ann was committed to engaging all stakeholders in the process of identifying, developing, and implementing a patient-centred care delivery system within the unique context of Seaview Home Health Care.

Would this be a suitable approach for you? Why or why not? Is there any group or individuals who Ann has not included as stakeholders? If so, who are they and why should they be included?

▌ THE EVIDENCE

- Nurses who are involved in collective action and who work in organizations where shared governance is practiced describe greater job satisfaction and empowerment.

- Nurses who experience a sense of empowerment in the workplace consider that their organization provides a higher quality of care and are more satisfied with the quality of their nursing practice.

✳ NEED TO KNOW NOW

- Validate how the professional practice, regulation, and socioeconomic welfare functions are implemented in your province or territory and by whom.
- Know the collective agreements of the unions active in your workplace as well as the unions' priority issues related to the socioeconomic welfare of nurses.
- Seek clarity from standards of practice and your nursing professional code of ethics about advocacy and the professional practice of nursing.

▌ CHAPTER CHECKLIST

Collectively, nurses possess the knowledge, skills, abilities, and numbers to influence policy and professional practice decisions. Collective action may take many forms. Nursing policy encompasses the three globally recognized functions of professional associations, regulatory bodies, and unions. They are important to nursing students, registered nurses, the nursing profession, and the people nurses serve around the world.

Geographical and organizational contexts influence the formal and informal structures in which nurses participate. An organization's structure establishes the parameters for participation in decision making.

Effective nurse managers employ participatory methods such as nursing professional practice councils and other democratic decision-making processes to engage and empower nurses in all settings of practice.

- The purposes of collective participation by nurses are as follows:
- To promote standards of practice of professional nursing.
- To establish and maintain standards of care.
- To allocate resources effectively and efficiently.
- To foster satisfaction and support in the practice environment.
- To advocate for the social determinants of health, public policy, and health equity in coalition with other organizations and associations.

- Collective bargaining is an effective, legal mechanism used by nurses to secure fair and satisfactory conditions of employment and obtain the right to participate in decisions regarding their practice.
- Nursing governance strategies dictate levels of participation. The type and level of participation in decision making influence job satisfaction.
- Professional governance is characterized by partnerships, equity, accountability, and ownership.
- The goal of workplace advocacy is to enable nurses to practice and make ethical decisions in a rapidly changing environment.

TIPS FOR TEAM BUILDING

- Know the issues, positions, and leadership of your province's or territory's nursing associations and the role of student nurses within the associations.
- As a new graduate nurse, be fully aware of what each union active in your workplace brings to the bargaining table and the level of awareness each union has regarding workplace issues for nurses.

- Understand that collective action is a professional responsibility of nurses and is most effective when nurses work together to bring an informed perspective to nursing, health, and public policy issues.
- Keep in mind that nurses have the opportunity to bring the experience of patient care and health issues in the community to bear on policy decisions.

Visit the Evolve website for suggested reading, Internet resources, and additional resources related to the content in this chapter: http://evolve.elsevier.com/Canada/Yoder-Wise/leading/

REFERENCES

Statutes
Canadian Labour Code, RSC c1-2 (1985) Retrieved from: https://laws.justice.gc.ca/eng/acts/L- 2/index.html.

Texts
Affara, F. A. (2005). Valuing professional self-regulation. *Journal of Advanced Nursing, 52*(6), 579. https://doi.org/10.1111/j.1365-2648.2005.03642.x.

Baldwin, M. A. (2003). Patient advocacy: A concept analysis. *Nursing Standard, 17*(21), 33–39. https://doi.org/10.7748/ns2003.02.17.21.33.c3338.

Buresh, B., & Gordon, S. (2006). *From silence to voice: What nurses know and must communicate to the public.* Ithaca, NY: Cornell University Press.

Canadian Federation of Nurses Unions. (n.d.). *Why unions.* Retrieved from: https://nursesunions.ca/why-unions.

Canadian Nurses Association (n.d.). *Vision and mission.* Retrieved from: https://www.cna-aiic.ca/en/about-cna/vision-and-mission.

Canadian Nurses Association. (2017). *Code of ethics for registered nurses (2008 centennial edition).* Toronto, ON: Author.

Canadian Nurses Association. (2018). *About CNA.* Retrieved from: http://www.cna-aiic.ca/en/about-cna.

Canadian Nurses Association. (2011). *National Expert Commission: Backgrounder.* Retrieved from: http://www.cna-aiic.ca/CNA/documents/pdf/publications/Expert_Commission_2011-2012_Backgrounder_c.pdf.

Chinn, P., & Kramer, M. (2011). *Integrated theory and knowledge development in nursing* (8th ed.). St. Louis, MO: Mosby.

Clavelle, J. T., Porter O'Grady, T., & Weston, M. J. (2016). Evolution of structural empowerment: Moving from shared to professional governance. *Journal of Nursing Administration, 46*(6), 308–312.

Doane, G. H., & Varcoe, C. (2015). *How to nurse: Relational inquiry with individuals and families in changing health and health care contexts*. Philadelphia, PA: Wolters Kluwer Health.

Donovan, D. J., Diers, D., & Carryer, J. (2012). Perceptions of policy and political leadership in nursing in New Zealand. *Nursing Praxis in New Zealand, 28*, 15–25.

Gadow, S. (1990). Existential advocacy: Philosophical foundations of nursing. In T. Pence & J. Cantrell (Eds.), *Ethics in nursing: An anthology*. New York, NY: National League for Nursing.

Geller, L. (2014). Feature article: Changing how the world thinks about nursing. *Canadian Nurse, 110*, 26–30.

International Council of Nurses. (n.d.). Pillars & programmes. Retrieved from: http://www.icn.ch/pillarsprograms/pillars-and-programmes/.

Kramer, M., Schmalenberg, C., Maguire, P., et al. (2008). Structures and practices enabling staff nurses to control their practice. *Western Journal of Nursing Research, 30*(5), 539–559.

Lachman, V. D. (2008). Whistleblowers: Troublemakers or virtuous nurses? *MedSurg Nursing; Pitman, 17*(2) 126–128, 134.

London Health Sciences (n.d.) Retrieved from: https://www.lhsc.on.ca/nursing/nursing-professional-practice-council.

MacDonald, H. (2007). Relational ethics and advocacy in nursing: Literature review. *Journal of Advanced Nursing, 57*(2), 119–126.

Mahlin, M. (2010). Individual patient advocacy, collective responsibility and activism within professional nursing associations. *Nursing Ethics, 17*, 247–254.

Mata, H., Latham, T. P., & Ransome, Y. (2010). Benefits of professional organization membership and participation in national conferences: Considerations for students and new professionals. *Health Promotion Practice, 11*, 450–454.

Mildon, B. (2013). A profession of leaders. *Canadian Nurse, 109*(5), 3.

Paul, P., & Ross-Kerr, J. (2011). Nursing in Canada, 1600 to the present: A brief account. In J. C. Ross Kerr & M. J. Wood (Eds.), *Canadian nursing: Issues and perspectives* (5th ed., pp. 18–41). Toronto, ON: Elsevier Canada.

Pittman, J. (2007). Registered nurse job satisfaction and collective bargaining unit membership status. *Journal of Nursing Administration, 37*(10), 471–476.

Porter-O'Grady, T. (2017). A response to the question of professional governance versus shared governance. *Journal of Nursing Administration, 47*(2), 69–71.

Porter-O'Grady, T. (2009). *Interdisciplinary shared governance: Integrating practice, transforming health care* (2nd ed.). Boston, MA: Jones & Bartlett.

Registered Nurses' Association of Ontario. (2006). *Healthy work environments best practice guidelines: Collaborative practice among nursing teams RNAO Nursing Best Practice Guidelines Program*. Retrieved from: http://rnao.ca/sites/rnao-ca/files/Collaborative_Practice_Among_Nursing_Teams.pdf.

Reutter, L., & Kushner, K. E. (2010). Health equity through action on the social determinants of health: Taking up the challenge in nursing. *Nursing Inquiry, 17*(3), 269–280.

Silas, L. (2012, March). The research to action project: Applied workplace solutions for nurses. *Nursing Leadership*, 9–20.

Spenceley, S., Reutter, L., & Allen, M. (2006). The road less travelled: Nursing advocacy at the policy level. *Policy, Politics and Nursing Practice, 7*, 180–194.

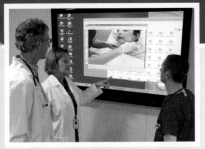

22

Understanding Quality, Risk, and Safety

Jocelyn Bennett, Judy Costello

This chapter explains key concepts and strategies related to quality, risk, and safety. All health care providers, including nurses, must be actively involved in the continuous improvement of patient care, promoting quality and safety and reducing risk.

OBJECTIVES

- Apply the principles of quality, safety, and high reliability to clinical situations.
- Use the six steps of the quality improvement process in practice.
- Understand the roles of leaders, managers, and followers in a culture of quality improvement.
- Describe the value of quality, safety, and process improvement activities at the unit level.
- Apply risk management strategies to a health care organization's work environment.

TERMS TO KNOW

benchmarking
high-reliability organization
hospital-acquired conditions
measurement
near miss
never events

nursing practice
nursing-sensitive outcomes
patient outcomes
patient safety
process improvement (PI)
quality improvement (QI)

quality management (QM)
risk management
root-cause analysis
sentinel event

❓ A CHALLENGE

Health care errors are a critical issue in safety, quality, and risk management. As a newly graduated registered nurse, Nadia has observed several near misses by colleagues on the orthopedic unit where she works. This is a source of anxiety for Nadia as she reflects on how she can ensure safety in her practice. Health care error was brought to the forefront through two key reports: a landmark US report by the Institute of Medicine, *To Err Is Human: Building a Safer Health System* (Medicine, 2000, p. 14); and *The Canadian Adverse Events Study* (Baker et al., 2004). Many policies or best practices, such as Positive Patient Identification (PPID), have been suggested to try to decrease the rate of adverse events in hospitals. However, a 2015 follow-up report to *The Canadian Adverse Events*

Study, entitled *Beyond a Quick Fix* (Baker & Black, 2015), identified that despite improvements in understanding, measurement, and practice, there continues to be limited improvement in patient safety. Increasing capacity pressures on hospitals and the higher demands placed on nurses mean that it is critical for organizations and clinicians to focus on ways they can advance quality care and prevent errors. Nadia wonders how to ease her anxiety related to concerns about the potential for errors in her practice and also how she can contribute to patient safety on her unit.

What do you think you would do if you were Nadia? What action would you take to reduce the potential for errors in your practice?

INTRODUCTION

Health care organizations and health care providers strive to provide high-quality, safe, efficient, and cost-effective care. Fundamental to these efforts is a deep understanding and commitment to the concepts of quality, safety, and risk in organizations. Historically, the terms *quality* and *safety* have been used together and have focused on incremental approaches to change through quality improvement activities. Reflection on improvements made in the health care system to date and continuing challenges in advancing patient safety and reducing health care error have led to a deeper focus on safety in organizations.

The philosophy of quality management (QM) and the process of quality improvement must shape health care culture and provide specific skills for assessment, measurement, and evaluation of patient care. The goal of an organization committed to quality care is a comprehensive, systematic approach that prevents errors or identifies and corrects errors so that adverse events are reduced and safety and quality outcomes are maximized. Despite a strong focus on quality improvement and safety, challenges remain in sustaining the reduction of health care errors. The concept of patient safety and the emergence of the principles of high reliability organizations have transformed the way health care leaders look at culture, teamwork, and how best to support and organize care to advance the safety agenda (Sutcliffe, Paine, & Pronovost, 2017). Hospital leaders, including nurses, must sharpen their expertise in patient safety and high-reliability principles to ensure structures and processes are aligned to result in effective outcomes for patients and the health care system (Oster & Deakins, 2018).

QUALITY AND SAFETY IN HEALTH CARE

Quality management (QM) in health care is about having a focus on improvement in patient care, patient safety, and resource use. Enabling and supporting quality, safety, and risk are key for staff, clinicians, and teams in hospitals and health care organizations.

Although there has been significant focus on improving patient safety and reducing health care error, little progress has been made, and there is a need to focus on organizational culture, high-performing teams, and effective work environments. Nurses have a unique role in patient safety and quality improvement as they deliver direct care to patients and have an understanding of the day-to-day issues involved in the delivery of care. The engagement of nurses in patient safety and patient care improvement efforts in a number of areas (e.g., patient flow problems, safe delivery of care during periods of low staffing or high patient census or high acuity, communication problems associated with complex patients, medication safety) not only promotes the quality and safety of patient care but creates a positive work environment for staff. In fact, nurses' perception of having access to empowering structures in their workplace is positively associated with nurse-assessed quality of care, patient safety climate, and work and unit effectiveness (Goedhart, van Oostveen, & Vermeulen, 2017). The results of this work call upon leaders to enable empowering work environments for all staff.

Baker and Black (2015) advocate that the creation of effective work environments and high-performing teams are fundamental for improving patient safety. The Canadian Patient Safety Institute (CPSI, 2008) identified six domains of safety competencies that can enhance patient safety across health care professions. The six competencies include: (1) contributing to a culture of patient safety, (2) working in teams for patient safety, (3) communicating effectively for patient safety, (4) managing safety risks, (5) optimizing human and environmental factors, and (6) recognizing, responding to, and disclosing adverse events. Quality necessitates maintaining safety in patient care and a continuous focus on clinical excellence by the entire interprofessional team. Although the safety competencies relate to individual practitioners in the environment, key organizational factors are also of importance to advance the safety agenda. One area that has emerged is the focus on high-reliability organizations. Various industries—airline, nuclear safety, and others—have demonstrated excellent performance outcomes for safety despite complex and risky work (Sutcliffe et al., 2017). The five principles of high-reliability organizations are outlined in Box 22.1.

Preoccupation with failure, the first principle, relates to the relentless focus of organizations on safety concerns in the work environment. Members of the interprofessional team (e.g., nurses, doctors, pharmacists, physiotherapists, etc.) and other team members (e.g., clerical staff, porters, housekeepers) are encouraged to identify any safety concerns as they may be part of

---

BOX 22.1 Five Key Principles of High-Reliability Organizations

1. Preoccupation with failure
2. Reluctance to simplify
3. Sensitivity to operations
4. Commitment to resiliency
5. Deference to expertise

Modified from Weick, K. S., & Sutcliffe K. M (2015). *Managing the unexpected: Sustained performance in a complex world* (3rd ed.). San Francisco, CA: Jossey-Bass.

---

a larger issue in the system or a gap in information or knowledge that may not be evident. Searching for potential failures and identifying them through safety huddles or reporting near miss safety events (good catches) that could be part of a larger system issue are important in high-complexity environments. The second principle, reluctance to simplify, focuses on the need for staff to look beyond the obvious and avoid jumping to potential quick-fix solutions. Asking questions about what is happening and potential drivers can help teams understand the issue more deeply, identify the root cause, and implement more effective solutions. Sensitivity to operations, the third principle, outlines the importance of situational awareness related to how systems and processes are working in the organization, so that potential risks to safety can be identified and actioned. Team members need to speak up for safety when they see an error or identify an issue or process that may affect safety for patients and staff. The fourth principle, commitment to resiliency, focuses on the ability of individuals and teams to address problems, implement solutions and bounce back from errors. Learning from errors and focusing on implementing change helps staff and organizations build knowledge, become learning organizations, and move forward to advance their safety agenda. The fifth and final principle of high-reliability organizations (HROs) is deference to expertise. Those who have the most knowledge about the situation are encouraged to speak up, voice concerns, and share ideas. The concept of hierarchy needs to be considered in that those who are delivering care or a service in an organization would be the experts in that area and could best identify gaps and opportunities (Weick, 2015). In high-reliability organizations, all team members play an important role in patient and staff safety.

Health care environments are complex and dynamic. The implementation of high-reliability principles can enhance quality and safety outcomes and reduce risk for patients and staff. Implementing HRO principles has been found to improve nursing-sensitive outcomes as measured by reductions in central line infections (CLI), catheter-associated urinary tract infections (CAUTI), falls, and pressure injuries (Oster & Deakins, 2018). Hospital-acquired conditions (e.g., CLI, fall, etc.) can have a substantial cost to the patient and health care system from a morbidity and mortality perspective, increased length of stay and costs of care, as well as reputational risk (negative public image, employee frustration, and employee turnover). A framework has been established based on HRO principles so as to build organizational capacity on the journey to high reliability, understanding that it is a journey and not a destination (Aboumatar et al., 2017). Steps to high reliability include having an organization-wide approach to managing risk through a relentless focus on safety. Tools that have been deployed in HROs include: standardized checklists, evidence-based practice bundles (e.g., a CLI prevention bundle), encouraging near miss reporting for trend analysis, and cascading daily safety huddles at all levels of the organization to ensure that unit or system safety concerns can be escalated and addressed in a timely manner. Also important is a requirement for standardized patient safety curriculum for all staff to understand their role in patient safety and use of tools to communicate clearly and effectively when concerns or risks are identified (i.e., SBAR: Situation, Background, Assessment, Recommendation). Fundamental to the shift to a high-reliability organization is transformational leadership to support the commitment to a culture shift and becoming a no-blame learning health care organization. All team members have the opportunity to lead for change in HROs and must understand their role in quality and patient safety. If they are actively involved in improving quality and patient safety and there is clear delineation in roles, a safety culture will be supported (Table 22.1).

Baker and Black (2015) conducted an analysis of the state of safety in Canada a decade after the Canadian Adverse Events study (Baker et al., 2004). The report outlined a number of recommendations for health care leaders to address the lack of sustained progress in safety. The recommendations evolved around how to

TABLE 22.1	**Roles and Responsibilities in Quality Improvement**	
Senior Leader	**Nurse Manager**	**Nurse**
• Leads cultural transformation • Sets priorities for house-wide activities, staffing effectiveness, and patient outcomes • Builds infrastructure, provides resources, and removes barriers for improvement • Defines procedures for immediate response to errors involving care, treatment, or services and contains risk • Assesses management and staff knowledge of the quality, risk, and safety activities regularly, and provides education as needed • Implements and monitors systems for internal and external reporting of information • Defines and provides support system for staff who have been involved in a sentinel event	• Is accountable for quality and safety indicator performance within areas of responsibility • Displays safety goals, performance metrics, and targets to staff on a quality board • Leads safety huddles at the quality board • Escalates safety concerns and risks to senior leader • Meets regularly with staff to monitor progress and help with improvement work • Uses data to measure effectiveness of improvement • Works with staff to develop and implement action plans for improvement of measures that do not meet target • Provides time for unit staff to participate in safety and quality improvement activities • Directly observes staff and coaches as needed • Consults patient safety specialist, quality management team, or risk management team as appropriate • Writes and submits to senior leaders a periodic action plan that includes performance metrics, successes, and plans for improvement • Shares information and benchmarks with other units and departments to improve organization's performance	• Follows policies, procedures, and protocols to ensure quality and safe patient care • Remains current in the literature on quality and safety specific to nursing; promotes evidence-informed practice standards • Communicates with and educates peers immediately if they are observed not following quality and safety standards • Reports quality and safety concerns and risks to supervisor/manager • Invests in patient safety by continually asking self, "What risks do I observe on the unit?" "What concerns should I bring up at the safety huddle? "What else do I need to do to meet our safety goal target?" • Participates actively in quality improvement activities

create more effective environments and high-performing teams (i.e., a patient safety and quality improvement strategy, adverse event reporting and analysis, strong teamwork and investment in work climate and processes, leadership capabilities, and engaging patients and caregivers in safety and quality improvement, among others). The recommendations align with the HRO principles outlined earlier.

In health care organizations, the approach to high-reliability processes can involve looking at structure, process and outcome elements: Structure (e.g.,

adequacy of staffing, effectiveness of computerized charting, availability of unit-based medication delivery systems), process (e.g., timeliness and thoroughness of documentation, adherence to critical pathways or care maps), and outcome (e.g., patient falls, hospital-acquired infection rates, medication errors, patient satisfaction).

The subsequent Literature Perspective expands the discussion of HROs in relation to ensuring quality and safety, while demonstrating the impact on the value of nursing services in health care organizations.

LITERATURE PERSPECTIVE

Resource: Oster, C. A, & Deakins, S. (2018). Practical application of high-reliability principles in healthcare to optimize quality and safety outcomes. *Journal of Nursing Administration*, 48 (1), 50–55.

In the current era of increasing accountability, nursing leaders are under pressure to demonstrate the value of nursing services to achieving organizational quality and safety objectives. Value is defined as the outcomes and impact of nursing care over the cost to deliver this care. Given that historical quality management and improvement approaches have demonstrated inconsistent impact on patient and staff outcomes, the emerging focus on high-reliability principles is showing promise for improving nurse sensitive outcomes, and thus reinforcing the value of nursing to health care. Focused on the reduction or elimination of preventable harm, consistent improvements have been demonstrated in nurse-sensitive indicators, such as pressure injury or falls with injury. This is achievable through the development of high-performing teams focused on the implementation of best-practice bundles through the use of process improvement activities. Improvements in patient outcomes and elimination of avoidable cost, such as hospital-acquired urinary tract infections related to indwelling catheter use, positively impacts both inputs in the value equation by improving patient outcomes while reducing the costs of care.

Implications for Practice

It is important that nursing leaders consider the processes and structures they build to improve nursing sensitive indicators and reduce practice variation within their organizations, programs or units. Focusing on the principles of high reliability can improve nurse-sensitive indicators and patient outcomes, as well as demonstrate the value of nursing care.

In Canada, the implementation of the accreditation process for health care organizations was a major influence on the evolution of quality processes. In 1958, the Canadian Council on Hospital Services Accreditation (CCHSA) was established to set standards for Canadian hospitals and monitor their adherence. The CCHSA acted as a key external stimulus for quality assessment programs in hospitals and community-based programs and services. In 2008, CCHSA launched the Qmentum Accreditation Program and changed its name to Accreditation Canada. This change reflected a shift to standards-based assessment of structures, processes, and outcomes in organizations, as well as identification of Required Organizational

Practice (ROPs) or key practices that must be present in organizations. More recently, following an extensive consultation of its service, Accreditation Canada launched an affiliate organization in 2017, called The Health Standards Organization (HSO). HSO will focus on standards development whereas Accreditation Canada will continue to deliver assessment programs that provide both accreditation and certification depending on the setting. As part of its transformation, Accreditation Canada strengthened patient and family engagement in program design and services as well as added patient surveyors to the survey team. The steps taken by Accreditation Canada reflect the continued evolution of the organization to advance the focus on safety, quality and continuous improvement.

Provincial and territorial professional associations and regulatory bodies in nursing have also been instrumental in the focus on quality processes in nursing by developing guidelines for implementing quality improvement programs, nursing practice standards and guidelines, and resources and tools for nurses to develop quality improvement (QI) competencies. The current emphasis in the health care system on improving patient safety has led many hospitals to hire patient safety specialists to work with clinical teams. The findings of the Canadian Adverse Events Study (Baker et al., 2004) were released shortly after the report by the US Institute of Medicine (IOM) (Medicine, 2000) report *To Err Human: Building a Safer Health System*. Finding of the study reported that in Canada, a 7.5% incidence rate for adverse events (of which 36.9% were highly preventable) accounted for 1.1 million additional hospital days. In 2003, the Canadian Patient Safety Institute (CPSI) was founded to provide a coordinating and leadership role across health care sectors and systems; promote leading practices; and raise awareness by stakeholders, patients, and the general public about patient safety. This not-for-profit organization works with governments, health organizations, health care leaders, and health care providers to inspire improvement in patient safety and quality by developing evidence-informed resources and working to deliver measurable results.

EXERCISE 22.1 Working in groups of 2 to 3 of your classmates, discuss the following questions:
1. What provincial/territorial bodies will govern your practice as a registered nurse?
2. What best practices or guidelines are available from these bodies?
3. How do these practice or guidelines relate to policy, safety or risk in your practice settings?

Public reporting of patient safety metrics is changing the way the public makes decisions about health care and is intended to improve care through easily accessible information. For example, Health Quality Ontario (n.d) reports to the public on quality metrics across all health sectors. Topics covered include patient safety and QI indicators, such as hospital-associated infections, hand-hygiene compliance, and hospital mortality rates. The public can access a searchable database and yearly reports on Ontario's health care system at the organization's Web site, as well as view a section on QI in health care delivery and is designed to assist the public to become informed users of Ontario's health care system. (http://www.hqontario.ca/Quality-Improvement).

Patient experience with health care can be assessed through the use of surveys, interviews, focus group discussions, or observation. Patients' perspectives should be a key component of any QI initiative. However, patients cannot always adequately assess the competence of clinical performance, and therefore patient feedback and patient experience surveys must serve as only one data source for QI initiatives.

Implementing process improvement changes must be based on data. The use of statistical tools enables nurse managers and staff to make objective decisions about QI activities. It is imperative that data are not merely collected to support a preconceived idea. Quality information must be gathered and analyzed without bias before improvement suggestions and recommendations are made.

However, recent mandates in some sectors to disclose publicly nosocomial infection rates highlight potential issues with disclosure of data. Specifically, simply reporting hospital infection rates is not enough to promote hand-hygiene practices and may do little to improve outcomes and reduce hospital-acquired infections. Unfortunately, the ability to compare data across health care sectors or organizations, such as hospital-acquired infection or hand-hygiene rates, may be hindered by differences in terminology. Information technology plays a vital role in QI by increasing the efficiency of data entry and analysis. A consistent information system that trends high-risk procedures and systematic errors would provide a useful database regarding outcomes of care and resource allocation. Efforts are underway to develop standardized indicators of performance so that true comparisons can be made across health care settings, provinces, and territories.

> **EXERCISE 22.2** What standardized performance indicators are being reported in your practice's settings?
> 1. How are they measured and monitored?
> 2. What targets for improvement have been set?
> 3. What changes can you implement in your practice to improve performance on these indicators?

THE QUALITY IMPROVEMENT PROCESS

Quality Improvement (QI) is a proven method to improve care for patients and processes for staff. QI involves the continuous analysis and evaluation of product, services, and approaches to optimize and improve processes to prevent errors and achieve consumer satisfaction. The QI process is continuous and should be part of everyone's activities because products and services can always be improved.

In health care, the QI process is a structured series of steps designed to plan, implement, and evaluate changes in care activities. Many models of the QI process exist, but most parallel the nursing process and all contain steps similar to those listed in Box 22.2 (HealthQualityOntario, 2012). Most improvement activities begin with a more general concern or thought about an area for improvement, and once a team is assembled, specific aims and measures can be identified.

These six steps are often integrated within the Model for Improvement and can easily be applied to clinical settings.

Assemble the QI Team

Once an opportunity is identified for possible improvement, an interprofessional team undertakes the QI process. QI team members should represent a cross-section

---

> ### BOX 22.2 Quality Improvement Process
>
> 1. Assemble the quality improvement team
> 2. Identify the aim: What are we trying to accomplish?
> 3. Identifying the measures: How will we know if a change is an improvement?
> 4. Defining the changes—what changes will result in an improvement?
> 5. Implement rapid cycle improvements
> 6. Sustain the improvements
>
> Modified from HealthQualityOntario. (2012). *Quality Improvement Guide*. Toronto ON: Queen's Printer for Ontario Retrieved from http://www.hqontario.ca/portals/0/Documents/qi/qi-quality-improve-guide-2012-en.pdf

of workers who are involved with the issue. This could include nurses, allied health professionals, physicians, as well as clerical and support staff and data and process improvement experts. Consideration should be given to including patients or consumers to the team. There is a growing recognition that quality care is possible only when patients are engaged in their own care. Sustainable changes in system performance are possible only through effective co-design: patients and family members working together with clinical teams and leaders (Baker, Judd, Fancott & Maika, 2016). To maximize success, team members may need to be educated about their roles before starting the QI process. Fundamental to effective unit-based QI teams is a workplace environment that promotes high-functioning, nonhierarchical teamwork. Some departments in health care facilities are more open to teamwork than others. Nursing students can use Exercise 22.3 to think about how they might develop a team on a project.

EXERCISE 22.3 You have been asked by the faculty to participate in the development of a committee to review the quality of clinical placements.
1. Who are the key people involved in clinical placements for students?
2. What are the skills sets and qualifications of the people who should be on your committee?
3. What information do committee members need to have to prepare for their committee participation?

Identify the Aim: What Are We Trying to Accomplish?

The QI process begins with the selection of a clinical activity or issue for exploration and improvement – what is the goal or aim of the improvement? Theoretically, any and all aspects of clinical care could be improved through the QI process. However, the aim of QI efforts should be concentrated on changes to patient care or systems that will have the greatest effect. The aim can be established in a number of ways but always involves a standard of practice. The improvement team should use accepted standards of care and practice whenever possible. Clinical practice guidelines and standards should reflect evidence-informed practice and should be updated as new research emerges. Sources that establish these standards include the following:

1. Provincial or territorial regulatory bodies, nurse practice acts, and standards of nursing practice
2. Accrediting bodies such as Accreditation Canada
3. Governmental bodies such as the Canadian Institutes of Health Research (CIHR), Canadian Institute for Health Information (CIHI), and Public Health Agency of Canada (PHAC)
4. Health care advisory groups such as Health Council Canada (HCC), Canadian Patient Safety Institute (CPSI), Institute for Safe Medication Practices (ISMP), National Quality Institute (NQI), Canadian Foundation for Health Improvement (CFHI), and the Canadian Centre for Occupational Health and Safety (CCOHS)
5. Policy statements and reports from nationally recognized professional associations, such as the Canadian Nurses Association (CNA)
6. Nursing evidence-informed Best Practice Guidelines
7. Health care organizational policies and procedures
8. Internal or external performance measurement data such as patient satisfaction surveys, employee opinion surveys, safety assessment surveys, patient or employee rounds, review of adverse event, or incident reporting to identify recurring or critical issues; identification of errors and/or near misses.

Identifying a clear aim provides the team with direction on how to address the issue or concern. Ideally, the aim statement is specific, including how much improvement is expected by when, and can be reviewed by the team and patients to ensure that it brings value to care.

The results of the research study in the Research Perspective below identified the importance of considering the literature in how to care for patients with unrecognized physiologic instability can result in failure to rescue by the clinical teams and nurses.

RESEARCH PERSPECTIVE

Resource: Sebat, F., Vandegrift, M., Childers, S., & Lighthall, G. (2018). A novel bedside-focused ward surveillance and response system. *Joint Commission Journal on Quality & Patient Safety, 44*(2), 94-100.

This study prospectively examined outcomes on adult medical wards at a community medical regional centre by exploring the effectiveness related to rapid response systems (RRSs) interventions with deteriorating patients. Outcomes under study include rapid response team (RRT) alerts,

Continued

RESEARCH PERSPECTIVE—cont'd

cardiac arrests, and patient mortality. By observing large numbers of patient encounters (N = 28,914 observation in the 24-month control period and N = 39,802 in the 33-month intervention period) the investigators were able identify opportunities for improvement. These include improving the education for ward nurses related to recognition of at-risk patients, system changes to empower staff to trigger RRTs, development of improved RRT treatment protocols, and improvised monitoring of overall outcomes. Overall outcomes demonstrated an increase in RRT calls and a significant decrease in cardiac arrests and patient mortality.

Implications for Practice
This study demonstrates the profound impact that nursing assessment and interventions have on significant

patient outcomes. Systematic measurement and understanding of outcomes can reveal safety issues and needed changes within a health care setting to improve patient outcomes. The interventions align with the Canadian Patient Safety Institute (Frank, 2008) domains of *The Safety Competencies* and highlight how teams working together can optimize patient safety and quality of care by sharing authority, leadership, and decision making for safer care (Domain 2: Work in Teams for Patient Safety). This is complemented by anticipating and recognizing situations that place patients at risk through the anticipation, identification, and management of high-risk situations (Domain 4: Manage Safety Risks).Resource:

Identifying the Measures: How Will We Know If a Change Is an Improvement?

Once the aim of the improvement activity is clarified, the team needs to identify what measures or outcomes would best be collected to explore the current status of the activity, service, process, or procedure identified for improvement. Nursing-sensitive outcomes are patient outcomes that are sensitive to nursing practice or interventions. *Nursing-sensitive indicators reflect the structure, process, and outcomes of nursing care.* The structure of nursing care is indicated by the supply of nursing staff, the skill level of the nursing staff, and the education/certification of nursing staff. Process indicators measure aspects of nursing care such as assessment, intervention, and nurse job satisfaction. Patient outcomes (the result of patient goals that are achieved through a combination of medical and nursing interventions with patient participation) are determined to be nursing sensitive if they improve with an increase in the quantity or quality of nursing care (e.g., pressure ulcers, falls, and intravenous [IV] infiltrations). Some patient outcomes are more highly related to other aspects of institutional care, such as medical decisions and institutional policies (e.g., frequency of primary Caesarean sections, cardiac failure), and are not considered nursing sensitive. Also important in the QI process are balancing measures or outcomes. Balancing measures may be Nurse Sensitive or Patient Outcomes and provide a differing view on the outcomes. An example of this includes: Patient Outcome Measure or Rate of Patient Falls; Process Measure

or Falls Best Practice Guideline (BPG) implementation; Balancing Measure or Rate of Patient Restraint Utilization. This reflects that the rate of patient falls is related to both BPG implementation and the degree to which patients at risk of falling are restrained. In an era of "least restraint," the application of physical or chemical restraints should not be used as a singular strategy to reduce patient falls.

Although individual health care organizations may have unique patient needs related to their specific population or environment, many targeted outcomes are similar. One way to evaluate the quality of outcomes is to compare one organization's performance with that of similar organization's. In a process called benchmarking, best practices, processes, or systems are identified and then compared with the practice, process, or system under review. Through this comparison, an organization identifies desired standards of quality performance. Examples of available data that can be used in benchmarking include all reported hospital-acquired infection rates in other institutions as well as specific data, such as postoperative infection rates in adult surgical critical care units of similar-size institutions.

Nursing has been a leader in the information system field by developing standardized nursing classification systems. The availability of standardized nursing data enables the study of health problems across populations and health care settings, and in relation to caregiving. The consistent use of standardized language enhances the QI process and also makes nursing's contributions clearer to regulators, health care policymakers, and the public. The use of standardized nursing terminology provides a means of collecting and analyzing nursing data and evaluating nursing-sensitive outcomes. In Canada, although there has been limited uptake of specific nursing classification systems in health care organizations, there has been a focus on measuring nursing-sensitive outcomes and implementing evidence-informed practice guidelines in nursing. Evidence-informed Best Practice Guidelines support decision making in the delivery of quality nursing care. Best Practice Guidelines are systematically developed statements based on the best available evidence to assist clinician and patient decision making about appropriate health care for specific clinical circumstances (Fleiszer, Semenic, Ritchie, et al., 2015). The Registered Nurses' Association of Ontario (RNAO) launched the nursing Best Practice Guidelines (BPGs) program in 1999 to support Ontario nurses by providing them with BPGs for patient care. To date, the program has developed and disseminated 50 guidelines covering clinical and nursing work environment topics. As well, a toolkit and an educator's resource kit for implementing these guidelines have been made available to the nursing community in all provinces and territories and have been translated into multiple languages and implemented globally in a number of jurisdictions. For more information on nursing-sensitive outcomes, see Chapter 5. For more information on quality indicators in nursing, see Chapter 3.

Defining the Changes—What Changes Will Result in an Improvement?

When the QI team has identified the aim and the measures for the improvement activity, it is time to engage in the generation of ideas of changes which may result in improvement. Change ideas can often be generated from the QI team who see opportunities for improvements in their work, or from best practices from other organizations or the literature. Students can actively contribute to change idea identification as they bring a differing perspective to clinical setting through their exposure to multiple different practices and policies across different clinical settings, and also bring an "outside" or fresh perspective to the improvement setting. They may also be more familiar with the most recent literature and best practices, because of learning in their programs. Nursing students can use Exercise 22.4 to think about the opportunities they observe.

EXERCISE 22.4 Ask yourself the following questions when thinking about your clinical experiences:

1. What activities have you observed that are focused on improving patient and/or staff outcomes?
2. What variations in practices have you observed across different clinical settings?
3. Are the practice variations based on evidence?
4. How might you engage staff in the clinical settings in discussions of the variations?

Teams may also use a variety of improvement tools to understand the current state and identify change ideas. Several useful tools for change idea generation include process maps and fishbone diagrams.

Process Maps

A detailed process map is used to understand all the different steps that take place in a process and is a basic tool for describing complex tasks in any QI project. The process map uses boxes and directional arrows to diagram all the steps of a process or procedure in the proper sequence. Sometimes, just diagramming a patient-care process in detail reveals gaps and identifies ideas for improvement.

Fishbone Diagrams

The fishbone diagram is an effective method of summarizing a brainstorming session. A specific problem or outcome is written on the horizontal line. All possible sub-causes leading to the main cases of the quality problem are written in a fishbone pattern.

Broader change concepts may also be useful to identify improvement activities. Non–health care industries have excelled in incorporating process improvement in their core operating strategies. Numerous business management philosophies have been expanded and modified for use in health care organizations. For example, Six Sigma, a data-driven approach targeting a nearly error-free environment, empowers employees to improve processes and outcomes. As health care organizations "go lean," nurses are challenged to eliminate unnecessary steps and reduce wasted processes (saving time and money) to improve the quality of care and the patient experience (Fine, Golden, Hannam, et al., 2009). Six Sigma uses a five-step methodology known as *DMAIC* (Box 22.3), which stands for *d*efine opportunities, *m*easure performance, *a*nalyze opportunity, *i*mprove performance, and *c*ontrol performance, to improve existing processes.

BOX 22.3 DMAIC

Define opportunities
Measure performance
Analyze opportunity
Improve performance
Control performance

BOX 22.4 Plan-Do-Study-Act Cycle

Plan
State the purpose of the PDSA (developing, testing, or
     implementing a change idea).
What is the change idea?
What indicator(s) of success will you measure?
How will data on these indicators be collected?
Who or what are the subjects of the test?
How many subjects will be included in the test and over
     what time period?
What do you hypothesize will happen?

Do
Conduct the test.
Document any problems or unintended consequences.

Study
Analyze the data and study the results.
Compare the data to your predictions.
Summarize and reflect on what was learned.

Act
Refine the change idea, based on the lesson learned
     from the test.
Prepare a plan for the next test.

© Queen's Printer for Ontario, 2012. Adapted and reproduced
with permission.

Testing Change Ideas—Implement Rapid Cycle Improvements

The cornerstone of process improvement is the implementation of Rapid Cycle Improvements to test change ideas. This is done through the use of the Plan-Do-Study-Act (PDSA) Cycle, which can be used to test both small scale change ideas and organizational wide initiatives. The activities within each step of the cycle are outlined in Box 22.4 (HealthQualityOntario, 2012, p. 9).

The PDSA Cycle enables a systematic approach to process improvement. The Plan Phase is the opportunity to articulate the approach developed from the Aim and Measure activities. The Do Phase involves testing out the idea with careful data collection of both intended and unintended outcomes. Analysis of the data occurs during the Study phase of the cycle using a variety of tools. Although QI teams should be able to use these basic statistical tools, analysis that is more complex is sometimes necessary. In many situations, a statistical expert, often in the form of a process or quality improvement expert, could be included on the QI team or the team may consult a statistician. Box 22.5 outlines some of the basic QI tools that nurses should learn to use and interpret.

Teams must consider that sometimes improvement in one part of a system presents new issues. For example, nurses implemented screening for suicide risk in adolescents and adults presenting to the emergency department. A result of this improvement in care was a greatly increased number of referrals for counselling, which overwhelmed the existing hospital and community resources. The improvement team may need to monitor balancing metrics to understand broader system impact and manage the inevitable obstacles that develop with the implementation of any new process or procedure.

Finally, in the Act Phase, the QI team is able to look to refine any results and move to the next PDSA. As is implied through this, Process Improvement should be an ongoing and continuous process of ever improving the quality of care. In some organizations, however, when a change is implemented successfully, the QI team disbands. Some organizations that have used the process improvement (PI) philosophy for several years establish permanent QI teams or committees. These QI teams do not disband after implementing one project or idea, but rather may meet regularly to focus on improvements in specific areas of patient care. The use of permanent QI teams or the adoption of a culture driven by principles of HROs and QM can provide continuity and prevent duplication of efforts within the quality teams.

Quality-focused organizations stress system-level change and the evaluation of outcomes. However, in recent years, the need for process and performance improvement, including individual performance appraisal, has reemerged within health care organizations. Self-review and peer evaluation are performance assessment methods that fit within the improvement philosophy. Many provincial and territorial regulatory bodies

---

BOX 22.5   Quality Improvement Tools

Line Graphs	Presents data by showing the connection among variables. The dependent variable is usually plotted on the vertical scale, and the independent variable is usually plotted on the horizontal scale. In quality improvement (QI), this technique is often used to show the trend of a particular activity over time, and the result may be called a *trend chart*.
Histograms	A histogram is a bar chart that shows the frequency of events.
Bar Charts	A bar chart that identifies the major causes or components of a particular quality control problem is called a *Pareto chart*. It differs from a regular bar graph in that the highest frequencies of occurrence of a factor are designated in the bar at the left, with the other factors appearing in descending order. Used often in QI, the Pareto chart helps the QI team determine priorities, allowing the most significant problem to be addressed first.

---

and professional associations have developed self-review tools and resources for performance appraisals. Any nurse can use the six steps of the QI process in a self-review to improve individual performance. For example, a nurse on a medical unit who wants to improve documentation skills might study past entries on patient records; review current institution policies, professional standards, and literature related to documentation; set specific performance improvement goals after consultation with the nurse manager and expert colleagues; devise strategies and a timeline for achieving performance goals; and, after implementing the strategies, review documentation entries to see whether self-improvement goals have been met.

Sustain the Improvements

Sustainability requires significant and ongoing attention and strategies to sustain a process should be built into ongoing improvement cycles at the very beginning. Planning a process improvement, concurrent with ideas and actions for sustainability, decreases the likelihood that performance drop off, or regression to previous

patterns of practice, will occur. Relentless and persistent actions for sustainability must accompany any improvement efforts. Fleiszer et al. (2015), p. 14 states, "Leaders may need to continually reflect on the successes and failures of their sustainability-oriented work, remaining attentive to the multiplicity of factors that accentuate or attenuate program sustainability, and to use those reflections as a basis for continued evolution and improvement." One of the crucial tasks of the nurse manager is to publicize and reward the success of each QI team. The nurse manager must also evaluate the work of the team and the ability of individual team members to work together effectively.

Although structured and frequent feedback on performance through regular data measurement is critical, it is this leadership engagement that is key to organizational performance and sustainability (Staines et al., 2017).

RISK MANAGEMENT

Quality, safety, and risk management are related concepts and emphasize the achievement of quality-outcome standards and the prevention of patient-care problems. Risk management is the systematic identification, assessment, and prioritization of risks and the development and implementation of strategies to reduce adverse events and liability associated with these risks. Chapter 7 also discusses risk management. Losses associated with risk include financial loss as a result of malpractice or absorbing the cost of an extended length of stay for the patient, negative public relations, and employee dissatisfaction. The inclusion of patient safety standards in accreditation programs further emphasizes the importance of risk management. For example, Accreditation Canada developed ROPs and tests for compliance for each ROP that organizations must meet to demonstrate meeting patient safety goals, which appear in Box 22.6.

A risk management department has several functions, which include the following:

- Defining situations that place the organization at some financial risk, such as medication errors and patient falls
- Determining the frequency of occurrence of those situations
- Intervening and investigating identified events
- Identifying potential risks or opportunities to improve care

> ### BOX 22.6 Accreditation Canada Patient Safety Goal Areas for Health Care Organizations
>
> Safety Culture: Create a culture of safety within the organization
>
> Communication: Promote effective information transfer with clients and team members across the continuum of care
>
> Medication Use: Ensure the safe use of high-risk medications
>
> Worklife/workforce: Create a worklife and physical environment that supports the safe delivery of care and service
>
> Infection Control: Reduce the risk of health care–associated infections and their impact across the continuum of care
>
> Risk Assessment: Identify and mitigate safety risks inherent in the client population
>
> © 2016. Accreditation Canada and its licensors.

A major focus of risk management programs in health care organizations is patient safety, which is the absence of preventable harm to a patient during the process of health care. The Canadian Adverse Events Study (Baker et al., 2004) reported the occurrence of 185,000 adverse events per year in Canada, with over one-third of these deemed potentially preventable. In a 2004 follow up to its 'To Err is Human Report' published in 2000, the Institute of Medicine (IOM) pointed to the critical role nursing plays in providing safe care and identified health care management practices necessary to create a positive patient safety culture. Those practices included creating and maintaining trust throughout the organization; actively managing the process of change, deploying health care providers in adenumbers; creating a culture of openness regarding reporting and preventing errors and involving health care providers in decision making regarding work design and workflow (Medicine, 2000). The IOM, 2004 emphasized that the quality of patient care is directly affected by the degree to which hospital nurses are active and empowered participants in decisions about their patients' plans of care and by the degree to which they have an active and central role in organizational decision making.

The CPSI created the Safer Healthcare Now! (SHN) program, which is a collaboration of people and organizations committed to improving patient safety. The program is founded on the principle that safe care is a top priority and that all organizations can make a difference when they partner and share information, strategies, and resources. The SHN program is supported by individual clinicians, teams, and health care organizations from across Canada that provide ongoing clinical expertise to SHN's work, including mentorship of health care providers working to implement SHN interventions on the front line. The CPSI has chosen a number of interventions to improve patient safety across Canada through the SHN program, including the prevention of central line–associated bloodstream infections, falls, surgical site infections, ventilator-associated pneumonia, and medication errors. The aim of these interventions is to improve health care delivery by focusing on patients and their safety to reduce the number of injuries and deaths related to adverse events. In addition to SHN, the CPSI established a 5-year plan (2013–2018) entitled Patient Safety Forward with Four to better align patient safety in Canada. A patient safety consortium including federal, provincial and territorial representation as well as key groups like the Academy of Canadian Executives Nurses, Accreditation Canada and Health Canada, among others, have been actively engaged in the development and implementation of an Integrated Patient Safety Action Plan for Canada. The priority areas identified are medication safety, surgical care safety, infection prevention and control, and home care safety. These are all important areas of focus for patient safety and risk management.

When considering risk management, the work environment is an important consideration. In a study on work environment and safety climate on patient deaths, Olds, Aiken, Cimiotti, et al. (2017) found that the work environment for nurses was more important than safety climate in reducing deaths. They suggest that to improve safety and quality, hospitals should focus on adequate staffing, management support for nurses, and good relationships among physicians and nurses.

Each individual nurse is a risk manager and has the responsibility to identify and report unusual occurrences and potential risks in their work. Participation in safety huddles and focusing on the principles of HROs can help nurse identify important safety issues to highlight to the unit leaders. However, active involvement in quality and risk management can be challenged by factors outside the control of the nurse or other staff. For example, Driscoll et al. (2018), identified that nurse-to-patient ratios impacted patient mortality and performance on other nurse sensitive indicators (e.g., pressure injury, use of restraints). Another study demonstrated that good work environment and reasonable nursing workload were associated with improved survival after in hospital cardiac arrest (McHugh et al., 2016). Findings from the Driscoll (2018) and McHugh (2016) studies are discussed further in The Evidence section.

Another barrier to improving patient safety is fear of blame or punishment, which inhibits people from acknowledging, reporting, or discussing errors. One way to minimize errors is to monitor threats to patient safety continually and to recognize that individual errors often reflect organizational and system failures.

Both risk management and QM deal with changing behaviour, prevention, focus on the customer, and attention to outcomes. The following clinical examples illustrate how QM and risk management complement each other. First, the implementation of lift teams reduces employee injuries associated with lifting heavy or fully dependent patients and simultaneously, for the patient, decreases adverse events associated with difficult transfers. The implementation of lift teams reflects managing both quality and risk. Second, adherence to the universal safety verification known as *time out* before the beginning of a surgical procedure ensures perioperative safety within a QM framework. Although nurse managers would prefer that all staff intrinsically embrace risk management practices aimed at patient and staff safety, accountability for safety can be one aspect of performance evaluations. Active involvement of staff in risk management activities is key to preventing adverse events. To support this engagement, nurse managers demonstrate leadership in quality and safety by holding daily safety huddles, conducting safety rounds, and recognizing staff for following best practice and speaking up for safety by identifying concerns and escalating risks for action. This approach reinforces that risk management not only benefits the patient but also works to keep individual employees safe in the workplace.

Adverse-event reduction is a key strategy for reducing health care mortality and morbidity because patients who suffer adverse events are more likely to die or suffer permanent disability. Nurses have always played a pivotal role in the prevention of adverse events and can reduce negative outcomes with a focus on accurate assessment, early identification, and correction of potentially adverse situations. Also adherence to best practice standards and ensuring quality standards for high-risk/high-volume practices (e.g., restraint use, medication reconciliation) can reduce adverse events. Never events are errors in medical care that are clearly identifiable, preventable, and serious in their consequences for patients and that indicate a real problem in the safety and credibility of a health care facility. Examples of never events include surgery on the wrong body part, a foreign body left in a patient after surgery, mismatched blood transfusion, major medication error, severe pressure ulcer acquired in the hospital, and preventable postoperative deaths. A comprehensive quality, safety, and risk program would proactively identify and reduce risks to patient safety by identifying and analyzing select high-risk situations. If an adverse event occurs, nurses should also be able to recognize near misses and sentinel events and participate with an interprofessional team in the root-cause analysis. A sentinel event is a serious, unexpected occurrence involving death or physical or psychologic harm, such as inpatient suicide, infant abduction, or wrong-site surgery. Similarly, a near miss is a clinical situation that resulted in no harm but highlights an imminent problem that must be corrected; it can provide useful lessons in terms of risk analysis and reduction. After a sentinel event is identified, a root-cause analysis is performed by a team that includes those directly involved in the event and those in leadership positions. A root-cause analysis, while similar to the QI process, involves a deeper review of an incident and the sequence of events that led to it with the goals of identifying and addressing the underlying causes to reduce the likelihood of reoccurrence.

Typically, risk or adverse events are communicated through electronic safety reporting systems or through incident reporting. Incident reports are kept separate from the patient's medical record and should serve as a means of communicating an incident that did cause or could have caused harm to patients, family members, visitors, or employees. Aggregated incident reports should be used to improve quality of care and decrease future risk. Trending data can illuminate system issues that need to be modified to reduce risk and achieve quality patient care. Organizations must institute mechanisms to ensure that nurses obtain feedback about the trends identified from analyzing the information gathered from error reporting. They should also establish policies and processes for reporting errors that include clear definitions for what constitute reportable errors.

The communication of errors through the appropriate chain of command is essential to improve quality.

Evaluating Risks

In gathering data about unusual occurrences, the risk management team, managers, and patient safety specialists may involve perspectives from numerous disciplines to discover underlying problems that a single discipline might miss. Risk managers also use multiple data sources, data collection techniques, and perspectives to collect and interpret the data. Quantitative methods, such as a questionnaire or records of medication administration, can be combined with qualitative methods, such as open-ended question interviews. Actionable plans for reducing the incidence of common preventable adverse events, such as medication administration errors (wrong patient, time, dose, drug, or mode of delivery), could result from assessment and analysis of both quantitative and qualitative data. Quality and risk management strategies aimed at high-volume and high-risk occurrences are essential. It is important to keep in mind that organizational accountability for quality efforts to provincial and territorial governments as well as public reporting, in which quality data are made available for comparison, have significant implications for nurses. Opportunities to contribute to quality efforts include participation on QI teams, data collection, and involvement in the implementation of quality initiatives. As members of the health care team, students play an important part and individual or group reflections on events in everyday practice can help uncover risks and opportunities to reduce harm (see Exercise 22.6).

> **EXERCISE 22.6** Describe an error that occurred in the health care organization where you practice that resulted in harm to one patient and did not result in harm to another patient. What would you suggest to avoid a reoccurrence? Decide under what circumstances you would disclose the information to the patient and family and under what circumstances you would not disclose the information.

CONCLUSION

Approaches to quality, risk, and safety require both organizations and health care providers to be preoccupied with the possibility of failure. This preoccupation must be coupled with a relentless focus on identification of the root causes of the complex system failures that can occur in health care, and a commitment to continuously improve systems, processes, teamwork, and work environment. QM principles and the process of QI must help shape a blame-free health care culture. Organizations committed to quality and safety will possess comprehensive, systematic approaches that prevent errors or identify and correct errors so that adverse events are reduced and safety and quality outcomes are maximized. Attention to quality processes is not sufficient in and of themselves. As Baker and Black (2015) comment, "Patient safety is a critical health system issue, but the fundamental basis for improving safety lies in creating more effective work environments and high performing teams, not just selectively introducing new interventions into poorly organized settings" (p. 23).

A SOLUTION

Nadia decided to actively participate in the daily "Safety Huddles," and through this process she gained confidence in her ability to speak up for safety, and she is pleased to see the action taken on the concerns and safety issues identified by herself and her colleagues. Nadia sees a call for safety coaches for the organization and she volunteers to be a coach. She attends the coach education and meets other nurses in the organization who share her passion for quality and safety. She learns how to educate and reinforces safe behaviours and use error prevention tools (e.g., SBAR). She also learns how to provide feedback and use safety stories to encourage and coach her colleagues to report incidents and good catches. At the monthly safety coach meeting, she is pleased to share unit successes, learning, as well as bring learning from other coaches back to her unit. Nadia now considers herself part of the organization's effort to improve quality and safety in their journey to high reliability.

Would this be a suitable approach for you? Why or why not?

THE EVIDENCE

A strong correlation has been established between nurse practice environments and patient outcomes. Driscoll et al. (2018) conducted a systematic review and meta-analysis of the impact of nurse-to-patient ratios on nurse-sensitive patient outcomes in specialist nursing units. Some 35 cross-country international studies that used large administrative data sets were included in the analysis. The impact of nursing care on primary outcome patient mortality was included in all studies reviewed. Fifteen of the studies also explore the impact on a variety of other Nurse Sensitive Indicators (i.e., pressure injury, physical restraints, sepsis). This analysis demonstrated a relationship between mortality and nurse-to-patient ratio with the authors identifying that "for every increase in one nurse, patients were 14% less likely to experience in hospital mortality" (Driscoll et al., 2018). However, because of the heterogeneous nature of the calculations of the ratios, the authors were unable to identify the exact "dose" of nursing required to achieve these outcomes.

McHugh et al. (2016) analyzed data from 11,160 patients across 75 hospitals in four states to explore the relationship of survival post in hospital cardiac arrest with nursing staffing and nursing work environment. Results demonstrated that on medical-surgical units, survival post in hospital cardiac arrest was improved by good work environments and reasonable nursing workloads with reduced nurse-to-patient ratios. Good work environments, as characterized by nurse participation, nurse manager ability, leadership, support of nurses, and physician–nursing relationships, were significantly associated with higher likelihood of survival regardless of staffing levels.

There is a consistent message in the literature that the amount of nursing care, coupled with the quality of the work environment, impacts nurse-sensitive outcomes and patient mortality. Nurse managers and leaders have several options for improving nurse practice environments and patient outcomes, including advocating for adequate nursing registered nurse staffing, moving to a more educated nurse workforce, and focusing on improving work environment and teamwork. Organizations with good work environments and adequate nursing staffing, coupled with strong safety cultures and a focus on the principles of high reliability, are associated with better nurse outcomes, as well as improved nurse sensitive outcomes that demonstrate the value of nursing care.

✳ NEED TO KNOW NOW

- Know how to access clinical practice guidelines and standards for quality and safety using sources such as Accreditation Canada, the Canadian Nurses Association, the Registered Nurses' Association of Ontario Best Practice Guidelines, other provincial or territorial nursing association's guidelines, resources from provincial quality councils/organizations, and the Canadian Patient Safety Institute resources.
- High-reliability principles and how they relate to patient care in your practice setting.

- Identify nursing-sensitive outcomes most pertinent to your practice area and identify evidence-informed practice literature that addresses managing patient safety, quality and risk.
- Know how to address any patient-care issue using the six steps of the quality improvement process, including the steps of the Plan, Do Study, Act (PDSA) Cycle.

CHAPTER CHECKLIST

Most health care organizations have implemented QM and patient safety programs. Many are in the process of striving to become HROs. Improving value in the health care system is the goal of implementing these programs. The QI process is continuous and should be part of everyone's activities because products and services can always be improved.

- Five key principles of HROs:
  - Preoccupation with failure
  - Reluctance to simplify

- Sensitivity to operations
- Commitment to resiliency
- Deference to expertise
- QM strives to prevent errors and improve value. Initial planning requires both time and money, but QM contributes to the bottom line in the long run.
- The steps in the QI process to evaluate and improve patient care are as follows:
  - Assemble the QI team
  - Identify the aim: what are we trying to accomplish?
- Identify the measures: how will we know if a change is an improvement?
- Define the changes: what changes will result in an improvement?
- Implement rapid cycle improvements
- Sustain the improvements
- Any process can be improved.
- The steps of the PDSA Cycle are: Plan, Do, Study, Act. Risk management focuses on ensuring safety and on minimizing loss after a patient-care error occurs.

▌ TIPS FOR QUALITY MANAGEMENT

- QM is based on data; anything measured and recorded can be improved.
- Concentrate QI energies on factors that are most important to patient quality and safety.
- Working together to prevent problems is more effective than fixing problems after they occur.

Visit the Evolve website for Suggested Readings, Internet Resources, and additional resources related to the content in this chapter: http://evolve.elsevier.com/Canada/Yoder-Wise/leading/.

REFERENCES

Aboumatar, H. J., Weaver, S. J., Rees, D., Rosen, M. A., Sawyer, M. D., & Pronovost, P. J. (2017). Towards high-reliability organising in healthcare: A strategy for building organisational capacity. *British Medical Journal Quality & Safety, 26*(8), 663–670.

Baker, G. R., Norton, P. G., Flintoft, V., Blais, R., Brown, A., Cox, J., et al. (2004). The Canadian Adverse Events Study: The incidence of adverse events among hospital patients in Canada. *CMAJ Canadian Medical Association Journal, 170*(11), 1678–1686.

Baker, R., & Black, G. (2015). *Beyond a Quick Fix: Strategies for improving Patient Safety*. Institute of Health Policy, Management and Evaluation. Toronto, ON: Institute of Health Policy, Management and Evaluation Dalla Lana School of Public Health. Retrieved from: http://ihpme.utoronto.ca/2015/11/beyond-the-quick-fix/.

Baker, R., Judd, M., Fancott, C., & Maika, C. (2016). *Creating "engagement-capable" environments in healthcare.*

Canadian Patient Safety Institute (CPSI). (2008). The safety competencies: Enhancing patient safety across the health professions. In J. R. Frank, & S. Brien (Eds.), *on behalf of The Safety Competencies Steering Committee* (1st ed). Retrieved from: http://www.patientsafetyinstitute.ca/en/toolsResources/safetyCompetencies/Documents/Safety%20Competencies.pdf#search=domains%20of%20safety%20competencies.

Driscoll, A., Grant, M. J., Carroll, D., Dalton, S., Deaton, C., Jones, I., et al. (2018). The effect of nurse-to-patient ratios on nurse-sensitive patient outcomes in acute specialist units: A systematic review and meta-analysis. *European Journal of Cardiovascular Nursing, 17*(1), 6–22.

Fine, B. A., Golden, B., Hannam, R., & Morra, D. (2009). Leading lean: A Canadian healthcare leader's guide. *Healthcare Quaterly, 12*(3), 32–41.

Fleiszer, A. R., Semenic, S. E., Ritchie, J. A., Richer, M. C., & Denis, J. L. (2015). An organizational perspective on the long-term sustainability of a nursing best practice guidelines program: A case study. *BMC Health Services Research, 15*, 535.

Goedhart, N. S., van Oostveen, C. J., & Vermeulen, H. (2017). The effect of structural empowerment of nurses on quality outcomes in hospitals: A scoping review. *Journal of Nursing Management, 25*(3), 194–206.

Health Quality Ontario. (n.d.). Public reporting. Retrieved from: http://www.hqontario.ca/public-reporting.

HealthQualityOntario. (2012). *Quality Improvement Guide*. Toronto, ON: Queen's Printer for Ontario. Retrieved from: http://www.hqontario.ca/portals/0/Documents/qi/qi-quality-improve-guide-2012-en.pdf.

Institute of Medicine. (2000). *To err is human: Building a safer health system*. Washington, DC: The National Academies Press.

Institute of Medicine. (2004). Keeping Patients Safe - Transforming the Work Environment of Nurses. Washington, DC: The National Academies Press.

McHugh, M. D., Rochman, M. F., Sloane, D. M., Berg, R. A., Mancini, M. E., Nadkarni, V. M., et al. (2016). Better nurse staffing and nurse work environments associated with increased survival of in-hospital cardiac arrest patients. *Medical Care, 54*(1), 74–80.

Olds, D. M., Aiken, L. H., Cimotti, J. P., & Lake, E. T. (2017). Association of nurse work environment and safety climate on patient mortality: A cross-sectional study. *International Journal of Nursing Studies, 74*, 155–161.

Oster, C. A., & Deakins, S. (2018). Practical application of high-reliability principles in healthcare to optimize quality and safety outcomes. *Journal of Nursing Administration, 48*(1), 50–55.

Sebat, F., Vandegrift, M., Childers, S., & Lighthall, G. (2018). A novel bedside-focused ward surveillance and response system. *Joint Commission Journal on Quality & Patient Safety, 44*(2), 94–100.

Staines, A., Amherdt, I., Lecureux, E., Petignat, C., Eggimann, P., Schwab, M., & Pittet, D. (2017). Hand hygiene improvement and sustainability: Assessing a breakthrough collaborative in Western Switzerland. *Infection Control & Hospital Epidemiology, 38*(12), 1420–1427.

Sutcliffe, K. M., Paine, L., & Pronovost, P. J. (2017). Re-examining high reliability: Actively organising for safety. *British Medical Journal Quality & Safety, 26*(3), 248–251.

Weick, K. S., & Sutcliffe, K. M. (2015). *Managing the unexpected: Sustained performance in a complex world* (3rd ed.). San Francisco, CA: Jossey-Bass.

23

Translating Research Into Practice

Barbara Campbell, Christina Murray

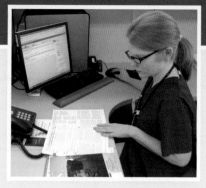

This chapter describes the importance of translating and applying research into nursing practice. The role of the nurse as a leader, manager, and member of a health care organization in applying research to practice is delineated using evidenced-informed data based on the best available research. This chapter describes the practical aspects of evaluation and translation of current research, the development of evidence-based practice (EBP) in nursing, and the integration of all forms of knowledge into practice. Strategies for translating research into practice that can be used by all nurses in the context of the organization are outlined.

OBJECTIVES

- Value each nurse's obligation to use research in practice.
- Distinguish between research utilization, evidence-based practice, and experiential knowledge.
- Formulate a clinical research question supported by the literature.
- Evaluate resources to access the best available evidence.
- Identify resources for critically appraising evidence.
- Assess organizational barriers to and facilitators of the implementation of research into practice.
- Identify strategies for translating research into practice within the context of an organization.

TERMS TO KNOW

clinical practice guidelines
diffusion of innovations
evidence-based practice
evidence-informed decision
making
evidence-informed practice
knowledge translation (KT)
metaanalysis
randomized controlled trial (RCT)
research
research utilization

❓ A CHALLENGE

Jade, a registered nurse with 7 years of surgical experience, works as a casual nurse on an orthopedic unit. At the beginning of one shift, shortly after midnight, Jade was told that they would receive an admission from the emergency department (ED). Jade prepared for the patient and received the verbal report from the ED nurse. Jade learned that the 58-year-old patient was being admitted with an open humerus fracture and a history of schizophrenia. The patient, Alex, also had a developmental delay and was considered to be a "difficult" patient who was described as "agitated" and "aggressive." The patient arrived on Jade's unit attempting to climb out of bed, grunting, and appearing to be distraught. The ED nurse failed to inform

Jade that the patient was deaf and nonverbal. The charge nurse immediately intervened with chemical restraints. She administered a large dose of haloperidol (Haldol) and morphine to the patient. Alex's eyes would continuously roll back in his head. Moreover, as Jade realized, Alex could not hear or speak besides making grunting sounds, and had been assigned a legal guardian through the province. How was Jade going to communicate and provide ethically responsible and responsive care to this patient over the next 12 hours?

What do you think you would do if you were Jade? What would be the first steps to take to provide nursing care for Alex?

INTRODUCTION

The challenge of translating research knowledge for use by practicing nurses is a daunting task. Canadian research has lacked innovation in the dissemination of health research information, particularly in clinical nursing practice. **Knowledge translation (KT)** is defined by the Canadian Institutes of Health Research (CIHR, 2016) "as a dynamic and iterative process that includes synthesis, dissemination, exchange and ethically-sound application of knowledge to improve the health of Canadians, provide more effective health services and products and strengthen the health care system" (p. 1). The *Canadian Nurse* interviewed leading nurse researchers to identify the importance of nursing research and how to build research capacity through translation and utilization of research to better health care and the profession (Edwards et al., 2015). In this interview, Porr, representing the Canadian Association for Nursing Research, states, "Nursing practice is evidence-informed so nurse researchers must uncover the best and most up-to-date ways for nurses to intervene to promote health and well-being (Edwards et al., p. 2). In addition, nurse researcher Nancy Edwards identifies that "research is a critical means of advancing the quality of nursing care we provide for patients, whether in hospitals or communities. We are all potential users of research; nurses, patients, their families and caregivers, and society are beneficiaries" (Edwards et al., 2015, p. 2). Although much evidence exists on the importance of nursing-related studies to advance nursing practice, strategies are needed to adopt and integrate this knowledge into nursing practice (Polit & Beck, 2017). Such strategies need to be articulated clearly and in detail.

If you or your family member required nursing care, you would want that care to be based on the best research evidence available. For example, if a family member needed to be on a ventilator, you would want to be sure that the nurses providing the care were using Best Practice Guidelines (BPGs) to prevent ventilator-associated pneumonia. You would want to know that communication and collaboration are excellent between nurses and physicians on the clinical unit where your family member has been placed. If that family member also had a central venous catheter, you would want to be sure that the nurse who removes that catheter is using an established current practice guideline that minimizes the risk for introducing an air embolism into the circulation. In addition, when that family member is discharged, you would want to know that the nurses are using evidence-based research and appropriate strategies to help that person transition to home, recover from his or her illness, and manage that illness. As a nurse manager or leader, you should be concerned about incorporating research not only into clinical practices but also into the management of systems of care. You know through research that teamwork and collaboration lead to lower mortality rates and fewer medication administration errors. The challenges, however, include how to: (1) find the best research evidence, (2) determine the appropriateness of that research for the practice setting, (3) incorporate the best evidence into practice in a meaningful and timely manner, and (4) motivate clinical nurses and organizational leaders to use research evidence in the midst of all the other challenges facing delivery of high-quality nursing care.

Research is an integral part of professional practice. *Research* is the "diligent, systematic inquiry or investigation to validate and refine existing knowledge and generate new knowledge" (Burns & Grove, 2009, p. 2). According to nurse researcher Marlene Smadu, "Research answers questions regarding all domains of practice and ensures that practices are current, effective, efficient, patient centred, appropriate, etc. The half-life of knowledge is decreasing rapidly, particularly in health care, and nurses must know how to get and create the kind of evidence they need to ensure high-quality practice in all domains" ("In Conversation," 2010). The Canadian Nurses Association (CNA, 2017) identifies that, "Nurses support, use and engage in research and other activities that promote safe, competent, compassionate, and ethical care, and they use guidelines for ethical research that are in keeping with nursing values" (p. 9). Nurses develop and implement research-informed BPGs, such as those disseminated through the Registered Nurses' Association of Ontario (RNAO) (http://www.rnao.ca). BPGs allow nurses to assess nursing and health care practices and implement recommendations where needed to enhance the quality of patient care (CNA, 2015). Nurses have the foundational knowledge to identify practice research questions and use research results to provide a scientific rationale for nursing interventions, thereby promoting quality patient care (CNA, 2015; College and Association of Registered Nurses of Alberta, 2011). CNA's latest research is related to nurse fatigue and its impact on patient care and professional health outcomes (Canadian Nurses Association & Registered Nurses Association of Ontario, 2010). Nurses are referred to as *knowledge navigators* who develop and implement research-based BPGs in the CNA (2015) document, *Framework for the Practice of Registered Nurses in Canada*. The CNA released a compendium of evidence-based practice (EBP) guidelines in the form of a Primary Care Toolkit, which offers a variety of resources to help Registered Nurses use evidence in making decisions regarding patient care, including information about theories, clinical judgements, ethics, legislation, and practice environments (CNA, 2014).

As professionals, nurses have an obligation to society that involves rights and responsibilities as well as accountability. The Code of Ethics for Registered Nurses is a "statement of the ethical values of nurses and of nurses' commitments to persons with health-care needs and persons receiving care" (CNA, 2017, p. 2). These values, developed by Canadian nurses for all nurses in any practice environment, are translated through the following CNA statement: "Nurses support, use and engage in research and other activities that promote safe, competent, compassionate, and ethical care, and they use guidelines for ethical research that are in keeping with nursing values" (CNA, 2017). Furthermore, the International Council of Nurses' (ICN, 2007) position statement on nursing research indicates that the organization "supports its national nurses associations (NNAs) in their efforts to enhance nursing research, particularly through: improving access to education which prepares nurses to conduct research, critically evaluate research outcomes and promote appropriate application of research findings to nursing practice" (p. 1).

The emphasis of translating research into practice is getting research into the hands of practitioners who can use it to improve patient care. Marlene Smadu suggested that nurse researchers partner with clinicians throughout the "whole research cycle, from working with them to formulate meaningful questions, to choosing appropriate methodologies, to sharing results, and to planning and implementing dissemination, translation and change" ("In Conversation," 2010). The translation of research into practice involves all health care disciplines. Gagnon and colleagues (2011) found that one-third of Canadians are affected by one of the six most common chronic conditions: heart disease, chronic obstructive pulmonary disease (COPD), diabetes, mood disorders,

cancer, and arthritis. However, the implementation of research-based practice guidelines has been incomplete, highlighting the difficulty of translating research into practice. For example, in the case of diabetes, even if several efficient strategies to prevent or delay diabetes complications exist, these strategies are suboptimally implemented in practice; that is, less than one-half of the patients received the recommended laboratory tests and procedures. Only 50% of Canadians suffering from heart disease receive proven therapies on a regular basis (Gagnon et al., 2011). We might believe that once a research study is published in a journal, clinicians read it immediately and then nurses or policymakers use it to improve practice. Often, that is not the case. The CIHR (2016) supports research, capacity building, and knowledge translation, and it is through its Evidence Informed Healthcare Renewal initiative that multiple researchers and decision makers work together to advance the current state of knowledge, generate novel and creative solutions, and contribute to evidence-informed decision making about health care renewal in Canada.

Research provides the foundation for nursing practice improvement. Examples include preoperative teaching, pain management, child development assessment, falls prevention, pressure-ulcer risk detection, incontinence care, and family-centred care in critical care units. Rycroft-Malone et al., (2004) proposed that research informed by evidence comes from local data, professional knowledge, experiential knowledge, and patient experience. In addition, various researchers suggest that the best evidence combines theoretical, experiential, and tacit knowledge derived from professional experience and patient preferences (Benner., 2008). According to Brownson and colleagues (2010), EBP involves integration of professional clinical expertise with best available clinical evidence from research. Nurses need to systematically evaluate nursing studies to decide what interventions should be implemented to improve the outcomes of care. Practices that were once thought to be the standard of care may quickly become outdated. Some practices may have been carried out for many years without ever being examined for their scientific basis or effectiveness. The latest research findings need to be incorporated into procedures and clinical practice guidelines (systematically developed statements of practice that assist practitioners and patients make appropriate clinical decisions) using an evidence-based model.

The integration of research into practice by knowledge users and practice into research by researchers bodes well for future implementation of EBP, and thus improved health care (Gagnon et al., 2011). The Evidence section at the end of the chapter illustrates how research can be incorporated into organizational practices.

> **EXERCISE 23.1** Identify a common activity that is part of your nursing practice, and determine whether any research supports that particular intervention or nursing care activity.

Nursing research designs can be categorized in several ways, such as basic versus applied, qualitative versus quantitative, cross-sectional versus longitudinal, experimental versus descriptive, and retrospective versus prospective. Regardless of the design, some research is ready for implementation and other research may not yet be ready to warrant a change in practice. Some decisions should not be based on the results of quantitative research alone, but instead should be integrated with data from qualitative research when applied to a particular practice situation. The quality of care and the quality of patient outcomes can be dramatically improved with the implementation of EBP. Patients, those entrusted to our care, are deserving of practices that are based on the best available evidence. Examining the evidence for a particular practice generally needs to go beyond examining the results of a single study. A single, well-designed study might be adequate for recommending and implementing a practice change at times. However, developing an EBP requires the development of a clearly written clinical question and a more thorough search of the literature including a comprehensive review of single studies, metaanalyses, metasyntheses, critically appraised topics, and systematic reviews.

All evidence must be critically appraised and placed in the context of patient, family, and community values. Nurse managers or leaders may not necessarily be the ones actually conducting research, evaluating research evidence, or developing clinical practice guidelines, but they will be facilitating the application of research findings in practice. Key concepts for facilitating improved nursing outcomes include research utilization, EBP, translating research into practice, evaluation of evidence, organizational strategies (for translating research into practice), and issues for nurse managers and leaders faced with implementing these processes.

RESEARCH UTILIZATION

Research utilization is the process of synthesizing, disseminating, and using research-generated knowledge to influence or change existing practices (Burns & Grove, 2009). Research utilization is different from, but complementary to, research. Although individual nurses may apply research findings to their own practice, nurses' broader responsibility to society includes activating the change process in translating research into practice. Research can be used for a variety of purposes: enlightenment, implementation of a research-based protocol, or the widespread adoption of standards based on research findings. Ultimately, multiple factors influence how a particular research finding is adopted, translated into practice, and sustained in practice.

Nurse researchers have a distinguished record of facilitating research utilization in clinical practice that has gone beyond dissemination through publication in research journals, but the gap of adapting research into practice still exists. Squires et al., (2011) recently conducted a systematic review to identify and analyze how nurses have used research findings in practice over the past 40 years. According to this review, nurses reported a moderate-high use of research, a level that remained relatively consistent over time until the early 2000s. The relatively unchanged self-reporting and the absence of studies to assess the effects of research use by nurses on patient outcomes is troubling with the increasing emphasis on EBP and easy access to electronic resources in research. Many research utilization models in nursing were developed in the 1970s and 1980s. One of the first was the Stetler-Marram model developed in 1976, which now includes the facilitation of EBP (Stetler, 2001).

Originally, research utilization consisted of evaluating research and determining its applicability to practice; in the 1990s, this focus changed to finding research-based solutions to a problem. Stetler's (2001) research utilization model provides direction for an individual and for group members. It has implications for nurses in leadership roles responsible for patient care management. According to Stetler, the preparatory steps of research utilization sustain EBP. Stetler's model consists of five phases: preparation, validation, comparative evaluation or decision making, translation or application, and evaluation (Fig. 23.1). The preparatory phase involves searching, sorting, and selecting sources of evidence, defining external factors influencing the

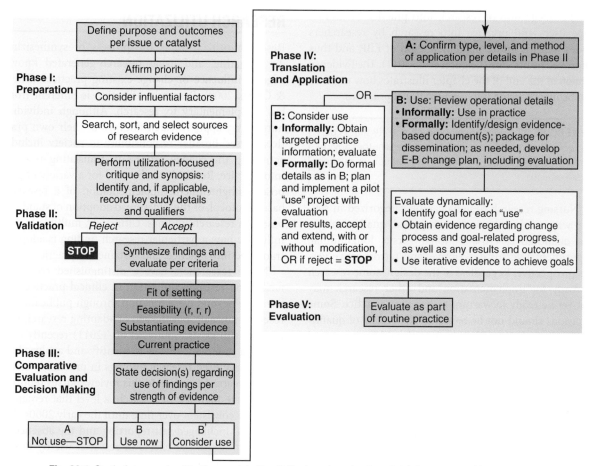

Fig. 23.1 Stetler's research utilization model. *Feasibility (r, r, r), evaluation of risk factors, need for resources, and readiness of others involved.*

application of a research finding, and defining internal factors diminishing objectivity. The second phase, validation, focuses on utilization with an appraisal of study findings rather than the critique of a study's design. This phase includes completing review tables to facilitate understanding of each study and to facilitate decision making. The third phase, comparative evaluation and decision making, involves making a decision about the applicability of the studies by synthesizing cumulative findings; evaluating the degree and nature of other criteria, such as risk, feasibility, and readiness of the finding; and actually making a recommendation about using the research. The fourth phase, translation and application, involves practical aspects of implementing the plan for translating the research into practice at the individual, group, department, or organizational level. Multiple

strategies are recommended for the implementation of change. It is important to be sure that translating the research finding into practice does not exceed what the evidence warrants. The last phase includes an evaluation, which can be informal or formal and may include a cost–benefit analysis. Evaluation can include whether the research innovation was implemented as intended and goal achievement. Stetler's model focuses heavily on the change process to facilitate the successful translation of research into practice.

The knowledge-to-action model (Fig. 23.2) developed by Straus and colleagues (2009) has been adopted by the CIHR as a model promoting the application of research and the process of knowledge translation in Canada. These authors suggest that this model is iterative, dynamic, and complex; it ranges from knowledge

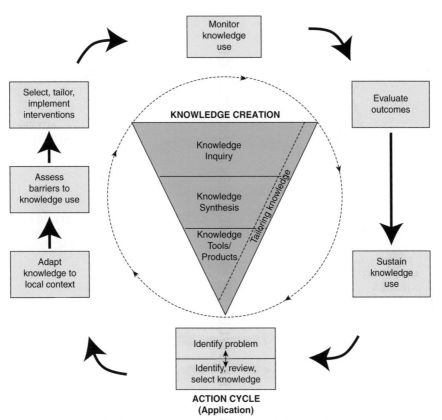

Fig. 23.2 Straus, Tetroe, and Graham's knowledge-to-action model.

creation through multiple stages of action toward implementation. The action cycle consists of seven key steps, commencing with the identification of the problem (gap). This critical element of the action cycle acts as the foundation for the remaining stages in the knowledge-to-action cycle, as programs will be tailored to address the specifics of the gap. The next step in the cycle (once the gap has been identified) is adapting the research to the local context. Localizing knowledge requires an assessment of the barriers and key facilitators to knowledge implementation as barriers and facilitators are analyzed and interwoven into the strategic initiative. Knowledge translation interventions need to be selected, tailored, and implemented based on the best research evidence or practices when dealing with a problem. Sustainability of knowledge through action ensures the continued implementation of innovative, evidence-based research in end-user programs and clinical practice guidelines. Adapting clinical practice guidelines for local use means that

knowledge and the best evidence have been translated into a set of specific recommendations for end users. This next section of the knowledge-to-action process deals with possible intervention directions one might face when determining the best possible approach in knowledge translation strategies. Therefore it is imperative that research findings be communicated to those who can use the research effectively through program implementation in specific practice settings. Linkages and exchange activities, such as face-to-face outreach visits and opinion leadership conferences, are based on social interactions, relationships, and networks (Straus et al., 2009).

In 2006, a CIHR-funded study used participatory action research to understand a rural East Coast community's knowledge about their children's health. A conceptual knowledge translation framework and the Ottawa Model of Research Use were applied to translate the knowledge gathered into action (Campbell, 2010). The graphical depiction of "applying knowledge to

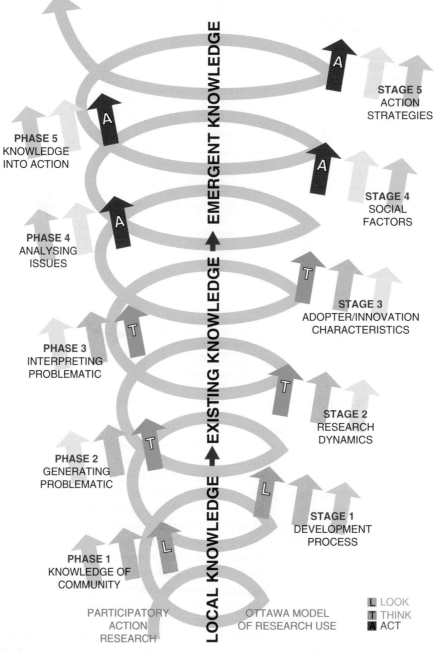

Fig. 23.3 Conceptual framework: applying knowledge to generate action. Influenced by: Logan & Graham (1998); Maguire (1987); Stringer & Genat (2004), © 2006 by Campbell.

generate action" (Fig. 23.3) incorporates the activities of community members and researchers working collaboratively to translate community knowledge and research into health promotion programs. The results indicated that the knowledge translated must be relevant, appropriate, applicable, timely, and reasonable to the needs of the users.

According to Straus and colleagues (2009), "Failures to use evidence from research to make informed decisions in health care are evident across all groups of decision-makers, including health care providers, patients, informal caregivers, managers and policymakers" (p. 165). A current Canadian example of this gap in research to practice is the extent to which patients with mood and anxiety disorders are using cannabis to self-medicate. Recently, a CNA national survey found that less than two-thirds of nurses considered themselves knowledgeable about the health risks associated with nonmedical cannabis use (Canadian Nurses Association, 2018). This lack of awareness is problematic, as nurses will likely have increased interactions with patients who regularly use cannabis, with the legalization of cannabis in Canada. Although knowledge gaps exist in nursing practice, Sarvet et al., (2018) discovered that self-medication of mood and anxiety disorders with cannabis was higher in jurisdictions that had passed medical marijuana legislation.

Think about the introduction of cannabis legislation and how this might look in your clinical nursing practice, for example, with older adults living in a long-term care facility. What research exists that addresses the use of cannabis in older adults? How can this research inform your practice in a long-term setting? Are there additional considerations that must be attended to as a result of the setting or context of care?

EVIDENCE-BASED PRACTICE

Evidence-based practice (EBP) is the integration of the best research evidence with clinical expertise and the patient's unique values and circumstances in making decisions about the care of individual patients (Straus et al., 2005). The Canadian Nurses Association asserts in their Code of ethics for registered nurses 2017 edition Canadian Nurses Association (2017), "Nurses support, use, and engage in research and other activities that promote safe, competent, compassionate and ethical care, and they use guidelines for ethical research that are in keeping with nursing values." (Part I.A. [10] p.15). Ingersoll (2000) developed one of the first definitions for evidence-based nursing practice: "the conscientious, explicit, and judicious use of theory-derived, research-based information on making decisions about care delivery to individuals or groups of patients and in consideration of individual needs and preferences" (p. 152). The definitions of EBP and evidence-based decision making have since become more varied (Canadian Nurses Association, 2018). However, as Karin Morin

(2010) excellently summarizes, "Irrespective of reference employed, key elements include addressing a clinical problem or question by examining the 'best available scientific evidence' and then integrating that evidence with patient preferences and practitioner expertise." Melynk and colleagues (2010) recently defined *evidence-based* in a nursing context as a "problem-solving approach to the delivery of health care that integrates the best evidence from well-designed studies and patient data, and combines it with patient preference and values and nurse expertise." Evidence-based decision making, also referred to as evidence-informed decision making, is defined by the CNA (2010) as "a continuous interactive process involving the explicit, conscientious and judicious consideration of the best available evidence to provide care." EBP integrates current research on best practices, clinical expertise, and patient values to optimize patient outcomes as well as quality of life (Finney et al., 2016). In EBP, clinical problems or gaps drive the search for solutions based on the best available evidence, which is then translated into practice. EBP is a broader, more encompassing view of research utilization. It is focused on searching for and evaluating the best evidence to address a particular clinical practice problem. A number of models exist for creating and implementing EBP, all based on the following five key essential elements (Moyer & Elliott, 2004): (1) ask a clinical question, (2) acquire the evidence, (3) appraise the evidence, (4) apply the evidence, and (5) assess the outcomes. Precisely articulating a clinical question is the first step in the process. Once the question is confirmed, an electronic literature search must be undertaken to acquire the existing evidence specific to the issue being researched. Critically analyzing the existing information on this topic is essential because of the volume of information available. At this time, a mechanism needs to be in place to disseminate the results of this research through communication and education to help identify necessary processes and outcome measures that should be assessed before any changes in a clinical practice site. Measuring process and outcome changes is a key step in the EBP model. Information systems play a key role in this process by measuring daily practice against evidence-based guidelines, standards, or protocols. The stage of evaluation is not a one-time activity with such changes, so it needs to be ongoing, reflective, and iterative. The role of an organization in adopting and implementing EBP is illustrated by Brown (2008) in the Literature Perspective.

LITERATURE PERSPECTIVE

Resource: Brown, S. J. (2008). Time to move on: definitions of evidence-based practice. *Journal of Nursing Care Quality*, 23, 201.

Using a definition of EBP based on definitions of evidence-based medicine is limiting because those definitions do not accommodate EBP as it is practised in clinical settings in which nurses work. Evidence-based medicine focuses on individual clinicians using research evidence for individual patients, whereas nurses typically practise within an organizational context and are part of an interdisciplinary team. Many nurses providing direct care have not had the educational preparation for the use of EBP. Workplace pressures may also affect the use of EBP.

Implications for Practice
EBP models in nursing need to include a broader-based organizational approach that more accurately reflects the use of evidence-based standards of care for patient populations and the nurse's use of research evidence for patient-care decisions.

BOX 23.1   Resources for Evidence-Based Health Care

Canadian Business and Current Affairs (CBCA): https://proquest.libguides.com/CBCAreference

Centre for Evidence-Based Medicine Toronto: http://ktclearinghouse.ca/cebm/

Centre for Reviews and Dissemination (CRD): http://www.york.ac.uk/inst/crd/

The Cochrane Collaboration: http://www.cochrane.org

Cochrane Database of Systematic Reviews (CDSR): https://www.cochranelibrary.com/

Database of Abstracts of Reviews of Effects (DARE): http://onlinelibrary.wiley.com/o/cochrane/cochrane_cldare_articles_fs.html

Government Information: MacOdrum Library, Carleton University: http://www.library.carleton.ca/find/government-information

Health Technology Assessment (HTA) Database: https://www.cadth.ca/resources/hta-database-canadian-search-interface

Knowledge Translation Canada: http://ktcanada.net/

National Guideline Clearinghouse: http://www.guideline.gov

National Institute for Health and Clinical Excellence: http://www.nice.org.uk

Scottish Intercollegiate Guidelines Network (SIGN): http://www.sign.ac.uk

---

EBP, including evidence-based medicine, is derived from the work of Archie Cochrane. He described the lack of knowledge about health care treatment effects and advocated for the use of proven treatments. Subsequently, the Cochrane Collaboration was established at Oxford University in 1993. About that time, Gordon Guyatt and his colleagues at McMaster University authored a series of articles in the *Journal of the American Medical Association* known as the *Users' Guides to the Medical Literature*. These articles provided a foundation for teaching evidence-based medicine. Since then, the EBP movement has grown exponentially with the establishment of centres, resources on the Web, and grants given specifically to advance the translation of research into practice. A number of evidence-based nursing centres have been established around the world. The Joanna Briggs Institute, based in Australia, has a network of collaborating centres and evidence-based synthesis and utilization groups around the world. These centres have teams of researchers who critically appraise evidence and then disseminate protocols for the use of evidence in practice. PubMed Central Canada provides free access to an online digital archive of full-text peer-reviewed research publications in health and life sciences.

Resources for evidence-based health care are listed in Box 23.1. Many nursing education programs incorporate EBP into their curricula.

Our understanding of how evidence is used in practice is evolving and, in response, associated terminology is changing. Increasingly, nursing and other health-based literature is using the phrase "evidence-informed" rather than "evidence-based" to describe decision making about the care of patients based on health-related research. Evidence-informed practice recognizes that decisions are not always made solely based on research and that other factors influence decision making, such as local indigenous knowledge, cultural and religious norms, and clinical judgments. You will notice in this textbook that we primarily use "evidence-informed" to convey that broader understanding of decision making. As the terminology evolves, you will find that sometimes terms are used interchangeably. For example, the CNA's NurseONE Web site discusses "strategies to promote evidence-based practice/evidence-informed decision making by nurses (https://www.nurseone.ca/ to promote evidence-based practice). The discussion of EBP in this chapter is important to enhance understanding of how the term entered nursing's language and how it is changing.

Various organizations have developed evidence-based standards of practice and clinical guidelines. The Oncology Nursing Society and the Registered Nurses' Association of Ontario have developed toolkits for EBP, whereas the CNA has a comprehensive Web site (https://www.nurseone.ca/) offering clinical practice guidelines for over 20 nursing-specific primary care topics. Societal factors such as the rising cost of health care, quality improvement initiatives, and the pressures to avoid errors have resulted in an increased emphasis on research as a basis for practice decisions. Nurses and other health care providers are called upon to use evidence in practice in the midst of an exponentially expanding scientific knowledge base.

Nursing research exists on a continuum, and not all research is ready for, or of a quality that is appropriate for, implementation, or it may not be ready for implementation in a particular setting. However, the quality of care and the quality of the outcomes of care can be dramatically improved with the implementation of evidence-based nursing practices. Nurses are heeding the call to develop EBPs. Burns and Grove (2011) suggest current research could be a systematic analysis of a treatment, a service, or an intervention to produce the most effective outcome. The steps toward engaging in effective research to inform a health practice context are similar to any decision-making process (including the nursing process):

1. Define the issue or the problem.
2. Search the appropriate research evidence efficiently.
3. Critically and efficiently appraise the available resources.
4. Interpret information and synthesize the evidence.
5. Adapt the evidence and the resources to the local context.
6. Implement the evidence into practice, program, policy development, or decision making.
7. Evaluate the effectiveness of implementation efforts (Ciliska et al., 2008).

The Ontario Public Health Association (2009) in collaboration with McMaster University developed a tool known as *Towards Evidence Informed Practice* (TEIP) in response to requests from Canadian health promoters for practical tools to facilitate the systematic search and

---

> **BOX 23.2 Resources for Evidence-Based/Evidence-Informed Nursing**
>
> **Canadian Nurses Association's Online Primary Care Toolkit**: Evidence-Based Practice: http://www.nurseone.ca/Default.aspx?portlet=StaticHtmlViewerPortlet&plang=1&ptdi=514
>
> **The Joanna Briggs Institute**: http://joannabriggs.org
>
> **The Sarah Cole Hirsch Institute for Best Nursing Practices Based on Evidence**: http://fpb.case.edu/Centers/Hirsh/
>
> **Oncology Nursing Society Evidence-Based Practice Resource Area (EBPRA)**: https://www.ons.org/practice-resources/pep
>
> **The Registered Nurses' Association of Ontario Nursing Best Practice Guidelines**: http://rnao.ca/bpg

application of reliable and relevant evidence to support programming in health promotion.

Nurse managers and leaders have a critical responsibility in promoting the use of the best evidence that informs practice. Resources for evidence-informed nursing are listed in Box 23.2.

> **EXERCISE 23.2** Select a clinical guideline appropriate for implementation in your clinical setting (see the Canadian Nurses Association Online Primary Care Toolkit (http://www.nurseone.ca). Identify as many strategies as possible for disseminating the guideline's key points to staff nurses at your facility or a facility where you have your clinical experiences. Compare your list of strategies with that of a colleague.

Widespread media attention to a particular finding can be instrumental in the adoption of a practice change. Extensive publicity accompanied the publication of a study about family presence during emergency procedures and resuscitation (Meyers et al., 2000). Publication of the study was accompanied by press releases and television news stories. Since then, the research has been replicated and expanded to other settings (Smith et al., 2007), thereby serving to strengthen the scientific basis for the innovation and facilitating the practice of allowing families to be present during resuscitation. In another example, Hatfield et al. (2008) found that the administration of oral sucrose to babies receiving their 2-month and 4-month immunizations reduced their pain scores. Their study received wide publicity in media outlets. Thus parents were alerted about the importance of asking that this simple pain management strategy be implemented for their infants when being immunized.

Nurse researchers write clinical articles in addition to research articles. Many journals that are directed toward clinicians provide nurses with easy-to-understand summaries of studies from the general health care and nursing research literature. Nursing schools develop press releases when researchers publish studies, which are then used by the media for their news articles. For example, Rachel Jones conducted research on the use of urban soap opera videos delivered on a handheld device to convey messages about human immunodeficiency virus (HIV) risk reduction in young adult urban women. Publicity in various media outlets in the community, her receipt of a *New York Times* award, and the Web site Stop HIV—Women's Power Against HIV/acquired immunodeficiency syndrome (AIDS) have increased the visibility of this important public health problem (Jones, 2008).

EXERCISE 23.3 Locate a research column in a clinical nursing journal. Identify one study that has implications for your practice. Retrieve the original article to learn more about the following: how the patient population is defined and the study design described, and how the results and any recommendations for practice are presented. Think about how you would summarize the article to your colleagues in clinical practice and what key points you would highlight.

The translation of research into practice requires that nurse managers and leaders understand group dynamics, individual responses to innovation and change, and the culture of their health care organization. Rogers (2003) categorized people according to how quickly they are willing to adopt an innovation. Box 23.3 describes these categories. Understanding the characteristics of innovation adopters is critical when planning to introduce new practices based on research evidence.

Nursing as a profession has an obligation to the public to condense the 17-year typical time frame from the discovery to the adoption of a research finding. Those committed to the EBP movement in nursing have attempted to speed up the adoption of innovations. Rogers' (2003) theory of diffusion of innovations is useful in helping us understand how research can be disseminated to the larger community. The diffusion of an innovation does

---

BOX 23.3   Characteristics of Innovation Adopters

Type	Characteristics
Innovators	They thrive on change, which may be disruptive to the unit stability.
Early adopters	They are respected by their peers and thus are sought out for advice and information about innovations and changes.
Early majority	They prefer doing what has been done in the past but eventually will accept new ideas.
Late majority	They are openly negative and agree to the change only after most others have accepted the change.
Laggards	They prefer keeping traditions and openly express their resistance to new ideas.

From Rogers, E. M. (1995). *Diffusion of innovations* (4th ed.). New York, NY: Free Press.

---

not necessarily follow a linear path. External factors may sometimes contribute to the adoption of an innovation. These may include the development of standards regarding the practice that are widely disseminated, cost-effectiveness studies, changes in the products or technology, the publication of clear and compelling evidence, and changes in staff members and leadership at an institution. A metaanalysis of the use of saline and the elimination of a low-dose heparin (Heparin) flush solution for capped angiocatheters is a well-known example of compelling evidence for innovation diffusion (Goode et al., 1991). A metaanalysis statistically combines the results of similar studies to determine whether the aggregated findings are significant. Although some institutions continued to use heparin flushes for a number of years, their use became less common and all but disappeared in the late 1990s. The decreased use of heparin flushes was considerably later than one would expect, given the compelling nature of the evidence. This example illustrates the particular challenges in implementing an EBP when more than one discipline is involved. The innovation needed to be communicated to nurses. Nurses also needed to convince physicians and the institutional hierarchy that using heparin was no longer appropriate. For some institutions, it was not until the costs were analyzed and concerns were raised about complications from small doses of heparin that the transition to saline flushes was finally accomplished. This research has been extended to central line catheters in adults and capped peripheral and central line catheters in children and neonates. A systematic review of heparin use in peripheral intravenous catheters in neonates indicated that because of variations in the neonates' clinical conditions and treatments, a recommendation to use heparin could not be made (Upadhyay et al., 2015). The American Society of Health-System Pharmacists (2012) concurred about the lack of clarity in using heparin in intravenous catheters placed in children and neonates. Unfortunately, heparin's continued use has led to several widely publicized serious and deadly errors. Thus careful analysis of research results, the timely implementation of important findings, and ongoing clinical research are critical to the nurse's role in promoting patient safety.

Another example of innovation diffusion is a review of the evidence for intramuscular injection technique conducted by Malkin (2008). The practice of administering intramuscular injections for pain management to adults in acute care settings has virtually disappeared with the use of the intravenous and epidural routes. Malkin rightfully emphasized that nurses learn the technique in their initial nursing program but may never subsequently question their practice in using this technique. Intramuscular injections are widely used in many settings throughout the world to deliver long-acting antibiotics; biologicals, such as immune globulins, vaccines, and toxoids; and hormonal agents. The use of the dorso-gluteal site is no longer recommended, yet we do not know what proportion of nurses who continue to use this technique. This review provides nurses with an evidence-based, research-based standard that takes on even more significance because of wide variation among nurses in injection technique.

Massey (2012) questioned the practice of listening to the bowel sounds of abdominal surgery patients to assess the return of gastrointestinal motility. They concluded that the presence or absence of bowel sounds was not associated with any interventions. The authors recommended that problems experienced by patients after abdominal surgery that indicate absent bowel motility (e.g., nausea, abdominal distention) can be treated with interventions such as administering an antiemetic or inserting a nasogastric tube. A practice guideline was developed and evaluated by the research team outlining the steps in gastrointestinal assessment.

Astute practitioners should observe for the subsequent adoption of these guidelines by nurses in other health care facilities and whether textbooks continue to mention the assessment of bowel sounds for patients after abdominal surgery.

Nursing students assigned to a public health office in Eastern Canada recently were alerted to a knowledge deficit regarding how to best prepare preschool children and their families for their comprehensive preschool assessment. This comprehensive assessment is offered to all preschool children between the ages of 4 and 5 years. During this clinic visit children are weighed and measured, have various vision and hearing exams, and receive immunizations. Guided by the Community-as-Partner model (Vollman et al., 2017), students worked in partnership with public health nurses and families to create an educational video that addressed this knowledge gap. The final video was uploaded to YouTube and showcased all phases of the preschool assessment. The students were attentive to using plain language and integrating images that would be appealing to a preschool child. Before posting the final video online, feedback was elicited from preschoolers.

Fetzer's (2002) metaanalysis of 20 studies demonstrated that the pain of venipuncture and intravenous line insertion could be reduced in 85% of the population (adults and children) with the use of an eutectic mixture of local anesthetics (EMLA) cream. This practice has not been widely adopted; this practice was illustrated by a study conducted in a large urban pediatric setting that indicated that minor procedures are commonly performed without pain management (MacLean et al., 2007). A stumbling block described by practitioners is the length of time required for the EMLA to take effect. This issue is also indicative of the relative value placed on patient comfort and patient satisfaction and the challenge in using research to change pain management practices.

TRANSLATING RESEARCH INTO PRACTICE

Research takes a long time to be translated into practice. Consider the classic example of scurvy. James Lancaster demonstrated that lemon juice supplements eliminated scurvy in sailors in 1601, and James Lind replicated that finding in 1747. However, it was not until 1795 that the British navy added a citrus juice supplement to the diet of its sailors (Brown, 2005). In nursing, medication tickets or small cards were first used in 1910 to facilitate the administration of medications. One hundred years later, some institutions are still using these tickets as reminders for some aspects of their medication-administration or treatment-administration systems despite evidence of the potential for error through their loss or duplication. This issue is indicative of a much broader problem related to the limited use of electronic health records. According to Geibert (2006), "Technology is the bridge to integrating EBP into patient care" (p. 132). As our world becomes ever more connected through the devices in our hands and homes, research no longer requires a trip to the library—rather, just a device connected to the internet. In one teaching hospital in Western Canada, all nurses and nurse practitioners carry personal digital assistants (PDAs) to assist them when providing up to date plans of care based on current research.

The actual translation of research into practice has not been as rapid. The seminal work of Funk and colleagues (1991) in categorizing barriers to research utilization according to the research itself, the nurse, the setting or organization, and presentation demonstrated that nurses perceived the most significant barrier to be organizational support, particularly time to use and conduct research. Nearly 10 years later, barriers to using research in Australia included access to research, anticipated outcomes of research use, organizational support, and support from others (Paramonczyk, 2005). Estabrooks et al., (2005) conducted surveys of 230 nurses from across various nursing practice settings in hospitals across Alberta and Ontario. They discovered that across all units, nurses preferred to use the knowledge they gained through personal experience and interactions with co-workers and patients rather than look to knowledge published in journal articles or textbooks.

Some of these same barriers continue to persist in nursing practice today.

When planning to translate a research finding into practice, nurses need to know what types of strategies have been most successful. It is also helpful to know how much time commitment was involved, how often the strategy was used, how long the treatment lasted, and whether the results were sustainable. Nurses are now testing the effectiveness of specific interventions within an organizational context and evaluating adherence to evidence-based guidelines. For example, although results may be good from a particular protocol used in a randomized controlled trial to decrease ventilator-associated pneumonia, those same results may not be as dramatic when the protocol is implemented at institutions with varying resources and degrees of commitment to implementing the protocol. Nurses need to pay careful attention to the development of a clinical protocol or an evidence-based guideline and also address the implementation process. For example, implementation of these guidelines with regard to pain management continues to be challenging. The implementation of an evidence-based pain management protocol for older adults with hip fractures not only improves the quality of pain management for these patients but also reduces hospital costs (Brooks et al., 2009; Titler et al., 2009). This evidence-based protocol used multifaceted strategies including practitioners' review and "reinvention" of the evidence-based guideline, quick reference guides, and clinical reminders. In addition, the use of opinion leaders and change champions, a 3-day train-the-trainer educational program, and educational outreach for physicians and nurses was incorporated into the protocol. The intervention had a strong effect on nurse practice but had less effect on physician practices (Titler et al., 2009).

Dobbins et al., (2005) evaluated the strength of the research evidence for various strategies that promote behavioural change among health care providers. Consistently, effective strategies included academic detailing or educational outreach visits (providing health care providers with accurate information in face-to-face visits), reminders, multifaceted interventions, and interactive education meetings and workshops. Strategies having mixed effects included audit and feedback, local opinion leaders, local consensus processes, and patient-mediated interventions. Strategies having little or no effect included the distribution of educational materials and didactic educational programs. The key point here is that active involvement leads to greater success. In a systematic review of interventions to increase nurses' research use, only four studies met inclusion criteria (Thompson et al., 2007). Educational meetings led by an opinion leader and formation of interdisciplinary committees were effective at increasing research use. Clearly, such limited evidence illustrates the need for additional research to examine best practices in increasing nurses' adoption of research.

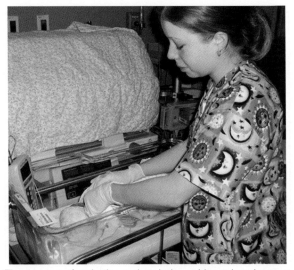

The purpose of gathering and analyzing evidence is to improve patient care.

BOX 23.4 **Steps in Evidence-Based Practice**

1. Cultivate a spirit of inquiry.
2. Ask the burning clinical question in PICOT (patient population, intervention or interest area, comparison intervention or issue of interest, outcome, and time) format.
3. Search for and collect the most relevant best evidence.
4. Critically appraise the evidence (i.e., rapid critical appraisal, evaluation, and synthesis).
5. Integrate the best evidence with one's clinical expertise and patient preferences and values in making a practice decision or change.
6. Evaluate outcomes of the practice design or change based on evidence.
7. Disseminate the outcomes of the EBP (evidence-based practice) decision or change.

From Melnyk, B. M., & Fineout-Overholt, E. (2011). Making the case for evidence-based practice and cultivating a spirit of inquiry. In B. M. Melnyk & E. Fineout-Overholt (Eds.), *Evidence-based practice in nursing and healthcare: A guide to best practice* (pp. 3–24). Philadelphia, PA: Lippincott, Williams & Wilkins.

The general public and government agencies will increasingly expect that research findings be implemented, particularly when that implementation can lead to significant improvements in patient outcomes and cost savings.

Evidence-based nursing involves a fundamental shift in philosophy. Rather than relying on nurses (be they clinicians, managers, or administrators) to read the research and apply it to practice, nurses are now expected to analyze practice problems and identify the research that will help them answer questions about how they should go about delivering care. There are generational differences between new graduates and senior nurses where the saying "we have always done it that way" impedes the use of current research-informed methods of care. As you think about your evolving nursing practice as a new graduate, how would you address a clinical challenge with a senior nurse who is in opposition of a skill when you are well aware of current evidence supporting this approach?

EVALUATION OF EVIDENCE

Evidence is best evaluated with a systematic process. The EBP steps are illustrated in Box 23.4. The first steps in the implementation of EBP are creating a spirit of inquiry and identifying the problem so that the relevant information can be obtained. The clinical question can be put into the widely used PICOT format of *patient population*, *intervention or interest area*, *comparison intervention or issue of interest*, *outcome*, and *time* to facilitate searching for the appropriate evidence (Melnyk et al., 2010; Thabane et al., 2009). These steps are illustrated in Box 23.5.

Identifying the question may be the most challenging part of the process. Different strategies can be used to identify practice problems. For example, one might conduct a survey of staff members or use a focus group methodology. Conducting a staff survey would necessitate that staff members have sufficient knowledge of research and EBP to understand what is desired. The data from surveys or focus groups, or even informal interviews with staff, can be examined along with patient outcome data for a particular setting to address relevant practice problems. Collaborating with nurses and extending that to collaboration with members of other disciplines to identify desired outcomes will enhance the ultimate success of an evidence-based project. This is because the staff members who will eventually be involved in implementing the practice are involved in its design and conception. Once the clinical question has been identified, writing it down will help in moving on to the next step of gathering evidence.

BOX 23.5 Asking the Right Question: the Picot Format

Patient population	What is the patient population or the setting? This could be adults, children, or neonates with a certain health problem; or home care versus an acute-care setting.
Intervention/ interest Area	What is the intervention? This can be an intervention or a specific area of interest (e.g., postoperative complications, the experience of postoperative pain).
Comparison	What is a comparison intervention? This is what the intervention might be compared with, such as a treatment, or the absence of a risk factor.
Outcome	What are the results? There might be multiple strategies to measure the results, such as complication rate, satisfaction, a nursing diagnosis, or a nursing quality indicator.
Time	What is the time frame for this intervention? Is time a relevant factor for this particular evaluation? For example, are you interested in short-term or long-term outcomes?

Modified from Thabane, L., Thomas, T., Ye, C., et al. (2009). Posing the research question: Not so simple. *Canadian Journal of Anaesthesia, 56*, 71–79.

EXERCISE 23.4 Here is an example of how to apply the PICOT format.

Example question: Can listening to sedative music for 45 minutes at bedtime over a 3-month period influence sleep duration and sleep quality among older adults in a long-term care facility?

Using the PICOT format this question can be broken up as follows:

P = Older adults in a long-term care facility

I = Listening to sedative music

C = Usual care (no music at bedtime)

O = Improved sleep duration and enhanced sleep quality

T = 45 minutes every day for 3 months

Now try to organize these research questions into the PICOT format.

1. Can the frequency and duration of visitation by family members influence recovery of older adult patients in critical care units?
2. Do compression stockings help prevent distension of veins in women over 65 years old who travel long distances?
3. Are pediatric patients who are rewarded for cooperating during nursing procedures more cooperative during subsequent nursing procedures than pediatric patients who are not rewarded?

Develop a clinical question using the PICOT format. Do a search in the Cumulative Index to Nursing and Allied Health Literature (CINAHL) (http://www.ebscohost.com/nursing/products/cinahl-databases) with the key PICOT terms.

The third step of the process is searching for and collecting evidence. A number of databases are available to search for evidence. Some databases contain preprocessed evidence, such as abstracts of studies and systematic reviews of evidence. Others contain citations for original single studies. Commonly used databases are listed in Box 23.6. Obtaining a librarian's assistance to navigate the databases is helpful because the databases are constantly being upgraded with new features. Several of the suggested readings that appear on the Evolve website (http://evolve.elsevier.com/Canada/Yoder-Wise/leading/) include more details on locating research evidence. Preprocessed evidence can also be located in the evidence-based/evidence-informed resources listed in Boxes 23.1 and 23.2.

The evidence for a particular practice problem can come from a single research study, an integrative review of the literature, a metaanalysis, a metasynthesis, a clinically appraised topic, a clinical guideline, or a systematic review. Sometimes a single research study might be appropriate for application to a particular problem. For other clinical questions, there might be multiple guidelines from different organizations on essentially the same clinical problem with slightly different recommendations. DiCenso and colleagues (2005) describe a hierarchy for rating the strength of evidence for treatment decisions as follows:

1. Unsystematic clinical observations
2. Physiologic studies (e.g., blood pressure, bone density)
3. Single observational study addressing important patient outcomes
4. Systematic review of observational studies addressing important patient outcomes
5. Randomized trial
6. Systematic review of randomized trials

BOX 23.6   Commonly Used Databases and Search Platforms for Nursing

CINAHL Cumulative Index to Nursing and Allied Health Literature
http://www.ebsco-host.com/cinahl/

A comprehensive nursing and allied health abstract database that includes some full-text material, such as state nursing journals, nurse practice acts, research instruments, government publications, and patient education material from 1982 to the present. A search platform for a variety of databases including CINAHL and MEDLINE. By institutional subscription.

EBSCO
http://www.ebscohost.com

NurseONE
http://www.nurseone.ca

A personalized interactive Web-based resource that provides nurses in Canada with access to current and reliable information to support their nursing practice, manage their careers, and connect with colleagues and health care experts.

OVID
http://www.ovid.com

A search platform for a variety of databases including CINAHL and MEDLINE. By institutional subscription and individual pay-per-view.

PsycINFO
http://www.apa.org/pubs/databases/psycinfo/index.aspx

Abstract database of the behavioural sciences and mental health literature from the 1800s to the present. By institutional subscription or individual article purchase.

PubMed
http://www.ncbi.nlm.nih.gov/pubmed

The abstract database of the National Library of Medicine, providing access to over 15 million citations from the 1950s to the present. Links to publishers' websites for many articles. Free.

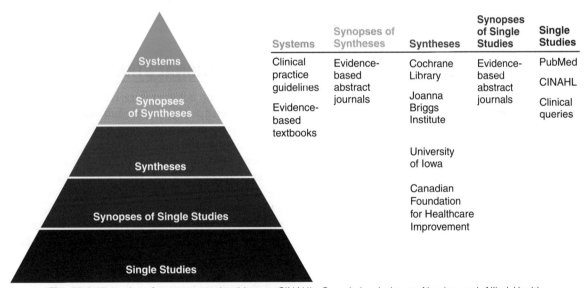

Systems	Synopses of Syntheses	Syntheses	Synopses of Single Studies	Single Studies
Clinical practice guidelines	Evidence-based abstract journals	Cochrane Library	Evidence-based abstract journals	PubMed
Evidence-based textbooks		Joanna Briggs Institute		CINAHL
				Clinical queries
		University of Iowa		
		Canadian Foundation for Healthcare Improvement		

Fig. 23.4 Hierarchy of preprocessed evidence. *CINAHL*, Cumulative Index to Nursing and Allied Health Literature.

A hierarchy of preprocessed evidence (i.e., evidence from a single research study to systems that integrate and regularly update EBP), originally developed by Haynes (2001) and adapted by Collins et al., (2005), is illustrated in Fig. 23.4. Researchers examining evidence and developing guidelines use a variety of different rating systems that include a hierarchy and key quality domains. Rating evidence is a rapidly growing field. No single established method of rating evidence is best for all situations. Ultimately, whoever conducts the analysis will have to make some decisions about the strength of the evidence and whether it can be applied to a particular patient population. What is important is that once the evidence has been located, an appropriate and systematic method for rating or appraising the evidence is used. This rating system should include an analysis of whether the evidence can be applied to a particular clinical situation.

Appraisal tools exist for evaluating different types of evidence from a single qualitative study, qualitative metasyntheses, descriptive studies, and randomized clinical trials to systematic reviews. The suggested readings provide examples. These appraisal tools generally include a series of steps for evaluating the quality of the research that is specific to the study design, type of review or guideline, or strategy for determining the applicability of the evidence to one's practice. The Appraisal of Guidelines for Research and Evaluation II, the AGREE II Collaboration (2009), an international collaboration of researchers and policymakers, provides a tool for evaluating clinical guidelines. Key elements of such appraisal tools include an assessment of the reliability and validity of the evidence.

Much of the EBP literature has been devoted to evaluating randomized clinical trials. A randomized controlled trial (RCT) includes at least two groups where study participants are randomly assigned to either the control group or the intervention group to test a treatment's effectiveness. In general, it is preferable that such studies are double-blinded, meaning that the participants and those who are evaluating the outcomes do not know who has received the treatment. Although this design is generally considered the gold standard in terms of ranking individual studies, the number of RCTs conducted in nursing remains limited. Also in certain clinical trials, blinding the recipients to a nursing intervention may be difficult—or ethically problematic—to accomplish. An RCT is not always an appropriate design for answering a particular research question. Hence it is important that the appraisal method examine the rigor or the quality of the research in accordance with standards for that type of study.

Once the evidence has been appraised, this information needs to be integrated with clinical expertise and the preferences and values of patients, families, and communities in making the change. For example, in evaluating a research-based protocol for teaching oncology patients about preparing for a bone marrow transplant, the amount and type of information that would be desired by the patient need to be considered. In this instance, a qualitative research study might provide guidance for decision making. For certain types of interventions, the inclusion of patient preferences might not be appropriate, as in the example of implementing a protocol for the reduction of ventilator-associated pneumonia. Determining patient preferences depends on the nature of the intervention or change that is proposed.

The sheer quantity and complexity of information available indicate that nurses in direct practice need to collaborate with researchers. Nurses bring their clinical expertise, their assessment of clinically relevant questions, and their understanding of the patient population. Researchers bring their capacity to appraise evidence to facilitate its application to the clinical setting. Patients or clients are the experts in their experiences and bring this personal knowledge to the forefront. Together, nurses, researchers, patients, and communities can forge a partnership in the development of evidence-based solutions to clinical practice problems, which can then be systematically evaluated and disseminated to the wider community.

ORGANIZATIONAL STRATEGIES

The partnership between nurses and researchers needs to be extended to top leaders and stakeholders within an organization. To implement EBPs, an organization needs to be committed to the process. Staff and management need to partner with researchers to identify the appropriate evidence. Key decision makers within the organization then need to receive the evidence in a usable format. For example, in deciding whether it is best for nurses to administer preprocedure sedation or for parents to administer sedatives to children before their arrival in a department for a procedure, one needs to consider the evidence, the safety of the procedure, and the risks of unmonitored or parent-administered sedation, particularly if the child is being transported to the procedure in the back seat of a car. Providing key organizational decision makers with evidence regarding the safety of such a practice would be critical for decision making.

Nurse managers and leaders need to understand the organizational context for using research evidence.

Lomas (2004) identifies the specific characteristics and competencies for creating the demand for research knowledge:

- Ability to understand the research and the decision-making environment
- Ability to find and assess relevant research
- Mediation and negotiation skills
- Communication skills
- Credibility

The RNAO (2012) released a comprehensive toolkit to assist nurses in the implementation of evidence-based guidelines. The toolkit describes strategies for working with key stakeholders and stresses their early involvement because of their understanding of the extent of the problem, unmet needs, and motivation required to address the problem. An environmental readiness assessment worksheet included in the toolkit appears in Box 23.7. Stetler (2007) emphasizes that to sustain EBP in an organization, the leadership needs to support a research culture, the organization needs capacity to engage in EBP, and an infrastructure needs to be created to facilitate EBP. The latter includes integrating research into key documents, creating expectations and roles, and providing recognition and technical support.

> **EXERCISE 23.5** Use the environmental readiness assessment worksheet in Box 23.7 to assess the capacity of your organization to implement an evidence-based guideline. Identify one strategy to address a specific barrier to implementation.

The adoption of EBPs ultimately depends on a complex interaction of individual and organizational factors. Outside of nursing, factors associated with the adoption of innovation include larger organizational size, presence of a research champion, less traditionalism, and uncommitted organizational resources. Organizational determinants that positively influence research utilization by nurses include staff development, opportunity for nurse-to-nurse collaboration, staffing, and support services; less research utilization has been associated with increased emotional exhaustion and higher rates of patient and nurse adverse events (Cummings et al., 2007). Nurse managers and administrators are increasingly called upon to support individual nurses, implement strategies to enhance individuals' use of evidence, and create an organizational infrastructure that promotes EBP.

CHALLENGES FOR NURSE MANAGERS AND LEADERS

Some of the challenges faced by nurse managers and leaders in acute and community-based clinical settings include lack of resources, excessive practice demands and time constraints, limited staffing and lack of expertise of staff members with respect to EBP, and lack of knowledge about nursing research and how to access current evidence in a timely manner in a limited time for researching and planning. Nurse leaders and managers are responsible for fostering effective clinical practice environments, but two major sources of uncertainty, the complexity of teamwork and variability in management, are apparent in today's environment. Strategies that could be used to decrease uncertainty arising from the complexity of teamwork include devising clear policies for nurses' scope of practice, wide distribution of specialized knowledge through introducing journal clubs and increased access to research-based information, and creating safe venues for multidisciplinary dialogue. Not all organizations can hire a full-time nurse researcher. Some organizations may choose not to employ clinical nurse specialists, which is shortsighted in view of the potential benefits of improved patient outcomes and cost savings because of a reduction in adverse outcomes. However, this resource limitation is a reality faced in many organizations. Regardless, it is important to remember that using the best available evidence can be most successful in a partnership model. Therefore working with nurse researchers at a local college or university should be mandatory. Box 23.8 provides an abstract on a study by Ford et al., (2011) on the process used to implement a Best Practice Guideline for patient-centred care through a partnership among clinical nurse specialists, primary health care nurse practitioners, and nurse educators in a Canadian teaching hospital. Faculty can partner with staff in a facility to provide consultation for a specific patient-care problem, and agencies can partner together to address a specific practice problem.

Collaboration is a critical organizational attribute ensuring that EBPs are incorporated into nursing care. Collaboration within the organization should involve the interdisciplinary health care team. For example, Lin et al., (2017) state that "frequent emergency department (ED) users often have complex medical, social, and behavioural health needs. They are more likely to have

BOX 23.7   Environmental Readiness Assessment for the Implementation of a Clinical Practice Guideline (CPG)

Element	Question	Facilitators	Barriers
Structure	To what extent does decision making occur in a decentralized manner? Is there enough staff to support the change process?		
Workplace culture	To what extent is the CPG consistent with the values, attitudes, and beliefs of the practice environment? To what degree does the culture support change and value evidence?		
Communication	Are there adequate (formal and informal) communication systems to support information exchange relative to the CPG and the CPG implementation processes?		
Leadership	To what extent do the leaders within the practice environment support (both visibly and behind the scenes) the implementation of the CPG?		
Knowledge, skills, and attitudes of target group	Does the staff have the necessary knowledge and skills? Which potential target group is open to change and new ideas? To what extent are they motivated to implement the CPG?		
Commitment to quality management	Do quality improvement processes and systems exist to measure results of implementation?		
Availability of resources	Are the necessary human, physical, and financial resources available to support implementation?		
Interdisciplinary relationships	Are there positive relationships and trust between and among the disciplines that will be involved or affected by the CPG?		

Data from Registered Nurses' Association of Ontario. (2002). Toolkit: implementation of clinical practice guidelines. Toronto, Canada: Registered Nurses Association of Ontario, p. 40. https://rnao.ca/sites/rnao-ca/files/BPG_Toolkit_0.pdf.

BOX 23.8   Implementing a Best Practice Guideline Through a Partnership Among Health Care Providers

Purpose	To implement the RNAO Best Practice Guideline (BPG) on Client-Centred Care (CCC) to make a positive impact on patient care through evidenced-based practice.
Background	In a Canadian teaching hospital, most practice guidelines are prescriptive, but this BPG was informed by elements of narrative theory, nursing models, and experiential learning from patients, families, and nurses.
Outcomes	This process resulted in a 12-week course: "The Telling of Our Practice-Client-Centred Care." Evidence of sustainability and the BPG were disseminated through research, patient safety workshops, nursing staff orientation, and professional development activities focusing on quality of work and falls prevention.
Conclusion	Linkages made from a variety of nursing practice sites under the CCC brought organizational mandates, specific subject matter, and current evidenced-based guidelines into a culture of caring and change, which helped form new relationships across all sectors in this teaching facility. Patient care improved, as did work life for all staff.

RNAO, Registered Nurses' Association of Ontario.
Ford, P. E. A., Rolfe, S., & Kirkpatrick, H. (2011). A journey to patient-centered care in Ontario, Canada: Implementation of a Best-Practice Guideline. *Clinical Nurse Specialist*, 25, 198–206.

chronic illness, report lower socioeconomic status, and use all health care services at higher rates, despite often having health insurance and identifying a usual source of care. Moe et al., (2017) found that although admissions among this population are low, the costs associated with these presentations are high. Interventions such as case management through multidisciplinary teams, including physicians, nurses, psychologists, social workers, and/or housing and community resource liaisons, who develop tailored care strategies for patients and link them to necessary services, care plans, and diversion strategies, have been found to be effective in reducing ED visits.

Another organizational issue is that many nurses might not have had research and/or statistics courses in their basic nursing education. It is also possible that nurses may have had research courses many years ago and have not since used their research knowledge. Even if they did take a statistics course, nurses, nurse managers, and administrators might not be familiar with the critical appraisal of evidence. Nurses on a clinical unit might not be familiar with reading research or with using advanced search strategies for locating evidence for a particular practice problem. This might be especially true for nurses who have been out of school for a long time and have not had the opportunity to develop computer literacy skills. Information on evidence-based nursing as an approach has only recently been incorporated into nursing research textbooks. Therefore a first step in developing the capacity to evaluate evidence for practice can be facilitated by starting a journal club that meets once a month. Journal clubs involve reading a relevant research article and discussing how it might be applied to the practice situation. Although a number of general and specialty nursing research journals exist, *Evidence-Based Nursing* and *Worldviews on Evidence-Based Nursing* are specifically devoted to evidence-based nursing practice. *Implementation Science* is a journal devoted specifically to the examination of strategies to promote the incorporation of research findings into routine health care.

In various parts of Canada, nurses are using personal devices at the bedside to access research and implement EBP. Researchers at the University of Alberta (Doran et al., 2012) conducted a study to evaluate front-line nurses' experiences in using mobile information technologies, such as PDAs, to access information electronically to support their clinical decision making.

In addition, they examined the role of organizations to support the use of PDAs in practice, as well as the characteristics of nurses to offer explanations for various patterns of use. Nurses in British Columbia are using PDAs in their everyday practice. The PDA has a pen-based interface, is able to synchronize data with a personal computer, and has clinical software. Nurses are able to take them home to do further research, look up medication in moments, and view research and BPGs at the bedside.

Doran et al., (2010) found that the initiative of the Nursing Secretariat, Ontario Ministry of Health and Long-Term Care, which provided nurses with PDAs and tablet PCs, to enable Internet access to information resources, such as drug and medical reference information, BPGs, and abstracts of recent research studies, showed a significant improvement in research awareness/values and in communication or research. It also showed a significant improvement over time in perceived quality of care and job satisfaction, but primarily in long-term care settings.

When translating research into practice, conduct an evaluation to document outcomes. It is preferable to collect outcomes data before implementing a protocol to have a basis for comparison. Collecting outcomes data is especially important when it is not possible to carry out an experimental design in which the intervention is implemented in one setting but not another. This may be the case because of sample size considerations or staff of different units casually talking with one another about the intervention. It is also important to consider whether the implementation of an EBP will turn into a research project. A research project is usually considered to be focused on generating new knowledge. Quality improvement activities and the adoption of EBPs might not meet the standards of a research project, and the results might not be generalizable to other settings (Newhouse, 2007). Regardless, nurses preparing to engage in an activity that might be considered a research project should consult with the organization's institutional review board early in the planning phase, regardless of whether data are collected directly from patients, medical records, or staff members.

Nurses, other health care providers, and the public might not be familiar with nursing research or evidence-based nursing. Therefore it is important to publicize key nursing research findings. When nursing research is publicized online, in the media, or through news alerts, be sure to communicate these findings to key organizational decision makers. Sending e-mails, posting articles, and providing resources helps people learn for themselves. Joining a professional association and a specialty association and signing up for alerts from key agencies provide nurses with access to the latest news, research, and standards. Research has a much better chance of being implemented if key stakeholders have the opportunity to understand its relevance.

It may be necessary to introduce concepts related to translating research into practice in small increments. For example, a first step might be incorporating research into the revision of procedures and employer guidelines as they come up for review. Subsequently, nurses and key stakeholders can be asked to identify clinical practice problems that create challenges in providing care to

develop an evidence-based solution. Multiple strategies are needed to implement research findings. Multiple strategies are needed to change a culture to one that is driven by research and evidence-based standards for practice. Finally, if one should have the opportunity to implement an EBP, as much consideration needs to be given to planning for implementation as protocol development. Advance planning should include a thorough and frank discussion of the barriers and facilitators, as well as how to minimize the barriers and maximize the facilitators. Also strategies to sustain the adoption of the practice over time need to be considered. Although the implementation of EBP is a very complex process, the increased emphasis on the use of scientifically based evidence creates an exciting opportunity for nurses to demonstrate the value of nursing in improving patient care and health care outcomes.

⟨?⟩ A SOLUTION

After an hour of trying to comfort Alex, it became clear to Jade that the patient was frightened of being in a strange place, scared of strangers hovering over, and scared about their physical situation. Alex would aggressively jump straight up in bed with his eyes bulging appearing to be barely able to catch their breath. Every time this happened, Jade would have to forcefully restrain Alex's body at the shoulders to protect the open fracture. After reflecting on the situation, Jade knew that there were nonpharmacologic interventions that could be helpful. After using multiple warm blankets, repositioning, and other nonpharmacologic comfort measures, Jade pulled up a chair and sat at Alex's bedside. Jade gestured to the patient to "try to get some sleep" and made the action of putting their head on their hands to signal sleeping. Alex then slowly reached over, grabbed Jade's hand, took a deep breath, and closed their eyes. Alex's breathing slowed and they, for once, looked somewhat relaxed. Jade sat there holding Alex's hand for 20 minutes until it appeared that Alex was asleep. Jade used their other

hand to remove Alex's tight grip and started to quietly tip-toe out of the room. Jade got to the door and was startled by a loud scream. It scared Jade, as well as her colleagues at the desk who came running over to help, thinking something was wrong. It was Alex communicating to Jade to "close the door." Alex *could* communicate and knew exactly what they wanted. There was nothing "difficult" about Alex, they were just trying to tell others how they were feeling. Before Jade left the room and closed the door, Alex repeated Jade's gesture of "try to get some sleep" and smiled. Jade smiled, turned off the light and closed the door.

Although this situation is not unique, it helped Jade reflect on how often we are too quick to judge and to rely heavily on categories or labels. Initially, the patient was labeled as "difficult" and "aggressive." It is not always easy to look beyond labels, but it is necessary to provide responsive, professional and ethically sound nursing care

Would this be a suitable approach for you? Why or why not?

▮ THE EVIDENCE

When providing nursing care, regardless of the setting of practice, there is a need to broaden the scope of EBP to include other forms of knowledge beyond explicit research knowledge. To apply scientific evidence-based

knowledge in practice, practitioners must contextualise and adapt explicit knowledge and make it relevant to local requirements. Knowledge gained through years of experience in a local context must be used to augment or adapt available research findings to enhance relevance and applicability in local settings (Kothari et al., 2012). When knowledge is translated into the realm of implementation, factors related to relevance, applicability, and context gain importance. These factors highlight the significance and importance of tacit experiential knowledge by synthesizing this tacit knowledge with explicit knowledge from research findings. Thus explication of tacit knowledge and its synthesis with explicit knowledge enables bridging of the know–do gap in context. The necessity of adapting knowledge to design and implement appropriate context-specific strategies renders tacit knowledge indispensable.

Peer-reviewed articles, printed and electronic books, formal assessments (surveys and interviews), legislation and regulations, and information available on the web come under the purview of explicit knowledge. Explicit knowledge has passed scientific rigour with established reliability and verifiability factors, and thus has sacrosanct value and is the dominantly accepted type of knowledge in the field of health. On the other hand, tacit knowledge in health settings represents knowledge derived from formal and informal discussions among health care professionals and persons involved in health settings and clinical observation. Thus knowledge obtained through discussions with, and observation of, experienced doctors, nurses, community health practitioners, and community Elders and Healers come under the purview of tacit knowledge. Kothari and colleagues found that tacit knowledge extended beyond needs assessment and illustrated the role of tacit knowledge during the program-planning process. In their study, tacit knowledge of front-line public health workers complemented explicit knowledge available in planning health care delivery (Kothari et al., 2012).

We need to follow the lead of our Indigenous peoples who have a decolonizing and rehumanizing experience when their tacit knowledge is acknowledged and validated. Indigenous ways of knowing are largely understood to be intangible, carried by Indigenous people within themselves and have been passed on orally from one generation to the next. Conversely, western ways of knowing are believed to be tangible, written or documented, peer reviewed and verified, and thus able to withstand tests of validity and reliability. When health care providers synthesize indigenous tacit knowledge with explicit knowledge, a heightened participation in one's own health care results. We have a lot to learn from our Indigenous Elders and Healers.

As we consider the future of nursing practice and how to best integrate evidence to practice, it is essential to recognize various challenges that exist when translating evidence-based knowledge into nursing practice. Resource limitations in health care systems may contribute to current evidence not being examined, appraised, or adopted. Nurses may not know where or how to access current evidence that could be integrated into practice. As we look at the future and the advancement of technology, opportunities exist for Canadian nurses to access evidence and integrate these directly into practice.

✴ NEED TO KNOW NOW

- Identify the most common practice problems in a clinical setting.
- Update practice by using the latest evidence.
- Work together with other nurses, key stakeholders, and colleagues across disciplines to adopt an evidence-based practice.
- Evaluate the results of a practice change.
- Communicate successes to colleagues, patients, families, and the public.

CHAPTER CHECKLIST

Society increasingly demands that health care be based on the best available evidence. Nurses have a societal obligation to use practices that are based on sound scientific evidence. The time from scientific discovery or publication of research to implementation in practice is lengthy and needs to be shortened. Nurses can speed up this process by using scientifically based strategies to facilitate the translation of research into practice.

The nurse manager needs to understand the organizational context for the implementation of evidence-based protocols. Multiple strategies need to be developed to enhance the use of evidence as the foundation for nursing care delivery. Ongoing engagement is needed with nurses, nurse managers, and nurse leaders to see the relevance and importance of translating research into practice. We cannot continue to "only do what we know" when the issue of life and death truly is determined by nurses at the bedside. Every nurse needs to foster the mantra that research does belong in the forefront of everyday practice.

- Research is an integral part of professional nursing practice and part of every nurse's obligation under the CNA's code of ethics (CNA, 2017).
- Research utilization is critical to an organization:
  - Synthesis, dissemination, and use of research are three distinct efforts.

Nurse researchers have a long history of developing demonstration or pilot projects to enhance research utilization.

  - Stetler's (2001) research utilization model incorporates elements of EBP and focuses heavily on the change process to facilitate translation of research into practice. The model's steps include preparation, validation, comparative evaluation or decision making, translation or application, and evaluation.
  - The knowledge-to-action framework is recognized by CIHR as the accepted model of knowledge translation.
- EBP is the driving force in today's health care approaches:
  - Research-based information is used to make decisions.
  - Patient needs and preferences are considered.
  - EBP is broad in scope in that it involves appraising the evidence to address a specific clinical practice problem, whereas research utilization involves applying the findings from a particular study in practice.
- Rogers' (2003) diffusion of innovations theory is a useful framework for understanding how innovations are diffused throughout an organization. The stages of the innovation adoption process are knowledge, persuasion, decision, implementation, and confirmation.

- According to Rogers (1995), innovation adopters can be classified as follows: innovators, early adopters, early majority, late majority, and laggards.
- Using research evidence should be done in a systematic manner:
  1. Ask the relevant clinical question.
  2. Acquire the evidence.
  3. Appraise the evidence.
  4. Integrate the evidence with clinical expertise; patient, family, and community preferences; and values.
  5. Assess the outcomes.
- Developing a relevant clinical question is enhanced by using the PICOT format.
- An organizational or environmental assessment of the capacity for evidence-based/evidence-informed practice will facilitate the translation of research into practice. An organizational assessment includes the following:
  - Access to resources for evidence
  - Capacity to appraise evidence
  - Adaptability in providing key leaders with summarized evidence
  - Capacity to demonstrate applicability of the evidence to key leaders
- Evidence-based/evidence-informed practice is a strategy to answer clinical practice questions in real-world settings.
- The characteristics and competencies required for creating the demand for research knowledge are as follows:
  - Ability to understand the research and decision-making environment
  - Ability to find and assess relevant research
  - Mediation and negotiation skills
  - Communication skills
  - Credibility
  - Collaboration
- Strategies to enhance individuals' abilities in using evidence, support for individual nurses' efforts to use research, as well the establishment of an organizational infrastructure will promote the use of EBPs.

TIPS FOR DEVELOPING SKILL IN APPLYING EVIDENCE TO PRACTICE

- Make a personal commitment to read and share research articles.
- Complete an online tutorial in EBP.
- Use your clinical experiences to develop relevant clinical questions.
- Collaborate and obtain assistance from researchers, advanced practice registered nurses, and nurse leaders.
- Use the patient population, intervention or interest area, comparison intervention or issue of interest,

outcome, and time (PICOT) format to search for evidence on a clinical practice problem.
- Create or join a journal club to encourage your colleagues to join you in learning about EBP and evaluating research evidence.
- Promote the use of personal devices to access research at the bedside.

Visit the Evolve website for Suggested Readings, Internet Resources, and additional resources related to the content in this chapter: http://evolve.elsevier.com/Canada/Yoder-Wise/leading/.

REFERENCES

AGREE Next Steps Consortium. (2009). The agree II instrument [electronic version]. Retrieved from http://www.agreetrust.org.

American Society of Health-System Pharmacist. (2012). Best practices for health-system pharmacy: positions and guidance documents of ASHP. Bethesda, MD.

Benner, P., Hughes, R. G., & Sutphen, M. (2008). Clinical reasoning, decision making, and action: thinking critically and clinically. In R. G. Hughes (Ed.), *Patient safety and quality: An evidence-based handbook for nurses*. Rockville, MD: Employer for Healthcare Research and Quality (US) Retrieved from http://www.ncbi.nlm.nih.gov/books/NBK2643/.

Brooks, J. M., Titler, M., Ardery, G., & Herr, K. (2009). Effect of evidence-based acute pain management practices on inpatient costs. *HSR: Health Services Research, 44*, 245–263.

Brown, S. J. (2008). Time to move on: Definitions of evidence-based practice. *Journal of Nursing Care Quality, 23*, 201.

Brown, S. R. (2005). *Scurvy: How a surgeon, a mariner, and a gentleman solved the greatest medical mystery of the age of sail*. New York, NY: St. Martin's Press.

Brownson, R. C., Baker, E. A., Leet, T. L., Gillespie, K. N., & True, W. R. (2010). *Evidence-based public health (eBook)*. n.p: Oxford University Press.

Burns, N., & Grove, S. K. (2009). *The practice of nursing research: Conduct, critique, and utilization* (6th ed.). St. Louis, MO: Saunders.

Burns, N., & Grove, S. K. (2011). *Understanding nursing research: Building an evidence-based practice* (5th ed.). Maryland Heights, MO: Elsevier Saunders.

Campbell, B. (2010). Applying knowledge to generate action: A community-based knowledge translation framework. *Journal of Continuing Education in the Health Professions, 30*(1), 65–71.

Canadian Institutes of Health Research. (2016). *About knowledge translation*. Retrieved from http://www.cihr-irsc.gc.ca/e/29418.html.

Canadian Institutes of Health Research. (2016a). *Evidence-informed healthcare renewal*. Retrieved from http://www.cihr-irsc.gc.ca/e/43628.html.

Canadian Nurses Association. (2018). *Definitions galore*. Retrieved from https://www.cna-aiic.ca/en/nursing-practice/evidence-based-practice/definitions-galore.

Canadian Nurses Association. (2018). Knowledge gap identified on non-medical cannabis risks. *Canadian Nurse, 114*(1), 10. Retrieved from https://proxy.library.upei.ca/login?qurl=http%3a%2f%2fsearch.ebscohost.com%2flogin.aspx%3fdirect%3dtrue%26db%3dc8h%26AN%3d128026451%26site%3dehost-live%26scope%3dsite.

Canadian Nurses Association. (2017). *2017 Edition Code of ethics for registered nurses*. Toronto, ON: Author. Retrieved from https://www.cna-aiic.ca/~/media/cna/page-content/pdf-en/code-of-ethics-2017-edition-secure-interactive.

Canadian Nurses Association. (2015). *Framework for the practice of registered nurses in Canada*. Ottawa, ON: Author. Retrieved from https://www.cna-aiic.ca/~/media/cna/page-content/pdf en/framework-for-the-pracice-of-registered-nurses-in-canada.pdf.

Canadian Nurses Association. (2014). *CNA's online primary care toolkit*. Retrieved from http://www.nurseone.ca/Default.aspx?portlet=StaticHtmlViewerPortlet&stmd=False&plang=1&ptdi=1798.

Canadian Nurses Association. (2010). *Position statement evidence-informed decision making and nursing practice.* Retrieved from https://www.cna-aiic.ca/-/media/cna/ page-content/pdf-en/ps113_evidence_informed_2010_e .pdf?la=en&hash=CF3FF9D11C714A1E1AC8A89B806B CF606698551.

Canadian Nurses Association & Registered Nurses Association of Ontario. (2010). *Nurse fatigue and patient safety.* Ottawa, ON: Author. Retrieved from http://www2 .cna-aiic.ca/CNA/practice/safety/full_report_e/files/ fatigue_safety_2010_report_e.pdf.

Ciliska, D., Thomas, H., & Buffett, C. (2008). *An introduction to evidence-based public health and a compendium of critical appraisal tools for public health practice.* Hamilton, ON: National Collaborating Centre for Methods and Tools.

College and Association of Registered Nurses of Alberta. (2011). *Scope of practice for registered nurses.* Edmonton, AB: Author. Retrieved from http://www.nurses.ab.ca/ content/dam/carna/pdfs/DocumentList/Standards/RN_ ScopeOfPractice_May2011.pdf.

Collins, S., Voth, T., DiCenso, A., et al. (2005). Finding the evidence. In A. DiCenso, G. Guyatt, & D. Ciliska (Eds.), *Evidence-based nursing: A guide to clinical practice* (pp. 20–43). St. Louis, MO: Mosby.

Cummings, G. G., Estabrooks, C. A., Midodzi, W. K., Wallin, L., & Hayduk, L. (2007). Influence of organizational characteristics and context on research utilization. *Nursing Research, 56*, S24–S39.

DiCenso, A., Ciliska, D., & Guyatt, G. (2005). Introduction to evidence-based nursing. In A. DiCenso, G. Guyatt, & D. Ciliska (Eds.), *Evidence-based nursing: A guide to clinical practice* (pp. 3–19). St. Louis, MO: Mosby.

Dobbins, M., Ciliska, D., Estabrooks, C., et al. (2005). Changing nursing practice in an organization. In A. DiCenso, G. Guyatt, & D. Ciliska (Eds.), *Evidence-based nursing: A guide to clinical practice* (pp. 172–200). St. Louis, MO: Mosby.

Doran, D., Haynes, B. R., Estabrooks, C. A., et al. (2012). The role of organizational context and individual nurse characteristics in explaining variation in use of information technologies in evidence based practice. *Implementation Science, 7*(122). https://doi: 10.1186/1748-5908-7-122.

Doran, D. M., Haynes, R. B., Kushniruk, A., Straus, S., Grimshaw, J., McGillis-Hall, L., & Jedras, D. (2010). Supporting evidence-based practice for nurses through information technologies. *Worldviews on Evidence-Based Nursing, 7*(1), 4–15.

Edwards, N., Porr, C., & Rieck Buckley, C. (2015). The practical side of research. *Canadian Nurse, 111*(7), 16–19.

Estabrooks, C. A., Chong, H., Brigidear, K., & Profetto-McGrath, J. (2005). Profiling Canadian nurses' preferred knowledge sources for clinical practice. *Canadian Journal of Nursing Research, 37*(2), 119–140.

Fetzer, S. J. (2002). Reducing venipuncture and intravenous insertion pain with eutectic mixture of local anesthetic: A meta-analysis. *Nursing Research, 51*(2), 119–124.

Finney, A., Johnson, K., Duffy, H., & Dziedzic, P. (2016). Critically Appraised Topics (CATs): A method of integrating best evidence into general practice nursing. *Practice Nurse, 46*(3), 32–34.

Ford, P. E. A., Rolfe, S., & Kirkpatrck, H. (2011). A journey to patient-centered care in Ontario, Canada: Implementation of a best-practice guideline. *Clinical Nurse Specialist, 25*, 198–206.

Funk, S. G., Champagne, M. T., Wiese, R. A., & Tornquist, E. M. (1991). Barriers: The barriers to research utilization scale. *Applied Nursing Research, 4*, 39–45.

Gagnon, M.-P., Labarthe, J., Légaré, F., Ouimet, M., Estabrooks, C. A., Roch, G., & Grimshaw, J. (2011). Measuring organizational readiness for knowledge translation in chronic care. *Implementation Science, 6*, 1–10.

Geibert, R. C. (2006). The journey to evidence: Managing the information infrastructure. In K. Malloch & T. Porter-O'Grady (Eds.), *Introduction to evidence-based practice in nursing and health care* (pp. 125–148). Boston, MA: Jones & Bartlett.

Goode, C. J., Titler, M., Rakel, B., et al. (1991). A meta-analysis of effects of heparin flush and saline flush: Quality and cost implications. *Nursing Research, 40*(6), 324–330.

Hatfield, L. A., Gusic, M. E., Dyer, A., & Polomano, R. C. (2008). Analgesic properties of oral sucrose during routine immunizations at 2 and 4 months of age. *Pediatrics, 121*(2), E327–E334.

Haynes, R. B. (2001). Of studies, syntheses, synopses, and systems: The "4S" evolution of services for finding current best evidence. *American College of Physicians Journal Club, 134*, A11–A13.

In conversation about Nursing Research (2010). *Canadian Nurse, 106*(2), 21–25.

Ingersoll, G. (2000). Evidence-based nursing: What it is and what it isn't. *Nursing Outlook, 48*, 151–152.

International Council of Nurses. (2007). *Nursing Research (position statement).* Retrieved from http://www.icn.ch/ images/stories/documents/publications/position_ statements/B05_Nsg_Research.pdf.

Jones, R. (2008). Soap opera video on handheld computers to reduce young urban women's HIV sex risk. *AIDS and Behavior, 12*, 876–884.

Kothari, A., Rudman, D., Dobbins, M., Rouse, M., Sibbald, S., & Edwards, N. (2012). The use of tacit and explicit knowledge in public health: A qualitative study. *Implementation Science, 7*(20).

Lin, M. P., Blanchfield, B. B., Kakoza, R. M., et al. (2017). ED-based care coordination reduces costs for frequent ED users. *American Journal of Managed Care, 23*(12), 762–766.

Lomas, J. (2004). *It takes two to tango: The importance of joint knowledge production for research use. Canadian Health Services Research Foundation.* Mexico City, Mexico: Presentation at the Ministerial Summit on Health Research and Global Forum.

MacLean, S., Obispo, J., & Young, K. D. (2007). The gap between pediatric emergency department procedural pain management treatments available and actual practice. *Pediatric Emergency Care, 23,* 87–93.

Malkin, B. (2008). Are techniques used for intramuscular injection based on research evidence? *Nursing Times, 104*(50–51), 48–51.

Massey, R. L. (2012). Return of bowel sounds indicating an end of postoperative ileus: Is it time to cease this long-standing nursing tradition? *MEDSURG Nursing, 21*(3), 146–150.

Melnyk, B. M., & Fineout-Overholt, E. (2011). Making the case for evidence-based practice and cultivating a spirit of inquiry. In B. M. Melnyk & E. Fineout-Overholt (Eds.), *Evidence-based practice in nursing and healthcare: A guide to best practice* (pp. 3–24). Philadelphia, PA: Lippincott, Williams & Wilkins.

Melnyk, B. M., Finehout-Overholt, E., Stillwell, S. B., & Williamson, K. M. (2010). Evidence-based practice: Step-by-step: The seven steps of evidence-based practice. *American Journal of Nursing, 110,* 51–53.

Meyers, T. A., Eichhorn, D. J., Guzzetta, C. E., et al. (2000). Family presence during invasive procedures and resuscitation: The experience of family members, nurses, and physicians. *American Journal of Nursing, 100*(2), 32–43.

Moe, J., Kirkland, S. W., Rawe, E., et al. (2017). Effectiveness of interventions to decrease emergency department visits by adult frequent users: A systematic review. *Academic Emergency Medicine, 24*(1), 40–52.

Morin, K. H. (2010). Evidence: Critical to practice and education. *Dean's Notes, 31*(4), 1–3.

Moyer, V. A., & Elliott, E. J. (2004). *Evidence-based pediatrics and child health* (2nd ed.). London, UK: BMJ Publishing Group.

Newhouse, R. (2007). Diffusing confusion among evidence-based practice, quality improvement, and research. *Journal of Nursing Administration, 37,* 432–435.

Ontario Public Health Association. (2009). *Towards evidence-informed practice: TEIP program evidence tool—revised June 2010.* Toronto, ON: Author. Retrieved from http://www.google.ca/search?q=Ontario+Public+Health+Association.+%282009%29.+Towards+Evidence-Informed+Practice.

Paramonczyk, A. (2005). Barriers to implementing research in clinical practice. *Canadian Nurse, 101*(3), 12–15.

Polit, D. F., & Beck, C. T. (2017). *Nursing research: Generating and assessing evidence for nursing practice.* Philadelphia, PA: Lippincott Williams & Wilkins.

Registered Nurses' Association of Ontario. (2012). *Toolkit: Implementation of Best Practice Guidelines* (2nd ed.). Toronto, ON: Author. Retrieved from http://rnao.ca/bpg/resources/toolkit-implementation-best-practice-guidelines-second-edition.

Rogers, E. M. (2003). *Diffusion of innovations* (5th ed.). New York, NY: Free Press.

Rogers, E. M. (1995). *Diffusion of innovations* (4th ed.). New York, NY: Free Press.

Rycroft-Malone, J., Seers, K., Titchen, A., Harvey, G., Kitson, A., & McCormack, B. (2004). What counts as evidence in evidence-based practice? *Journal of Advanced Nursing, 47*(1), 81–90.

Sarvet, A. L., Wall, M. M., Keyes, K. M., Olfson, M., Cerdá, M., & Hasin, D. S. (2018). Self-medication of mood and anxiety disorders with marijuana: Higher in states with medical marijuana laws. *Drug & Alcohol Dependence, 186,* 10–15.

Smith, A. B., Hefley, G. C., & Anand, K. J. (2007). Parent bed spaces in the PICU: Effect on parental stress. *Pediatric Nursing, 33*(3), 215–221.

Squires, J., Hutchinson, A. M., Boström, A., O'Rourke, H. M., Cobban, S. J., & Estabrooks, C. A. (2011). To what extent do nurses use research in clinical practice? A systematic review. *Implementation Science, 6,* 1–17.

Stetler, C. B. (2001). Updating the Stetler model of research utilization to facilitate evidence-based practice. *Nursing Outlook, 49,* 272–279.

Stetler, C. B., Ritchie, J., Rycroft-Malone, J., Schultz, A., & Charns, M. (2007). Improving quality of care through routine, successful implementation of evidence-based practice at the bedside: An organizational case study protocol using the pettigrew and whipp model of strategic change. *Implementation Science: IS, 2*(1), 3.

Straus, S. E., Richardson, W. S., Glasziou, P., & Haynes, B. (2005). *Evidence-based medicine: How to practice and teach EBM* (3rd ed.). Edinburgh, UK: Churchill Livingstone.

Straus, S. E., Tetroe, J., & Graham, I. (2009). Defining knowledge translation. *Canadian Medical Association Journal, 181,* 165–168.

Thabane, L., Thomas, T., Ye, C., & Paul, J. (2009). Posing the research question: Not so simple. *Canadian Journal of Anaesthesia, 56,* 71–79.

Thompson, D. S., Estabrooks, C. A., Scott-Findlay, S., Moore, K., & Wallin, L. (2007). Interventions aimed at increasing research use in nursing: A systematic review. *Implementation Science, 2,* 1–16.

Titler, M. G., Herr, K., Brooks, J. M., et al. (2009). Translating research into practice intervention improves management of acute pain in older hip fracture patients. *Health Services Research, 44,* 265–287.

Upadhyay, A., Verma, K. K., Lal, P., Chawla, D., & Sreenivas, V. (2015). Heparin for prolonging peripheral intravenous catheter use in neonates: A randomized controlled trial. *Journal of Perinatology, 35*(4), 274–277.

Vollman, A., Anderson, E., & McFarlane, J. (2017). *Canadian community as partner: Theory and multidisciplinary practice* (4th ed.). Philadelphia, PA: Lippincott Williams & Wilkins.

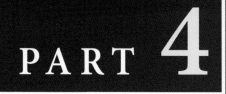

PART 4

Interpersonal and Personal Skills

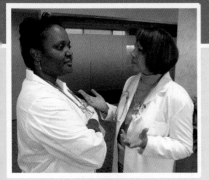

Understanding and Resolving Conflict

Shannon Dames

Conflict management skills are essential in professional nursing practice because conflict is a natural product of work environments that embrace diverse ways of being and doing. For nurse managers to promote effective conflict resolution, they must be able to determine the nature of a particular issue, choose the appropriate approach for each situation, and implement a course of action. This chapter focuses on maximizing the nurse manager's ability to deal with conflict by providing effective strategies for conflict resolution. In this chapter, the term manager *represents all forms of formal nurse leadership/supervisory roles.*

OBJECTIVES

- Determine the nature and source of perceived and actual conflict.
- Understand how congruence and self-compassion impact one's ability to address conflict.
- Determine which of the five approaches to conflict is the most appropriate in different situations.
- Identify conflict management techniques that will prevent lateral violence from occurring.
- Assess your preferred approach and your commitment to addressing conflict rather than avoiding it.

TERMS TO KNOW

accommodating	compromising	mediation
avoidance	conflict	negotiation
bullying	congruence	organizational conflict
collaborating	interpersonal conflict	self-compassion
competing	intrapersonal conflict	social dominance

Mark worked as a care aid in a long-term care facility for 5 years before deciding to go to school to become a registered nurse (RN). Once he graduated, he left his role as a care aid and accepted a position as an RN in the same facility. The facility had 100 beds with varying degrees of care required, including a handful of hospice beds. The RN role was to supervise the care aids and licensed practical nurses and to manage the more complex tasks as they arose. Mark was excited to stay at the facility where he had developed many relationships over the years, believing that staying in the familiar environment would be an asset during his transition into his new nursing role.

On Mark's first shift as the RN, where his role was now to oversee the rest of the nursing team, he noticed that the colleagues he had worked with were now avoiding eye contact with him. In addition, when he overheard news of a staff gathering, he was ignored when he took interest in being included. Later in the shift, Mark brought some of the team members together to inform them about an incoming resident. He delegated the initial assessment to a licensed practical nurse (LPN) so that they would have the paperwork completed by shift change. When the time came to report off to the oncoming team, Mark noticed that no documentation had been completed on the new admission. When he asked the LPN about the lack of documentation, they reacted defensively, claiming that they were not told to do so and that Mark should complete the assessment himself. As a result of this experience, Mark felt attacked and emotionally unsafe, making it difficult to assert himself in their new role. He avoided the LPN for the rest of the shift and called in sick for the rest of the set. He was afraid to face the conflict, and as a result, he felt he could not fulfill the RN leadership functions that were required of him.

What conflict resolution strategies could Mark use to effectively manage this situation?

INTRODUCTION

Conflict is a disagreement in values or beliefs within oneself or between people or organizations. When addressed respectfully and assertively, it has the potential to strengthen relationships and stimulate beneficial changes in the practice environment. Conversely, when it is avoided or used as vehicle to dominate others, it erodes trust and fuels hostile work environments. In homogenizing cultures, whereby diverse ways of being and doing are perceived as a threat to the professional image, conflict can be highly threatening because those who challenge the status quo are often the target of workplace hostility (Porath & Pearson, 2012). However, if avoided, it also has a negative impact on the individual and the organization (Mitchell, Ahmed, & Szabo, 2014). When conflict is managed in a collaborative fashion, empowering individual voices and working toward solutions that honor the diverse perspectives within the team, then relationships are strengthened and congruence is promoted.

Congruence is described as an alignment of one's real and ideal selves, resulting in a greater ability to be authentic and self-actualize/thrive in one's life roles (Rogers, 1959). Conversely, if one primarily identifies with the ideal self, which is socially prescribed, they will lose touch with their authentic/real self. This separation between the ideal and the real selves results in feelings of shame when one's ability to meet their idealistic standards is threatened. As a result, they have a greater tendency toward maladaptive perfectionism, emotional dissociation, and avoidance of conflict.

When a work environment is populated with more congruent employees, conflict is viewed as an opportunity to explore differences and to collaborate. In addition, intraprofessional relationships can be strengthened, making for higher-functioning teams. Some of the first authors on organizational conflict (e.g., Blake & Mouton, 1964; Deutsch, 1973; Duffy, 1995) claimed that a complete resolution of conflict might, in fact, be undesirable because conflict can stimulate growth, creativity, and change. Furthermore, conflict, which often stirs emotions, can be the motivating force for individuals to explore areas of incongruence and to clarify their core values and goals in the process.

Conflict is inherent in clinical environments that are driven by patient needs that are complex, often unpredictable, and frequently changing (Latham et al., 2013; Sherman & Pross, 2010). Furthermore, when nurses operate in a state of survival, feeling little control/autonomy in their workday, they are more likely to react from a place of threat when unpredictable events or opposing opinions present. Adding to this, highly stimulating work environments leave little time for employees to be proactive because of constant distractions, which can be a barrier to engaging in thriving or self-actualizing activity. Health care providers are exposed to these high stress levels because of increased demands on an ever-limited and aging or inexperienced workforce, a decrease in available resources, a more acutely ill patient population, and a rapidly changing practice environment. In professional practice environments, unresolved conflict among nurses is a significant issue resulting in job dissatisfaction, absenteeism, and turnover. Furthermore, the complexity of the health care workplace compounds the impact that caregiver stress and unresolved conflict have on patient safety.

Successful organizations are proactive in anticipating the need for conflict resolution and innovative in developing conflict resolution strategies that apply to all members (Berwick, 2011; Mitchell et al., 2014). Nurses employed in healthy practice environments report more positive job experiences and fewer concerns about quality care. In addition, health care settings with positive nurse–physician relations are associated with better patient outcomes and increased satisfaction with nursing (Friese & Manojlovich, 2012). Finally, when employees have positive views of self, including self-compassion, self-esteem, self-efficacy, and emotional congruence, they are more likely to engage in constructive conflict management, which contributes to team effectiveness (Mazurek et al., 2013).

Self-compassion correlates with one's ability to receive and respond constructively to feedback and is a necessary element toward attaining congruence. It occurs when one extends kindness to themselves in response to suffering and during times of perceived inadequacy. It promotes one's ability to effectively cope with intrapersonal and workplace stressors, mitigates declines and well-being, and, as a result, buffers them from maladaptive perfectionism and burnout (Dames et al., 2018; Gunnell et al., 2017; Montero-Marin et al., 2016). Similarly, a positive view of one's self is also a predictor of quality leader–staff relationships, empowerment, and job satisfaction for nurse managers (Canadian Nurses Association [CNA], 2009; Roche et al., 2010). The diverse workforce in health care settings today reveals varying characteristics and work values, which is an opportunity for creative and synergizing teamwork but can also stimulate conflict. To successfully manage stress and conflict in the work environment, managers need to understand their unique context. For instance, in environments where diversity is feared, conflict is often avoided, as employees do not want to be viewed in a negative light by their peers. Given the tribalistic culture of many nursing environments, whereby nurses often have informal assumptions and loyalties within their work teams, these fears are quite common, especially for students and novice nurses who feel the need to earn their place on the team. Nurse managers and leaders have a growing responsibility to effectively manage the nursing workforce by creating cultures that embrace diversity (Wolff et al., 2010). Unfortunately, homogenization, often presenting as socially prescribed perfectionism, is first introduced in nursing school, whereby students are immersed in a binary curriculum

that prescribes idealistic standards, as opposed to encouraging an exploration and integration of one's authentic self with nursing values and goals (Dames et al., 2018; Gazelle et al., 2015). Review Chapters 30 and 31 to clarify your own values and beliefs about nursing and yourself. Although the profession of nursing will always strive to operate by black-and-white best-practice principles, there must also be recognition that the reality of nursing is full of complexities that make decision making far grayer in nature. This recognition can diffuse binary ways of thinking, working toward creative solutions that use practice principles as a guide in the critical thinking process.

Nurses tend to avoid conflict, compromise, and even withdraw in hopes of spontaneous resolution (Jackson et al., 2013). The stereotypical self-sacrificing behaviour seen in avoidance and accommodation is strongly supported by the altruistic nature of nursing (Blair, 2013). However, it erodes the ability for coworkers to be authentic and to establish relationships of trust. Conversely, high-functioning relationships intertwine empathy and compassion with assertive communication. Furthermore, when employees are authentic, making their values and goals clear, it enables them to take on roles that align with their passions. Although avoidance may be a temporary leadership strategy during times of high stress and may seem relatively harmless, it can leave employees with the perception that the manager is abstaining from active leadership (Jackson et al., 2013). When leaders avoid conflict, it impacts the well-being of nurses and diminishes their commitment to the organization. It is important that nurse leaders lead by example and strive to challenge the status quo by co-constructing a climate of shared work goals and outcomes with the common purpose of creating a work environment were nurses can be authentic, delivering safe and high-quality nursing care (CNA, 2009; Wolff et al., 2010).

TYPES OF CONFLICT

The recognition that conflict is a part of everyday life suggests that mastering conflict management strategies is essential for overall well-being and personal and professional growth. Determining the type of conflict present in a specific situation is important because the more accurately conflict is defined, the more likely it will be resolved. The three types of conflict are as follows: intrapersonal, interpersonal, or organizational; a combination of types can also be present in any given conflict.

Intrapersonal conflict occurs within a person when confronted with the need to think or act in a way that seems at odds with one's personality, goals, and/or values, resulting in emotional incongruence. Questions often arise that create a conflict over priorities, ethical standards, and values. When a nurse manager/formal leader decides what to do about the future (e.g., *Do I want to pursue an advanced degree or start a family now?*), conflict arises between personal and professional priorities. Some issues present a conflict over comfortably maintaining the status quo (e.g., *I know my operating room [OR] nurse leader prefers the OR over the surgical day care centre; Should I ask them to manage the centre anyway, because I need someone with their skills at the centre?*). Taking risks to confront people when needed (e.g., *Would recommending a change in practice that I learned about at a recent conference offend my manager?*) can resolve intrapersonal conflict, but because it involves other people, it may lead to interpersonal conflict. In professions, like nursing, which are heavily identified by best-practice ideals, intrapersonal conflicts are likely to be triggered when the reality of their nursing role falls out of alignment with the ideals they have been taught to adhere to. This tension between nursing ideals and the reality of the role can produce chronic intrapersonal conflict, especially for those who lack self-compassion. Furthermore, while nurses learn about the impact of trauma on patients, it is equally important to also recognize the impact trauma has in their own professional practice. For instance, those who have unresolved emotional trauma are more likely to experience emotional transference in the practice setting; this too can provoke and intensify intrapersonal conflict.

Interpersonal conflict occurs between and among patients, family members, nurses, physicians, and members of other departments. Conflicts occur that focus on a difference of opinion, priority, or approach with others; these conflicts can become heavily subjective when involved parties feel that their sense of belonging, esteem, or moral/ethical values are threatened. A nurse manager may be called upon to assist two nurses in resolving a scheduling conflict or issues surrounding patient assignments. Members of health care teams often have disputes over the best way to treat particular cases or disagreements in determining how much information is necessary for patients and families to have about their illness. Interpersonal conflicts are the most common type of conflict experienced by nurses in the workplace (Johansen, 2012).

Organizational conflict arises when discord exists about policies and procedures, personnel codes of conduct, or accepted norms of behaviour and patterns of communication. Some organizational conflict is related to hierarchical structure and role differentiation among employees. Nurse managers and their staff often become embattled in institution-wide conflict concerning staffing patterns and how they affect the quality of care, resulting in moral/ethical dissonance. Complex ethical and moral dilemmas may arise over the allocation of limited resources and funding for health care delivery (e.g., access to health care resources in remote areas vs. densely populated urban centres, or discharging patients earlier because of capacity issues). A major source of organizational conflict stems from strategies that promote more participation and autonomy of staff nurses. Increasingly, nurses are charged with balancing direct patient care with active involvement in organizational initiatives surrounding quality patient care. Nurses who perceive themselves as working in a healthy environment that promotes collaboration are more likely to report enhanced employee well-being and effective conflict management strategies (Bennett & Sawatzky, 2013). The following are other forces that contribute to effective conflict management in the practice environment:

- Organizational structure (nurses' felt empowerment in shared decision making)
- Management style (nursing leaders create an environment empowering leadership opportunities among employees, encourage and value feedback, and demonstrate effective communication with staff)
- Personnel policies and programs (efforts to promote nurse work–life balance)
- Protecting the image of nursing while also promoting authenticity and a diversity of ideas (nurses effectively influencing system-wide processes)
- Promoting autonomy by empowering nurses to be leaders and providing opportunities to engage in organizational governance.

> **EXERCISE 24.1** Recall a situation in which you had an interpersonal conflict with someone. Describe verbal and nonverbal communication and how each person responded. What was the outcome? Was the conflict resolved? Were any issues left unresolved? How might you handle this situation in the future?

STAGES OF CONFLICT

Conflict proceeds through four distinct stages: frustration, conceptualization, action, and outcomes (Thomas, 1992). The ability to resolve conflicts productively depends on understanding these stages (Fig. 24.1) and concurrently addressing thoughts, feelings, and behaviours that form barriers to resolution. As one navigates through the stages

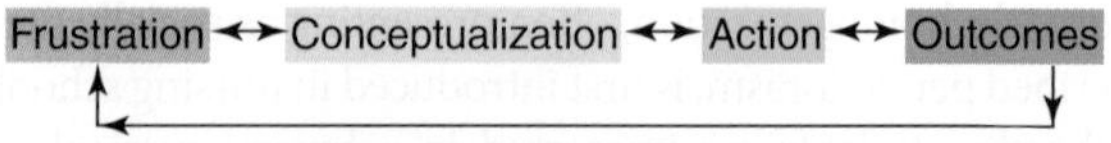

Frustration ↔ Conceptualization ↔ Action ↔ Outcomes

Fig. 24.1 Stages of conflict.

of conflict, moving into a subsequent stage may lead to a return to and change in a previous stage. To illustrate, consider the example of nurses in a medical unit who are asked to pilot a new protocol surrounding the process that is followed when the offgoing nurse hands off patient care information to the oncoming nurse. The pilot stimulates intense emotions because the unit is already inadequately staffed (frustration). Two of the medical unit nurses interpret this conflict as a battle for control with the nurse educator, and a third nurse thinks it is all about professional standards (conceptualization). A nurse manager facilitates a discussion with the three nurses (action); she listens to the concerns and presents evidence about the potential effectiveness of the shift change protocol. All agree that the real conflict comes from a difference in goals or priorities (new conceptualization), which resolves negative emotions and ends with a much clearer understanding of all the issues (diminished frustration). The nurses agree to pilot the shift change protocol after their ideas are incorporated into the plan (outcome).

Frustration

When people or groups perceive that their goals may be blocked, frustration results. This frustration may escalate into stronger emotions, such as anger and deep resignation, which often distracts employees from thriving in their role. For example, a nurse may perceive that a postoperative patient is uncooperative, when in reality the patient is afraid, or has a different set of priorities at the start from those of the nurse. At the same time, the patient may view the nurse as controlling and uncaring, because the nurse repeatedly asks if the patient has used his incentive spirometer as instructed. When such frustrations occur, it is a cue to stop and clarify the nature and cause of the differences.

Conceptualization

Conflict arises when there are different interpretations of a situation, including a different emphasis on what is important and what is not, and different thoughts about what should occur next. Everyone involved develops an idea of what the conflict is about, and individual views may or may not be accurate. Viewpoints are influenced by past experiences, which can lead one to jump to an instant conclusion or may be developed by observed patterns that have formed over time. Everyone involved has an individual interpretation of what the conflict is and why it is occurring. Most often, these interpretations are dissimilar and involve the person's own perspective, which is based on emotional transference based on past experiences, values, beliefs, and attitudes.

- Regardless of the accuracy of variously held viewpoints, the root of employee frustrations is differing conceptualizations. One's orientation to events influences their problem-solving approach and resulting outcomes. Differences in conceptualization that go unidentified can block the ability to resolve it; therefore clarifying how each person views the event or conflict enables differences to be navigated and for a shared conceptualization to develop. The following questions can help advance to shared conceptualization and a resolution:
- What is the nature of our differences?
- What are the reasons for those differences?
- Does the current manager and culture endorse ideas or behaviours that add to or diminish the conflict?
- Do I need to be mentored by someone, even if that individual is outside my own department or work area (to avoid triangulated communication), to successfully resolve this conflict?

Action

A behavioural response to a conflict follows the conceptualization. This may include seeking clarification about how another person views the conflict, collecting additional information that informs the issue, or engaging in dialogue about the issue. As actions are taken to resolve the conflict, the way that some or all involved conceptualize the conflict may change. Successful resolution frequently stems from identifying a common goal that unites individuals (e.g., quality patient care, good working relations). It is important to understand that people are always taking some action regarding the conflict, even if that action is avoidance, deliberately delaying action, or choosing to do nothing. The longer that ineffective actions continue, the more likely that frustration, resistance, and hostility will fester. The more appropriately the actions match the nature of the conflict, the more likely that the conflict will be resolved in a timely manner with desirable results.

Outcomes

Tangible and intangible consequences result from actions taken and have significant implications for the work setting. Either the conflict is approached with a goal of resolving or at minimum collaboratively managing, or it is avoided and therefore unresolved; the outcomes are then highly dependent on the approach, which may be conscious or subconsciously chosen
(1) The conflict is resolved/managed, which results in:
- Growth; professional and organizational
- Resolution or collaborative management of the problem

- Unification of groups and improved relationships and team functioning
- Productivity increases
- Enhanced employee commitment and satisfaction

(2) The conflict is unresolved/avoided, which results in:

- Frustration festers, increasing negativity and resistance to resolution
- Stagnation as opposed to growth
- Group divisions and weakened relationships and team functioning
- Productivity decreases
- Decreased employee commitment and satisfaction

Assessing the degree of conflict resolution is useful for improving individual and group skills in resolutions. Two general outcomes are considered when assessing the degree to which a conflict has been resolved: (1) the degree to which important goals were achieved, and (2) the nature of the subsequent relationships among those involved (Box 24.1; J. Hurst & Kinney, 1989).

CATEGORIES OF CONFLICT

Categorizing and determining the root cause of a conflict can help define an appropriate course of action toward its resolution. Conflicts arise from discrepancies in four areas: facts, goals, approaches, and values. Sources of fact-based conflicts are external written sources and include job descriptions, hospital policies, and provincial and territorial standards of practice. Objective data can be provided to resolve a disagreement generated by discrepancies in information. Goal conflicts often arise from competing priorities (e.g., desire to empower employees vs. control through micromanagement); often, focusing on a common goal (e.g., quality patient care) can aid conflict resolution. Even when agreement exists on a common goal, different ideas about the best approach to achieve that goal may ignite conflict. For example, if the unit goal is to reduce costs by 10%, one leader may target overtime hours and another may eliminate the budget for continuing education. Values, opinions, and beliefs are much more personal, thus generating disagreements that can be threatening and adversarial. Because values are subjective, value-based conflicts sometimes remain unresolved. In these circumstances, professionals should find ways for competing values to coexist, such as agreeing to disagree.

A pessimist sees the difficulty in every opportunity; an optimist sees the opportunity in every difficulty.
Winston Churchill

APPROACHES TO CONFLICT RESOLUTION

Understanding the ways in which health care providers respond to conflict and the current states of incivility and moral distress in various health care domains is an essential first step in identifying effective strategies to help nurses constructively handle conflicts in the practice environment. Five distinct approaches can be used in conflict resolution: avoiding, accommodating via obliging, competing via dominating, compromising, and collaborating via integrating. These approaches can be viewed within the dimensions of assertiveness (satisfying one's own concerns) and cooperativeness (satisfying the concerns of others). Most people tend to use a combined set of actions that are appropriately assertive and cooperative, depending on the nature of the conflict situation and their preferred and natural patterns of behaviour when responding to conflict (Barsky, 2016; Thomas, 1992). See the conflict self-assessment in Box 24.2.

BOX 24.1 Assessing the Degree of Conflict Resolution

1. Quality of decisions?
   a. How creative are resulting plans?
   b. How practical and realistic are they?
   c. How well were intended goals achieved?
   d. What surprising results were achieved?
2. Quality of relationships?
   a. How much understanding has been created?
   b. How willing are people to work together?
   c. How much mutual respect, empathy, concern, and cooperation has been generated?

Modified from Hurst, J., & Kinney, M. (1989). *Empowering self and other.* Toledo, OH: University of Toledo Press.

EXERCISE 24.2 Self-assessment of preferred conflict-handling approaches is important. As you read and answer the 30-item conflict survey in Box 24.2, think of how you respond to conflict in professional situations. After completing the survey, tally, total, and reflect on your scores for each of the five approaches. Consider the following questions:

- Which approach do you prefer? Which do you use least?
- What determines if you respond in a particular manner?
- Considering the reoccurring types of conflicts you have, what are the strengths and weaknesses of your preferred conflict-handling styles?
- Have others offered you feedback about your approach to conflict?

BOX 24.2 Conflict Self-Assessment

Directions: Read each of the following statements. Assess yourself in terms of how often you tend to act similarly during conflict at work, at clinical placements, and at school. Place the number of the most appropriate response in the blank in front of each statement. Put *1* if the behaviour is never typical of how you act during a conflict, *2* if it is seldom typical, *3* if it is occasionally typical, *4* if it is frequently typical, or *5* if it is very typical of how you act during conflict.

_____ 1. Create new possibilities to address all important concerns.

_____ 2. Persuade others to see it and/or do it my way.

_____ 3. Work out some sort of give-and-take agreement.

_____ 4. Let other people have their way.

_____ 5. Wait and let the conflict take care of itself.

_____ 6. Find ways that everyone can win.

_____ 7. Use whatever power I have to get what I want.

_____ 8. Find an agreeable compromise among people involved.

_____ 9. Give in so others get what they think is important.

_____ 10. Withdraw from the situation.

_____ 11. Cooperate assertively until everyone's needs are met.

_____ 12. Compete until I either win or lose.

_____ 13. Engage in "give a little and get a little" bargaining.

_____ 14. Let others' needs be met more than my own needs.

_____ 15. Avoid taking any action for as long as I can.

_____ 16. Partner with others to find the most inclusive solution.

_____ 17. Put my foot down assertively for a quick solution.

_____ 18. Negotiate for what all parties value and can live without.

_____ 19. Agree to what others want to create harmony.

_____ 20. Keep as far away from others involved as possible.

_____ 21. Stick with it to get everyone's highest priorities.

_____ 23. Argue and debate over the best way.

_____ 23. Create some middle position everyone agrees to.

_____ 24. Put my priorities below those of other people.

_____ 25. Hope the issue does not come up.

_____ 26. Collaborate with others to achieve our goals together.

_____ 27. Compete with others for scarce resources.

_____ 28. Emphasize compromise and trade-offs.

_____ 29. Cool things down by letting others do it their way.

_____ 30. Change the subject to avoid the fighting.

Conflict Self-Assessment Scoring

Look at the numbers you placed in the blanks on the conflict assessment. Write the number you placed in each blank on the appropriate subsequent line. Add up your total for each column and enter that total on the appropriate line. The greater your total is for each approach, the more often you tend to use that approach when conflict occurs at work. The lower the score is, the less often you tend to use that approach when conflict occurs at work.

Collaborating	Competing	Compromising	Accommodating	avoiding
1. _____	2. _____	3. _____	4. _____	5. _____
6. _____	7. _____	8. _____	9. _____	10. _____
11. _____	12. _____	13. _____	14. _____	15. _____
16. _____	17. _____	18. _____	19. _____	20. _____
21. _____	22. _____	23. _____	24. _____	25. _____
26. _____	27. _____	28. _____	29. _____	30. _____
Total _____	Total _____	Total _____	Total _____	Total _____

Throughout the rest of this section, there are descriptions of each approach and related self-assessment and commitment-to-action activities. Use the scores you received above to think about how you do and could handle conflict at work. Most important, consider if your pattern of frequency tends to be consistent or inconsistent with the types of conflicts you face. That is, does your way of dealing with conflict tend to match the situations in which that approach is most useful?

Hurst, J. B. (1993). *Conflict self-assessment.* Toledo, OH: Human Resource Development Center, University of Toledo.

Avoidance

Avoidance is a fear-based approach to conflict management. Most people do not consciously choose avoidance, but rather, from a place of fear, they will subconsciously distract themselves from acknowledging the conflict and the impact it has on themselves and others. It is passive and typically unproductive because people who avoid conflict deny their own needs and goals and also fail to contribute to the goals and needs of others in the process. Avoidance ensures that conflict is postponed or prolonged, which may escalate frustration and discord among team members. That is not to say that all conflict must be addressed immediately, as some issues require considerable reflection before strategies can be selected and action taken. The positive side of withdrawing may be postponing an issue until a better time or simply walking away from a "no-win" situation.

Avoidance can be effective when:

1. Facing trivial and/or temporary issues, or when other far more important issues are pressing
2. There is no chance to obtain what one wants or needs, or when others could resolve the conflict more efficiently and effectively
3. The potential negative results of initiating and acting on a conflict are much greater than the benefits of its resolution
4. People need to "cool down," distance themselves, or gather more information

The self-assessment in Box 24.3 will help you recognize your own avoidance behaviours and use them more effectively.

Accommodating via Obliging

When accommodating, people neglect their own needs, goals, and concerns (passive) while trying to satisfy those of others (cooperative). This approach has an element of being self-sacrificing and simply obeying orders or serving other people. For example, a co-worker requests that you cover her weekends during her children's holiday break. You had hoped to visit friends from college, but you know how important it is for her to have more time with her family, so you agree.

Accommodation via obliging can be effective when:

1. Other people's ideas and solutions appear to be better, or when you have made a mistake.
2. The issue is far more important to the other(s) person than it is to you.

> ### BOX 24.3 Avoidance: Self-Assessment and Commitment to Action
>
> **If You Tend to Use Avoidance Often, Ask Yourself the Following Questions:**
> 1. Do people have difficulty getting my input into and understanding my view?
> 2. Do I block cooperative efforts to resolve issues?
> 3. Am I distancing myself from significant others?
> 4. Are important issues being left unidentified and unresolved?
>
> **If You Seldom Use Avoidance, Ask Yourself the Following Questions:**
> 1. Do I find myself overwhelmed by a large number of conflicts and a need to say "no"?
> 2. Do I assert myself even when things do not matter that much? Do others view me as an aggressor?
> 3. Do I lack a clear view of what my priorities are?
> 4. Do I stir up conflicts and fights?
>
> **Commitment to Action**
> What two new behaviours would increase your effective use of avoidance?
> 1.
> 2.

---

3. You see that accommodating now "builds up some important credits" for later issues.
4. You are outmatched and/or losing anyway; when continued competition would only damage the relationships and productivity of the group and jeopardize accomplishing major purpose(s).
5. Preserving harmonious relationships and avoiding defensiveness and hostility are very important.
6. Letting others learn from their mistakes and/or increased responsibility is possible without severe damage.

As discussed, there are situations where accommodation is the most effective approach; however, individuals who habitually accommodate others are more likely to suffer from emotional incongruence (defined earlier) by frequently denying their authentic needs and wants, resulting in feelings of disappointment and resentment. Developing a subconscious habit of accommodating is no longer a strategic choice, and often ends in feeling taken advantage of. A self-assessment in Box 24.4 asks you to examine your current use of accommodation and challenges you to think of new ways to use it more effectively.

BOX 24.4 **Accommodation: Self-Assessment and Commitment to Action**

If You Use Accommodation Often, Ask Yourself the Following Questions:
1. Do I feel that my needs, goals, concerns, and ideas are not being attended to by others?
2. Am I depriving myself of influence, recognition, and respect?
3. When I am in charge, is "discipline" lax?
4. Do I think people are using me?

If You Seldom Use Accommodation, Ask Yourself the Following Questions:
1. Am I building goodwill with others during conflict?
2. Do I admit when I have made a mistake?
3. Do I know when to give in, or do I assert myself at all costs?
4. Am I viewed as unreasonable or insensitive?

Commitment to Action
What two new behaviours would increase your effective use of accommodation?
1.
2.

BOX 24.5 **Competing: Self-Assessment and Commitment to Action**

If You Use Competing Often, Ask Yourself the Following Questions:
1. Am I surrounded by people who agree with me all the time and who avoid confronting me?
2. Are others afraid to share themselves and their needs for growth with me?
3. Am I out to win at all costs? If so, what are the costs and benefits of competing?
4. What are people saying about me when I am not around?

If You Seldom Compete, Ask Yourself the Following Questions:
1. How often do I avoid taking a strong stand and then feel a sense of powerlessness?
2. Do I avoid taking a stand so that I can escape risk?
3. Am I fearful and unassertive to the point that important decisions are delayed and people suffer?

Commitment to Action
What two new behaviours would increase your effective use of competing?
1.
2.

Competing via Dominating

When competing, people tend to come from blueprint of scarcity or survival, whereby they pursue their own needs and goals at the expense of others; this is often a subconscious projection or habit that develops from incongruence (described earlier). From this perspective, they use their personal and professional resources to position themselves in a place of superiority over their peers; the end goal is to 'win.' Although this approach tends to be harmful to work environments that promote the thriving of all employees, there are circumstances that may be best addressed with this more black-and-white approach. For example, it may take the form of standing up for one's basic rights or defending important principles, as when opposition to mandatory overtime is voiced.

Competing via dominating can be effective when:
1. Quick, decisive action is necessary.
2. Important, unpopular action needs to be taken, or when trade-offs may result in long-range, continued conflict.
3. An individual or group is right about issues that are vital to group welfare.

4. Others have taken advantage of an individual's or group's noncompetitive behaviour and now are mobilized to compete about an important topic.

People whose primary approach to addressing conflict is through competition often react by feeling threatened, acting defensively or aggressively, or even resorting to cruelty in the form of cutting remarks, deliberate gossip, or hurtful innuendo. Competition within work groups can generate ill will, favour a win–lose stance, and compel people to a stalemate. Such behaviours force people into a corner from which there is no easy or graceful exit. Use Box 24.5 to help you learn to use competing more effectively.

Compromising

Compromising is assertive and cooperative and requires maturity and confidence. Negotiation is a learned skill that is developed over time. A give-and-take relationship results in conflict resolution, with the result that each person can meet his or her most important priorities as much of the time as possible. Compromise is very often the exchange of concessions as it creates middle ground. This is the preferred means of conflict resolution during union negotiations, in which each side is appeased to some degree. With this approach, nobody gets everything they think they need, but a sense of energy exists that is necessary to build important relationships and teams.

Negotiation and compromise are valued approaches and tend to be a middle-ground approach, whereby both self and others can be heard and responded to, recognizing that neither party may achieve their ideal outcome. Compromising is a blend of both assertive and cooperative behaviours, although it calls for less finely honed skills for each behaviour than does collaborating. Negotiation, which involves conferring with others to bring about a settlement of differences, is somewhat like trading (e.g., "You can have this if I can have that" as in "I will chair the regional committee on improving morale if you send me to the hospital's leadership training classes next week, so I can have the skills I need to be effective"). Compromise is one of the most effective behaviours used by nurse managers because it supports a balance of power between themselves and others in the work setting.

Compromise can be effective when:

1. Two powerful sides are committed strongly to perceived mutually exclusive goals.
2. Temporary solutions to complex issues need to be implemented.
3. Conflicting goals are "moderately important" and not worth a major confrontation.
4. Time pressures people to expedite a workable solution.
5. Collaborating and competing fail.

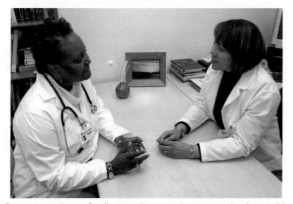

Documentation of all meetings and communication with employees is an important aspect of the nurse manager's role.

The self-assessment in Box 24.6 will help you become more aware of your own use of negotiation and compromise and improve it.

Collaborating via Integrating

Collaborating refers to a group of people working together to achieve a common goal, whereby the focus is on sharing ideas and experiences to produce the best outcome. Although the most time-consuming approach to conflict resolution, it is the most creative. It is both assertive and cooperative because people work creatively and openly to find a solution that most fully satisfies all important concerns and goals to be achieved. Collaboration involves analyzing situations and defining the conflict at a higher level where shared goals are identified and commitment to working together is generated. When nurses use cooperative conflict management approaches, decision making becomes a collective process in which action plans are mutually understood and implemented. For example, when nurses and physicians work together, they can collaborate by asking, "What is the best thing we can do for the patient and family right now?" and "How does each of us fit into the plan of care to meet their needs?" This requires discussion about the

---

BOX 24.6   Negotiation/Compromise Self-Assessment and Commitment to Action

If You Tend to Use Negotiation Often, Ask Yourself the Following Questions:

1. Do I ignore large, important issues while trying to work out creative, practical compromises?
2. Is there a "gamesmanship" in my negotiations?
3. Am I sincerely committed to compromise or negotiated solutions?

If You Seldom Use Negotiation, Ask Yourself the Following Questions:

1. Do I find it difficult to make concessions?
2. Am I often engaged in strong disagreements, or do I withdraw when I see no way to get out?
3. Do I feel embarrassed, sensitive, self-conscious, or pressured to negotiate, compromise, and bargain?

Commitment to Action

What two new behaviours would increase your compromising effectiveness?

1.
2.

plan, how it will be accomplished, and who will make what contributions toward its achievement and proposed outcomes.

Collaboration/integration is most effective when:

1. Seeking creative, integrative solutions in which both sides' goals and needs are important, thus developing group commitment and a consensual decision.
2. Learning and growing through cooperative problem solving, resulting in greater understanding and empathy.
3. Identifying, sharing, and merging vastly different viewpoints.
4. Being honest about and working through difficult emotional issues that interfere with morale, productivity, and growth.

At the onset of conflict, involved collaborating individuals can analyze situations to identify the source of the conflict and choose an appropriate approach. For example, a conflict arises when a staff nurse and a charge nurse on a psychiatric unit disagree about how to handle a patient's complaints regarding the staff nurse's delay in responding to the patient's requests. At the point that they reach an agreement that it is the staff nurse's responsibility and decision to make, collaboration has occurred. The nurse leader might say, "I didn't realize your plan of care was to respond to the patient at predetermined intervals or that you told the patient that you would check on her every 30 minutes. I can now inform the patient that I know about and support your approach." Or the staff nurse and nurse leader might talk and subsequently agree that the staff nurse is too emotionally involved with the patient's problems and that it may be time for her to withdraw from providing care and enlist the support of another nurse, even temporarily. Discussion can result in collaboration aimed at allowing the staff nurse to withdraw appropriately. Another, less desirable choice could be to compete and let the winner's position stand (e.g., "I'm in charge; I'm going to assign another nurse to this patient to preserve our patient satisfaction scores" or "I know what is best for this patient; I took care of them during her past two admissions"). The self-assessment tool in Box 24.7 will assist you to see how you engage in collaboration.

DIFFERENCES OF CONFLICT-HANDLING STYLES AMONG NURSES

The way in which nurses respond to conflict has changed very little in the past 20 years. Previous studies suggest that avoidance and accommodation remain the predominant choices for staff nurses and that the prevalent style for nurse managers is compromise, despite the emphasis placed on collaboration as an effective strategy for conflict management (Iglesias & Vallejo, 2012; Mahon & Nicotera, 2011). See the Research Perspective for a discussion about the correlation between emotional intelligence and the preferred conflict-handling styles among nurses. Professional nurses often avoid conflict when they fear a consequence (Johansen, 2012). Nurses sometimes choose to avoid conflict because they fear that engaging in conflict or even attempting to resolve conflict may jeopardize their career advancement (Johansen, 2012; Mahon & Nicotera, 2011). Adding to this, nursing culture tends to be homogenizing in nature, whereby diversity is perceived as a threat; it produces implicit fears of conflict, which then further pushes differences into shadows and makes them all the more divisive found that diversity (Palmer et al., 2010). It is interesting to note that newly graduated nurses are

---

BOX 24.7 Collaboration: Self-Assessment and Commitment to Action

If You Tend to Collaborate Often, Ask Yourself the Following Questions:

1. Do I spend valuable group time and energy on issues that do not warrant or deserve it?
2. Do I postpone needed action to get consensus and avoid making key decisions?
3. When I initiate collaboration, do others respond in a genuine way, or are there hidden agendas, unspoken hostility, and/or manipulation in the group?

If You Seldom Collaborate, Ask Yourself the Following Questions:

1. Do I ignore opportunities to cooperate, take risks, and creatively confront conflict?
2. Do I tend to be pessimistic, distrusting, withdrawing, and/or competitive?
3. Am I involving others in important decisions, eliciting commitment, and empowering them?

Commitment to Action

What two new behaviours would increase your collaboration effectiveness?

1.
2.

especially vulnerable to workplace conflict as they strive for acceptance, a fundamental part of the human condition (Dickerson et al., 2009), and report being unprepared to effectively address conflict (Latham et al., 2013). Students most frequently use avoidance and compromise as strategies to manage conflict (Pines et al., 2012); this results in unresolved emotional dissonance, which is a key distractor from thriving (Dames et al., 2018). See also Chapter 28 for how these student approaches coincide with role transition.

RESEARCH PERSPECTIVE

Resource: Chan, J. C. Y., Sit, E., N. M. & Lau, W. M. (2014). Conflict management styles, emotional intelligence, and implicit theories of personality of nursing students: A cross-sectional study. *Nurse Education Today*, 34(6), 934–939.

The purpose of this study was to examine undergraduate nursing students conflict management styles when navigating conflicts with their overseeing nurse/instructor in practicum settings. They also aimed to explore the association between emotional intelligence and personality with conflict management styles.

The study is relevant to all nurses, novice and otherwise, because conflict management, as opposed to avoidance, is an essential nursing skill that enables oneself to engage, despite differences, in authentic connection to self, patients, and colleagues in the work setting.

The research design was a cross-sectional quantitative survey with 568 undergraduate nursing students.

As for styles of conflict management, results demonstrated that when students faced conflict with their instructor/senior nurse they often resorted to obliging, collaborating, and dominating the least. Emotional intelligence was a significant predictor of which style was employed. Those with higher emotional intelligence were more likely to use integrating, compromising, and dominating. Those with less emotional intelligence were more likely to avoid the conflict. Furthermore, personality was significantly associated with compromising. Those with stronger personalities were less likely to compromise, compared with their more malleable peers.

Implications for Practice

The results of the study further enable nurses and nurse leaders to navigate conflict, even seeing the benefits, without being disabled by it. Emotional intelligence is significant in terms of which style of conflict management they will use. Personality was only associated with one's tendency to compromise.

Researchers have generally found that nurses and physicians do not routinely collaborate with each other during conflict situations (Brooks et al., 2014). Conflicts between nurses and physicians may be intensified because of communication breakdowns that prevent clarification of roles and issues where practice domains overlap (Brooks et al., 2014). Furthermore, when asked to describe working relationships with physicians, nurses frequently reported power imbalance as a dominant theme that supported major impediments to improving nurse–physician collaborative behaviours (Nair et al., 2012). Compromising strategies were found to be the most common conflict-handling approach to nurse–physician interactions. Finally, improving physician–nurse collaboration will likely enhance job satisfaction and reduce turnover among nurses (Zhang et al., 2016). These findings further emphasize that conflict is disruptive and influences clinical practice environments and patient safety (Brooks et al., 2014). Health care organizations need to strengthen healthy professional relationships and foster an organizational culture that embraces collaborative practice to promote flourishing work environments and, as a result, to safeguard positive patient outcomes.

THE ROLE OF THE LEADER

All nurses are leaders in their work environment, and in fact, informal leadership has a significant impact on work culture. Encouraging positive working relations among health care providers requires effective conflict management as an integral part of the practice environment (Lachman et al., 2012). The role of the manager or formal nurse leader is to foster a practice environment that empowers nurses to develop their capacity to lead, encourages open communication, collaborative practices for achieving mutual goals, and constructive approaches to conflict management (Ceravolo et al., 2012).

Many front-line nurses report feeling unprepared to take on leadership roles and have identified the need for organizations to provide ongoing education and competency development to enhance leadership abilities in front-line nurses (Sherman et al., 2011). Nurses at the front line are often change agents. They coordinate, integrate, and facilitate interprofessional and intraprofessional teamwork to ensure that quality patient care is provided (Porter-O'Grady, 2011). Front-line nurse leaders must have strong communication and organizational skills and must be approachable, emotionally intelligent, and have an ability to embrace others who may have different opinions and ways of being.

Nurse leaders promote positive clinical practice environments by promoting conflict prevention and supporting conflict resolution (Ceravolo et al., 2012). Nurse leaders model professionalism and empower employees by coaching nurses to think strategically about conflict resolution strategies and to respond to conflict in a timely manner and with carefully selected approaches. Disrespectful communications or miscommunications are common elements of conflict that can often be resolved with collaboration, active listening, and respectful assertive communication (Ceravolo et al., 2012). Furthermore, triangulated communication has become common practice in many nursing settings, where nurses avoid working out their conflicted feelings with the colleague that triggered them, going instead to other nurses or to the nurse manager. Nurse leaders can encourage collaboration by modeling direct, open, honest communication and demonstrating commitment to address conflict in a timely fashion (Spence Laschinger et al., 2014). Furthermore, work environments that promote authenticity and diversity tend to be less threatened by conflict, enabling employees to feel accepted and a sense of belonging despite differences in opinions and ways of being (Dames et al., 2018; Palmer, 2008).

The health care workforce today is made up of individuals from four generations, and generational differences in values, traits, expectations, communication style, and behaviour influence professional relationships (Leiter et al., 2010). These intergenerational tensions can sometimes lead to conflict. In nursing, individuals with a higher status, such as senior nurses, often from an older generation, tend to set emotional display rules and determine when these displays are appropriate (Porath & Pearson, 2012). Individuals that question these power imbalances, disturbing the status quo, are a risk of becoming targets of shaming and incivility. This pattern is often subtly supported by nurse leaders who fear diversity by discrediting the disturbers in a variety of ways, which eventually silences them (Jackson et al., 2002). Leaders can help establish workplace cultures that acknowledge generational differences by highlighting and building on the strengths this diversity brings while concurrently emphasizing common goals (Keepnews et al., 2010). Healthy work environments do not fear conflict; rather, they see it as a healthy component of authentic

relationships that honors diversity, and as a result, they are committed to productive and respectful resolution. To have employees that are willing to engage in conflict, as opposed to avoiding it, they must experience a sense of unconditional regard from their colleagues (Rogers, 1959). Unconditional positive regard is evident in environments that empower authenticity, seeing beauty in the mosaic of diverse backgrounds and personalities and an ability to navigate differences with compassion and respect. Employees must believe that they will not be shamed for bringing forward new ideas that challenge the status quo.

RESEARCH PERSPECTIVE

Resource: Almost, J., Doran, D. M., McGillis Hall, L., & Spence Laschinger, H. K. (2010). Antecedents and consequences of intra-group conflict among nurses. *Journal of Nursing Management, 18*(8), 981–982.

This study recognized that job dissatisfaction was linked to the negative impacts of conflict in nursing work settings, which has important implications for a workforce that is dealing and will continue to deal with a nursing shortage. To develop effective strategies aimed at mitigating the negative impact of conflict in the workplace, a greater understanding of the causes and outcomes is necessary.

The aim of this predictive, nonexperimental study was to test a theoretical model, which links antecedent variables (Fig. 24.2) to intragroup conflict, conflict management styles, and job stress among nurses.

The researchers recruited a random sample of 277 acute-care nurses, and the analysis revealed that self-evaluations, complexity of care, and their relationships with their nurse manager and colleagues correlated with the perceived degree of conflict they experienced. Furthermore, their conflict management style partially buffered them from job dissatisfaction, and job stress was directly tied to job satisfaction. Finally, self-evaluation directly affected one's perceived degree of job stress.

Implications for Practice

Conflict is complex and is tied to one's disposition, context, and interpersonal factors. Conflict cannot and should not be prevented, as it is a natural part of a culture that embraces diversity. However, learning to manage it via collaboration and accommodation can improve job satisfaction among nurses. The implications for nursing management is that strategies that aim to manage and reduce the negative impacts of conflict include promoting work cultures that promote interactional justice practices and celebrate positive interpersonal relationships.

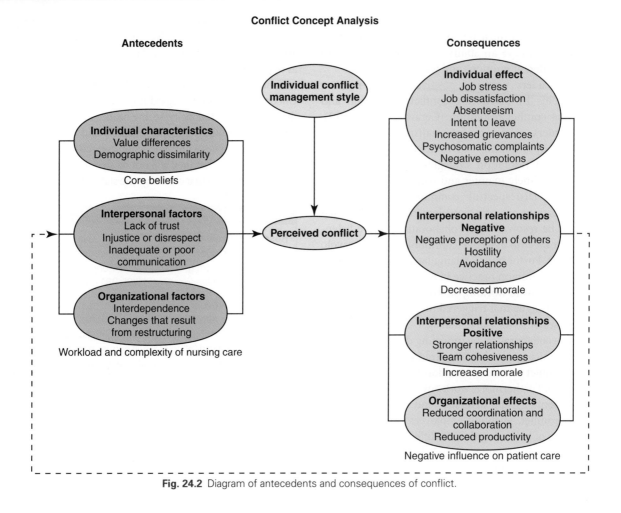

Fig. 24.2 Diagram of antecedents and consequences of conflict.

Nurse managers often do not invest enough time into assessing the workplace culture, and specifically the conflict management habits of employees. Many do not feel qualified or sufficiently experienced to deal with conflict (Becher & Visovsky, 2012). Moreover, some staff can be difficult to work with, so managers must remain focused on the problem and not the personalities of the team members. Nurse managers must quickly address and intervene in conflict and lateral violence. They must also remain cognizant of other pitfalls of effective conflict resolution. For example, nurse managers commonly avoid conflict in the workplace by delaying responding to colleagues' concerns voiced in staff meetings, not replying to voice mails or e-mail messages, or cancelling or postponing important meetings. Equally harmful, they may encourage

triangulated communication, whereby employees report their grievances about one another to the manager instead of addressing each other directly. However, if this behaviour is known and continues, conflict remains, and the avoiding behaviour becomes acceptable and leads to poor outcomes for the individuals involved, patients, and the organization (Johansen, 2012). To reduce conflict and the incidence of workplace violence, the leader must empower employees to create a respectful practice climate while at the same time set acceptable standards of behaviour (Spence Laschinger et al., 2014). Zero-tolerance policies can be helpful to underscore certain organization values, ensuring that employees are aware that certain behaviors will not be tolerated. However, this methodology tends to work by instilling fear in employees, which can be detrimental to

BOX 24.8   Leadership Principles Behind Strong Indigenous Communities

Indigenous women from Canada, the United States, and New Zealand wrote this book, representing a variety of influences. It explores the leadership principles behind strong Indigenous communities. For the purpose of this chapter, only conflict management styles will be addressed.

The first nations Indigenous leadership model honors the process from which people move from awareness to interaction to mastery. It encourages one to go inside first and then to exercise goodness when relating to others. Conflict is viewed as a normal and productive part of interpersonal relationships, which when used in positive fashion can birth creative solutions and greater group cohesiveness. Furthermore, leadership, whether formal or informal, requires one to risk that conflict may occur, but the priority focus is to reach an outcome that is for the good of all. This is couched in the principle that one above all stays focused on the whole, as opposed to a western tendency to focus on the individual.

Source: Kenny, C., Fraser, T. N. (2012). *Living Indigenous leadership: Native narratives on building strong communities.* Vancouver, BC: University of British Columbia Press.

BOX 24.9   Core Indigenous Ethics: Reciprocity and Interconnectedness

Reciprocity is a core principle within indigenous ways of knowing and being, taking only what one needs with a focus on giving back. Being in relationship includes how one interacts with the land, the water, and all objects and beings, which is celebrated and honored through spiritual traditions and ceremonies. It is believed that hardship will follow if one deviates from practicing reciprocity, whereby they do not honor and respect the interdependent nature of kin, indigenous neighbors, and all of creation.

Source: McNeil-Seymour, J. (2017). Two-spirit resistance. In *Whose land is it anyway? A manual for decolonization.* Retrieved from http://www.fpse.ca/sites/default/files/news_files/Decolonization%20Handbook.pdf.

feelings of emotional safety and a willingness to be authentic in the workplace.

Working in teams is an important part of health care delivery. Negative relationships among colleagues can disrupt team performance, ultimately compromising patient safety (Becher & Visovsky, 2012). For teams to be successful, they need to work independently of managers, receiving direction and interventions when needed. Functional teams working together will initiate meetings and implement decision-making procedures (actions emphasizing participatory management) that promote the sharing of ideas, a sense of ownership, and are able to self-direct. When teams begin to lose focus and cohesiveness, they may be signaling the need for further support and direction from a manager (Boxes 24.8 and 24.9).

MEDIATION VIA NEGOTIATION

When those close to its source cannot manage the conflict, mediation—a process using a trained third

party to assist with conflict resolution—may occur. Mediation is a learned skill for which advanced training and/or certification is available. Principled negotiation can produce mutually acceptable agreements in every type of conflict. The method involves separating the people from the problem; focusing on interests, not positions; inventing options for mutual gain; and insisting on using objective criteria. The mediator is an impartial individual who assists those involved in the conflict to better hear and understand one another. Mediation helps reduce the focus on who can control whom and on a "winner." In clinical practice environments, negotiating conflicts may be more difficult when at least one of the parties is on an unequal or uneven playing field. These inequalities are made worse when they are not acknowledged as part of the problem.

MANAGING SOCIAL DOMINANCE

A significant source of interpersonal conflict in the workplace stems from social dominance, which in nursing is often referred to as *lateral, horizontal violence,* or *bullying.* Social dominance is exercised through shaming and intimidation, verbal abuse, overreporting, excluding behavior, less favorable work assignments, denying career opportunities, and withholding information. Social dominance typically stems from subconscious projections, whereby one's insecurities motivate them to establish a dominant position over the peers they feel threatened by (Dames et al., 2018). The literature identifies several common forms of lateral violence, such as criticizing a colleague, belittling or making hurtful comments to or about a colleague in front of others, complaining about a colleague, rolling eyes, or simply ignoring a colleague (Mitchell et al., 2014). **Bullying** is another form of social dominance, closely related to lateral or horizontal violence, but a real or perceived power differential between the instigator and recipient must be present in bullying. Acts of bullying are associated with psychologic and physical stress, underperformance, professional disengagement, increased job turnover, and the potential for diminished quality of care (Vessey et al., 2009). Finally, it is important to remember that social dominance occurs because hurt people hurt people (Wilson, 2015). Therefore it is best diffused via a compassionate response that enables those who are instigating the lateral violence to address the roots of their insecurity.

Gordon et al., (2013) found that transitioning from one nursing role to another could precipitate intraprofessional conflict between nursing colleagues. Mutual respect is imperative, including embracing as opposed to being threatened by others who have different opinions and values; an absence of this produces work cultures that are perfectionistic and often rampant with implicit shaming aimed at snuffing out diversity. Nursing students and inexperienced nurses are especially vulnerable to social dominance and are generally not prepared to effectively handle it (Latham et al., 2013). Newly graduated nurses and students depend on collegial support because of their lack of familiarity with the work environment and work tasks, which makes them especially vulnerable to conflict horizontal/lateral violence (Johnson, 2010; King-Jones, 2011). Unfortunately, this scenario lays the groundwork for a victim–perpetrator cycle, which is a well-established pattern in many nursing cultures. This is evident in that those who are most vulnerable, such as students and novice nurses, become accustomed to being treated as "less than" in nursing environments. Overtime, as they move from novice to expert and begin to garner social capital and as a result, they climb the hierarchy, and subconsciously many will perpetuate the same pattern by treating students and novice nurses in the same manner they were treated. See Chapters 28 and 32 for further discussion on student transition.

Many nurses who suffer from emotional exhaustion and burnout become chronically hostile and remain in the field. When employees continued to work in a burned-out condition, it causes ripple effects of adverse consequences for themselves, work teams, and clients. This scenario perpetuates lateral violence, with more nurses hurting each other and perpetuating the cycle of hostility in the workplace (Spence Laschinger et al., 2014). The CNA and the Canadian Federation of Nurses Unions (2015) jointly affirmed that workplace violence includes actual and attempted incidents of verbal and psychologic abuse (including bullying), and that such violence negatively affects all health care providers, patients, and organizations. They recommend that leaders in health care organizations address these behaviours, advocate for collaborative and all-inclusive practice environments, and seek to eliminate violence.

Conflict resolution must be encouraged and supported, avoiding triangulated communication whenever possible, as this erodes trust and a sense of emotional safety in the workplace. However, there are certain situations where direct communication has not been effective, or when the risks of confronting a colleague directly may outweigh the benefits; for these situations, a mechanism for confidential reporting is also necessary.

A primary factor that influences one's ability to engage in authentic relationships at work and frequent moments of thriving is the habitual practice of self-compassion, which is described earlier. Self-compassion acts as a buffer against the stress produced from making mistakes, role ambiguity, and negative feedback from co-workers. Ultimately, those that can view themselves in a compassionate might appear to be better able to resolve workplace stimuli and to prevent rumination on negative self-talk before it became disabling. Those who habitually practice self-compassion naturally demonstrate compassion toward others, as opposed to gravitating toward social dominance in times of uncertainty.

Increased awareness of the types and sources of conflict and the development of emotional intelligence/congruence and self-compassion are imperative to improve conflict resolution efforts in professional practice environments. Ultimately, healthy work environments require a committed, compassionate, emotionally intelligent leader and organizational supported training. Leadership training is essential in building competencies in how to recognize and defend against lateral violence (Johansen, 2012).

> **EXERCISE 24.3** Consider a conflict you would describe as "ongoing" in a learning or clinical setting. Reflect on the issue in terms of the concepts presented in this chapter. Consult with people involved in the conflict to get their perspective on this issue. Once you have gathered the details, consider the following questions:
> - What are their positions and years of experience?
> - How are resources, time, and personnel wasted on mismanaging this issue?
> - What blocks the effective management of this issue?
> - What currently aids in its management?
> - What new things and actions would add to its management in the future?

ⓘ A SOLUTION

Conflict can be uncomfortable, but learning about conflict and developing conflict resolution strategies can build your skills and confidence to effectively handle these situations. Furthermore, conflict has benefits, as it provides an opportunity to reflect on values and often reveals unresolved dissonance from the past, which if embraced, can potentially be resolved. Mark analyzed the way he was dealing with the negativity in the workplace and, after completing a conflict self-assessment, he realized that he was avoiding the conflict. His ability to care for patients was being impacted by the resulting hostility, and because his attempts to address the conflict directly were not successful, he knew he needed to get help. He approached his nurse manager and, without naming individuals, described the conflict he was having. The nurse manager first ensured that he made an attempt to address the situation directly to avoid triangulation, which can erode trust and fuel hostility in work teams. She assured Mark that he had a right to a workplace free of psychological violence and that the hospital was committed to preventing such a workplace. The nurse manager referred him to free counseling through the human resources department and assured him that his concerns would be followed up on. Mark felt that he had been heard and that his feelings and thoughts were important to the nurse manager. He is seeing a counselor, who is supporting him in processing his emotions and developing the self-compassion and self-efficacy required to be more assertive in the workplace. These practices are helping Mark develop the skills and willingness to address and better manage the conflict.

Was this approach effective in this situation? How does this approach to handling conflict align with your preferred conflict management style? Why or why not?

▮ THE EVIDENCE

Conflict is inherent in the professional practice environment and has both positive and negative outcomes for nurses and other health care providers, organizations, and even patients. Lateral violence is toxic to the profession. Lateral violence is often rampant in perfectionistic and homogenizing cultures (Dames et al., 2018; Palmer, 2008) and causes physical and psychologic effects on nurses, as well as negative outcomes for patients. Lateral violence festers in environments of fear, where employees feel they must put on an image that is not authentic to their genuine values and emotions. Real change occurs by promoting authenticity, developing a culture where nurses feel a sense of unconditional positive regard for one another (Rogers, 1959). Nurses must explore their own emotional dissonance with self-compassion, which also prevents them from socially ascribing perfectionistic standards on their colleagues. Addressing lateral violence starts by addressing the incongruence individual nurses first; congruent nurses naturally produce congruent work settings. As described previously, congruence describes an alignment between one's real and ideal selves. The further apart one's real self is from one's ideal self, the less authentic they feel they can be. Adding to this, incongruence is perpetuated by low levels of self-compassion and high levels of perfectionism (Dames et al., 2018). Furthermore, when cultures promote humility, whereby individuals begin by reflecting on their own dissonance and related projections, there is a reduction in the tendency to blame and shame others.

Finally, the need for a culture change to take lateral violence seriously has been endorsed by a number of professional organizations, including the CNA, the Canadian Federation of Nurses Unions, and the International Council of Nurses. Nurses must first address their own developmental vulnerabilities related to gaining emotional congruence/intelligence (Dames et al., 2018) to eliminate hostile work environments, workplace intimidation, reality shock for new graduates, and accepted notions of "nurses eating their young."

❋ NEED TO KNOW NOW

- Know how to assess conflict and its circumstances to determine which approach to conflict resolution is potentially most effective.
- Take an inventory of your own emotional vulnerabilities and how they may impact your willingness to address conflict among your colleagues.

- Identify and offer appropriate behaviours to prevent or resolve conflict in your practice environment.
- Evaluate your practice environment for situations reflecting lateral violence. Be proactive and know how to respond to a colleague who demonstrates lateral violence.

CHAPTER CHECKLIST

A more thorough understanding of conflict within the professional practice environment will enable the nurse to prevent or successfully manage nonproductive conflict. Navigating desirable conflict within the work environment will promote change, resulting in organizational growth and personal and professional enrichment of nurses.

- The three types of conflict are as follows:
  - Intrapersonal
  - Interpersonal
  - Organizational
- The conflict process progresses through four stages:
  - Frustration:
    - Blocked goals lead to frustration.
    - Frustration is a cue to stop and clarify differences.
  - Conceptualization:
    - The way a person perceives a conflict determines how he or she reacts to the frustration.
    - Differences in conceptualizing an issue can block resolution.
  - Action:
    - Intentions, strategies, plans, and behaviour are formulated.
  - Outcomes:
    - They include both tangible and intangible consequences.

- When assessing how well a conflict has been resolved, one must consider the following:
  - The quality of decisions, including the degree to which important goals were achieved by assessing the outcomes
  - The quality of relationships, including how willing people involved in the conflict are to work together
  - The five modes of conflict resolution are as follows:
    - Integrating/collaborating (respect of self and others)
    - Dominating/competing (less respect for others)
    - Obliging/accommodating (less respect for self)
    - Avoiding (less respect for self and others)
    - Compromising (moderate respect for both)
- Each mode of conflict resolution can be viewed along two dimensions:
  - From uncooperative to highly cooperative
  - From unassertive to highly assertive
- The role of the nurse manager is to foster a practice environment that encourages open communication, collaborative practices for achieving mutual goals, and constructive approaches to conflict management.

▐ TIPS FOR ADDRESSING CONFLICT

- Remember that conflict is a naturally and beneficial process toward developing individuals and improving organizations.
- Acknowledge that frustration and different conceptualizations are normal and that there are a variety of approaches to resolving it.
- Assess the work environment to see what behaviours are endorsed and fostered by the manager. Determine if these behaviours align with your goals and values.
- Determine any similarities and differences in facts, goals, methods, and values in sorting out the different conceptualizations of a conflict situation.
- Assess the degree of conflict resolution by reflecting on the quality of the decisions (e.g., creativity, practicality, achievement of goals, productive results) and the quality of the relationships (e.g., understanding, willingness to work together, mutual respect, cooperation).
- Reflect on your preferred strategies for resolving conflict. For example, which of the five approaches do you not use often enough and which do you overuse?

- Assess each situation to match the best approach for that type of conflict regardless of which is your favourite approach.
- Model collaborative conflict resolution practices and assist others to do the same, while careful to avoid triangulated communication.
- Commit to addressing and confronting disruptive behaviours.
- View conflict as an opportunity to grow as a person and a professional, recognizing that conflict often illuminates areas of unresolved emotional dissonance from previous life events. Do your part in fostering a healthy work environment that embraces diversity and inclusion.
- Speak out about violence to help increase awareness and knowledge.
- Consider "zero tolerance" policies to underscore the commitment to addressing violence and hostility in the workplace. These need to be implemented in an informed and compassionate manner, as opposed to perpetuating cultural shaming.

Visit the Evolve website for Suggested Readings, Internet Resources, and additional resources related to the content in this chapter: http://evolve.elsevier.com/Canada/Yoder-Wise/leading/.

REFERENCES

Almost, J., Doran, D. M., McGillis Hall, L., & Spence Laschinger, H. K. (2010). Antecedents and consequences of intra-group conflict among nurses. *Journal of Nursing Management, 18*(8), 981–982.

Barsky, A. (2016). *Conflict resolution for the helping profession: Negotiation, mediation, advocacy, facilitation, and restorative justice* (3rd ed.). Oxford: Oxford University Press.

Becher, J., & Visovsky, C. (2012). Horizontal violence in nursing. *MEDSURG Nursing, 21*(4), 210–232.

Bennett, K., & Sawatzky, J. A. (2013). Building emotional intelligence: A strategy for emerging nurse leaders to reduce workplace bullying. *Nursing Administration Quarterly, 37*(2), 144–151.

Berwick, D. (2011). Preparing nurses for participation in and leadership of continual improvement. *Journal of Nursing Education, 50*(6), 322–327.

Blair, P. (2013). Lateral violence in nursing. *Journal of Emergency Nursing, 39*(5), e75–e78.

Blake, R. R., & Mouton, J. S. (1964). *Solving costly organization conflict.* San Francisco, CA: Jossey-Bass.

Brooks, A. M. T., Polis, N., & Phillips, E. (2014). The new healthcare landscape: Disruptive behaviors influence work environment, safety and clinical outcomes. *Nurse Leader, 12*(1), 39–44.

Canadian Nurses Association (CNA). (2009, October). *Position statement: Nursing leadership.* Retrieved from http://www.nanb.nb.ca/PDF/CNA_Nursing_Leadership_2009_E.pdf.

Canadian Nurses Association & Canadian Federation of Nurses Unions. (2015). *Joint position statement: Workplace violence.* Retrieved from https://cna-aiic.ca/policy-advocacy/policy-support-resources/policy-support-tools/cna-position-statements.

Ceravolo, D. J., Schwartz, D. G., Foltz-Ramos, K. M., et al. (2012). Strengthening communication to overcome lateral violence. *Journal of Nursing Management, 20*(5), 599–606.

Chan, J. C. Y., Sit, E. N. M., & Lau, W. M. (2014). Conflict management styles, emotional intelligence, and implicit theories of personality of nursing students: A cross-sectional study. *Nurse Education today, 34*(6), 934–939.

Dames, S., Groen, J., Raffin-Bouchal, S., & Kawalilak, C. (2018). *A study of the interplay between new graduate life experience, context, and the experience of stress in the workplace: Exploring factors towards self-actualizing as a novice nurse.* Calgary: Werklund School of Education.

Deutsch, M. (1973). *The resolution of conflict: Constructive and destructive processes.* New Haven, CT: Yale University Press.

Dickerson, S. S., Gruenewald, T. L., & Kemeny, M. E. (2009). Psychobiological responses to social self-threat: Functional or detrimental? *Self and Identity, 8*(2), 270–285.

Duffy, E. (1995). Horizontal violence: A conundrum for nursing. *Journal of the Royal College of Nursing, 2*(2), 5–17.

Friese, C. R., & Manojlovich, M. (2012). Nurse–physician relationship in ambulatory oncology settings. *Journal of Nursing Scholarship, 44*(3), 258–265.

Gazelle, G., Liebschutz, J. M., & Riess, H. (2015). Physician burnout: Coaching a way out. *Journal of General Internal Medicine, 30*(4), 508.

Gordon, K., Melrose, S., Janzen, K. J., et al. (2013). Licensed practical nurses becoming registered nurses: Conflicts and responses that can help. *Clinical Nursing Studies, 1*(4), 1–8.

Gunnell, K. E., Mosewich, A. D., McEwen, C. E., Eklund, R. C., & Crocker, P. R. E. (2017). Don't be so hard on yourself! Changes in self-compassion during the first year of university are associated with changes in well being. *Personality and Individual Differences, 107*, 43–48.

Hurst, J., & Kinney, M. (1989). *Empowering self and others.* Toledo, OH: University of Toledo Press.

Hurst, J. B. (1993). *Conflict self-assessment.* Toledo, OH: Human Resource Development Center, University of Toledo.

Iglesias, M. E. L., & Vallejo, R. B. B. (2012). Conflict resolution styles in the nursing profession. *Contemporary Nurse, 43*(1), 73–80.

Jackson, D., Clare, J., & Mannix, J. (2002). Who would want to be a nurse? Violence in the workplace – a factor in recruitment and retention. *Journal of Nursing Management, 10*(1), 13–20.

Jackson, D., Hutchinson, M., Peters, K., et al. (2013). Understanding avoidant leadership in healthcare: Findings form a secondary analysis of two qualitative studies. *Journal of Nursing Management, 21*(3), 572–580.

Johansen, M. L. (2012). Keeping the peace. Conflict management strategies for nurse managers. *Nursing Management, 43*(2), 50–54.

Johnson, M. (2010). The bullying aspect of workplace violence in nursing. *JONA's Healthcare Law, Ethics and Regulation, 12*(2), 36–42.

Keepnews, D. M., Brewer, C. S., Kovner, C. T., et al. (2010). Generational differences among newly licensed registered nurses. *Nursing Outlook, 58*(3), 155–163.

Kenny, C., & Fraser, T. N. (2012). *Living indigenous leadership: Native narratives on building strong communities.* Vancouver, BC: University of British Columbia Press.

King-Jones, M. (2011). Horizontal violence and the socialization of new nurses. *Creative Nursing, 17*(2), 80–86.

Lachman, V., Murray, J. S., Iseminger, K., et al. (2012). Doing the right thing: Pathways to moral courage. *American Nurse Today, 7*(5), 24–29.

Latham, C. L., Ringl, K., & Hogan, M. (2013). Combating workplace violence with peer mentoring. *Nursing Management, 44*(9), 30–38.

Leiter, M. P., Price, S. L., & Spence Laschinger, H. K. (2010). Generational differences in distress, attitudes and civility among nurses. *Journal of Nursing Management, 18*(8), 970–980.

Mahon, N. M., & Nicotera, A. M. (2011). Nursing and conflict communication: Avoidance as preferred strategy. *Nursing Administration Quarterly, 35*(2), 152–163.

Mazurek Melnyk, B., Hrabe, D. P., & Szalacha, L. A. (2013). Relationships among work stress, job satisfaction, mental health and healthy lifestyle behaviors in new graduate nurses attending the nurse athlete program. *Nursing Administration Quarterly, 37*(4), 278–285.

McNeil-Seymour, J. (2017). Two-spirit resistance. In *Whose land is it anyway? A manual for decolonization* Retrieved from http://www.fpse.ca/sites/default/files/news_files/Decolonization%20Handbook.pdf.

Mitchell, A., Ahmed, A., & Szabo, C. (2014). Workplace violence among nurses, why are we still discussing this? Literature review. *Journal of Nursing Education and Practice, 4*(4), 147–150.

Montero-Marin, J., Zubiaga, F., Cereceda, M., et al. (2016). Burnout subtypes and absence of self-compassion in primary healthcare professionals: A cross-sectional study. *PloS One, 11*(6), e0157499.

Nair, D. M., Fitzpatrick, J. K., McNulty, R., et al. (2012). Frequency of nurse–physician collaborative behaviors in acute care hospital. *Journal of Interprofessional Care, 26*(2), 115–120.

Palmer, P. J. (2008). *A hidden wholeness: The journey toward an undivided life: Welcoming the soul and weaving community in a wounded world.* San Francisco, CA: Jossey-Bass.

Palmer, P. J., Zajonc, A., & Scribner, M. (2010). *The heart of higher education: A call to renewal.* Retrieved from https://ebookcentral.proquest.com.

Pines, E. W., Rauschhuber, G. H., Norgan, J. D., et al. (2012). Stress resiliency, psychological empowerment and conflict management styles among baccalaureate nursing students. *Journal of Advanced Nursing, 68*(7), 1482–1493.

Porath, C. L., & Pearson, C. M. (2012). Emotional and behavioral responses to workplace incivility and the impact of hierarchical status. *Journal of Applied Social Psychology, 42*, 326–357.

Porter-O'Grady, T. (2011). Leadership at all levels. *Nursing Management, 42*(5), 32–37.

Roche, M., Diers, D., Duffield, C., et al. (2010). Violence toward nurses, the work environment, and patient outcomes. *Journal of Nursing Scholarship, 42*(1), 13–22.

Rogers, C. (1959). A theory of therapy, personality and interpersonal relationships as developed in the client-centered framework. In S. Koch (Ed.), *Psychology: A study of a science* (Vol. 3). New York: McGraw Hill.

Sherman, R., & Pross, E. (2010). Growing future nurse leaders to build and sustain healthy work environments at the unit level. *Online Journal of Issues in Nursing, 15*(1), Manuscript 1. https://doi.org/10.3912/OJIN.Vol15No01Man01.

Sherman, R., Schwarzkopf, R., & Kiger, A. J. (2011). Charge nurse perspectives on frontline leadership in acute care environments. *International Scholarly Research Network Nursing, 2011.* https://doi.org/10.5402/2011/164052.

Spence Laschinger, H. K., Cummings, G. C., Wong, C. A., et al. (2014). Resonant leadership and workplace empowerment: The value of positive organizational cultures in reducing workplace incivility. *Nursing Economics, 32*(1), 5–16.

Thomas, K. W. (1992). Conflict and conflict management: Reflections and update. *Journal of Organizational Behavior, 13*(3), 265–274.

Vessey, J. A., DeMarco, R. F., Gaffney, D. A., et al. (2009). Bullying of staff registered nurses in the workplace: A preliminary study for developing strategies for the transformation of hostile to healthy workplace environments. *Journal of Professional Nursing, 25*(5), 299–306.

Wilson, S. D. (2015). *Hurt people hurt people: Hope and healing for yourself and your relationships.* Grand Rapids, MI: Discovery House Publishers.

Wolff, A. C., Ratner, P. A., Robinson, S. L., et al. (2010). Beyond generational differences: A literature review of the impact of relational diversity on nurses' attitudes on work. *Journal of Nursing Management, 18*(8), 948–969.

Zhang, L., Huang, L., Liu, M., Yan, H., & Li, X. (2016). Nurse–physician collaboration impacts job satisfaction and turnover among nurses: A hospital-based cross-sectional study in Beijing. *International Journal of Nursing Practice, 22*(3), 284–290.

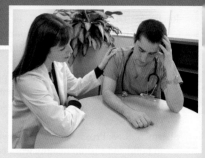

25

Managing Personnel Challenges

Shannon Dames

This chapter discusses various personnel obstacles that nurses in formal leadership roles are tasked with navigating. It provides insights and tools to better understand the roots of employer-employee conflict and how it can be proactively managed. Emphasis is placed on effective communication, both written and verbal. In this chapter, the term "manager" represents all formal nurse leadership/supervisory roles.

OBJECTIVES

- Describe common personnel obstacles to navigate.
- Describe how clarifying role expectations can help resolve personnel conflicts.
- Understand strategies that are useful in approaching specific personnel challenges.
- Understand the steps involved in nonpunitive and progressive discipline.
- Describe the guidelines that should be followed when terminating an employee.
- Describe how to document performance concerns.
- Recognize the implicit leadership role that all nurses hold.

TERMS TO KNOW

absenteeism	grievance	role strain
chemical dependency	nonpunitive discipline	role stress
congruence	progressive discipline	

❓ A CHALLENGE

Tanya started their new job as a resource float pool nurse with a shift on the mother baby unit. While taking care of the mother and her newborn, Tanya noticed that the newborn was jittery, irritable, and having difficulties with breastfeeding, even after several attempts. Tanya was focused on caring for the mother and used most of their time to reassure her and to assist her with positioning the newborn at the breast. Later in the shift, the nurse manager was checking in on Tanya and their patients and noticed that the newborn was jittery. After discussing the progress of the newborn's breastfeeding and reviewing the birth weight with Tanya, the manager inquired about the newborn's blood glucose level. Tanya had not checked the newborn's blood glucose level, as they were unaware of the protocol. They felt terrible and questioned their competency to continue working on the mother baby unit.

Consider this scenario from the viewpoint of nurse manager. What are your thoughts about this situation, and how might you manage it?

INTRODUCTION

Novice nurses often need an extensive orientation, mentoring, and a period of reduced workload that acknowledges inefficiencies. In addition, they often require coaching for ongoing knowledge development and determining when to ask for guidance and when to directly involve their more experienced colleagues to ensure patient safety. (See Chapter 32 for further discussion on the student-to-resistered-nurse transition experience). If nurses fear they will be criticized for requiring support for practice competency or labeled as incompetent if they ask a question or make a mistake, they will be less likely to reach out for help during times of uncertainty. These conditions lead to what has been termed *imposter syndrome*, preventing one from being authentic, and resulting in an increased risk of mistakes and emotional burnout. Novice nurses often feel this tension between their fears of being authentic in work environments that feel critical or perfectionistic, and wanting to ensure they are practicing safely. Maslow's hierarchy of needs (1943) illustrates this tension, whereby a sense of belonging and esteem are requirements of being human; thereby nurses will subconsciously avoid situations that put these basic needs at risk. When basic needs are met via working conditions where unconditional positive regard is felt, workers and work cultures promote emotional congruence (Rogers, 1959), whereby employees feel safe to be their authentic/real self. Congruency occurs when one is accepted for one's 'real' self as opposed to an 'ideal' self that lacks authenticity and which acts as a barrier to their ability to self-actualize or thrive in their novice nurse role.

Nursing teams work collaboratively with a multitude of specialties to address the complexities of acute and community health care delivery in Canada. Most settings will include Registered Nurses (RN), Licensed Practical Nurses (LPN), and care aids, all of which take on different roles within the care setting. Nurse managers also assume responsibility for other staff members, such as housekeeping staff, dietary service workers, and other allied health professionals. The role of the nurse manager spans a plethora of duties that requires advanced critical thinking capacity and emotional congruence. When emotionally charged issues or events occur, the nurse manager must find the balance of honoring their own emotions while navigating the challenge from a relatively objective perspective; this may require outside counsel.

Effective nurse managers empower employees to thrive by providing safe and nurturing communities of practice that support authentic and diverse ways of being, a sense of acceptance and belonging, and respectful communication norms (Dames et al., 2018; Palmer, 2008). As a natural outcome of flourishing work environments, the team will work together to maintain a high standard of patient care in a supportive, safe environment that enables nurses to ask for help when needed, and connect with and fulfill their calling as a nurse. As a result, they are more likely to preserve the dignity of all and promote justice even when addressing difficult issues and taking action that potentially creates moral distress about participants' perceptions, observations and experiences of nurses who are impaired at work. (Canadian Nurses Association [CNA], 2017). Finally, nurse managers who invest time on the frontline will have a greater understanding of nurse vulnerabilities, which makes them more likely to be *pro*actively addressed, as opposed to *re*acting to quality care issues, toxic work cultures, and other downstream consequences that occur as a result.

Some common personnel challenges experienced by nurses include absenteeism, uncooperative or unproductive employees, clinical malpractice, lack of competence, and mental and physical health challenges. These challenges must be carefully managed while providing a safe space for employees to be authentic, honoring their personhood, and minimizing the impact on patient care and staff morale. Finally, documentation is essential to ensure continuity of care and regulation of practice, both of which are critical aspects of quality nursing care. Accurate and thorough documentation of performance problems or any conflict within the professional practice environment is imperative when formal actions need to be taken to address personnel issues and workplace safety concerns (College of Nurses of Ontario, 2013; Longo, 2010). In this chapter, it is from this perspective that management challenges and the roles and responsibilities of the novice nurse are examined.

PERSONNEL OBSTACLES: ABSENTEEISM

The term absenteeism describes the rate at which nurses miss work because of unplanned events. Because most absences are last minute in nature, managers are often left scrambling to fill vacancies. Although absenteeism cannot be eliminated altogether, it can be minimized by managing workloads, proactively addressing unusually high rates of absenteeism, and working toward an authentic and respectful work environment. When nursing teams work short, nurses must take on additional patients to cover the absent member, which impacts staff morale and potentially compromises patient care. Furthermore, even when nurses are redeployed from other areas, they are often unfamiliar with the workplace routines, which also impacts morale, productivity, and patient care.

With the current and impending threat of a nursing shortage in Canada, absenteeism is especially concerning because inadequate staffing leads to fatigue, which then leads to an increase in absenteeism. Once the cycle has begun, it is difficult to control, and it has significant impact on morale relating to working short staffed. In addition, absenteeism has steep financial costs because of having to fill vacancies with nurses on overtime, which compromises support for other creative efforts of the unit, such as staff education or the ability to purchase new equipment. Finally, nurses who miss breaks, stay late, and pick up additional shifts in response to staffing needs have a higher likelihood of fatigue, which can lead to calling in sick for future shifts, and so the cycle is perpetuated.

Research indicates that nurse managers tend to avoid taking meaningful action because of fears of conflict, providing an ambivalent response and as a result, the problem is frequently left to fester (Jackson et al., 2013). However, nurse managers can compassionately address absenteeism by discussing the situation directly with the employee (refer to Chapter 25), by seeking understanding as to why the absenteeism is occurring, and by clearly communicating concerns:

- "I am concerned about you. You seem to be more stressed at work and I see that you have been absent 3 days this month."
- "I think there is a way to support your self-care, while also ensuring that we have enough staff on the unit to manage the workload of other team members and the safety of patients."
- "How can we work together to proactively reduce these absences?"

There will always be unplanned illnesses, accidents, bad weather, sick family members, a death in the family, and even jury duty, all of which are legitimate reasons for missing work and that are beyond the control of management. Adding to this, difficult personal situations can cause nurses to experience **role stress**, feeling unable to adequately manage stressors and a perceived inability to fulfill an important life role. Because nurses have a diversity of life roles, role stress can occur inside or outside of their nursing role, both of which impact their ability to thrive at work. Absenteeism may also indicate an employee's dissatisfaction with work; this is of particular concern because a disengaged nurse often has to put on an emotional display that does not align with their authentic feelings, making them more at risk for burnout (Hochschild, 2012). Furthermore, it prevents one's ability to authentically connect with their patients and co-workers, which impacts patient care and morale. If the nurse manager believes that an issue is related to work dissatisfaction, team meetings and one-on-one discussion may lead to insight about the source of the issue. These discussions are an opportunity to illuminate whether a stressor can be removed or better managed, and whether there are other underlying issues that need to be addressed. Doing so may help the organization implement strategies to prevent the loss of dissatisfied employees. Some employees who remain chronically dissatisfied may require outside counsel to better understand the roots of their discontentment. Ultimately, challenges and solutions will be unique to each situation, but if the manager can remain compassionate and open, as opposed to feeling threatened by the situation and/or the employee, it can deescalate the power battles that often get in the way of meaningful resolution.

When the root of a stressor is revealed, one must then determine if the stressor can be removed, and if it cannot be removed, if employees and managers can work together to manage and mitigate the impact. Essentially, the goal is to transform a perceived stressor into stimuli that can be managed. Although removal is ideal in terms of the most effective way to manage stress, the second-best option is to reorient oneself, whereby the stimuli is optimistically viewed as a challenge that they have the skills to navigate (Troy, 2015). The Serenity Prayer, written in 1943 by Reinhold Niebuhr, is a widely adopted frame of mind and reflects this timeless sentiment, "God, give us the grace to accept with serenity the things that cannot be changed, the courage to change the things that should be changed, and the wisdom to distinguish one from the other" (Sifton, 1998).

When workplace stimuli are perceived as threatening to the nurses' esteem, it often relates to incongruence, or a misalignment between one's nursing reality and their nursing ideals; this results in role stress, which is fueled by shame and anxiety. Other threatening stimuli can relate to unmet physiologic needs, such as missing food/water/rest breaks, and a sense of belonging on the nursing team. Furthermore, those who are less congruent in nature are more prone to perfectionism; therefore they are apt to perceive workplace changes/events/stimuli as threatening stressors, as opposed to their more congruent counterparts, who navigate the stimuli before it becomes a stressor (Dames et al., 2018).

Role strain is the emotional dissonance or anxiety experienced as a result of role stress; it often leads to: (1) withdrawal from interaction with patients, colleagues, and the organization, (2) decreased commitment to the mission and the team, and (3) job dissatisfaction. All of these factors could also be manifested through absenteeism, whereby nurses call in sick to avoid the strain they are experiencing in the workplace. For employees to continue thriving as a nurse, they must feel authentically called and connected to their role, which enables them to remain present, and to sustain energy stores by tapping into their passion throughout the day. Furthermore, role strain correlates with incongruence, low levels of self-compassion, risks of maladaptive perfectionism, and rumination on self-destructive thoughts. To adequately address the root of absenteeism, individually or within a nursing team, the nurse manager needs to understand the culture, the current situation, the context surrounding the situation, and what is needed to better support change. When employees are congruent and satisfied with their work, they are more likely to thrive in their role and are more committed to their co-workers and their employer.

> **EXERCISE 25.1** Interview a nurse who supervises other employees in your clinical placement or local health region and inquire about their experience with absenteeism. Find out what strategies and processes the nurse manager uses when dealing with chronic absenteeism. What are the possible consequences for employees who are chronically absent from work?

PERSONNEL OBSTACLES: LACK OF COOPERATION AND PRODUCTIVITY

Nurse managers are often faced with situations where certain employees appear to resist change efforts or are less productive than their peers. Two major dimensions of job performance that relate to this problem are motivation and ability (Hersey et al., 2008). Employee motivation is a significant element in organizational performance.

Motivation springs from the need to have one's basic needs met, followed by a desire to meet one's higher goals, which then evolves into a calling to help others attain their goals. If one's basic needs are not met (Maslow, 1943), they will often be distracted, or even disabled from working toward their goals and those of their organization. Nurse managers enable motivation by first ensuring that the work environment is meeting the basic needs of the employee(s); for example, physiologic needs, such as rest and nutrition breaks, belonging to a work community that provides unconditional positive regard, and honoring diversity so that all nurses can feel a 'real' sense of esteem in their nursing role. Once these primary needs are met, the nurse manager can assist the employee to create goals and foster an environment that enables them to be reached.

Seminal research on the topic of self-efficacy, which continues to be relevant today, found that the degree of self-belief/self-efficacy and ownership of one's goals correlates with one's motivation and ability to reach them (Zimmerman et al., 1992). In addition, those with greater self-efficacy are more committed, use better task strategies to attain goals, and respond more positively to negative feedback than do people with lower self-efficacy (Locke & Latham, 2002). Relating to the process of effective goal setting, leaders who set high goal standards from a top-down approach negatively impact motivation and goal achievement (Zimmerman et al., 1992), and negative feedback leads to higher career stress and a lower motivation to set and reach goals (Hu et al., 2018). Nurse managers can support motivation and ability by being visible and engaged in the work environment. They have a significant influence on work ethic, mutual respect, and interpersonal relationships that promote diverse ways of being and doing. Furthermore, by being present in the work environment, they will have a sense of who is thriving and who is merely surviving, which provides an opportunity to further support employees.

If an employee is uncooperative or unproductive because of a lack of knowledge or ability, education is an appropriate intervention. Through observations and conversations with employees, the nurse manager can observe and determine the employee's strengths and opportunities for growth. Frequent errors are often an indication of lack of knowledge, skill, and critical thinking. Nurse managers must document all variances or untoward events after discussing them with the employee. Tracking errors and problematic behaviours enables nurse managers to identify potential trends. To prevent errors, is important for managers to lead with a strength-based approach, which creates an emotionally safe space, whereby nurses freely ask for help. Conversely, when work environments feel emotionally unsafe because of frequent scrutiny, employees may be too embarrassed to ask for help, because they believe doing so shows weakness or reflects negatively on their work identity and relationships.

All nurses and employees have a right to clear expectations, appropriate supervision, and ongoing feedback with the opportunity to demonstrate improvement (CNA, 2009). Nurse managers can provide coaching and mentoring to enhance skills, abilities, and attitudes in their employees (Batson & Yoder, 2012). When the problem is the result of a need for more education or training, the nurse manager can work with various educational resources, such as the clinical nurse educator to help the employee improve his or her skills. Most employees are receptive in such situations because they want to improve and meet job expectations.

PERSONNEL OBSTACLES: EMOTIONALLY INCONGRUENT EMPLOYEES

Sometimes an unproductive employee simply lacks emotional **congruence** (Rogers, 1959). Carl Rogers, a seminal clinician and researcher in the field of psychology and counseling, described congruence as one's ability to be 'real' or their authentic self, enabling them to acknowledge and process dissonance as it arises. Conversely, those who have not developed emotional congruence tend to deny their 'real' self. Incongruence leaves nurses feeling compelled to display a socially prescribed 'ideal' self and are prone to emotional dissociation, perfectionism, and a lack of self-compassion (Dames et al., 2018). Relationships of unconditional positive regard enable nurses to feel accepted for their 'real' self, as opposed to feeling compelled to adhere to a socially prescribed 'ideal.' Those who are congruent tend to be more open to feedback. They are not threatened by shortcomings because they have a deep sense of self-integrity and emotional security. They have learned to embrace all parts of themselves and naturally practice self-compassion when knowledge gaps or errors occur. Congruence may also be described as *emotional intelligence,* which enables one to form relationships with healthy boundaries, manage one's emotions, and a desire to collaborate with co-workers.

Emotional incongruence affects all care providers in any given challenge; however, whereas some are distracted by it, others can be completely disabled by it. Incongruence often leads to a lack of insight into their behaviour and how their behaviours impact others. Humans are emotional beings; thereby staying connected to, acknowledging, and reflecting one's emotions is imperative to thrive in one's life roles. Given that nursing environments are often wrought with emotional stressors, managing these emotions amongst a plethora of competing tasks is a challenge. It takes a compassionate and supportive work environment to enable nurses to process dissonance/emotional cues, without feeling the need to dissociate from them to survive their workday (Dames et al., 2018; Palmer, 2008). Another factor that can challenge nurses in the practice environment is emotional transference from past trauma. Although many nurses learn about how trauma impacts their patients, often referred to as *trauma informed care*, they may overlook how the same principle applies to them. When emotions are avoided, because of incongruence or transference, they become unmanaged, which produces subconscious projections that can trigger hostility toward others, addictive tendencies, and maladaptive perfectionism.

Emotional incongruence in an employee may not be readily apparent, particularly because it is often masked with perfectionism. However, it may manifest in the following actions: defiance, testing of workplace guidelines, passivity or hostility, or a lack of support for management decisions. The challenge for the nurse manager is to remain objective, as opposed to reacting to a subjective feeling of threat. This can be done through personal reflection, acknowledging their own emotions, and managing how they may impact their decisions. This awareness and honoring of emotion enables it to be more objectively managed from a compassionate space and often prevents subconscious projections. If the nurse manager focuses on identifying the root cause of the undesirable behaviour, he or she will be better able to find the right solution and be better prepared to address the issue as a whole. For example, if an employee states, "Administration is always making decisions to make our jobs harder," rather than making a hostile or defensive comment in reply, the nurse manager could take the employee aside and say, "I notice that you seem to be angry about this new policy. Let's talk about it some more." Emotional incongruence is often most evident when employers and employees are under stress. It is important to keep in mind that an employee may be displaying dynamics rooted in unresolved personal matters and that the behaviour is not a personal attack on the nurse manager. The employee may also be illuminating a frustration that is shared among other team members, which the manager could deescalate if they had a better understanding of the issue. A collaborative strategy to manage this, is to jointly discuss the specific problem, outline potential solutions, define acceptable behaviour expectations, and if necessary, to outline consequences for nonadherence to policies and procedures. Some employees may comply with specific performance expectations but push boundaries and test management in other areas. As this testing occurs, the nurse manager must continue to communicate performance expectations clearly and frequently and offer suggestions for improvement.

Emotional incongruence often leads to challenges in the workplace because of maladaptive perfectionism, or a desire to control everything, a lack of self-worth, black and white thinking, and an inability to control their emotions and behaviours (Dames et al., 2018). Research indicates that nursing can take a toll on the psychosocial and physical health of the nurse (Sabo, 2011), including a broad range of problems associated with emotional exhaustion, posttraumatic stress disorder, and burnout (CNA, 2010; CNA, 2012; Czaja et al., 2012). Facilitating goal accomplishment, providing compassion when employees are struggling, fostering an environment that supports relationships of unconditional positive regard, and offering praise when appropriate, are empowering strategies that promote the development of congruence. Finally, emotional incongruence amongst nursing personnel may affect not only the individual involved but also co-workers and, indirectly, patients. The nurse manager must be aware that certain behaviours, such as poor judgment, increased errors, increased absenteeism, decreased productivity, and a negative attitude, may be manifestations of emotional problems in employees.

For example:

A nurse manager began hearing complaints from patients about a nurse named Ryan. Patients were saying that Ryan was abrupt and uncaring with them. The nurse manager had not received any complaints about Ryan before this time, which led to questions about why this was occurring. Ryan reported that his mother was very ill and he was so worried about her and so upset that he could not sleep and was extremely tired lately. He went on to say that he was having trouble being sympathetic with complaining patients when they did not seem to be as sick as his mother.

When an employee's behaviour changes significantly, personal problems with which the person cannot cope may be the cause. The nurse manager is not, and should not be, a counselor to the staff but must intercede, not only to support the staff member but also to maintain the adequate functioning of the unit. In dealing with the employee who exhibits behaviours that indicate unresolved emotional problems that clearly extend beyond the work context, the nurse manager assists the individual to obtain professional help to address the root of the emotional dissonance. The individual's work setting and schedule may need to be adjusted, which may necessitate support from other nurses and staff to minimize negative effects on the care team and on patient care. The nurse manager acknowledges that an employee is experiencing emotional difficulties and yet the standards of practice for quality patient care must be upheld. It is reassuring for staff to witness the care and concern shown to a co-worker who is in a difficult situation. Staff can interpret that similar support would be given to them if they were in a difficult situation.

It is important for the nurse manager to be supportive, caring, empathic, and encouraging with an emotionally troubled employee. Many organizations have employee assistance programs (EAPs) to which the nurse manager should refer employees. Throughout the process, nurse managers must consult with human resources about any potential legal implications. Nurse managers should always remember that various resources are available to assist employees who experience personal problems. They should never feel required to know all of the legal implications regarding employment policies. Rather, they must know that help is available and how to access it.

EXERCISE 25.2 As a nurse manager in a community health centre, you have just attended a meeting that was requested by several of your staff nurses. They expressed concern regarding another nurse colleague, Christine, who has been coming to work looking disheveled and who has been tearful several times during the past week. They report that Christine spends a lot of time in the bathroom when they are at work, and their eyes are red and swollen as if they have been crying when they comes out of the bathroom. Their co-workers have offered to support them, but they have refused to discuss their distress with their colleagues. Christine's colleagues express concern and ask you to help them.

Take a moment to reflect on the role of the nurse manager in this situation. What is your response to the group of concerned colleagues? How would you manage this situation?

PERSONNEL OBSTACLES: NOVICE CHALLENGES VERSUS CLINICAL INCOMPETENCE

Clinical incompetence is possibly one of the most complex problems that nurse managers encounter. Because of the complex, and often subjective, nature of these types of situations, the nurse manager usually requires the support and consultation services of human resources personnel and the local professional regulatory body. Clinical incompetence may present immediately after hire, or over a period of time it may become evident that the nurse is unable to meet the expected practice competencies (CNA, 2015). Moreover, although the term incompetence appears to be black and white in nature, this is often not the case. Nurses move from novice to expert and then back to elements of novice practice throughout their career and assume new and/or more advanced roles. As lifelong learners, self and other compassion is imperative to enable employees to flourish, even in the face of mistakes and perceived inadequacies. Balancing the need for patient safety with an environment that supports the novice reality, whereby a majority of learning occurs through experience, is a tension that is important for nurse managers to learn and navigate.

Some nurses may be reluctant and unwilling to report instances when they witness clinical incompetence because they fear repercussions. Nurses may feel ambivalent about their loyalties in these types of

situations, feeling pressure to choose between collegial relationships and their patient safety concerns. The hierarchy of needs (Maslow, 1943) illustrates this intrapersonal conflict, whereby the primal need for belonging and esteem/self-integrity feels at odds. To be specific, one's sense of esteem may be threatened when self-integrity is compromised, and one's sense of belonging and approval from peers may be threatened if an unfavorable report is made about a colleague.

When a nurse manager becomes aware that one nurse covers for the mistakes of another, the nurse manager must offer support, guidance, and resources, such as additional education, but ultimately must encourage employees to honor their self-integrity and uphold professional standards. Bowen & Weil (2011) reported that less than 10% of nurse leaders use the CNA code of ethics (2017) to counsel their employees/colleagues. The nurse manager has a responsibility to create an environment where ethical issues are openly discussed and addressed (Bowen & Weil, 2011). The nurse manager can guide and support employees to reflect on morally and ethically distressing situations so that they can be managed, as opposed to avoiding the dissonance, which leads to habitual emotional dissociation. All RNs have a professional responsibility to address and report inappropriate and unprofessional behaviour (College of Registered Nurses of British Columbia [CRNBC], 2012a, 2012b). However, when colleagues make mistakes or are clearly challenged because of hardships that are compromising their professional practice, it is important to remember that using shame, a commonly tactic in nursing culture, to address professional practice issues only fuels fear-based, perfectionistic, and hostile work environments. One can be assertive, addressing professional conduct issues, and still come from a place of care and compassion.

The CNA code of ethics (2017) outlines ethical issues, and a nursing regulatory body practice advisor can be an excellent resource to support nurses through difficult situations. Ignoring and avoiding practice violations contributes to unsafe nursing practice, which jeopardizes patient care and ultimately patient safety. Canadian nursing regulatory bodies take practice violations very seriously; a practice violation can lead a nurse to be reprimanded or, in some cases, have his or her nursing license revoked.

Most health care organizations use skills checklists or a competency evaluation program to ascertain that their employees have and maintain essential skills and abilities necessary for their position. A skills checklist is one way to determine basic clinical competency (Table 25.1). This checklist typically includes a list of basic skills and essential skills for safe nursing practice. Any type of skills review should be directly linked to quality-improvement indicators. Moreover, the purpose and process of the skills review should be explained to the staff nurse, which may increase the staff nurse's motivation and commitment. When

---

TABLE 25.1 Example of a Skills Checklist

Purpose

1. The clinical skills inventory is a three-phase tool to enable the newly hired registered nurse (RN) and the nurse manager to determine individual learning needs, verify competency, and plan performance goals.
2. The RN will complete the self-assessment of clinical skills during the first week of employment. The RN will use the appropriate scale to document current knowledge of clinical skills.
3. The nurse manager will document observed competency of the orientee or delegate this to a peer. All columns must be completed on the inventory level.
4. At the end of orientation, the new RN and the manager will use the inventory to identify performance goals on the plan sheet. The skills inventory will be in a specified place on the nursing unit so that it is available to the manager and other RNs. It should be updated at appropriate intervals as specified by the manager.

Scale for Self-Assessment

1 = Unfamiliar/never done
2 = Able to perform with assistance
3 = Can perform with minimal supervision
4 = Independent performance/proficient

Score for Validation of Competency

1 = Unable to perform at present
2 = Able to perform with assistance
3 = Progressing/repeat performance necessary
4 = Able to perform independently

Clinical Skills (Examples)	SELF-ASSESSMENT		Comment	VALIDATION			Comment
	Scale	Date		Score	Date	Initials	
Epidural catheter care							
Nasogastric tube Insertion Management							
Preoperative care/teaching							
Postoperative care/teaching							

Plan Sheet for Skills Inventory

Name _____Date _____

Goals   **Date to Be Completed**

_____

_____

_____

_____

_____

_____

_____

Orientee's signature _____
Manager's signature _____
Date _____

the nurse manager explains the purpose and process of the skills review, he or she demonstrates respect for the staff nurse; a nurse manager who engages the staff nurse in the process may help motivate the employee. The skills review may require the employee to undertake a self-assessment of specific skills or competencies and then perform a return demonstration for the nurse educator or manager to validate adequate competency of the skills. If the nurse manager determines that an employee is having difficulty meeting performance expectations and cannot perform a skill adequately, he or she may choose to work alongside the nurse while delivering direct patient care, giving the nurse manager a chance to observe the nurse's strengths and support areas requiring growth. It can be helpful for the staff nurse to develop a learning portfolio to document the strengths and areas requiring growth, not just skills (CNA, 2013a). For example, some nurses struggling with time management or medication administration may benefit from coaching, formal mentoring, or other more formal education. The nurse manager must document and keep detailed records of all meetings with the staff nurse to have a paper trail and clear documentation for future reference should further counsel and/or reprimand or termination be necessary. When managing ancillary personnel, the nurse manager supports the team by being present in the clinical environment, being available, and being approachable.

EXERCISE 25.3 You are a nurse manager of a 32-bed medical unit, which is over capacity because of a lack of long-term care beds to discharge patients to. As a result, on top of an already acute patient load, nurses are challenged to manage patients with advanced dementia who would be best served on a low stimulus and locked unit. Although those at highest risk are assigned a one-to-one care aid, those viewed as moderate risk are often left unattended. One of the RNs, Tara, reports to you that another nurse, David, who is struggling to stay on top of their assigned workload, is inappropriately using restraints on one of the patients because the patient, who has a history of falling, is continually trying to get out of bed and disrupting the other patients in the four-bed room. Tara had not talked to David about their concern.

   As the nurse manager, how would you navigate this scenario? Would you consider this a professional practice issue?

PERSONNEL OBSTACLES: CHEMICAL DEPENDENCY

Chemical dependency among nurses and other health care providers is a serious global problem that puts patients and co-workers at risk (Berg et al., 2012). Chemical dependency is a psychophysiologic state in which an individual requires a substance, such as medications or alcohol, to deal with emotional transference/dissonance, and to prevent the onset of symptoms of abstinence. An employee who is working impaired adversely affects morale and may add stress to other staff members who have to assume additional responsibilities to compensate for the impaired or absent member. Patient safety is also at risk for many reasons; for example, nursing colleagues and staff are often focusing more on the problems of a co-worker than on those of the patients (New, 2014). Novice nurses must be aware of their professional and ethical responsibility to report incidents in which peers or team members exhibit signs of chemical dependency. According to professional nursing standards throughout Canada, nurses have a responsibility to identify, report, and address actual or potential unsafe practices, such as when nurses are under the influence of a chemical substance (CNA, 2015; Saskatchewan Registered Nurses Association, 2013). This responsibility includes taking action in all situations where patient safety and the well-being of any other group of people are potentially compromised (CNA, 2017; Edmonson, 2010). The nurse manager must professionally intervene and handle the situation while abiding by organization policies and professional practice standards that are aligned with ethical and morally responsible care and ensure that situations are handled consistently (Edmonson, 2010; New, 2014). It is important to understand that trauma-informed care, which is typically focused on patients, is equally relevant to nurses. Nurses are not immune to the impacts of trauma. Normalizing this fact within the culture of nursing promotes congruence by enabling nurses to get 'real' about their humanity, as opposed to feeling the need to put on a socially prescribed 'ideal' image that fuels the need for substances to cope.

   Substance use is often a result of past trauma, unresolved emotional dissonance, and low sense of coherence (Antonovsky, 1979); these are developmental vulnerabilities that are triggered in high stress environments, making it highly relevant to nurses

> **EXERCISE 25.4** We are continually exposed to stories in the news about nurses, physicians, and other health care providers. Media stories are nonacademic resources, but they can be useful learning tools for health care providers to further develop critical-thinking skills and better understand issues and concepts that affect health care workers.
>
> Search for a media story on a health care provider's experience with substance abuse. How would you view the matter from the perspective of a nurse manager, a co-worker, and a patient? Reflect on the professional, ethical, and moral obligations of the health care provider involved in the media story.

(Dames & Javorksi, 2018). Sense of coherence, coined by Aaron Antonovosky, is a concept used to understand why, in the same environments, some people are able to thrive and others succumb to disease or dis-*ease*. Those with higher sense of coherence scores are more apt to thrive and to effectively manage stimuli before they become stressors. The need to use substances is often related to a low sense of coherence, a developmental vulnerability, and, as a result, a great deal of unresolved emotional pain that causes a variety of dysfunctions. When managers and colleagues understand this, they can address the issue with compassion and be more likely to connect them with the resources they need.

The *Health Professions Acts* and professional nursing standards and competencies vary across Canada. The underlying expectation is that members of any health care profession recognized in Canada will always act to protect the public's interest (CNA, 2009). Some of Canada's provinces and territories have a mandatory "duty to report" clause, which imposes reporting requirements on registrants of the health professional regulatory body (see also Chapter 7). As is true of all nurses, nurse managers must uphold the nursing practice standards of the province or territory in which they practice. Also, they should be familiar with the legal and safety risks associated with employing a nurse who has a chemical dependency (CNA, 2009). Nurse managers handle situations involving the chemical dependency of unregulated care providers according to organizational policies. Consultation with human resources personnel is critical to ensure adherence with organizational expectations.

In Canadian health care organizations, and most unionized environments, there is a concerted effort to support affected individuals by offering support in seeking treatment versus immediately terminating the employee (CNA, 2009). Identifying an employee with a chemical dependency is usually difficult, as one of the primary symptoms is denial. Employees may also display obvious behavioural changes that are different from the behaviours the employee normally exhibited (New, 2014). Those different behaviours include lying, stealing, sudden and unusual neglect of personal appearance, an unusual interest in patients' pain control, frequent changes in jobs and shifts, and an increase in absenteeism and tardiness (College of Registered Nurses of Nova Scotia, 2017; New, 2014).

Nurse managers have a responsibility to use due diligence and address concerns and suspicions of chemical dependence in all employees (CNA, 2009). Open and supportive leadership is critical, but the nurse manager must consider the legal, ethical, and potential regulatory aspects of these situations. Referring an employee who is struggling with chemical dependency for treatment demonstrates supportive action. In addition, the nurse manager must consider if a report should be made to the provincial or territorial nursing regulatory body about the matter. For example, if a nurse is terminated for ongoing substance abuse and the nursing regulatory body of that province or territory is not notified, the nurse may be able to continue to practice nursing and put patients and colleagues at risk. Nursing regulatory bodies have a responsibility to protect the public, but they also have an obligation to support nurses in meeting standards of practice (CNA, 2009; Nurses Association of New Brunswick, 2011).

Canada has rehabilitation programs available for nurses who suffer from an addiction so that they may return to nursing once rehabilitated. Nurse managers are sometimes involved with monitoring the return-to-work process once the rehabilitative therapy is complete. Action plans, monitoring guidelines, and follow-up expectations are collaboratively established with the employee, the health care organization, and the nurse manager (Angres et al., 2010). Sometimes, provincial or territorial nursing regulatory bodies impose sanctions on the nurse who suffers from an addiction. For example, a nurse who has been through rehabilitation for narcotics substance abuse may be allowed to work in a setting in which narcotics are never used, or the nurse may have a restricted nursing license and not be permitted to administer any controlled substances or narcotics. This type of

LITERATURE PERSPECTIVE

Resource: Kunyk, D. (2015). Substance use disorders among registered nurses: prevalence, risk, and perceptions in a disciplinary jurisdiction. *Journal of Nursing Management, 23*(1), 54-64.

The purpose of this Canadian research study was to investigate substance use, health risks, and impaired practice amongst nurses and the effectiveness of using a disciplinary process to address the issues. The research is relevant because substance use/chemical dependency amongst nurses impacts patient safety, and the health of the nurse. Furthermore, the effectiveness of using discipline to address substance use issues is lacking in the literature.

Regarding methodology, the study used a convenience sample of 4064 nurses in Alberta, Canada via an internet survey. Participants self-reported about their use of substances, their health status, and their perception of organizational support. In addition, they inquired about their perceptions on how substance use treatment and their observations or experiences about the disposition of nurses who are impaired at work.

Study results demonstrated that chemical dependency amongst nurses was similar to the general population. Furthermore, those who self-reported as chemically dependent were not in treatment and continued to work,

which was unknown to their employer. The primary reason for people not seeking treatment was that they were too embarrassed to tell anyone and that some felt that they could not be helped. Most nurses in the study felt that the employer had a responsibility to regulate when impairment becomes evident and to assist in aiding the employee to access treatment. Furthermore, the majority of the participants felt that chemical dependency was treatable; that such employee issues should be kept confidential, and that once treated they could be trusted and productive in their nursing role. As for responding via a disciplinary pathway, this study demonstrated that nurses did not feel that discipline, feeling punitive, was an effective approach for risk mitigation, nor helpful in supporting nurses with substance use issues.

Implications for Practice

This study has implications for nurse manager who play an important role in responding to substance use issues in the workplace. The nurse manager may be the one person who provides the necessary support for the employee to feel safe enough to reach out and to accept the help they need. Using a disciplinary approach is ineffective course of action as it only perpetuates fears of self-reporting and related fears of being further shamed.

---

situation can be difficult for health care teams, colleagues, and nurse managers; however, if handled positively, professionally, and openly, it can further enhance the team's cohesiveness and have minimal impact on patient care. If the nurse manager models professional ethics while offering empathy, he or she can deescalate the associated distress and disorganization (National Business Group on Health, 2009; Tanga, 2011). It is always prudent for the nurse manager to seek guidance from other senior leaders and human resources consultants when faced with such challenges. The nurse manager is responsible for establishing and fostering an environment that supports professional practice.

EMPLOYEE DISCIPLINE APPROACHES

Nonpunitive

For less serious personnel issues, many employers have moved from a progressive discipline approach to a nonpunitive approach; this shifts the responsibility to act from the manager to the employee, enables both parties

to attain their dignity, and minimizes ambiguity-related *role stress*. Nonpunitive discipline minimizes power battles, focuses on objective measures, and puts the choice in the hands of the employee.

The nonpunitive disciplinary process begins with a verbal discussion, whereby the agency's standards and employment expectations that were agreed to at the time of hiring, or are part of one's professional nursing requirements, are reiterated, as is the gap between what is expected of the employee and the employee's current performance. It is imperative to ensure that organizational policies on termination, as well as collective agreements, are transparent early on in the disciplinary process; ambiguity and resulting miscommunications must be minimized. There should be no surprises during the process.

If the first verbal discussion is unsuccessful, the manager will then call another meeting. This meeting acts as a check in and includes a written reminder of the performance issue, again reiterating the gap. This meeting acts as a formal warning where specific behaviours are noted, as is the gap between professional expectations and current performance. It clearly communicates that if behaviours do not come into compliance with agency standards, then the employee will be terminated. The language of the written warning needs to be clear, outlining the exact problems, and how they fail to meet agency standards. At this point, whereby a more formal warning has been issued, an employee has a right to support and guidance while striving to meet the performance expectations, and the organization must collaboratively determine the supportive measures required.

Once a written warning has been issued, it is at this point that some employers may offer a 'decision-making leave.' This paid day off may be given for the employee to take the time to reflect on whether they can meet the standards required of them, followed by a meeting the following workday, whereby the employee either agrees to the agency standards or offers a letter of resignation.

If they agree to meet the agency's standards, but it becomes apparent that the employee fails to make the necessary changes, then a consultation with human resources is in order. The human resources department is typically well versed to ensure the path toward termination is in line with the agency and the collective bargaining agreement, which varies between professionals and provinces. Collective agreements vary from province to province and health region to health region, and there are different collective agreements within each profession. The human resources department will also ensure that adequate documentation exists to support the decision to terminate. All contracts and written agreements must be maintained and copies provided to the employee, employer, and the organization's human resources department. A model for behavioural change using nonpunitive discipline appears in Fig. 25.1. This model demonstrates how behaviours, such as absenteeism, can be successfully altered.

Progressive Discipline

Progressive discipline consists of evaluating performance and providing feedback within a specified structure of increasing sanctions. Harassment, abuse of a patient, and working while impaired are examples of professional misconduct that usually involve progressive discipline. Progressive discipline must be handled according to organizational policies. Inappropriate discipline is not only detrimental to the relationship between the supervisor and the employees but can directly contravene collective agreements. The sanctions, which progress from least severe to most severe, are described in Box 25.1.

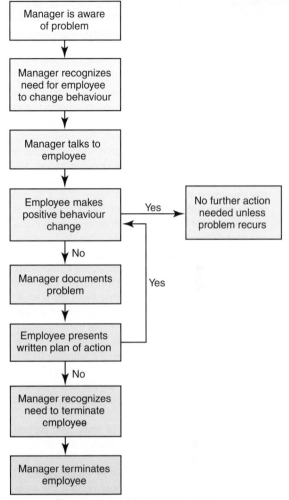

Fig. 25.1 Model for behavioural change.

TERMINATION

In some situations, despite the best efforts of the nurse manager, the employee issue or disruptive behaviour may continue. In such cases, sometimes no choice exists but to terminate the employee. Terminating an employee is one of the most difficult functions of the manager role. The following guidelines should be followed when terminating an employee:

1. The provisions of human resources policies and procedures and relevant collective agreements must be followed.
2. All communication between the employee and employer and incidents must be accurately documented in detail and show evidence of due process.

BOX 25.1   Steps in Progressive Discipline

1. Discuss the problem in detail with the employee.
2. Reprimand the employee. A verbal reprimand usually precedes a written one, but some organizations issue both a verbal and a written reprimand simultaneously, depending on the issue. Documentation must include evidence that the wrongdoing or misconduct was brought to the attention of the employee, and best practices would indicate that both the nurse manager and employee sign the documentation (Crigger & Godfrey, 2014). By signing the documentation, the employee is not stating that he or she agrees with the reprimand but, rather, that he or she is aware of the reprimand. It is important that the process is transparent and that all documentation is kept in the employee's human resources file.
3. Suspend the employee if the problem persists (depending on the corresponding collective agreement). The consequences vary according to the collective agreement but might include time away from work, mandatory education courses, and possibly the need to report to the provincial or territorial nursing regulatory body (for registered nurses and licensed practical nurses) (Brous, 2012). Explain the rationale for the disciplinary action so that there is no surprise for the employee. At this point, the employee often realizes the magnitude and seriousness of the problem based on the resulting discipline.
4. Allow the employee to return to work with written conditions regarding problem behaviour and strict follow-up.
5. Terminate the employee (subject to the guidelines of the corresponding collective agreement) if the problem recurs following rehabilitation. Human resources must be consulted regarding this process.

Documentation provides a paper trail of the specifics of the incident and details of conversations between the employer and employee and should be considered a legal document. When nurse managers do not maintain relevant documents or their documentation lacks specificity and clarity, there is a lack of evidence to support management decisions regarding discipline or termination. Documentation should include evidence that the employee was aware of the position expectations, was offered guidance on how to meet expectations, and was given opportunities to improve. It should also include specific examples of how the employee was not meeting performance expectations. Documentation is time consuming, but it is a necessary aspect of management.

3. Throughout the disciplinary process, and in the event of termination, human resources personnel must be consulted, and legally binding collective agreements must be followed.

Terminating an employee follows extensive investigation and due process. Situations that may warrant immediate dismissal include theft, violence in the workplace, and willful abuse of a patient. The following example illustrates an incident that led to the immediate termination of an employee.

> *Ben, a new graduate nurse, worked at a community mental health clinic. They recently completed the new employee orientation, which included the agency's standards and the professional regulations and obligations surrounding social media use.*
>
> *Two months following the session, Ben posted several pictures on their Facebook page of a patient they cared for at the community mental health clinic. The pictures were accompanied by derogatory, demeaning comments. Ben's postings had a nasty tone and contained inappropriate vulgar terms. Management became aware of the Facebook postings and deemed them as an unethical use of social media. The nurse manager consulted with the regional human resources department, and the nurse was immediately terminated.*
>
> *In this example, the nurse did not abide by the CNA code of ethics (2017) and contravened one of the primary values, to preserve the dignity of all. Ben's inappropriate use of social media also violated a very basic organizational policy by breaching the confidentiality of the patient. Ben did not act as a moral agent nor did they act in the best interest of the patient.*

As illustrated in the earlier example, the termination of employees should be vetted with human resources, and the infraction should be an obvious deviation from agency policies. Steps should be taken to avoid the possibility of miscommunications, and potentially violent reactions, while the notice of termination is given. Furthermore, formal and clear delivery of the notice is imperative, avoiding engaging in argument or negotiation. The dignity of the employee should be preserved, minimizing embarrassment by carefully planning who is present, ensuring privacy, and strategically choosing the time and place of the meeting. The person being terminated should not be blocked from accessing the exit door. Formal paperwork and severance pay should be available at the termination meeting. Arrangements to gather their personal belongings should be planned before the meeting, ensuring that there is no reason that the employee needs to return to the work site. Managers should be prepared for multiple potential outcomes, including potentially needing security nearby, and counseling options.

Grievances

Occasionally, grievances are filed against organizations. A grievance describes the process that occurs when an individual believes that the collective bargaining agreement has not been followed. Collective agreements provide employees with the right to grieve most decisions against them, and the union supports the employee throughout the grievance process (see Chapter 7 for more information on collective agreements). Typically, in these types of situations, the human resources department will consult with legal services, whose recommendations are taken into account throughout the termination process. Disciplinary and termination processes are complex, and nurse managers should not attempt to handle them in isolation.

> **EXERCISE 25.5** Explore your provincial or territorial nursing regulatory body website. Locate and examine the professional nursing practice standards and identify what potential incidents might call for immediate termination from a nursing position.

Disciplinary meetings can be used as an opportunity to gain a sense of control by understanding the expectations of their role and the resources in that area available to meet them. Although most organizations provide orientation to novice nurses so that they can learn organizational policies, procedures, and performance expectations, it should also be recognized that they will come to know many of the agency expectations through work experience and mentorship. To ensure that the basic skills and expectations are understood, many employers will use policy and skills checklists like the example in Table 25.1. However, all nurses, including novice nurses, have a responsibility to ask questions when they do not understand or when they need support and guidance. When mistakes occur or shortcomings become evident, it is important to remember that for one to be able to stay open to teachable moments, as opposed to feeling threatened and defensive which blocks learning, they must feel a sense of grace, compassion, and acceptance

for their 'real' self from their colleagues. If senior nurses model this to novice nurses, they too will model the same compassionate behaviours when they mentor newer nurses.

DOCUMENTATION

Documentation of all conversations and meetings with employees regarding their work performance challenges should be accurately documented in detail and kept in employees' human resources file. From a regulatory and legal perspective, it is imperative that nurse managers maintain detailed documentation logs. Mooney (2013) suggested that writing reports and documentation is the most important step in the process of dealing with an employee who is unable to navigate their emotional dissonance and related substance abuse issues.

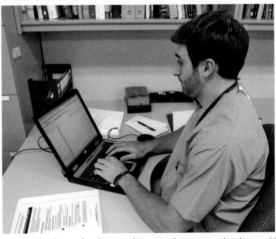

Documentation of all meetings and communication with employees is an important aspect of the nurse manager's role.

Documentation cannot be left to memory! At the time that an employee is involved in a difficult situation or when an employee receives a compliment or exceeds expectations, a notation should be made and kept in the employee file. This entry must include the date, time, and a brief description of the incident. Along with this information, the nurse manager should keep a log or summary sheet of all reported errors, unusual incidents, and wrongdoings/mistakes. This documentation can reveal patterns of individual's problem areas, areas of excellence in individual performance, and overall organizational problematic areas. The nurse manager who engages with employees and carefully keeps

---

BOX 25.2   Documentation of Performance Problems

- Description of incident—an objective statement of the facts related to the incident
- Actions—statements describing the plan to correct and/or prevent future problems
- Follow-up—dates and times that the plan is to be carried out, including required meeting with the employee

Example

Several patients reported that Rebecca, one of the registered nurses, was "curt" and "gruff" and seemed uncaring with them. I called Rebecca into my office and reiterated the complaints that I had received, including the specifics of times and incidents. I reminded Rebecca about what my expectations were relating to patient care, emphasizing the importance of a caring attitude with all patients. We discussed what the possible cause of Rebecca's behaviour might be, such as problems at home or lack of sleep. Rebecca denied being curt or gruff but

agreed that some of her mannerisms might be misinterpreted. I suggested to Rebecca that perhaps she needed to be particularly aware of her body language and to soften her tone of voice. After discussing this incident and reminding Rebecca of the importance of caring in nursing, I cited the policy regarding behaviour and told Rebecca that this behaviour would not be tolerated. I told Rebecca we needed to meet once a week to discuss how the week had gone and to determine how she was interacting with the patients assigned to her. I also told Rebecca I would be checking with patients to see what they had thought of Rebecca, pointing out that I do this routinely.

These weekly meetings are to be conducted for 6 weeks, followed by monthly meetings for a 3-month period. If problems do not recur, the meetings will be discontinued after this time.

Jean-Paul Martin, RN, MSN, Hospital Nurse Manager

---

records about organizational functioning has greater control and influence in the management of employee problems. Box 25.2 describes the content and format for such documentation and provides an example.

CONCLUSION

All employees, including nurse managers, need to support and foster a positive and healthy work environment. Organizations must implement a zero-tolerance policy for unethical or disruptive behaviour among co-workers. However, running parallel to this policy, it is equally important to remember that socially dominant behaviour often referred to as *bullying*, which is detailed in Chapter 16, festers in perfectionistic environments that lack self and others compassion (Dames et al., 2018). Meeting social dominance with more of the same, does not address the cultural roots of the problem. Conversely, work environments filled with employees who regularly practice self and others compassion, as opposed to maladaptive perfectionism, are far less likely to deal with social dominance issues (Dames et al., 2018; Jahromi et al., 2012). Employees require an emotionally safe work environment where they feel empowered to address areas of moral and ethical dissonance in relation to themselves, their co-workers, and their patients (see Boxes 25.3 and 25.4).

BOX 25.3   Principles of Indigenous Leadership

Tewa Scholar, Gregory Cajete describes western leadership models and indigenous leadership models as significantly different in terms of their epistemologies, or ways in which they believe one comes to know. Perhaps the most profound difference is that indigenous communities come to know, come to lead, come to be from a relational context. Indigenous leadership cannot be theorized nor understood outside of its relational context.

Communal forms of leadership that honor cultural traditions are an imperative. Furthermore, leaders are developed within a relational community of affection, affiliation, and education. Affection describes the unconditional positive regard that flows between the leader and those who follow, which is held together via a shared set of values. Affiliation describes how one comes to know via relationship with all life forces, including nature and spirit. These affiliations are reflected through rituals and symbolism. Education informs how one comes into their identity, guided by the community, honoring their passions while staying grounding in their core values.

Source: Wolfgramm, R., Spiller, C. & Voyageur, C (2016). Special issue: Indigenous leadership – editors' introduction. *Leadership, 12*(3), 263–269.

BOX 25.4   Recognizing the Value of Indigenous Ways of Knowing and Being

The current economic and political structures are often divisive in nature, leading to competitive environments fueled by power and social domination. Because many of us are incubated in these structures, we often become accustomed to them and are prone to perpetuate the harmful aspects within our communities, our families, workplaces, and close personal relationships. Awareness of these structures is necessary to enable us to take a step back so we can view the harmful aspects more objectively. The side effects of colonial structures, often embedded within capitalism, are hierarchies, social dominance, fixation on material wealth, and immediate gratification, despite the wider societal impacts. Challenging these systems will require us to work together to deconstruct and then reconstruct them, based on shared values that can put a stop to the spiritual and psychological violence that is perpetuating ongoing divisiveness and moral injury within our communities. If we do nothing, we will continue to be driven by colonial ways, not recognizing the inherent value and wisdom of Indigenous ways of knowing and being.

Source: Laboucan-Massimo, M. (2017). Lessons from Wesahkecahk. In *Whose land is it anyway? A manual for decolonization.* Retrieved from http://www.fpse.ca/sites/default/files/news_files/Decolonization%20Handbook.pdf

---

❓ A SOLUTION

The nurse manager determined that the root cause of Tanya's error was a lack of knowledge regarding the specific needs and protocols on the specialized hospital unit. They collaborated with Tanya and the unit's nurse educator to compile a specific skills checklist and develop a professional development module for new hires and nurses from the resource float pool that occasionally work on the mother baby unit. The manager followed up by having float nurses, newly hired nurses, and regular staff nurses complete a questionnaire to determine their knowledge about unit policies and procedures as well as maternal child nursing.

Would this be a suitable approach for you? Why or why not? Reflecting on this scenario, consider other strategies to support casual float nurses who provide nursing care on units that they are not familiar with.

▌THE EVIDENCE

Davey et al. (2009) sought to identify predictors of short-term absenteeism in staff nurses. Such absenteeism contributes to lack of continuity in patient care and decreases staff morale, which is costly to a health care organization. A systematic review of studies conducted from 1986 to 2006 led to the inclusion of 16 peer-reviewed research studies. The authors found that individual nurses' "history of prior absences," "work attitudes" (e.g., job satisfaction, organizational commitment, and work involvement), and "retention factors" (e.g., shared governance) reduced absenteeism. By contrast, poor leadership, "burnout," and "job stress" increased absenteeism. It became clear that the reasons underlying absenteeism are still poorly understood and that a robust theory for nurse absenteeism is lacking. Further theory development and research are needed.

✳ NEED TO KNOW NOW

- The human resources department is an essential resource for nurse managers. The collaborative problem solving and decision making between nurse managers and human resources personnel are critical to consistent and effective management and leadership.
- Successful nurses
  - Habitually demonstrate compassion toward self and others, work through areas of dissonance to remain connected to their authentic selves, and as a result, are able to maintain a positive outlook toward their patients and families.

- Demonstrate respect and compassion for all co-workers, from housekeeping staff to the Chief Executive Officer.
- Participate in open discussion and decision making that is fair and reflects the organizational mission.
- Recognize and celebrate the contributions of co-workers.
- Practice according to organizational policies and their professional code of ethics.

▌ CHAPTER CHECKLIST

To obtain satisfaction from working with people, a nurse manager must be knowledgeable about employee and personnel issues that are common in the work setting. The nurse manager must be able to detect, prevent, and correct problems that affect nursing care and staff morale. Accurate and factual documentation and follow-up actions are key elements in the successful management of all personnel issues.

- Absenteeism's detrimental effects are as follows:
  - Patient care may be below standard.
  - Replacement personnel require additional supervision.
  - Absenteeism may increase among the entire staff.
  - Financial management of the unit suffers adverse effects.
- Effective strategies to reduce absenteeism include the following:
  - Enhance nurses' job satisfaction.
  - Undertake nonpunitive discipline.
- When employee behaviours are uncooperative or unproductive, the problem is often rooted in motivation and ability.
- Praise and affirmation are often the most effective strategies for an employee who lacks maturity.
- Clinical incompetence is a correctable problem for nurse managers:
  - Clinical incompetence may be masked by coworkers' enabling behaviour.
  - A skills checklist helps determine basic clinical competency and pinpoint the need for additional training and education.
  - A comprehensive competency program may include not only a skills checklist but also a means for evaluating the critical-thinking ability of the employee.
- When mental health concerns arise, the nurse manager must assist the employee in getting professional help.

- The nurse manager is responsible for early recognition of chemical dependency and referral for treatment when appropriate.
  - The nurse manager must do the following:
    - Uphold the professional standards for nursing practice.
    - Be familiar with the laws of the province or territory regarding chemical dependent employees.
    - Know the health care organization's personnel policy on chemical dependency.
  - Possible warning signs of chemical dependency are as follows:
    - Behavioural changes, such as mood swings
    - Lying and theft
    - Sudden and unusual neglect of personal appearance
    - Unusual interest in patients' pain control
    - Increased absenteeism and tardiness
- Documentation of problems must include the following:
  - A description of the incident
  - A description of the manager's actions
  - A plan to correct/prevent future occurrences
  - Dates and times of follow-up measures
- Progressive discipline may be used when other corrective measures have failed. Steps in progressive discipline (subject to collective agreements) are as follows:
  - Discuss the problem in detail with the employee, clearly identifying the concern.
  - Reprimand the employee (first verbally, then in writing).
  - Suspend the employee if the problem persists.
  - Allow the employee to return to work, with written stipulations regarding problem behaviour.
  - Terminate the employee (subject to the guidelines of the corresponding collective agreement) if the problem continues or recurs following rehabilitation.

▌ TIPS FOR DOCUMENTING PROBLEMS

- Identify the incident and related facts. Avoid the temptation to water down the facts with niceties, as this can cause ambiguity, resulting in a greater risk of miscommunicating the severity of the situation.
- Describe the actions taken by the nurse manager when the problem was identified.

- Develop an action plan for everyone involved.
- Schedule a follow-up meeting to evaluate the progress of the action plan.

Provide detailed, objective, and accurate information in documentation.

Visit the Evolve website for Suggested Readings, Internet Resources, and additional resources related to the content in this chapter: http://evolve.elsevier.com/Canada/Yoder-Wise/leading/.

REFERENCES

Angres, D. H., Bettinardi-Angres, K., & Cross, W. (2010). Nurses with chemical dependency: Promoting successful treatment and reentry. *Journal of Nursing Regulation, 1*(1), 16–20. Retrieved from https://jnr.metapress.com.

Antonovsky, A. (1979). *Health, stress and coping.* San Francisco: Jossey-Bass.

Batson, V. D., & Yoder, L. H. (2012). Managerial coaching: a concept analysis. *Journal of Advanced Nursing, 68*(7), 1658–1669.

Berg, K. H., Dillon, K. R., Sikkink, K. M., et al. (2012). Diversion of drugs within health care facilities, a multiple-victim crime: Patterns of diversion, scope, consequences, detection and prevention. *Mayo Clinic Proceedings, 87*(7), 674–682.

Bowen, D. J., & Weil, P. A. (2011). ACHE's code of ethics highlights challenges faced by healthcare leaders. *Healthcare Executive, 26*(4), 39–42. Retrieved from http://issuu.com/healthcareexecutive.

Brous, E. (2012). Common misconceptions about professional licensure. *American Journal of Nursing, 112*(10), 55–59.

Canadian Nurses Association. (2017). *Code of ethics for registered nurses.* Toronto, ON: Author. Retrieved from https://www.cna-aiic.ca/500Error.html?aspxerrorpath=/~/media/cna/page-content/pdf-en/code-of-ethics-2017-edition-secure-interactive.pdf.

Canadian Nurses Association. (2015). *Framework for the practice of registered nurses in Canada.* Ottawa, ON: Author. Retrieved from https://www.cna-aiic.ca/~/media/cna/page-content/pdf-en/framework-for-the-pracice-of-registered-nurses-in-canada.

Canadian Nurses Association. (2013a). *Building my online portfolio.* Retrieved from http://www.nurseone-inf-fusion.ca/Default.aspx?portlet=StaticHtmlViewerPortlet&&ptdi=1304.

Canadian Nurses Association. (2012). *Fact sheet: Nurse fatigue.* Retrieved from https://www.cna-aiic.ca/~/media/cna/page%20content/pdf%20en/2013/07/26/10/39/fact_sheet_nurse_fatigue_2012_e.pdf.

Canadian Nurses Association. (2010). *Position statement: Taking action on nurse fatigue.* Retrieved from http://www.nanb.nb.ca/PDF/CNATaking_Action_on_Nurse_Fatigue_E.pdf.

Canadian Nurses Association. (2009). *Position statement: Nursing leadership.* Retrieved from http://www.cna-aiic.ca/~/media/cna/page%20content/pdf%20en/2013/07/26/10/52/ps110_leadership_2009_e.pdf.

College of Nurses of Ontario. (2013). *Professional conduct, professional misconduct.* Toronto, ON: Author. Retrieved from http://www.cno.org/Global/docs/ih/42007_misconduct.pdf.

College of Registered Nurses of British Columbia. (2012a). *Assisting nurses with significant practice problems.* Vancouver, BC: Author. Retrieved from https://www.crnbc.ca/Standards/Lists/StandardResources/354AssistingNursesPracticeProblems.pdf.

College of Registered Nurses of British Columbia. (2012b). *Professional practice standards for registered nurses and nurse practitioners.* Vancouver, BC: Author. Retrieved from https://crnbc.ca/Standards/Lists/StandardResources/128ProfessionalStandards.pdf.

College of Registered Nurses of Nova Scotia. (2017). *Problematic substance use in the workplace: A resource guide for registered nurses.* Halifax: NS: Author. Retrieved from https://crnns.ca/publication/problematic-substance-use-in-the-workplace-practice-guideline/.

Crigger, N., & Godfrey, N. S. (2014). Professional wrongdoing: Reconciliation and recovery. *Journal of Nursing Regulation, 4*(4), 40–45. Retrieved from http://jnr.metapress.com.

Czaja, A. S., Moss, M., & Mealer, M. (2012). Symptoms of post-traumatic stress disorder among pediatric acute care nurses. *Journal of Pediatric Nursing, 27*(4), 357–365.

Dames, S., Groen, J., Raffin-Bouchal, S., & Kawalilak, C. (2018). *A Study of the interplay between new graduate life experience, context, and the experience of stress in the workplace: Exploring factors towards self-actualizing as a novice nurse.* Werklund School of Education.

Dames, S., & Javorski, S. (2018). Sense of coherence, a worthy factor toward nursing student and new graduate satisfaction with nursing, goal setting affinities, and coping tendencies. *Quality Advancement in Nursing Education, 4*(1).

Davey, M. M., Cummings, G., Newburn-Cook, C. V., et al. (2009). Predictors of nurse absenteeism in hospitals: A systematic review. *Journal of Nursing Management, 17*(3), 312–330.

Edmonson, C. (2010). Moral courage and the nurse leader. *Online Journal of Issues in Nursing, 15*(3).

Hersey, P., Blanchard, K., & Johnson, D. E. (2008). *Management of organizational behavior: Utilizing human resources* (9th ed.). Englewood Cliffs, NJ: Prentice Hall.

Hochschild, A. R. (2012). *The managed heart: Commercialization of human feeling (Update, with a new preface.* Berkeley: University of California Press.

Hu, S., Hood, M., & Creed, P. A. (2018). Negative career feedback and career outcomes: The mediating roles of self-regulatory processes. *Journal of Vocational Behavior, 106*, 180–191.

Jackson, D., Hutchinson, M., Peters, K., et al. (2013). Understanding avoidant leadership in health care: Findings from a secondary analysis of two qualitative studies. *Journal of Nursing Management, 21*(3), 572–580.

Jahromi, F. G., Naziri, G., & Barzegar, M. (2012). The relationship between socially prescribed perfectionism and depression: The mediating role of maladaptive cognitive schemas. *Social and Behavioral Sciences, 32*, 141–147.

Kunyk, D. (2015). Substance use disorders among registered nurses: Prevalence, risk, and perceptions in a disciplinary jurisdiction. *Journal of Nursing Management, 23*(1), 54–64.

Locke, E., & Latham, G. P. (2002). Building a practically useful theory of goal setting and task motivation: A 35-year odyssey. *American Psychologist, 57*(9), 705–717.

Longo, J. (2010). Combating disruptive behaviors: Strategies to promote a healthy work environment. *Online Journal of Issues in Nursing, 15*(1).

Maslow, A. H. (1943). A theory of human motivation. *Psychological Review, 50*(4), 370–396.

Mooney, D. H. (2013). Investing and making a case for drug diversion. *Journal of Nursing Regulation, 4*(1), 9–13. Retrieved from http://jnr.metapress.com.

National Business Group on Health. (2009, August). *An employer's guide to workplace substance abuse: Strategies and treatment recommendations.* Retrieved from https://www.businessgrouphealth.org/pub/f3151957-2354-d714-5191-c11a80a07294.

New, K. (2014). Preventing, detecting, and investigating drug diversion in health care facilities. *Journal of Nursing Regulation, 5*(1), 18–25. Retrieved from http://jnr.metapress.com.

Nurses Association of New Brunswick. (2011). *Recognition and management of problematic substance use in the nursing profession.* Fredericton, NB: Author. Retrieved from http://www.nanb.nb.ca/downloads/Recognition%20and%20Management%20of%20Problematic%20Substance%20Use%20in%20the%20Nursing%20Profession_E_New%20Cover.pdf.

Palmer, P. J. (2008). *A hidden wholeness: The journey toward an undivided life: Welcoming the soul and weaving community in a wounded world.* San Francisco: Jossey-Bass.

Rogers, C. (1959). A theory of therapy, personality and interpersonal relationships as developedin the client-centered framework. In S. Koch (Ed.), *Psychology: A study of a science. Vol. 3).* New York: McGraw Hill: Formulations of the person and the social context.

Sabo, B. (2011). Reflecting on the concept of compassion fatigue. *Online Journal of Issues in Nursing, 16*(1).

Saskatchewan Registered Nurses Association. (2013). *Standards and foundation competencies for the practice of registered nurses.* Regina, SK: Author. http://www.srna.org/images/stories/Nursing_Practice/Resources/Standards_and_Foundation_2013_06_10_Web.pdf.

Sifton, E. (1998). The serenity prayer. *Yale Review, 86*(1), 16.

Tanga, H. Y. (2011). Nurse drug diversion and nursing leaders responsibilities: Legal, regulatory, ethical, humanistic and practical considerations. *JONA's Healthcare Law, Ethics & Regulation, 13*(1), 13–16.

Troy, A. S. (2015). Reappraisal and resilience to stress: Context must be considered. *The Behavioral and Brain Sciences, 38*, e123.

Zimmerman, B., Bandura, A., & Martinez-Pons, M. (1992). Self-Motivation for personal attainment: The role of self-efficacy beliefs, and personal goal setting. *American Educational Research Journal, 29*(3), 663–676.

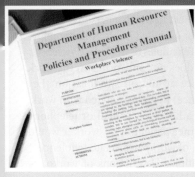

26

Workplace Violence and Incivility

Yolanda Babenko-Mould

Nurses working in hospitals and other health care facilities are at a disproportionally high risk for physical violence because of the very nature of their job. Health care workers screen patients and their visitors to the best of their ability, but one never knows who will walk through the door and in what mental state. To maintain personal safety and an environment free from the potential of physical violence, nurses must be alert to signs of trouble. Not all health care workplace violence is of a physical nature or from patients or their families; like any other workplace, health care settings are subject to horizontal violence and incivility. Horizontal violence includes intimidating or derisive behaviour between and among staff, managers, or physicians; it interferes with optimal job performance and negatively affects the delivery of high-quality patient care. Research suggests that incivility can be prevented if organizations ascribe to and uphold civility norms where incivility is not tolerated. Further, if organizations maintain policies and procedures to address workplace violence and incivility, leaders and staff could be provided with opportunities to learn about how to create positive work conditions and how to effectively deal with potentially problematic situations. No organization can completely prevent or eliminate workplace violence and incivility, but with proper planning and effective programs, the opportunities for such occurrences can be dramatically reduced.

OBJECTIVES

- Categorize the types of violence and incivility that can occur in the workplace.
- Understand the risk factors for potential violence or disruption.
- Understand how to conduct an organizational workplace violence assessment.
- Describe interventions that can help prevent horizontal violence and incivility.

TERMS TO KNOW

bullying
horizontal violence

incivility
interpersonal conflict

lateral violence
toxic workplace

❓ A CHALLENGE

Sophie, a fourth year nursing student, had been recording a report for the change of shift in the reporting room on a medical–surgical unit at approximately 6:00, when Sophie heard loud yelling and what sounded like smashing metal. Sophie immediately ran out into the dimly lit hallway to see a colleague, Louisa, at the end of the hall, standing just inside the brightly lit entrance of the clean utility room, wearing a uniform that was now covered in blood. Next to Louisa was a male who had been admitted to the unit from the emergency department moments before while Sophie was recording the report. The male patient turned away from Louisa and glared at Sophie. Then the patient began to run at Sophie. The patient was not wearing a hospital gown. Louisa yelled at Sophie to back up against the wall. Sophie did just that, but in doing so was helpless as the patient came closer. The patient approached Sophie, looked into Sophie's eyes, but it seemed that they were not really seeing Sophie. The patient kept running down the hall. Louisa ran after them.

What do you think you would do if you were Sophie?

INTRODUCTION

Workplace violence and incivility in health care have emerged as important safety issues over the past decade. Workplace violence is seen on a continuum from threats or intimidation to its most extreme form, homicide. Violence, whether by persons outside or within an organization, has been shown to have negative effects including increased job stress, reduced productive work time, decreased morale, increased staff turnover, and loss of trust in the organization and its management. The purpose of this chapter is to increase awareness of the risk factors for violence and incivility in health care facilities and to enhance consideration of strategies for decreasing or preventing those events in the workplace.

DEFINING WORKPLACE VIOLENCE AND INCIVILITY

The Canadian Centre for Occupational Health and Safety (CCOHS, 2014a) conducts research, carries out projects, and publishes information on workplace health and safety to carry out a vision of "creating a work world without pain, loss, or tragedy." The CCOHS works with industry and labour organizations to understand and improve worker safety and health in Canada. Although one might assume that workplace violence is related specifically to acts that cause physical injury, the CCOHS (2014c) defines

---

> ### BOX 26.1   Types of Violence
>
> Workplace violence includes these broad categories:
> - **Threatening behaviour:** For example, shaking fists, destroying property or throwing objects; verbal or written threats and any expression of an intent to inflict harm
> - **Harassment:** Any behaviour that demeans, embarrasses, humiliates, annoys, or alarms a person and is known or would be expected to be unwelcome. It includes verbal abuse (swearing, insults, or condescending language), disrespectful gestures, intimidation, bullying, or other inappropriate activities
> - **Physical attacks:** The act of hitting, shoving, pushing, or kicking someone
>   Rumours, pranks, arguments, property damage, vandalism, sabotage, theft, psychologic trauma, anger-related incidents, rape, arson, and murder are also examples of workplace violence.

From Canadian Centre for Occupational Health and Safety. (2014b). Violence in the workplace: Awareness, p. 9. Retrieved from http://author.vubiz.com/fModules/5595EN/LMS-Start.html?vModId=5595EN.

---

workplace violence as "any act in which a person is abused, threatened, intimidated or assaulted in his or her employment." Box 26.1 provides examples of workplace violence.

Workplace violence does not only occur in the work setting. It can take place at any off-site location (i.e., home, business conference) that is associated with work. For instance, receiving a harassing e-mail or telephone call at home from a former patient or co-worker would be considered as a form of workplace-related violence.

In recent years, additional descriptions of workplace violence have been added. Horizontal violence is "an act of aggression that is perpetuated by one colleague toward another colleague" (Longo & Sherman, 2007, p.35). Lateral violence, which is often used interchangeably with *horizontal violence*, refers to "psychologic harassment evidenced by verbal abuse, intimidation, exclusion, unfair assignments, denial of access to opportunities, and withholding of information" (Morse, 2008, p. 4). Other terms associated with this type of violence include bullying, which is a practice closely related to lateral or horizontal violence, but a real or perceived power differential between the instigator and recipient must be present in bullying (Public Service Alliance of Canada, 2015). The CCOHS (2018) defines workplace bullying as "usually seen as acts or verbal comments that could 'mentally' hurt or isolate a person in the workplace. Sometimes, bullying can involve negative physical contact as well. Bullying usually involves repeated incidents or a pattern of behaviour that is intended to intimidate, offend, degrade or humiliate a particular person or group of people. It has also been described as the assertion of power through aggression". Interpersonal conflict occurs between and among patients, family members, nurses, physicians, and members of other departments. These behaviours exist in what has been termed toxic workplaces, which are organizations in which people feel devalued or dehumanized and in which disruptive behaviour often flourishes. Incivility includes a wide range of behaviours from ignoring, to rolling one's eyes, to yelling, and eventually to personal attacks, both physical and psychological. The term *bullying* is often subsumed under the term *incivility*. Workplace violence and incivility can also occur from patients, or from members of the public who do not have a direct connection to the organization.

Scope of the Problem

The true scope of workplace violence in health care is difficult to determine. Violence against health care providers is a serious problem throughout the world. The International Council of Nurses (2009) has indicated that nurses are the health care workers most at risk for workplace violence;

female nurses are most vulnerable to experiencing violence in the workplace. In the United Kingdom, over 56,000 incidents of violence against health care workers was reported in 2016 to 2017, which was an increase of almost 10% in one year (HSJ, 2018; Stephenson, 2018). A Statistics Canada report on workplace violence (Shields & Wilkins, 2009) noted that, in 2005, 34% of nurses in Canada who were employed in acute or long-term health care organizations reported being physically abused by a patient, whereas 47% reported that they had experienced emotional abuse at work. Nurses who reported abuse were often male, had less experience, usually worked nonday shifts, and perceived staffing or resources as inadequate, nurse–physician relations as poor, and co-worker and supervisor support as low. This report raises questions about why incidents of violence are on the rise, why male nurses might be reporting workplace violence more often than female nurses, and what contributes to underreporting of such issues in the health care sector. It is important to consider if violence is being normalized in some settings, such as emergency departments, mental health settings, and long-term care (Angharad Ashtonet al., 2018).

According to the Government of Ontario, Ministry of Labour health care report (2017), workplace violence "accounted for 12% of all lost-time injuries in the health care sector in 2015". This data was drawn from Workplace Safety and Insurance Board (WSIB) data published in 2016. In a 2014 analysis by the WSIB regarding claims, it is noted that there was an increase of 6.4% in reports of workplace violence from 2013 to 2014 in the health care sector. The Ontario Nurses' Association (ONA) states that "Health care is dangerous work, especially when it comes to workplace violence. In 2014 health care workers had more lost-time injuries because of violence than manufacturing, construction and mining combined. Six hundred and eighty lost-time WSIB claims were accepted for health care workers in Ontario" (2018). Further, ONA notes that in 2016, lost-time injuries attributed to violence in the workplace increased by 27% over 4 years (2017). Clancy (2015), a journalist with the Canadian Broadcasting Corporation, reported statistics from WorkSafe BC, which highlighted that between 2005 and 2012 almost 4000 health care workers reported injuries as a result of violence in the workplace. WorkSafe BC highlights that "health care and social services are disproportionately represented in time-loss claims because of acts of violence; 62 percent of all violence-related time-loss claims arise out of the health care and social services" (2018). An older, but still relevant Statistics Canada report (de Léséleuc, 2004) noted that of the 356,000 incidents of workplace violence that took place in the provinces, 33%

were reported by health care or social assistance workers. A shortage of national data on workplace violence exists, which means that accurate data for health care alone and nursing in particular, are hard to determine in Canada. In its position statement about incivility, bullying, and workplace violence, The American Nurses Association (ANA) (2015) notes that the financial cost is difficult to measure because of similar issues experienced in Canada related to estimating organizational and individual level costs. The ANA (2015) suggests that challenges in estimating cost could be attributed to various measures used to assess productivity in health care settings, treatment costs for workplace violence injuries, and expenses accrued by organizations to educate employees about, and to manage, issues related to violence, bullying, and incivility. Nonetheless, workplace violence, bullying, and incivility in health care facilities is unsettling

A key concern is that the true rate of workplace violence is much higher because many incidents might not be reported, especially when violence does not result in physical injury or is verbal in nature (e.g., intimidation or bullying). In many instances, workplace insurance boards do not fully recognize psychologic injuries. As such, psychologic injuries, such as posttraumatic stress disorder often go unrecognized, which can lead to an undervaluing of such injuries by the employer and even colleagues. Underreporting is thought to be related to nursing perceptions that assaults with or without injuries are "part of the job." According to the Canadian Federation of Nurses Unions (CFNU), health care worker lost-time related to violence between 2006 to 2015 resulted in 16,617 claims. This is over double the rate reported by police and correctional service officers in the same time period (CFNU, 2017). A CFNU national poll of nurses found that 61% have experienced violence in the workplace, as compared with 15% of employees in other occupational sectors over two years (2017). What is troubling, is that the rates of violence do not appear to have decreased, as is evidenced by a review conducted by Hader (2008) who found that 80% of the 1377 nurse respondents from the United States and 17 other countries reported having experienced some form of violence within the work setting. Verbal rather than physical forms of violence were reported most often. According to the survey, the perpetrator was a patient 53.2% of the time, with nurse colleagues a close second at 51.9% of the time. The ranking of those who experienced violence was as follows: physicians (49%), visitors (47%), and other health care workers (37.7%). Nearly eight out of 10 (79.7%) nurses observed their colleagues being the primary target of this violence, and well over half (56.1%)

had personally been the target. Many earlier studies with similar findings demonstrate the need to examine the causes of workplace violence and develop programs and strategies to improve personal safety in the workplace. In particular, attention needs to be paid to the causes and remedies for lateral violence issues.

Ensuring a Safe Workplace

Although legislation or regulations to address the prevention of workplace violence exist in each province and territory, their content is not consistent across Canada. Most recently, Bill 168 gained royal assent by the Legislative Assembly of Ontario as an amendment to the *Occupational Health and Safety Act* in relation to violence and harassment in the workplace. The CCOHS has published voluntary guidelines for workers in health care and several other high-risk professions. Although not all employers across Canada are legally obligated to follow the CCOHS guidelines, the *Canada Occupational Health and Safety Regulations*, and any derivative of the acts that exist in the provinces or territories, generally mandate employers to comply with workplace hazard-specific standards. Employers have a general duty to provide their employees with a workplace free from recognized hazards likely to cause death or serious physical harm. Consequences can occur if such measures are not adhered to. For instance, an organization can be cited if its leaders fail to address such hazards. The CCOHS (2013) developed a *Violence in the Workplace Prevention Guide* to help organizations develop violence-prevention plans. Several provinces are also enacting or developing laws, standards, or recommendations that address health care workplace security and safety. Recently, WorkSafe BC published a report with strategies to help employers decrease workplace injuries in sectors including health care (2018).

The Canadian Nurses Association (CNA, 2009) position statement on leadership in nursing calls for nurse leaders to create and sustain practice environments that are free of violence for patients, families, and health care providers. The position statement cites studies that suggest intimidating and disruptive behaviours contribute to poor patient satisfaction and preventable adverse outcomes. The CNA's *Code of Ethics for Registered Nurses* (2017) includes the following core responsibilities central to ethical nursing practice: promoting health and well-being; preserving dignity; promoting justice; being accountable; and providing safe, compassionate, competent, and ethical care. Provincial and territorial nursing associations and regulatory bodies have developed practice standards that are drawn from the CNA code of ethics. These standards articulate the role of nurses in promoting safe and healthy practice environments for those who are in their care and for their nursing colleagues. For instance, the College of Nurses of Ontario (2018) practice standards include accountability, continuing competence, ethics, knowledge application, leadership, and relationships. Thus when nurses engage in any form of workplace violence toward patients or other health care providers, they are in effect breaching the ethics and standards of their profession. Further, if nurses are the victims of or witnesses to workplace violence, they have a duty and right to report the situation and to seek support to address the incident, as required. Given the profession's standards and code of ethics, it is evident that nurses' and patients' well-being are to be considered a priority in all health care settings.

The Cost of Workplace Violence

Our knowledge of the scale of workplace violence remains incomplete because no consistent system of data collection exists in Canada (de Léséleuc, 2004). Data regarding less severe forms of workplace violence nationally are particularly sparse. Even less clear is the financial toll workplace aggression exacts on businesses. The annual direct and indirect costs in the United States of workplace incivility and violence are US$23.8 billion (Sheehan et al., 2001, as cited in Laschinger et al., 2013). Speroni and colleagues (2014) conducted a study of a hospital with 5000 nurses that spends almost USD 100,000 each year on treatment related to nurses who have experienced workplace violence. Of the 762 nurse participants in their study, 76% reported experiencing violence in the workplace, including physical and verbal abuse by patients and visitors (Speroni et al., 2014). Given reports of the incidence of workplace violence and incivility rising across years, it is likely that both direct and indirect costs have also increased in the United States. Although Canadian figures for the overall costs of workplace violence in health care are not currently available, if one applies the US per capita costs to the Canadian population, then the costs of workplace violence to Canadian health care organizations are similarly exorbitant. The costs from lost work time and wages, reduced productivity, medical costs, workers' compensation payments, legal and security expenses, and the costs to patients may be difficult to estimate but are clearly excessive when compared with the cost of prevention.

Gates et al. (2011) found that workplace violence led to costs associated with nurses' health and well-being. Gates et al. (2011) noted that, of the 230 emergency department nurses who participated in their study, 94% experienced at least one episode of posttraumatic stress disorder in relation to an incident of violence in the practice setting. Gates et al. (2011) also stated that nurses' levels of stress in the workplace were associated with decreased productivity. Rees and colleagues (2018) found that nurses and midwives in Australia who experienced workplace violence had higher rates of burnout and lower levels of resilience than colleagues who had not experienced such violence.

Other costs of workplace violence include increased staff turnover rates. In China, researchers found that nurses who experienced workplace violence reported lower job satisfaction and increased turnover intention (Zhao et al., 2018). A metaanalysis of 66 studies on bullying in nursing found that workplace violence was associated with "both job-related and health- and well-being–related outcomes, such as mental and physical health problems, symptoms of posttraumatic stress disorder, burnout, increased intentions to leave, and reduced job satisfaction and organizational commitment" (Nielsen & Einarsen, 2012, p. 309). Loss of the organizational investment required to train qualified staff, as well as the departure of experienced existing staff, can increase operating expenses and reduce the quality of care. Pearson and Porath (2009) suggest that cost estimates should consider how many times people report they are sick when they are really avoiding bad behaviour, as well as decreases in productivity because employees no longer feel comfortable in the environment. The costs of absenteeism alone mount rapidly. When nurses begin to stay away from the practice setting because of workplace violence issues, it is plausible that they are considering leaving the setting altogether. Research has demonstrated that stress, burnout, and incidences of incivility in the workplace are linked with intentions to leave the practice setting (Oyeleye et al., 2013). Studies have yet to capture the full cost of workplace violence in its many forms. More measurement is also needed to assess the cost and effectiveness of known intervention strategies.

Making a Difference

So what is the nurse in a leader, manager, or follower role to do, given the serious and complex issue of violence in the workplace? Making a difference includes promotion of an organizational culture of safety, developing and implementing a safety strategy, providing training programs, predicting problems, and using technology (e.g., to monitor isolated places) to reduce the incidence of violence. A culture of safety includes health care providers, patients, and their families. When workplace violence occurs in the practice setting, both nurses' and patients' health and well-being are at risk. If nurse leaders' and nurses' time and

energy are being directed away from patient care because of workplace violence issues, then the implications for patients could range from decreased attention to patient pain control needs, lack of or receipt of incorrect treatments, and potentially even death (Emergency Care Research Institute, 2009). When considering the issue of workplace violence from a nurses' perspective, given the gravity of the issue and the myriad of negative personal and professional outcomes it can have, strategies to prevent being victimized by violence in any practice setting are critical.

PREVENTION STRATEGIES

The old adage "an ounce of prevention is worth a pound of cure" is particularly relevant when dealing with workplace violence. Preventing even one act of violence can save money and time and diminish the possible negative psychological impact of such an event (Ostrofsky, 2012). By taking a proactive approach that includes preventing violence, organizations can also avoid being victimized. To address the issue of violence, it is necessary to recall that violence can be perpetuated by co-workers, managers, patients, former employees, or members of the public not aligned with the organization (CCOHS, 2014b). Thus the types of violence that may be encountered, and the signs that portend a potentially violent situation, might differ depending on who is the perpetrator. In short, prevention is the right thing to do for people and for the organization.

Identifying Risk Factors

Although anyone working in health care is at risk of becoming a victim of violence, those with direct patient contact are at a higher risk. Violence is also a frequent occurrence in psychiatric and geriatric settings. Hospital-based violence can take place either horizontally, among nurses, or can be directed at nurses by patients or their families, as a result of feeling frustration or anger. Such acts are usually related to feelings of vulnerability, stress, and loss of control that accompany illness (College of Nurses of Ontario [CNO], 2017). Many factors have been identified that can increase the risk of violence erupting in health care facilities. The Occupational Safety and Health Administration (OSHA, 2016) report *Guidelines for preventing workplace violence for health care and social service workers* identifies risk factors for workplace violence in health care facilities that occur between a nurse and a client, among colleagues, or management and nurses. These factors are listed in Box 26.2. Other risk factors for violence in the workplace relate to the organization itself, and include the location of the

BOX 26.2   Risk Factors for Violence in Health Care Facilities

- Low staff levels, especially during visiting hours and meal times
- Transportation of patients between areas within a facility
- Long wait times for patient care
- Overcrowded, uncomfortable waiting areas
- Solo work in an area isolated from other staff
- Solo work in an area with no backup or way to get assistance, such as communication devices or alarm systems
- Poor environmental design
- Inadequate security
- Lack of staff training in handling potentially violent situations
- Lack of policies for preventing and managing crises with potentially violent individuals
- Unrestricted movement of patients or visitors
- Poorly lit corridors, rooms, parking lots, or other areas
- Prevalence of handguns or other weapons among patients, their families, or friends
- Increasing presence of gang members, drug or alcohol abusers, trauma patients, or distraught family members
- Use of hospitals or health care facilities for holding criminals, violent individuals, and the acutely mentally disturbed
- An increase in the number of chronically mentally ill patients being released without adequate resources for follow-up care
- Availability of money or medications within the facility

Modified from Occupational Safety and Health Administration. (2016). *Guidelines for preventing workplace violence for health care and social service workers* (OSHA Publication No.3148-06R 2016). Washington, DC: U.S. Department of Labor. Retrieved from https://www.osha.gov/Publications/osha3148.pdf

facility, its size, the type of care provided, lack of policies and education about how to assess for and manage escalating behaviours, high rates of staff turnover, limited security, and less than optimal numbers of staff during peak times, long wait times, crowded treatment or waiting areas, and a sense that there are limited consequences when violence occurs (OSHA, 2016).

Similar to the nursing process, prevention of workplace violence begins with a systematic assessment. Assessing risk and planning for prevention of workplace violence call for input and expertise from a variety of staff. A risk assessment based on a multidisciplinary team approach to workplace violence prevention is often the most effective. A team with representation from administration, staff, security, facilities, engineering, human resources, legal counsel, and risk management is needed to address risks from all perspectives. The *Violence in the Workplace Prevention Guide* developed by the CCOHS (2013) provides readers with a step-by-step, common-sense approach to assessing and reducing existing and potential areas of workplace violence. The Ontario Ministry of Labour has also developed an online resource to assist individuals and groups to create programs and policies to support a healthy work environment free of workplace violence called *Developing Workplace Violence and Harassment Policies and Programs: A Toolbox* (2013). Similar to other regulatory bodies in Canada, the CNO (2017) outlines key factors that can lead to conflict in the workplace, along with prevention strategies that are focused at various levels—nurse and client, nurse and nurse, nurse and management, and organizational. In addition, in the United States, the Department of Labor, OSHA's *Guidelines for Preventing Workplace Violence for Health Care and Social Service Workers* (2016) provides a comprehensive assessment with detailed checklists (Box 26.3).

When looking at possible threats or hazards, those from within an organization must also be considered. Determining if current employees pose a danger in the workplace is a critical factor that is often overlooked. In addition to personal and psychologic factors, behaviours can be observed in employees that may be related to violence or aggression in the workplace (Paludi et al., 2006). The most obvious of these is a previous history of aggression and substance abuse. Screening potential employees through background inquiries and references can help reduce these risks. Paludi et al. (2006) also advise of warning signs that can alert employers of problems with current employees that warrant intervention to prevent a violent incident.

No profile or litmus test exists to identify whether a current employee might become violent. It is important for employers and employees alike to remain alert to problematic behaviour that, in combination, could point to possible violence. Because no one behaviour in and of itself suggests a greater potential for violence, behaviours must be looked at in totality. Problem situations and circumstances that may heighten the risk of violence can involve a particular event or employee or the workplace as a whole.

BOX 26.3   Workplace Violence Program Checklists

The Occupational Safety and Health Administration (OSHA) has provided a comprehensive checklist that can help "Health and Safety, Crime/Workplace Violence Prevention Coordinator, or joint labor/management committee" to conduct an organizational workplace violence assessment. The checklist titles are provided here. The checklists provide detailed step-by-step instructions to conduct an in-depth assessment and establish a monitoring program.

To see the complete document, go to https://www.osha.gov/Publications/osha3148.pdf

Checklist 1: Risk factors for workplace violence.
Checklist 2: Inspecting work areas.
Checklist 3: Inspecting exterior building areas.
Checklist 4: Inspecting parking areas.
Checklist 5: Security measures.

The Occupational Safety and Health Administration. (2016). *Guidelines for preventing workplace violence for health care and social service workers* (OSHA Publication No. 3148-06R 2016). Washington, DC: U.S. Department of Labor. https://www.osha.gov/Publications/osha3148.pdf

---

EXERCISE 26.1 Assess several practice settings for workplace violence risks. Can you identify any of the risks listed in Box 26.2? What security measures are currently in place? Can any of the identified risks be improved? How? How safe would you feel in the different geographic areas?

Once the risk assessment is completed, the next step is to analyze the data and prioritize the problems that need to be addressed. Priorities can be established by asking a few basic questions: What are the risks? Who might be harmed and how? What is the level of risk? What measures need to be taken to reduce or eliminate risk? Do changes need to be implemented now or later? Once the priorities are set, the business of designing or improving prevention programs can begin.

EXERCISE 26.2 What elements do you think represent a healthy workplace or practice environment? Consider a practice setting where you were employed or where you were a student that you feel represents such "healthy" elements. What was it like to work and learn in such a setting? What were the relationships like among health professionals, among nurses, and among nurses and the nursing leadership? In what ways do you think that such a healthy practice environment ultimately influenced the quality of patient care and patient outcomes? What is your role as a student or new graduate nurse in contributing to the development and sustainability of a healthy practice environment?

HORIZONTAL VIOLENCE: THE THREAT FROM WITHIN

Horizontal violence includes a wide variety of behaviours, from verbal abuse to physical aggression between co-workers. This term, although commonly used, may be limiting because it suggests that the violence is perpetrated between those at the same level of authority. It may be better termed *relational aggression*, which involves bullying using psychologic and social behaviours between people at the same or different levels (Dellasega, 2009).

Horizontal violence and its effects have been reported in nursing literature for more than 20 years. A review of five research studies published between 2003 and 2004 on horizontal violence found that horizontal violence is experienced by all nurses, regardless of their degree of work experience (Woelfle & McCaffrey, 2007). Many of the research studies found infighting and a general lack of support among nurses to be common occurrences. The studies also indicated that new graduates were likely to experience horizontal violence, which resulted in high absentee rates and thoughts of leaving nursing after the first year. *Nursing2011* conducted a survey to identify how often nurses experience or witness horizontal violence. In all, 82% or 778 of survey respondents reported having witnessed or experienced horizontal violence either daily or weekly (Dumont et al., 2012). Nurse peers were most often cited as the perpetrators of horizontal violence, and supervisors were cited as next to highest (Dumont et al., 2012). Findings from this survey caused the researchers to ask this question: How can nurses treat patients kindly and give them the respect they need when they treat each other so poorly? In light of the looming nursing shortage, these consistent findings among nurses were cause for concern.

Many theories exist as to why horizontal violence takes place in nursing. Historically, horizontal violence in nursing was considered to be a result of nursing's traditional hierarchical structure, the oppression of nursing as a profession, or feminism (Farrell, 2001). However, because workplace aggression is common in other professions as well, it is most likely the result of a complex myriad of individual, social, and organizational characteristics (Farrell, 2001; Hutchinson et al., 2006). More recently, bullying in the workplace has been linked to worker burnout and decreased access to empowering structures in the work environment, including access to information, resources, supports, and opportunities (Laschinger et al., 2010). When nurses are more structurally empowered, they report fewer incidents of bullying (Laschinger et al., 2010), which supports the proposition that empowering work environments have the potential to decrease incidents of workplace violence of the horizontal type (see the Research Perspective for more on building empowering work environments). Regardless of the reasons why it happens, the concerns are that impaired intrapersonal relationships between nurses at work can cause errors, accidents, and poor work performance (Gates et al., 2011) and that those relationships may play a significant role in attrition (Johnson, 2009). In a classic survey on workplace intimidation published by the Institute for Safe Medication Practices (2003), almost half of the 2095 respondents recalled being verbally abused when questioning or clarifying medication prescriptions. This intimidation led some health care providers to refrain from questioning a medication order to avoid confrontation with the prescriber. The results of the survey had professional health care and nursing organizations issue calls to action to address all types of workplace violence in the interest of promoting a safe and respectful work environment that promotes the delivery of high-quality care instead of threatening it. Shortly after the release of the Institute's report, the International Council of Nurses (ICN, 2006) published a position statement on health care workplace violence, which included the following assertion:

> *Violence in the workplace threatens the delivery of effective patient services and, therefore patient safety. If quality care is to be provided, nursing personnel must be ensured a safe work environment and respectful treatment. Excessive workloads, unsafe working conditions, and inadequate support can be considered forms of violence and incompatible with good practice.*

RESEARCH PERSPECTIVE

Resource: Laschinger, H. K. S., Leiter, M. P., Day, A., et al. (2012). Building empowering work environments that foster civility and organizational trust. Testing an intervention. *Nursing Research, 61*(5), 316–235.

The authors studied the impact of a workplace intervention (a Civility, Respect, and Engagement in the Workplace [CREW] program) on nurses' empowerment, experiences of incivility, and trust in nursing management. The 6-month-long CREW program was instituted in eight acute care hospital units across two provinces. A total of 33 units were control groups. The CREW program involved weekly unit meetings that were facilitated by a CREW "expert." At the meetings, management and nursing staff would develop goals to achieve positive interpersonal relationships, and strategies were selected from the CREW toolkit to support the achievement of the goals. The process for enacting strategies was also outlined in the weekly planning meetings. Participants in the control and intervention groups completed measures to assess perceptions of structural workplace empowerment, rates of supervisor and co-worker incivility, and trust in management. Initially, it appeared that the intervention and control group measurement scores were similar. However, in-depth statistical analysis demonstrated that over time, in comparison to the control group, the intervention group scores were significantly improved for overall empowerment and trust in management, and reported rates had significantly decreased over time for supervisor and co-worker incivility.

Implications for Practice
The authors noted that the CREW program showed promising results in supporting management and staff to foster and sustain positive professional relationships. The authors underscored that empowering work environments are associated with decreased levels of incivility. Empowering environments have been associated with enhanced psychologic empowerment, which in turn influences nurses' use of empowering behaviours, job satisfaction, and nurse-assessed quality of care (Purdy et al., 2010). Therefore managers who make a concerted effort to enhance access to support, resources, opportunities for growth and learning, and information related to the broader organization give nurses a greater opportunity to find more meaning and self-efficacy in their role. Further, managers who engage in empowering behaviours, such as involving nurses in decision making and problem solving on the unit and provide timely feedback about performance foster greater job satisfaction for nurses. Finally, when nurses partner with management to create and sustain strategies to enhance relationships, such as those in the CREW program, the number of incidents of workplace incivility will decrease, which can ultimately lead to better patient outcomes.

LITERATURE PERSPECTIVE

Resource: Anthony, M., & Yastik, J. (2011). Nursing students' experiences with incivility in clinical education. *Journal of Nursing Education, 50*(3), 140–144.

A qualitative study was conducted with 21 nursing students in focus group settings to explore students' experiences of incivility in the clinical setting and to understand their views about how nursing programs should attend to the topic and issue of incivility. Students' comments reflected themes of exclusion and being dismissed by nursing staff, along with being subjected to rude and hostile behaviour from staff. Students also shared positive experiences, such as when staff took the initiative to include students in learning opportunities involving patient care. Students felt that they would benefit from more preparation about the challenges they might face in the practice setting related to incivility. They also felt that nursing programs could better liaise with nurse leaders and nursing staff in the practice setting so that staff are aware of students' course goals and level of knowledge and skill at the outset of the clinical experience. Students also felt that when clinical instructors were respected by nursing staff, by extension, they were treated well by staff.

Implications for Practice
The findings of the study suggest that healthy work environments exist when nursing staff, nurse leaders, educators, and nursing students recognize that their individual and collective efforts are contributing factors to such environments. Finally, when organizational structures support a healthy work environment, then opportunities can exist for staff nurses to practise in a more inclusive and civil manner.

In 2008, the Center for American Nurses published a position paper stating that no place exists in a professional practice environment for horizontal violence and bullying among nurses or health care providers overall. These disruptive behaviours are toxic to the nursing profession and have a negative impact on retention of quality staff. Horizontal violence and bullying should never be considered as a normal part of socialization in nursing or be accepted in professional relationships. The subsequent Literature Perspective discusses nursing student experiences with incivility. The Center for American Nurses asserts that all health care organizations should implement a zero-tolerance policy on disruptive behaviour, as well as a professional code of conduct, and educational and behavioural interventions to assist nurses in addressing disruptive behaviour. The CNA partnered with the CFNU (2008) to publish a joint position statement about workplace violence, noting that "it is the right of all nurses to work in an environment that is free from violence" (p. 1). With professional groups in both Canada and the United States calling for change from within nursing, we must examine how to implement that change.

CONCLUSION

Workplace violence and incivility affect us all. The burden is borne not only by victims but also by their co-workers, their families, their employers, and every worker at risk of such acts. Workplace violence and incivility also have real consequences for patients and patient safety. Although we know that, each year, workplace violence in Canada results in deaths, injuries, and financial costs, our understanding of workplace violence in health care is still in its infancy. Much remains to be done in the area of research, particularly in data collection and interventions for horizontal violence. Without basic information on who is most affected and which prevention measures are effective in what settings, we can expect only limited success in addressing these problems. The first steps have been taken, but a number of key issues have been identified that require future research. All nurses and health care leaders need a broader understanding of the scope and impact of workplace violence and incivility to reduce the human and financial burden of these significant public health problems.

📍 A SOLUTION

Sophie ran to the nurses' station and called for security and for the emergency department physician to come to the unit. Then, they ran back down another hall where they could hear the man yelling at Louisa in a patient room. When Sophie entered the room, the patient was in what had been an empty bed, and Louisa and another nurse, Beth, were standing close to him. The patient was holding the bed linens up to their chest and was yelling incoherently at the two nurses. Louisa, who had blood all over the front of her uniform, had not been seriously physically injured. Beth's hair was dishevelled and they were not wearing their glasses. The nurses were speaking calmly to the patient, trying to reassure them that they were safe and that nobody was going to harm them. Within what felt like mere seconds, security personnel had entered the room with the emergency department physician. The physician had a copy of the patient's blood work that had been drawn just before they were admitted to the unit. The patient's blood glucose was dangerously low. The physician verbally ordered medication to increase the patient's blood glucose level. While waiting in the room with the patient, the physician and one of the nurses kept responding to the patient in a calm manner. Louisa, Beth, and Sophie stepped away from the patient's bed to offer a feeling of space. The ordered medication arrived very quickly and was administered by the physician via injection. Within less than 1 minute, the patient's behaviour was completely altered. They were confused about where they were and what was going on. The patient apologized profusely, as they came to realize that they were not wearing clothing, saw that security personnel were in the room, and saw the blood on Louisa's uniform. Beth explained to the patient that their blood glucose had been very low, which caused them to act out of character, but that the nurses would continue to provide the care necessary for the patient to feel safe, and they were not moved to another room, as that was felt to be too disruptive for the patient at the time.

After the incident, Sophie learned how the situation unfolded. When the patient was admitted to the unit, Beth was starting an intravenous (IV) and they accused Beth of taking their glasses. The patient believed that Beth's glasses were their own. Thus, they grabbed Beth's hair. Beth was in pain from having their hair severely torn at, so they called for help. That is when Louisa entered the patient's room and tried to move the patient's hand from the hold they had on Beth's hair. Next, the patient began to tear the IV catheter out, which caused what looked like the loss of a lot of blood on Louisa's uniform. The patient then leapt out of bed, tore off their hospital gown, and began chasing Louisa down the hallway. That was the point when Sophie observed the patient and Louisa down the hall.

At the time of this situation, Sophie was a student nurse. What they learned from this experience is that the situation was addressed effectively by the collaboration amongst the team of health care providers. The patient's dignity was respected throughout the incident, and they were never physically restrained. Communication techniques and body language skills were used to deescalate the situation, while a medically therapeutic intervention was enacted. When the patient's behaviour returned to normal, the nursing staff did not demean nor cast blame on the patient. Instead, they took even more time with the patient to ensure they felt safe and respected. Recognizing the patient's humanity in this situation helped make a tangible difference in the outcome.

How might you have dealt with this situation in the practice setting?

▌ THE EVIDENCE

Workplace violence is recognized as a significant problem within health care. Reviews of nursing literature indicate that violence in the workplace is a significant reason for nurses to leave their jobs and, in some cases, the nursing profession. With growing concern about a nursing shortage, nurse leaders need to implement effective intervention programs to foster a healthier workplace. To date, education has been the main intervention strategy, however, there is a paucity of published research focused on evaluating the efficacy of education alone in addressing workplace violence.

Lamont and Brunero (2018) conducted a quasi-experimental study with 78 nurses employed at a 440-bed referral hospital in Australia who attended a one-day workshop about workplace violence "in relation to risk assessment and management practices, deescalation skills, breakaway techniques, and confidence levels" (p. 45). The researchers found a statistically significant difference

■ THE EVIDENCE—cont'd

from pretest to posttest on nurses' clinical behaviour intentions related to the workshop training objectives, and on nurses' confidence to cope with patient aggression. The results highlight the relevance of education about workplace violence management in building coping and confidence among nursing staff. The researchers note that such education is but one factor in addressing workplace violence, incivility, and bullying, and that organizations have a "duty of care to ensure employee safety" (p. 51).

✴ NEED TO KNOW NOW

- Know how to access the workplace safety plan in your area of practice.
- Be aware of your surroundings at all times, keeping in mind that you are at increased risk for violence.

- Use an assessment tool to help you identify behaviours that predict violence.
- Practise what to say to stop workplace bullying.

■ CHAPTER CHECKLIST

Nursing research indicates that violence in any form can drain nurses of their enthusiasm for their work and undermine efforts to create a satisfied workforce. At a time when we are facing a nursing shortage, it is imperative to prevent or eliminate workplace violence and incivility in health care.

- All nurses—leaders, managers, and followers—must be aware of the potential for all forms of violence and incivility. They must also strive to not participate in horizontal violence, which weakens nursing as a profession. The key to preventing violence is understanding the potential for it and implementing interventions to minimize that potential.
- Workplace violence and incivility in health care are important safety issues.
- Workplace violence includes threatening behaviour, harassment, and physical attacks. It can be perpetuated by co-workers, managers, patients, former employees, or members of the public not aligned with the organization.
- Key organizations are calling for action to reduce workplace violence, including the following:
  - Canadian Centre for Occupational Health and Safety (CCOHS)
  - Canadian Nurses Association (CNA)
  - International Council of Nurses (ICN)
  - Institute for Safe Medication Practices
- The risk factors for violence in health care facilities must be assessed when planning for prevention.
- Horizontal violence is experienced by all nurses, regardless of their degree of work experience.
  - Regardless of why it happens, the concerns are that impaired intrapersonal relationships can cause errors, accidents, and poor work performance.
- When nurses are more structurally empowered, they report fewer incidents of bullying.

■ TIPS FOR PREVENTING WORKPLACE VIOLENCE

- Take advantage of education offered on workplace violence. If education is not offered, ask your employer to consider providing it.
- Make a personal commitment not to participate in any behaviours that perpetuate horizontal violence.

- Practise precautionary strategies and analyze workplaces for safety risk factors.

Visit the Evolve website for Suggested Readings, Internet Resources, and additional resources related to the content in this chapter: http://evolve.elsevier.com/Canada/Yoder-Wise/leading/.

REFERENCES

Statutes

Canada Occupational Health and Safety Regulations, SOR/86-304.

Occupational Health and Safety Act, RS0 1990, c. O.1.

Texts

American Nurses Association. (2015). *Position statement on incivility, bullying, and workplace violence.* Retrieved from: https://www.nursingworld.org/practice-policy/ nursing-excellence/official-position-statements/id/ incivility-bullying-and-workplace-violence/.

Angharad Ashton, R., Morris, L., & Smith, I. (2018). A qualitative meta-synthesis of emergency department staff experiences of violence and aggression. *International Emergency Room Nursing, 39,* 13–19.

Anthony, M., & Yastik, J. (2011). Nursing students' experiences with incivility in clinical education. *Journal of Nursing Education, 50*(3), 140–144.

Canadian Centre for Occupational Health and Safety. (2013). *Violence in the workplace prevention guide.* Retrieved from: http://www.ccohs.ca/products/publications/violence.html.

Canadian Centre for Occupational Health and Safety. (2014a). *About CCOHS.* Retrieved from: http://www. ccohs.ca/ccohs.html.

Canadian Centre for Occupational Health and Safety. (2014b). *Violence in the workplace: Awareness.* http:// sauthor.vubiz.com/fModules/5595EN/LMSStart.html?v-ModId=5595EN.

Canadian Centre for Occupational Health and Safety. (2014c). *Violence in the workplace: Warning signs.* Retrieved from: http://www.ccohs.ca/oshanswers/ psychosocial/violence_warning_signs.html.

Canadian Centre for Occupational Health and Safety. (2018). *Bullying in the workplace fact sheet.* Retrieved from: https:// www.ccohs.ca/oshanswers/psychosocial/bullying.html.

Canadian Federation of Nurses Unions. (2017). *Enough is enough: Putting a stop to violence in the health care section – A discussion paper.* Author. Retrieved from: https:// nursesunions.ca/wp-content/uploads/2017/05/CFNU_ Enough-is-Enough_June1_FINALlow.pdf.

Canadian Nurses Association. (2017). *Code of ethics for registered nurses.* Toronto, ON: Author. Retrieved from: https:// www.cna-aiic.ca/~/media/cna/page-content/pdf-en/ code-of-ethics-2017-edition-secure-interactive.

Canadian Nurses Association. (2009). *Position statement: Nursing leadership.* Retrieved from: http://cna-aiic. ca/~/media/cna/page-content/pdf-en/ps110_leadership_2009_e.pdf.

Canadian Nurses Association & Canadian Federation of Nurses Unions. (2008). *Joint position statement: Workplace violence.* Retrieved from: https://nursesunions.ca/sites/ default/files/workplace_violence_position_statement_ cna-cfnu_0.pdf.

Center for American Nurses. (2008). *Policy statement on lateral violence and bullying in the workplace.* Retrieved from: http://www.mc.vanderbilt.edu/root/pdfs/nursing/ center_lateral_violence_and_bullying_position_statement_from_center_for_american_nurses.pdf.

Clancy, N. (2015). *Nurse attacks: are bruises and black eyes the new face of B.C. health care.* CBC News. Retrieved from: http://www.cbc.ca/news/canada/british-columbia/ nurseattacks-are-bruises-and-black-eyes-the-new-face-of-b-c-health-care-1.2980754.

College of Nurses of Ontario. (2017). *Practice Guideline: Conflict Prevention and Management.* Author. Retrieved from: https://www.cno.org/globalassets/docs/prac/47004_conflict_prev.pdf.

College of Nurses of Ontario. (2018). *Professional Standards, Revised 2002.* Author. Retrieved from: http://www.cno.org/ Global/docs/prac/41006_ProfStds.pdf?epslanguage=en.

de Léséleuc, S. (2004). *Criminal victimization in the workplace (Canadian Centre for Justice Statistics Profile Series).* Ottawa, ON: Statistics Canada. Retrieved from: http://www. statcan.gc.ca/pub/85f0033m/85f0033m2007013-eng.pdf.

Dellasega, C. (2009). Bullying among nurses. *American Journal of Nursing, 109*(1), 52–58.

Dumont, C., Meisinger, S., Whitacre, M. J., et al. (2012). Horizontal violence survey report. *Nursing 2012,* 44–49.

Emergency Care Research Institute. (2009, March). Disruptive practitioner behavior. *Healthcare Risk Control.* Retrieved from: https://www.ecri.org/Documents/PSA/ May_2009/Disruptive_practitioner_behavior.pdf.

Farrell, G. (2001). From tall poppies to squashed weeds: Why don't nurses pull together more? *Journal of Advanced Nursing, 35*(1), 26–33.

Gates, D., Gillespie, G., & Succop, P. (2011). Violence against nurses and its impact on stress and productivity. *Nursing Economics, 29*(2), 59–66.

Hader, R. (2008). Workplace violence survey 2008. *Nursing Management, 39*(7), 13–19.

HSJ. (2018). *Exclusive: Dramatic rise in attacks on hospital staff.* United Kingdom: Author. Retrieved from: https:// www.hsj.co.uk/7022150.article#.

Hutchinson, M., Vickers, M., Jackson, D., et al. (2006). Workplace bullying in nursing: towards a more critical organizational perspective. *Nursing Inquiry, 15,* 118–126.

Institute for Safe Medication Practices. (2003). *Survey on workplace intimidation*. Retrieved from: http://www.ismp.org/Survey/surveyresults/Survey0311.asp.

International Council of Nurses. (2006). *Position statement: Abuse and violence against nursing personnel*. Retrieved from: http://www.icn.ch/images/stories/documents/publications/position_statements/C01_Abuse_Violence_Nsg_Personnel.pdf.

International Council of Nurses. (2009). *Violence: A worldwide epidemic. [Fact sheet]*. Geneva, Switzerland: Author. Retrieved from: http://www.icn.ch/images/stories/documents/publications/fact_sheets/19k_FS-Violence.pdf.

Johnson, S. (2009). Workplace bullying: Concerns for nurse leaders. *Journal of Nursing Administration, 39*(2), 84–90.

Lamont, S., & Brunero, S. (2018). The effect of a workplace violence training program for generalist nurses in the acute hospital setting: A quasi-experimental study. *Nurse Education Today, 68*, 45–52.

Laschinger, H. K. S., Grau, A., Finegan, J., et al. (2010). New graduate nurses' experiences of bullying and burnout in hospital settings. *Journal of Advanced Nursing, 66*(12), 2732–2742.

Laschinger, H. K. S., Leiter, M. P., Day, A., et al. (2012). Building empowering work environments that foster civility and organizational trust. Testing an intervention. *Nursing Research, 61*(5), 316–325.

Laschinger, H. K. S., Wong, C., Regan, S., et al. (2013). Workplace incivility and new graduate nurses' mental health: The protective role of resiliency. *The Journal of Nursing Administration, 43*(7/8), 415–421.

Longo, J., & Sherman, R. O. (2007). Levelling horizontal violence. *Nursing Management, 34–36*, 50+.

Morse, K. J. (2008). Lateral violence in nursing [Editorial]. *Nursing2014 Critical Care, 3*(2), 4.

Nielsen, M. B., & Einarsen, S. (2012). Outcomes of exposure to workplace bullying: A meta-analytic review. *Work and Stress, 26*(4), 309–332.

Occupational Safety and Health Administration. (2016). *Guidelines for preventing workplace violence for health care and social service workers (OSHA Publication No. 3148–06R 2016)*. Washington, DC: U.S. Department of Labor. Retrieved from: https://www.osha.gov/Publications/OSHA3148/osha3148.html.

Ontario Ministry of Labour. (2013). *Developing workplace violence and harassment policies and programs: A toolbox*. Author. Retrieved from: https://www.labour.gov.on.ca/english/hs/pubs/wvps_toolbox/index.php.

Ontario Ministry of Labour. (2017). *Inspection focus: Major hazards and key issues in health care*. Author. Retrieved from: https://www.ontario.ca/document/health-care-sector-plan-2017-18/inspection-focus-major-hazards-and-key-issues-health-care#foot-8.

Ontario Nurses Association. (2016). *Workplace violence and harassment. A guide for ONA members*. Author. Retrieved from: https://www.ona.org/wp-content/uploads/ona_guide_workplaceviolenceandharassment.pdf.

Ontario Nurses Association. (2018). *The Statistics*. Author. Retrieved from: http://violence.ona.org/the-statistics/.

Ontario Nurses Association. (2017). *Workplace violence and harassment: Not part of your job-infographic*. Author. Retrieved from: https://www.ona.org/wp-content/uploads/ona_workplaceviolenceinfographic_20171127.pdf.

Ostrofsky, D. (2012). Incivility and the nurse leader. *Nursing Management*, 18–22.

Oyeleye, O., Hanson, P., O'Connor, N., et al. (2013). Relationship of workplace incivility, stress, and burnout on nurses' turnover intentions and psychological empowerment. *Journal of Nursing Administration, 43*(10), 536–542.

Paludi, M., Nydegger, R., & Paludi, C. (2006). *Understanding workplace violence: A guide for managers and employees*. Westport, CT: Praeger.

Pearson, C., & Porath, C. (2009). *The cost of bad behavior: How incivility is damaging your business and what to do about it*. London, UK: Portfolio.

Public Service Alliance of Canada. (2015). *Violence and bullying prevention*. Author. Retrieved from: http://psacunion.ca/violence-and-bullying-prevention.

Purdy, N., Laschinger, H. K. S., Finegan, J., et al. (2010). Effects of work environments on nurse and patient outcomes. *Journal of Nursing Management, 18*, 901–913.

Rees, C., Wirihana, L., Eley, R., Ossieran-Moisson, R., & Hegney, D. (2018). The effects of occupational violence on the well-being and resilience of nurses. *Journal of Nursing Administration, 48*, 452–458.

Shields, M., & Wilkins, K. (2009). Factors related to on-the-job abuse of nurses by patients. *Health Reports, 20*(2), 1–13. Retrieved from: http://www.statcan.gc.ca/pub/82-003-x/2009002/article/10835-eng.pdf.

Speroni, K. G., Fitch, T., Dawson, E., Dugan, L., & Atherton, M. (2014). Incidence and cost of nurse workplace violence perpetrated by hospital patients or patient visitors. *Journal of Emergency Nursing, 40*, 218–228.

Stephenson, J. (2018). *Sharp spike in number of physical assaults on NHS staff. Nursing Times*, 1–3. Retrieved from: https://www.nursingtimes.net/news/workforce/sharp-spike-in-number-of-physical-assaults-on-nhs-staff/7024106. article.

Woelfle, C., & McCaffrey, R. (2007). Nurse on nurse. *Nursing Forum, 42*(3), 123–131.

Workplace Safety and Insurance Board (WSIB). (May 2014). *Enterprise Information Warehouse (EIW) Claim Cost Analysis Schema*. data snapshot.

data snapshot. *Workplace Safety and Insurance Board Enterprise Information Warehouse (EIW) Claim Cost Analysis Schema.* (June 2015). courtesy of Public Services Health and Safety Association.

data snapshot. *Workplace Safety and Insurance Board (WSIB) Enterprise Information Warehouse (EIW) Claim Cost Analysis Schema.* (June 2016). courtesy of Public Services Health and Safety Association.

WorkSafeBC. (2018). *WorkSafeBC releases three-year strategy to reduce serious injuries in the health care sector.* Author. Retrieved from: https://www.worksafebc.com/en/about-us/news-events/news-releases/2018/February/health-care-high-risk-strategy?origin=s&returnurl=https%3A%2F%E2%80%A6.

Zhao, S.-H., Shi, Y., Sun, Z.-N., et al. (2018). Impact of workplace violence against nurses' thriving at work, job satisfaction and turnover intention: A cross-sectional study. *Journal of Clinical Nursing, 27,* 2620–2632.

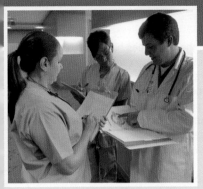

27

Inter- and Intraprofessional Practice and Leading in Professional Practice Settings

Erin Wilson

Nurses are integral members of inter- and intraprofessional teams. Although effective collaboration is a complex process, the outcomes can positively impact patients, health care providers, organizations, and the health care system overall. This chapter presents the nursing role in interprofessional diverse settings and reviews how legislation and regulation of nurses can influence interprofessional collaboration. It identifies a framework for interprofessional collaboration, as well as barriers and facilitators of collaboration. It also examines how nursing leadership can provide the backbone for effective teams.

OBJECTIVES

- Define interprofessional team and intraprofessional team.
- Understand the role and boundaries of nurses' scope of practice in your province or territory, as well as how the scope of practice overlaps with that of other health care providers.
- Understand the complexity of effective interprofessional collaboration and nurses' role on an interprofessional team in providing patient-centred care.

- Identify the purpose of the National Interprofessional Competency Framework.
- Describe strategies to enhance collaboration.
- Understand how team leaders can facilitate successful collaboration.
- Understand how structures and processes influence the function of interprofessional teams.

TERMS TO KNOW

accountability
collaboration
collaborative practice
delegation

interprofessional team
intraprofessional team
patient-centred care
role clarity

scope of practice
unregulated care providers
(UCPs)

? A CHALLENGE

Thomas is a student nurse on a general surgery ward. He is speaking with the physiotherapist about Mrs. Haley's progress with walking and reviewing medications that might interfere with her balance. Suddenly, a breathless porter approaches Thomas asking why Mrs. Haley isn't in X-ray for her fluoroscopy-guided procedure. Thomas was unaware this procedure had been booked. Just then, Mrs. Haley begins retching and her daughter is asking when her mother last received Gravol (dimenhydrinate). Thomas thinks his preceptor Layla, a registered nurse (RN), gave Mrs. Haley a p.r.n. dose while Thomas was on his break, but when he checks the medication administration record, nothing is recorded. The physiotherapist would like to know when Mrs. Haley might attend a phys-

iotherapy appointment, the porter has his hands on Mrs. Haley's chair ready to wheel her to radiology, and her daughter is holding Mrs. Haley's head over a kidney basin while she vomits. Thomas feels overwhelmed: should he search for Layla to see if Mrs. Haley had any dimenhydrinate, try to find out what procedure Mrs. Haley has booked in radiology, assist Mrs. Haley while she is sick, or direct the physiotherapist as to when Mrs. Haley might attend physiotherapy?

Identify the interpersonal, organizational, and systemic components of this scenario that could be improved by better interprofessional collaboration. What would you do if you were Thomas?

INTRODUCTION

In 1978 the Declaration of Alma-Ata identified that primary health care and improvement in health of the world's populations would rely in part on the ability of health care providers to work in teams (World Health Organization, 1978). In the intervening decades, policymakers in Canada have identified effective interprofessional collaboration as a national priority (Curran, 2007; Laschinger, 2007), and interprofessional research demonstrates the impact of interprofessional collaboration at patient, organizational, and system levels (Regan et al., 2015). The benefits of interprofessional care include improved health care delivery, while reducing patient morbidity and mortality (World Health Organization, 2010). The implementation and integration of interprofessional teams within Canada's health care system can allow health care providers to work to their full scope of practice and create innovative, sustainable ways of providing high-quality health care for all Canadians.

Despite the laudable benefits of interprofessional collaboration, it is a concept that can be difficult to implement and measure (Pullon et al., 2016). Barriers to collaboration include macrolevel restrictions impacting microlevel processes (Munro et al., 2013), such as outdated legislation, regulatory mechanisms, and practice protection (Regan et al., 2015). For example, nurses, physicians, and social workers may all have the necessary skills to assess patients to sign forms for income benefits. Yet adding titles to the forms, so that professionals other than physicians may sign, can require opening of legislative acts,

which can take months or even years. Issues of role clarity and understanding the scope and function of various roles can also be barriers to enacting collaborative practice (Orchard et al., 2017). In this chapter, we will examine the nurse's role as an interprofessional team member and leader, and discuss how some of the barriers to effective collaboration might be most effectively addressed.

CONCEPTS AND DEFINITIONS

Interprofessional Team

Working as part of an interprofessional team requires additional skills and knowledge compared with working as part of an interdisciplinary team. Although an interdisciplinary team requires members to work alongside one another, an **interprofessional team** comprises "different health care disciplines working together toward common goals to meet the needs of a patient population. Team members divide the work based on their scope of practice; they share information to support one another's work and coordinate processes and interventions to provide a number of services and programs" (Virani, 2012, p. 3). Increased knowledge of different professionals' roles and functions, and how they can be optimized for patient care, is required of interprofessional team members.

An **intraprofessional team** is composed of different nurses collaborating with one another. Intraprofessional teams have been studied less than interprofessional teams, yet we do know that collaboration among nurses is noted to be complicated and does not necessarily occur spontaneously (Moore & Prentice, 2012).

Interprofessional team-based care can take time to develop (Kotecha et al., 2015). Team members who are able to engage in clear and frequent communication, treat others with respect, demonstrate the ability to resolve conflict, articulate a shared understanding of "health," share protocols or best practices, and understand all members' roles within the team can be more effective in achieving the competencies of interprofessional collaboration (Canadian Interprofessional Health Collaborative [CIHC], 2010; Laschinger, 2007; Sargeant et al., 2008).

Although interprofessional teams are more recognizable in health care service provision in Canada today, nurses must be leaders in advancing interprofessional teams for their synergistic effects and potential to reorient health care services, versus maintaining the status quo.

Collaborative Practice and Collaboration

Collaborative practice is "an interprofessional process for communication and decision making that enables the separate and shared knowledge and skills of the care providers to synergistically influence the client/patient care provided" (Way et al., 2000, p. 3). Collaboration has been described as a complex, voluntary, and dynamic process with underlying concepts of power, interdependency, sharing, partnership, and process (D'Amour et al., 2005). Through collaboration, interprofessional teams should be able to accomplish more than individuals working alone or in tandem. Care for patients could occur more seamlessly between institutions and communities, health promotion and illness prevention could be included for all patient encounters, health care providers could be able to stay informed of new evidence, and health outcomes could be improved (CIHC, 2010; Jones & Way, 2007).

THE RISE OF DISTINCT DISCIPLINES

Historically, professions developed through craft guilds first formed in the 1500s "to protect and promote their members' interests through the ownership of knowledge" (Reeves et al., 2010, p. 259). Noticeably, this approach is contrary to interprofessional collaboration. From these guilds arose the health care professions. Nursing did not professionalize until almost a century after medicine; thus the division of work was not intentionally determined but developed over time through the influence of political and economic factors (Reeves et al., 2010).

Today, health care providers continue to be educated in disciplinary silos, although interprofessional opportunities are increasingly sought in educational approaches. Educational programs might offer interprofessional rounds or lectures, simulation opportunities, and role modelling of collaborative practice in clinical practice (Moore & Prentice, 2012; Pfaff et al., 2014). Interprofessional education can help students in the health professions learn about one another's disciplines, core principles, or philosophies (Moore & Prentice, 2012) to identify collaborative methods for solving problems, develop a shared vision of health, and facilitate common documentation practices.

SCOPE OF PRACTICE

The Canadian Nurses Association (CNA, 2015) defines scope of practice as "activities nurses are authorized, educated and competent to perform" (p. 14). Grounded in provincial or territorial legislation and regulations, "the registered nurse (RN) scope of practice is complemented by standards, guidelines, policy positions and ethical standards from jurisdictional nursing regulatory bodies" (CNA, 2015, p. 14).

The scope of practice for nursing does not outline an exclusive role. Rather, the idea that sharing access to controlled acts with other health professionals based on overlapping scopes of practice is expected and accepted (CNA, 2015; Lahey & Fierlbeck, 2016; Regan et al., 2015). Recognizing where roles and functions may overlap with other members of an interprofessional team requires identifying common ground and striving for mutual understanding of team members' roles (CNA, 2015).

Within nursing, distinctions can be made between many overlapping practices of RNs, licensed practical nurses, and registered psychiatric nurses by regulatory bodies (CNA, 2015). In Nova Scotia and British Columbia, the regulatory bodies of each nurse type are in the process of amalgamating to co-create one nursing regulatory body for all nurse types to reduce complexity, promote consistency of professional standards, and bridge professional differences, while supporting the contributions of different nurse types to the profession (College of Registered Nurses of British Columbia [CRNBC], 2017b). Amalgamating nursing regulatory bodies is perhaps just beginning in Canada, but this is a model that is already used in Australia and the United Kingdom (CRNBC, 2017b).

RNs and nurse leaders can enhance safe collaborative practice by understanding overlap and distinctions in the scope of practice of all nurse types. On an intraprofessional team, RNs are responsible to make decisions about what functions team members perform in relation to providing high quality patient care. In various staff mix models, there are ratios of RNs to practical nurses, as well as unregulated care providers, such as health care assistants or aides who are commonly employed in settings such as long-term care, home care, and nursing stations. In such settings, RNs are often responsible for delegating tasks regarding patient care to these team members. Delegation refers to achieving performance of care outcomes for which you are accountable and responsible by sharing activities with other individuals who have the appropriate authority to accomplish the work. To delegate safely, an RN must be aware of the scope of practice and ability of the delegatee, communicate effectively, and seek a degree of trust in the delagator-delagatee relationship. Delegation is an entry-level competency of an RN (CNA, 2015). The regulatory bodies of several provinces (e.g., Nunavut and Northwest Territories, Nova Scotia, New Brunswick, Ontario, Manitoba, Alberta, British Columbia) provide registrants with frameworks, or practice guidelines, for delegation to unregulated care providers as well as other nurse types.

> **EXERCISE 27.1** Visit your provincial or territorial nursing regulatory body or professional association website. Read the professional and practice standards and scope of practice statements, then ask two or more preceptors or instructors how they stay current with the requirements of the regulatory body, and what is required for continuing competence once in practice.

Widespread concern persists over the clarity of scopes of practice in a number of health professions (Baranek, 2005). Such concerns promise to be increasingly complex as nursing scopes of practice are expanding rapidly, with appeals for nurses to work to full scope of practice (Orchard et al., 2017). Certified practice in British Columbia, and legislation permitting nurse prescribing are two recent examples.

Over time, several provinces have replaced the model of professional licensing (which allowed only professions with a particular license to perform particular services or functions within the scope of practice) with a "restricted activities" or "controlled acts" model. The controlled acts model is structured so that those outside a particular profession are not necessarily restricted from performing that function (Lahey & Fierlbeck, 2016). For example, suturing a simple laceration or performing cervical cancer screening (pap smears) is a restricted activity that physicians and RNs can perform in many jurisdictions via legislation, with standards, limits, and conditions applied at the regulatory level. If an act is not restricted (or controlled), it can be performed by anyone (Baranek, 2005).

The controlled acts model has several benefits over the licensure model: it allows professionals to perform to the range of their competency and abilities; it recognizes that scope of practice is not static and does not have firm boundaries; it places greater emphasis on standards and competence; and it increases flexibility in allowing patients more choice in providers and employers more innovation in optimal skill mix, while protecting the public from harm (CNO, 2014; CRNBC, 2017a). Although each of these benefits is important, the legislative reform to recognize overlapping competencies can contribute to role confusion, further competition over "turf" for various health care providers, and difficulty in optimizing skill mix (Baranek, 2005). In addition, legal reporting requirements must be exceptionally clear to members of an interprofessional team. Numerous legislative acts (e.g., those that relate to the reporting of child abuse, gunshot wounds, and adverse events) (see also Chapter 7) identify several health professions as having a legal obligation to report occurrences of these events. Health care providers (including nurses), employers, and patients can be uncomfortable with the nuance and varying levels of accountability (the obligation to account for one's actions) that accompany competency-based practice. It can lead to diminished professional identity (Orchard et al., 2017) that, in turn, can undermine role clarity, which is essential in understanding inclusion on an interprofessional team.

A FRAMEWORK FOR INTERPROFESSIONAL COLLABORATION

If nurses and other team members are going to be successful collaborators, it is essential to understand their own and others' roles and also strive to use common terminology to establish a strong platform for communication. To facilitate a common understanding of interprofessional collaboration amongst disciplines, the Canadian Interprofessional Health Collaborative (CIHC) has produced a National Interprofessional

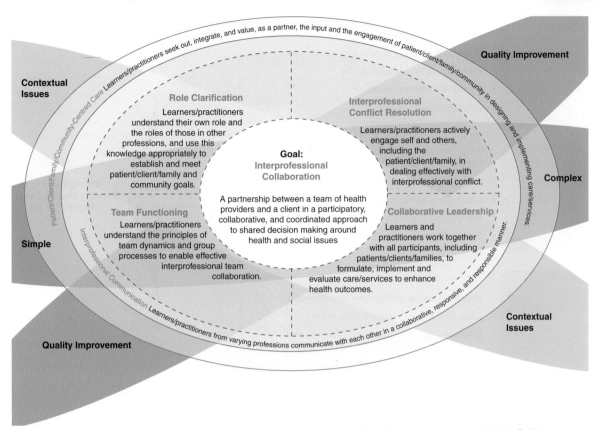

Fig. 27.1 The National Interprofessional Competency Framework. (Canadian Interprofessional Health Collaborative. (2010). A national interprofessional competency framework. p. 11. Retrieved from http://www.cihc.ca/files/CIHC_IPCompetencies_Feb1210.pdf. Thanks to the Canadian Interprofessional Health Collaborative for permission to use the CIHC Competency Framework.)

Competency Framework (Fig. 27.1). The framework consists of six competency domains that "highlight the knowledge, skills, attitudes and values that together shape the judgments that are essential for interprofessional collaborative" (CIHC, 2010, p. i). The six competency domains are as follows: interprofessional communication; patient/family/community-centred care; role clarification; team functioning; collaborative leadership; and interprofessional conflict resolution (CIHC, 2010). In every situation, the domains of patient/family/community-centred care and interprofessional communication are relevant and consistently influence and support the other four domains (CIHC, 2010). This framework was designed so that any professional can learn and apply the competencies, regardless of skill or practice setting. The CIHC views interprofessional learning as an additive and continuous process that begins prelicensure (CIHC, 2010).

> **EXERCISE 27.2** Ask three staff nurses to identify the top three team members they communicate with most frequently (i.e., unit clerks, social workers, physicians), and then ask which team member is easiest to talk with, and why they think that is so.

When considering the competencies required to achieve interprofessional collaboration, it is also important to identify the factors that influence collaboration. Martin-Misener and Valaitis (2012) described the factors influencing collaboration between primary care and public health, which can be organized in three separate layers: interactional, organizational, and systemic (Fig. 27.2). Leaders, managers, and followers have important roles in facilitating interprofessional collaboration at the organizational and interpersonal levels of their health care settings (for further discussion, see Chapters 1–3).

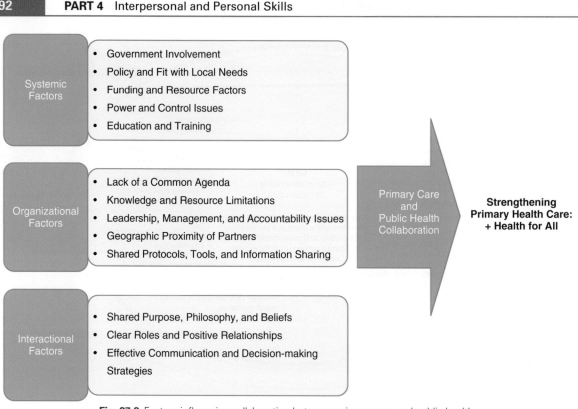

Fig. 27.2 Factors influencing collaboration between primary care and public health.

Nurses are integral members of any team, regardless of the setting. Whether they are part of a palliative care team in a hospice, an operating room team in an acute care setting, or a public health team in the community, nurses have an important role. By incorporating the framework reviewed here, nurses and other members of the interprofessional team can identify common ground, name the barriers and facilitators facing their particular team, and progress toward effective collaboration that can be beneficial to patient outcomes, health care providers, and their organization.

MOVING FORWARD IN COLLABORATIVE PRACTICE

When collaboration is ineffective or unsuccessful, disciplinary silos are reinforced and turf protection escalates. Turf protection can be identified when one profession insists that a particular function falls within their scope only, such as physicians opposing midwife practice or pharmacist prescribing. Environments that do not foster collaboration contribute to workplace stress and affect patient care (Laschinger, 2007). Consider the example of the pediatric cardiac surgery inquest of 12 deaths in 1994 at a Winnipeg hospital. Nurses raised serious and legitimate concerns about problems they had noticed, but were not taken seriously (Grinspun, 2007).

Even when a series of deaths occurred in rapid succession, there was not a timely and appropriate response within the surgical team, the Child Health program, the medical and administrative structures of the hospital, the death review processes of the Office of the Chief Medical Examiner, and the complaints/investigation processes of the College of Physicians & Surgeons of Manitoba (p. 87).

In the report of the inquest, Justice Sinclair clarified that the nurses were not treated as full, equal members of the surgical team in the pediatric surgery program (Sinclair, 2000). Nurses have a role and responsibility in addressing unsafe practices in the context of a team, and to facilitate this, Justice Sinclair (2000) recommended policy to allow staff to report concerns about patient care without risk to themselves or their job. Justice Sinclair (2000) also recommended the province of Manitoba pass "whistle blowing" legislation to protect health care professionals from reporting legitimate concerns about unsafe practices.

EXERCISE 27.3 Find out whether your current place of practicum or work has a "whistle-blower" policy. If it does, describe the policy's purpose and who it protects. If it does not, provide reasons why an organization can benefit from a mechanism to allow nurses and other professionals to report unsafe care.

Although most instances of ineffective collaboration do not lead to as serious and tragic an outcome as described previously, we are reminded that working collaboratively can be challenging (D'Amour et al., 2005). Role clarification is one strategy to enhance collaboration and can be addressed by defining scopes of practice. When a nursing function overlaps with the functions of a pharmacist, a physician, or a physiotherapist, role clarity can be ambiguous. Role clarity is when an individual understands his or her own role and that of others and applies this understanding while performing the role, communicating within the role, collaborating with others, and delivering care (CIHC, 2010). When role clarity is lacking, health care providers tend to retreat to what is familiar, which is often their own disciplinary silos (Baranek, 2005; Curran, 2007; Hills et al., 2007; Laschinger, 2007).

Health care providers can avoid following a silo approach in at least two ways: by providing patient-centred care and by evaluating their role in the local context. Patient-centred care is an approach in which the patient is viewed as a whole person; it is not just about delivering services and involves advocacy, empowerment, and respecting the patient's autonomy, voice, self-determination, and participation in decision making. Innovative and practical solutions to patient care can be found if nurses and other members of the interprofessional team consistently ask themselves, *What is best for the patient?* This approach requires operationalization of the concept of "working with" versus "taking care of" patients (Lasker & Weiss, 2003). Thus it requires acceptance of the patient's choice of provider and the patient's values and beliefs regarding treatment choices, as well as the incorporation of the patient's health care agenda with the professional's agenda of providing high-quality evidence-informed care.

Nurses on interprofessional teams can evaluate their role and professional identity within their own team and reevaluate when team composition or vision changes. All team members should be clear about what they bring to the health care and team process (Baranek,

2005; Laschinger, 2007). This clarity can be facilitated by co-location and engagement in effective communication practices. Although simply grouping a variety of health care providers together in the same building will not create a team (Koetcha et al., 2015), co-location can have many benefits, including timely and personal consultations or referrals regarding patient care, increased understanding and respect for all members' roles, and informal opportunities to connect, whether personally or regarding patients (Curran, 2007; Sargeant et al., 2008). Moreover, nurses can clarify their role and reinforce professional identity by engaging team members during regular team meetings in some simple thought exercises. An example of an activity a nurse might use to draw out niches of expertise appears in Exercise 27.4.

EXERCISE 27.4 During postconference, each student identifies one discipline to represent on a team relevant for the practice setting (e.g., interprofessional team on a rehabilitation unit). Together, students review a patient report. It might be an emergency department form, a consult letter, or a discharge summary. Ask each "team member" to describe what would stand out to them from their particular disciplinary standpoint. Is there information that is particularly striking? What information is missing that is relevant to their represented discipline? Allow 5 minutes for everyone to read the report and make notes, then ask your peers to read out what they wrote down. Encourage discussion by asking: Who took note of the social history? The vital signs? The course of the hospital stay? Who wrote down that they would update the patient chart when they noticed a new medication was added for the patient's blood pressure? Who wrote down that they would follow up with the patient regarding the strong family history of breast cancer? In this fashion, subtle differences to professional roles can be appreciated, and it is possible to recognize synergy, as it becomes clear to appreciate the different contributions each professional makes to patient care.

Undoubtedly, the tension between maintaining one's professional identity and participating in collaborative care in an interprofessional setting will remain for some time. However, in practice, nurses and other team members must strive to reduce this tension. Maintaining teams that are co-located in flexible, innovative environments can foster supportive relationships and shared goals to offset challenges of interprofessional collaboration and improve team functioning (Pullon et al., 2016). Effective interprofessional communication includes transparency and disclosure with all team members, as well as patients (CIHC, 2010). Finally, nurses advocate for integration of an internationally recognized framework, such as the National Interprofessional Competency Framework (CIHC, 2010) to help all team members understand the domains they might work on together to achieve the synergy of effective collaboration that can improve patient care and outcomes.

EXERCISE 27.5 At your clinical placement or place of work, reflect on the unregulated care providers and clerical staff (e.g., unit clerks, administrative assistants, porters) you interact with daily. Do you know everyone's name? Do you know the boundaries of their roles and responsibilities? How frequently and in what ways are they involved as part of the interprofessional team? Input from clerical or unregulated care providers can be invaluable, and ensuring they are valued and heard as team members is an important step toward effective collaborative care.

LEADING INTERPROFESSIONAL TEAMS

Providing leadership within an interprofessional team is complex (Reeves et al., 2010), and requisite abilities include knowledge of the competencies of nurses as set out by regulation and employers (Lankshear & Rush, 2016), a willingness to share leadership roles and functions (Kotecha et al., 2015), role modelling of collaborative behaviours (Pfaff et al., 2014), strong skills in change management, and implementing processes to resolve disagreements (Orchard et al., 2017). The Research Perspective provides an example of the complexities involved in leading teams.

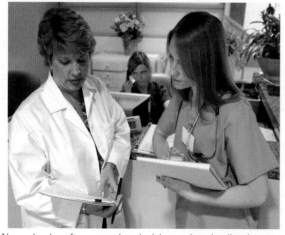

Nurse leaders face complex decisions when leading interprofessional teams.

To facilitate successful collaboration, team leaders must be able to inspire, engage, and motivate; they must be able to establish and articulate a vision and purpose to the team and greater community, and be open and inclusive in their language and actions (French, 2004; Lasker & Weiss, 2003).

In interprofessional practice, leadership might be more effective when it is shared. For example, one team member might lead others to carry the work forward, whereas another team member might ensure that patients and families are staying connected to the team and that the work of the team has meaning and impact for the key team player—the patient (CIHC, 2010). Teams might also choose to rotate leadership or choose leaders in different situations based on the contextual or experiential knowledge of the proposed leader. Either of these leadership models may help redistribute the hierarchical power that is common in health care settings. Regardless, leaders must be able to apply principles that will support and enhance successful collaborative efforts, as well as anticipate conflicts such as power hierarchies, role ambiguity, and competing priorities (CIHC, 2010). Team leaders may or may not be part of management. Leadership and management, although not the same, are interdependent (French, 2004).

Followers have a symbiotic relationship with leaders (Whitlock, 2013). Followers are not subordinates but individuals who use their judgement to decide which leader they feel motivated to help be successful (Thomas, 2012). An exemplary follower has strong critical-thinking skills, is participative and competent, and feels motivated when engaged in interesting and challenging work (Thomas, 2012). The effectiveness of leaders depends on relationships between leaders and followers that develop through motivating and inspiring others, as opposed to managing and controlling them (Batcheller, 2012).

Leadership development can begin in nursing prelicensure programs (French, 2004; Oandasan, 2007). Guided by the National Interprofessional Competency Framework (CIHC, 2010) and the principles outlined by the CNA position statement on interprofessional collaboration (2011), collaborative leadership could be included as a competency to prepare future graduates with skills and knowledge to collaborate and lead in interprofessional practice settings.

RESEARCH PERSPECTIVE

Resource: Lingard, L., McDougall, A., Levstik, M., et al. (2012). Representing complexity well: a story about teamwork, with implications for how we teach collaboration. *Medical Education*, 46, 869–877.

Researchers in this ethnographic study aimed to produce a rich description of how teamwork happens in a distributed team. The setting was a solid-organ transplant unit of a tertiary care hospital in Canada. Thirty-nine team members consented to participate, and data collection involved 162 hours of observation, 30 field interviews, and 17 formal interviews. The study employed activity theory and the concept of "knotworking" to explore how the team worked through challenges or barriers. It also employed the concept of "boundary" to examine how interactions within the team are shaped by organizational and professional boundaries. The results identified the different challenges faced by different parts of the team: the "core" transplant team, the "interservice" team (where challenges were identified between the core transplant team and other clinicians or services within the hospital), and "outside" challenges between the core team and clinical or administrative or social supports outside the hospital. The results of this study are

presented in a nontraditional manner in that a patient story is related to the reader with supporting observational and interview data to highlight the complexities and challenges of the team involved in a transplant patient's care.

Implications for Practice

This study revealed the difficulty faced by interprofessional teams and the type of emerging challenges that need to be addressed and resolved daily in health care settings to provide timely, safe patient care. The division of labour can be fluid, as can the authority and roles of team members, who may be distributed across time and space in a single setting. Most important, this study highlighted how roles are sometimes fluid or blurred within teams. The intricacies of working within an interprofessional team as described in this article can help nurses in novice and leadership roles alike better understand the different priorities and motives of team members, which can help resolve everyday tensions and conflict in any patient care setting. Skills in assessing and addressing competing priorities and motives are helpful for nurses with leadership roles in interprofessional teams.

The structures and processes that nursing leaders can influence underpin successful team function. Structures, such as administrative support, adequate meeting space, dedicated times for team members to meet, a culturally safe practice environment, and even the practice location (Curran, 2007; LeClerc et al, 2008; Pullon et al., 2016) can be barriers or levers for collaborative practice (Lahey & Fierlbeck, 2016). Processes nurse leaders can help develop, implement, or evaluate include articulating shared goals, assisting all members to work to full scope of practice, building relationships among team members, helping team members to learn about one another's scope of practice, provide opportunities for team members to socially interact, and address concerns for professional sustainability and safety (Kotecha et al., 2015; Moore & Prentice, 2012; Munro et al., 2013; Orchard et al., 2017; Regan et al., 2016).

In some environments, leaders are responsible for human resources planning or implementing care delivery models. This can be challenging; however the nursing literature can provide guidance to nurse leaders so that

evidence can inform nursing practice at a macro level. One example of this kind of research is found in a study by LeClerc et al. (2008), who described the implementation of a care delivery model based on an optimal skill mix at a continuing-care facility. This example is illustrative of leadership in action, whereby the facility went from delivering care according to a traditional model of nursing service where nurses spent too much time and effort "coordinating, delegating and supervising" (p. 67) to an autonomous–collaborative model, in which the time spent by nurses in a 24-hour period on nonnursing duties was reduced from 9.75 hours to 2.85 hours. The autonomous–collaborative model allowed team members to work together while maintaining accountability for care provision, making each nurse "responsible for determining his or her own level of knowledge, skill and judgment" (LeClerc et al., 2008, p. 69). As this example indicates, patients, health care providers, and the health care system benefit when leaders have a clear understanding of team members' scope of practice and can integrate overlapping skills and functions of team members in an appropriate, safe, and effective manner.

EXERCISE 27.6

Scenario A

Three months ago, you accepted your first job as a registered nurse (RN) in a community-based, long-term care facility in Moncton, New Brunswick. Yesterday, you delegated the administration of a heparin injection and a dressing change for a leg ulcer to a patient care aide. Today, you delegate the same tasks to a different patient care aide who was also hired about 3 months ago. She tells you she has only ever given one injection before and has never cared for someone with a leg ulcer. What do you do?

Scenario B

You are a RN in northern Saskatchewan. Your job requires you to spend 1 week in one community and the following week in a different community that is a 45-minute drive away. You are available by phone for the community health representative when you are not in the community. Today, the community health representative calls you to say a mother has brought her child to the clinic with a rash and she is pretty sure it is chicken pox. The community health representative asks you if she may dispense calamine lotion and acetaminophen (Tylenol©) to the mother. What do you do?

WORKING "WITH" VERSUS "ALONGSIDE" OTHERS

Understanding the "what" of interprofessional collaboration does not address the "how" to achieve implementation of collaboration, shared decision making, and effective leadership into practice. Many health care team members have collegial relationships, and some have real partnerships that can be attributed to multiple factors, not the least of which is sustained effort. However, for these working partnerships to be fully realized, issues of power and hierarchy require further examination and action.

Although the health care literature is dominated by nurse–physician interactions and power differentials (Moore & Prentice, 2012), "turf" protection is evident within intra- and interprofessional teams whereby some professions prevent others from being able to fully practice (Regan et al., 2016). The traditional top-down or "lead decision-maker" approach may not be the best fit for successful interprofessional collaboration (Kotecha et al., 2015). Today, it remains common within interprofessional teams, for nonphysician team members to judge their contributions in relation to the physician's practice (Hills et al., 2007, p. 131). For example, Hills et al. (2007) found nonphysician team members who spent time reviewing medications and providing health education to a patient did not consider their contribution to comprehensive, high-quality patient care; instead, "these activities were valued for saving the physician's time" (p. 131).

In Canada, nurses are included in almost every interprofessional team across a wide variety of practice settings, interacting with patients from birth to death. All nurses, and particularly those in leadership positions, can advocate for moving beyond recurring debates of professional competition to focus on the opportunities afforded by linking interprofessional care to improved patient outcomes. Bringing the focus back to what is best for the patient can be an excellent catalyst for change to structures, processes, and values, and propel nurses to act beyond the walls of their organizations to research, educate, and lead reforms at organizational, policy, and systems levels.

CONCLUSION

Practising and leading in an interprofessional setting is complex but necessary to meet the health care needs of Canadians in the twenty-first century. Nurses can advocate and lead change in areas of interprofessional education, practice, and research. Nurses are integral to championing the implementation and integration of innovative, sustainable collaborative teams that have a shared goal of providing high-quality patient-centred care to all Canadians.

? A SOLUTION

Interpersonal components: Keeping Mrs. Haley's well-being at the centre of Thomas's decisions, he helps the daughter tend to her, tells the physiotherapist he will phone her in 30 minutes, and asks the porter to quietly get Layla so that he can ask about the last dose of dimenhydrinate. Thomas communicates to Mrs. Haley and her daughter that he will be getting medication for her nausea and emesis as soon as he establishes a safe dose for an antiemetic based on the last dose she received. Thomas apologizes for the wait and provides reassurance that it will be sorted quickly. This addresses themes of shared purpose, maintaining good relationships, and effective communication and decision making (Martin-Misener & Valaitis, 2012).

Organizational components: A clear structure exists for reporting when one leaves and returns from breaks, with attention to prompt documentation in addition to a verbal report. Although uncertainty regarding Layla's medication administration to Mrs. Haley may be an oversight, consistent use of a reporting structure can decrease this and other oversights.

In addition, if dimenhydrinate is not controlling Mrs. Haley's symptoms, there should be a clear and easy way to obtain an order for a different, more suitable medication. This addresses themes of accountability, common agendas, and shared protocols (Martin-Misener & Valaitis, 2012).

Systemic components: With regards to the X-ray that has been booked in radiology, interorganizational electronic booking systems should be accessible to direct-care providers so that they can check these databases along with other appointments to ensure patients are ready for their appointments in a timely manner. Such systems should be programmed so that cross referencing is allowed; that is, to ensure the patient does not have an appointment booked with another department at the same time, such as physiotherapy. This addresses themes of information infrastructure, education and training, funding, and government involvement; in fact, most of these themes are interconnected (Martin-Misener & Valaitis, 2012). *What other components would you address and how?*

THE EVIDENCE

A pilot project assigned seven students from different health care educational programs to the same site for clinical rotations and included organized case-based discussions between the students of different professions. Cragg and colleagues (2010) described the opportunity given to students to share different perspectives and appreciate the contributions of other professions at a clinical site that was already known to have supportive administration and good communication channels. The participating students represented four professional groups that included nursing, physiotherapy, medicine, and spiritual care, and the program ran for 12 weeks, with weekly sessions attended between 5 and 12 times. Pre- and postqualitative and quantitative data were collected through semi-structured interviews and a scale to measure interprofessional attitudes was also applied.

At the end of the pilot project, the students reported that they would practise differently as a result of the project. They also noted important learning outcomes, including the recognition of different approaches, values, and terminology of different professions.

This pilot project, although small, highlighted how prelicensure exposure to other health care providers can increase understanding of roles on an interprofessional team, and can be a cost-effective way to promote interprofessional education. As a result of this project, weekly interprofessional rounds were started on an inpatient unit and continued after the students completed their rotation.

✳ NEED TO KNOW NOW

- Understand the elements of successful collaboration.
- Be familiar with provincial or territorial legislation that impacts nursing practice and how your regulatory body or professional association regulates this legislation for nurses. Know whether the legislation is designed to affect several health professions or just nursing.
- Consider what you bring to the health care process. What aspects of care do others on your team contribute?

What is missing? Who should provide the "missing pieces"?
- Reflect on how you will add your voice to those of other nurses across Canada. Be aware of the role of the Canadian Nurses Association and how its mission, vision, and mandate might be different from that of your regulatory body.

CHAPTER CHECKLIST

Practising and leading in interprofessional settings is a dynamic process throughout which nurses play a critical role. In some settings, nurses may be the health care providers who not only see patients the most but also interact with the greatest variety of professionals who are also involved in patient care. For this reason, nurses must step forward and take a leadership role in interprofessional care. They must also demonstrate the competencies of interprofessional practice and educate others in how to apply them. At the interpersonal, team, organizational, and systemic levels, nurses must seek to bring clarity to their roles, acknowledge what other health care providers and staff bring to patient care, families, and communities, and be comfortable with the shades of grey in overlapping scopes of practice.

- Practice in interprofessional settings requires flexibility and knowledge.
- Nurses must be prepared to enact power redistribution, as effective collaboration cannot occur within an imbalanced hierarchy.
- Interprofessional teams must work toward a shared goal or purpose to be effective. This goal should include patient-centred care.
- Regular meetings, open communication, and orientation of all team members are essential to effective collaboration.
- Building a trusting relationship takes time and has tremendous value in working effectively.
- Legislation and regulation provide the legal structure for nurses; the Canadian Nurses Association's *Code of Ethics for Registered Nurses* provides the ethical structure.

TIPS FOR PRACTISING AND LEADING IN INTERPROFESSIONAL SETTINGS

- Be knowledgeable of all team members' roles and competencies.
- Use the National Interprofessional Competency Framework to identify and apply competencies for interprofessional practice.
- Be sure to engage in evaluation to assess the team's accomplishments.
- Maintain open and respectful communication practices.

- Pay attention to employee retention and what keeps professionals happy and healthy in their work environment.
- Keep the patient at the centre of your decisions in an effort to provide high-quality patient care and decrease professional competition.

Visit the Evolve website for Suggested Readings, Internet Resources, and additional resources related to the content in this chapter: http://evolve.elsevier.com/Canada/Yoder-Wise/leading/.

REFERENCES

Baranek, P. M. (2005). *A review of scopes of practice of health professions in Canada: A balancing act.* Toronto, ON: Health Council of Canada.

Batcheller, J. (2012). Learning how to dance: Courageous followership: A CNO case study. *Nurse Leader, 10*(2), 22–24.

Canadian Interprofessional Health Collaborative. (2010). *A national interprofessional competency framework.* Retrieved from: http://www.cihc.ca/files/CIHC_IPCompetencies_Feb1210.pdf.

Canadian Nurses Association. (2015). *Framework for the practice of registered nurses in Canada.* Ottawa, ON: Author. Retrieved from: https://www.cna-aiic.ca/~/media/ cna/page-content/pdf-en/framework-for-the-pracice-of-registered-nurses-in-canada.pdf.

Canadian Nurses Association. (2011). *Interprofessional collaboration.* Ottawa, ON: Author. Retrieved from: https://www.cna-aiic.ca/en/nursing-practice/the-practice-of-nursing/health-human-resources/interprofessional-collaboration.

College of Nurses of Ontario. (2014). *RHPA: Scope of practice, controlled acts model.* ON: Toronto. Retrieved from: http://ltctoolkit.rnao.ca/node/1851.

College of Registered Nurses of British Columbia. (2017a). *Overview of Health Professions Act, Nurses (Registered) and Nurse Practitioners Regulation, CRNBC bylaws.* Vancouver, BC: Author. Retrieved from: https://www.crnbc.ca/crnbc/documents/324.pdf.

College of Registered Nurses of British Columbia. (2017b). *Declaration of intent to form a single nursing regulator in British Columbia.* Vancouver, BC: Author. Retrieved from: https://www.crnbc.ca/crnbc/ONR/Pages/Default.aspx.

Cragg, B., Hirsh, M., Jelley, W., et al. (2010). An interprofessional rural clinical placement project. *Journal of Interprofessional Care, 24*(2), 207–209.

Curran, V. (2007). *Collaborative care. Synthesis series on sharing insights.* Ottawa, ON: Health Canada.

D'Amour, D., Ferrada-Videla, M., San Martin Rodriguez, L., et al. (2005). The conceptual basis for interprofessional collaboration: Core concepts and theoretical frameworks [Review]. *Journal of Interprofessional Care, 19*(Suppl. 1), 116–131.

French, S. (2004). Challenges to developing and providing nursing leadership. *Canadian Journal of Nursing Leadership, 17*(4), 37–40.

Grinspun, D. (2007). Healthy workplaces: The case for shared clinical decision making and increased full-time employment. *Healthcare Papers, 7,* 85–91 special issue.

Hills, M., Mullett, J., & Carroll, S. (2007). Community-based participatory action research: Transforming multidisciplinary practice in primary health care. *Pan American Journal of Public Health, 21*(2/3), 125–135.

Jones, L., & Way, D. (2007). Healthy workplaces and effective teamwork: Viewed through the lens of primary healthcare renewal. *Healthcare Papers, 7,* 92–97 special issue.

Koetecha, J., Brown, J. B., Han, H., et al. (2015). Influence of a quality improvement in learning collaborative program on team functioning in primary healthcare. *Families, Systems, & Health, 33*(3), 222–230.

Lahey, W., & Fierlbeck, K. (2016). Legislating collaborative self-regulation in Canada: A comparative policy analysis. *Journal of Interprofessional Care, 30*(2), 211–216.

Lankshear, S., & Rush, J. (2016). Enhancing role clarity for the practical nurse. *Journal of Nursing Administration, 46*(6), 300–307.

Laschinger, H. K. (2007). Building healthy workplaces: Time to act on the evidence. *Healthcare Papers, 7,* 42–45 special issue.

Lasker, R. D., & Weiss, E. S. (2003). Creating partnership synergy: The critical role of community stakeholders. *Journal of Health and Health Services Administration, 2003*(Summer), 119–139.

LeClerc, C. M., Doyon, J., Gravelle, D., et al. (2008). The autonomous–collaborative care model: Meeting the future head on. *Canadian Journal of Nursing Leadership, 21*(2), 63–75.

Lingard, L., McDougall, A., Levstik, M., et al. (2012). Representing complexity well: A story about teamwork, with implications for how we teach collaboration. *Medical Education, 46,* 869–877.

Martin-Misener, R., & Valaitis, R. (2012). *A scoping literature review of collaboration between primary care and public health: a report to the Canadian Health Services Research Foundation.* Retrieved from: http://fhs.mcmaster.ca/nursing/documents/MartinMisener-Valaitis-Review.pdf.

Moore, J., & Prentice, D. (2012). Collaboration among nurse practitioners and registered nurses in outpatient oncology settings in Canada. *Journal of Advanced Nursing,* 1574–1583.

Munro, S., Kornelsen, J., & Grzybowski, S. (2013). Models of maternity care in rural environments: Barriers and attributes of interprofessional collaboration with midwives. *Midwifery, 29,* 646–652.

Oandasan, I. (2007). Teamwork and healthy workplaces: strengthening the links for deliberation and action through research and policy. *Healthcare Papers, 7,* 98–103 special issue.

Orchard, C. A., Sonibare, O., Morse, A., Collins, J., & Al-Hamad, A. (2017). Collaborative leadership, part 2: The role of the nurse leader in interprofessional team-based practice – Shifting from task- to collaborative patient-family-focused care. *Nursing Leadership, 30*(2), 26–38.

Pfaff, K. A., Baxter, P. E., Jack, S. M., & Ploeg, J. (2014). Exploring new graduate nurse confidence in interprofessional collaboration: A mixed methods study. *International Journal of Nursing Studies, 51,* 1142–1152.

Pullon, S., Morgan, S., Macdonald, L., McKinlay, E., & Gray, B. (2016). Observation of interprofessional collaboration in primary care practice: A multiple case study. *Journal of Interprofessional Care, 30*(6), 787–794.

Reeves, S., Macmillan, K., & van Soeren, M. (2010). Leadership of interprofessional health and social care teams: A socio-historical analysis. *Journal of Nursing Management, 18*(3), 258–264.

Regan, S., Laschinger, H. K. ,S., & Wong, C. A. (2016). The influence of empowerment, authentic leadership, and professional practice environments on nurses' perceived interprofessional collaboration. *Journal of Nursing Management, 24,* E54–E61.

Regan, S., Orchard, C., Khalili, H., Brunton, L., & Leslie, K. (2015). Legislating interprofessional collaboration: A policy analysis of health professions regulatory legislation in Ontario, Canada. *Journal of Interprofessional Care, 29*(4), 359–364.

Sargeant, J., Loney, E., & Murphy, G. (2008). Effective interprofessional teams: "Contact is not enough" to build a team. *Journal of Continuing Education in the Health Professions, 28*(4), 228–234.

Sinclair, C. M. (2000). *Report of the Manitoba pediatric cardiac surgery inquest: An inquiry into twelve deaths at the Winnipeg Health Sciences Centre in 1994.* Winnipeg, MB: Provincial Court of Manitoba.

Thomas, S. (2012). Followership: Leadership's partner. *Canadian Journal of Medical Laboratory Sciences*, *74*(4), 8–10.

Virani, T. (2012). *Interprofessional collaborative teams*. Ottawa, ON: Canadian Health Services Research Foundation. Retrieved from: http://www.cfhi-fcass.ca/Libraries/Commissioned_Research_Reports/Virani-Interprofessional-EN.sflb.ashx.

Way, D., Jones, L., & Busing, N. (2000). *Implementation strategies: "Collaboration in primary care—family doctors & nurse practitioners delivering shared care*. Ottawa, ON: Ontario College of Family Physicians. Retrieved from: http://www.eicp.ca/en/toolkit/hhr/ocfp-paper-handout.pdf.

Whitlock, J. (2013). The value of active followership. *Nursing Management*, *20*(2), 20–23.

World Health Organization. (2010). *Framework for action on interprofessional education and collaborative practice*. Geveva: World Health Organization. Retrieved from: http://apps.who.int/iris/bitstream/handle/10665/70185/WHO_HRH_HPN_10.3_eng.pdf;jsessionid=B87019ED-5354B31E4FA82B25E2E9604E?sequence=1.

World Health Organization. (1978). *Declaration of Alma-Ata*. Alma-Ata, USSR: International Conference on Primary Health Care, 6–12. Retrieved from: http://www.who.int/publications/almaata_declaration_en.pdf.

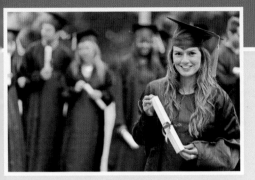

28

Role Transition

Judy Boychuk Duchscher

Role transition in nursing is the process of moving from one role, embedded within a framework of knowledge, to another. Managing the work done by others requires a fundamental understanding of the challenges inherent in making a role transition. The exercises in this chapter offer opportunities to recognize and build on your abilities to facilitate the evolution of the professionals under your direction.

OBJECTIVES

- Describe the stages of role transition for the new nursing graduate (NGN) in the first year of practice.
- Describe what "ROLES" stands for and how each of its elements applies to role transition.
- Understand the phases of the professional role transition model: role preparation, role orientation, role integration, and role stabilization.
- Identify the challenges posed by role transition.
- Define strategies that can help promote role transition.

TERMS TO KNOW

mentorship
preceptorship
role discrepancy
role expectations

role integration
role negotiation
role orientation
role preparation

role stabilization
role strain
role stress
role transition

🔆 A CHALLENGE

On her first day, Claire walked into the nurses' report room, and all eyes zeroed in on her. She was absolutely certain that she had "NEWBIE" written across her forehead. One nurse turned to another and asked, "Who is she?" There were no more chairs in the room, so Claire stood throughout the entire report. She knew the routine from her student days, but this was different; now they EXPECTED her to know what she was doing! Everyone spoke quickly and used many abbreviations that she did not understand. She could not keep up and got lost. Claire said to herself, "*Whatever you do, don't look stupid*". Following report, Claire mustered up enough confidence to ask, "*Who am I with today?*" In response, Claire heard individual nurses say, "*I took the last one, I need a break,*" "*I have a really heavy patient load today, it wouldn't be a*

good shift with me," "*I don't want her.*" And then, finally, like a breath of fresh air, one of the more senior nurses, Alexis, said, "*She can come with me today.*" With a wink at Claire, Alexis said, "*You ready to roll?*"

Alexis was wonderful about explaining tasks to Claire, however she found it odd that Alexis never asked her a single question about where she had come from, what experience she had, or what skills she wanted to work on. Nonetheless, she offered Claire all kinds of advice, some of which Claire retained and some of which she did not understand. During the shift, some nurses asked who Claire was and some did not. Alexis introduced Claire to some patients and not to others. Claire hoped that Alexis would not ask her something that she did not know as she desperately wanted to look like she knew what she was doing.

continued

? **A CHALLENGE—cont'd**

Claire had been a strong student in school and looked forward to the challenge of her new role, even though she was a bit nervous about it. Although she was merely observing on her first day, she was beyond exhausted when her shift ended. She never met the nurse manager or educator. Alexis must have been busy because she did not say goodbye to Claire at the end of the shift. Even though the day had been full,

Claire never got the opportunity to say "*Good morning, my name is Claire and I will be the registered nurse working with you today*" to her patients. She was really looking forward to that; maybe tomorrow.

What more could the nurse manager, educator, and Alexis have done to support Claire's transition into her new role?

INTRODUCTION

Role transition occurs when one moves from a role that is familiar (e.g., nursing student) to one that is unfamiliar (e.g., novice professional nurse). Necessarily, changes to the way a person interacts with and is perceived by others in a new role challenges his or her established professional identity. During the initial days and weeks of a formal role transition, that which was consistent, predictable, familiar, and stable is disrupted, inviting uncertainty and, with it, anxiety.

New graduates are making their first truly significant professional transition as they move from being a student role to being a practicing nurse. Although the expectations of students are clearly specified by course and clinical objectives, and feedback from instructors and preceptors is consistent and explicit, the expectations for a new nurse may not be so clear. The Literature Perspective and Research Perspectives found in this chapter provide further information on role transitions for new nursing graduates (NGNs).

RESEARCH PERSPECTIVE

Resource: Rheaume, A., Clement, L., & LeBel, N. (2011). Understanding intention to leave amongst new graduate Canadian nurses: a repeated cross-sectional survey. *International Journal of Nursing Studies*, 48, 490–500.

This study described a 5-year repeated survey that explored the correlations between demographics, employment, and orientation programs, as well as mentorship quality and availability and the new nursing graduates (NGNs) initial 12 to 16 months of practice. The authors used Menon's (2002) definition of empowerment as:

"A cognitive state characterized by perceptions of control regarding one's own health and health care; perceptions of competence regarding one's ability to maintain good health and manage interactions with the health care system; and internalization of health ideals and goals at the individual and societal level" (p. 34).

Employment and orientation programs varied significantly (2–10 days) with 67% of NGNs rating the length of time as adequate to meet their needs. Although the majority of NGNs expressed high levels of empowerment consistently throughout data collection, 45.5% of the NGNs (those with the lowest levels of empowerment) considered leaving their current employer; this value remained stable throughout the 5 years. The other variables explaining the intent to leave variance included the quality

of the work environment (workload and staffing resources), the quality of care the NGNs were able to provide, their perceptions of input into hospital affairs, as well as the leadership support offered them while transitioning.

Implications for Practice

New graduates who felt able to enact the practice goals they had internalized during their education, and those able to practice quality care were the least likely to leave their workplace. An interesting finding was that 76% of the variance of the NGNs intent to leave remained unexplained. It is worth noting that generational characteristics, and the "natural mobility" tendencies of the millennials, may be inadvertently contributing to this exit data. Possibly related to generational theory, the authors conclude that the ability of NGNs to enact their professional values in the quality of care they are supported to deliver, was identified as a factor feeding intent to leave or remain with their current employer. The influence of nurse managers and unit educators on the care environment and professional culture of the workplace, should be neither underestimated nor overstated. Leaders who are visible, authentic in their approach to practicing nurses, and willing to advocate for a positive and productive work environment may well be a defining factor in our ability to recruit NGNs and retain and develop quality senior practitioners.

LITERATURE PERSPECTIVE

Resource: Dwyer, P.A. & Revell, S.M.H. (2016). Multilevel influences on new graduate nurse transition. *Journal of Nurses in Professional Development*, 32(3), 112–121.

This review of data from 42 articles suggested that a significant interplay exists between intrapersonal, interpersonal, and organizational factors as they relate to the NGN transition experience. Most interesting was the paucity of demographic variables shown to consistently influence transitional outcomes. Equally impressive, and perhaps even concerning, were the multitude of studies demonstrating that those NGNs "with higher educational preparation being associated with undesirable outcomes, such as higher perceptions of job difficulties, lower perceptions of job control, and turnover intent" (Dwyer & Revell, p. 113). The concept of *PsyCap* (an individual's positive psychologic state as characterized by level of confidence, anticipation of making a positive contribution, perseverance, and resilience) was introduced as strongly correlative with job satisfaction and work engagement. Workplace ties and relationships were identified as highly instrumental in a successful NGN transition whereas inci-

vility was found to be highly detrimental to the same. Not surprisingly, challenging workloads and staffing shortages were considered to be significant barriers to NGN transition.

Implications for Practice
Strategies that strengthen workplace relationships while at once supporting practice environments conducive to quality care (is there an echo in here?) are highlighted as advantageous to NGN transition (and we would suggest to the workplace satisfaction and outcomes for ALL nurses). Researchers offered insight into the PsyCap instrument, suggesting the utility of 2 to 3 hour workshops spread throughout the initial year of transition, emphasizing hope, optimism, resilience, and efficacy as it related to the practice of NGNs. It was further noted that, while "arming" NGNs to respond to incivility through approaches such as cognitive rehearsal therapy is important, actually changing the culture to render such responses unnecessary is the preferred goal. Finally, offering authentic leadership training programs and supporting engagement of nurse managers with their direct-care nurses would go a long way to changing cultures within the hospital environment.

LITERATURE PERSPECTIVE

Resource: Edwards, D., Hawker, C., Carrier, J., & Rees, C. (2015). A systematic review of the effectiveness of strategies and interventions to improve the transition from student to newly qualified nurse. *International Journal of Nursing Studies*, 52(7), 1254–1468.

This systematic review evaluated 30 articles published between 2000 and 2011; it aimed to determine the effectiveness of strategies used to support newly qualified nurses during the transition into the clinical workplace and to evaluate the impact of these on individual and organizational level outcomes. There were four different support strategies identified: nurse internship/residency programs, graduate nurse orientation programmes, mentorship/preceptorship, and simulation-based graduate programmes. Although this systematic review found it difficult to draw firm conclusion about the effectiveness of such strategies limiting because of the poor methodologic quality of the studies, it did suggest that the type of support strategy is less important; it is the focus upon and investment in easing new graduate nurses' transition by organizations that is important.

Implications for Practice
Nearly all forms of intervention lead to successful outcomes. Transition programs for new graduate nurses are generally effective in increasing retention and improving their overall experience. This would suggest that a well-organized attempt by a health organization to smooth the transition period will have an impact on a number of organizational outcomes and individual outcomes for newly qualified nurses. Studies indicated that an increase in competency, knowledge, confidence, and job satisfaction occurred when support strategies were implemented. Furthermore, internship/residence programs and mentorship/preceptorship programs were found to be effective in reducing levels of stress and anxiety of graduate nurses. A number of studies mentioned the importance of structured support from colleagues, as well as the organization to aid in the successful journey from graduate student to competent qualified nurse.

LITERATURE PERSPECTIVE

Resource: Rush, K. L., Adamack, M., Gordon, J., Lily, M., & Janke, R. (2013). Best practices of formal new graduate nurse transition programs: an integrative review. *International Journal of Nursing Studies, 50*, 345–356.

This integrative review looked at 47 articles published between 2000 and 2011 that identified best practices of formal new graduate nurse transition programs, in an attempt to provide useful information for organizations who are developing a formal transition program for newly hired nurses. Using Cooper's (1989) five-stage approach to integrative review, the literature was examined according to four themes: Education, Support/Satisfaction, Competence and Critical Thinking, and Workplace Environment. A strong theme throughout the literature was that a formal transition program improved retention rates and that new graduates benefited from mentors who could provide them support. Transition programs should provide support for at least 9 months and there should be a level of formal training for those who work with new graduates.

Implications for Practice

Support of new graduates across the transition period is critical. Length of a new graduates' orientation time plays a significant part in the new graduates' integration to practice; increase in retention, job satisfaction, and comfort with skills are outcomes that have been reported when lengthier orientation is given. In fact, one US study (*n* = 329) showed that longer orientations decreased turnover rates. Another study showed that new graduates who had already left their first nursing job had on average an orientation 2 weeks less than new graduates who had not left their first nursing job. Although the initial stage of transition is trying for the new graduate, there is evidence to suggest that new graduates struggle with high levels of stress and low levels of job satisfaction at the 6- to 9-month posthire period; therefore it is important to provide support to new graduates throughout the entire transitional process. Some form of "people support"—a mentor, clinical coach, or transition program coordinator to name a few, is necessary to reduce the stress of the new graduate and to provide guidance and support. New graduates value the moral support provided by peer-support opportunities as well. The work environment was identified as a significant variable impacting new graduate transition; healthy work environments decrease a new graduates' reality shock and aide in facilitating a successful transition.

New graduates are not the only professional nurses facing role transition. The direct care nurse who decides to advance his or her education or scope of practice, or perhaps branch out into the role of clinical educator or nurse manager is making a role transition. The same is true for the staff nurse who becomes a nurse manager, or the staff nurse who moves from an acute care setting to a home health care agency. Regardless of the kind of transition, organizations play a key role in assisting employees through role transitions. Changes in roles can be either painful or exciting, depending largely on the work culture and support provided. According to Meleis (2010), "human beings always face many changes throughout the lifespan that trigger internal processes . . . [and] are characterized by different dynamic stages, milestones, and turning points" (p. 11). Knowing what to expect during a transition can reduce stress and facilitate a healthy acceptance of the change over time.

TYPES OF ROLE TRANSITIONS

From Nursing Student to Practicing Nurse

Duchscher's (2012) theory outlines the transition from nursing student to practicing nurse as a journey of *becoming*, where new graduates progress through stages of *doing, being,* and *knowing.* The stages of role transition that occur for NGNs during the initial 12 months of professional practice appear in Table 28.1. Stage 1, which takes place in the first 3 to 4 months of the NGNs journey, is often an exercise in adjusting and adapting to the realities of the new workplace, professional life, and personal life. New professionals have little energy or time to lift their gaze from the very immediate issues or tasks set before them, and their "shock" (Fig. 28.1) state demands a concerted focus on simply "surviving" the experience, without revealing their feelings of overwhelming anxiety or exposing their self-perceived incompetence.

Stage 2 of professional role transition for NGNs takes place over the next 4 to 5 months of the postorientation period and is characterized by a consistent and rapid advancement in their thinking, knowledge level, and skill competency. As this period progresses and the new graduates gain a comfort level with their professional role and responsibilities, they are often confronted by inconsistencies and inadequacies within the health care system that serve to challenge their somewhat idealistic pregraduate notions of the profession. An increased

TABLE 28.1	Stages of Role Transition for the New Nursing Graduate	
Stage	**Processes**	**The Experience**
Stage 1: Doing (3–4 months)	Learning Performing Concealing Adjusting Accommodating	• Is most comfortable in a *learning* role and least comfortable applying theory to practice • Often defaults to theory as that is what the new graduate knows • Feels that everything is new—even the familiar looks different • Is most concerned with the ability to *perform* tasks required; the objective is not to "stand out" but to focus on "what" and "how" • Is motivated by a desire for acceptance, so the new graduate *conceals* insecurities or feelings of inadequacy from colleagues • *Adjusts* to new roles, responsibilities, and relationships • Takes practice cues from surrounding nurses—more vulnerable to poor modelling and may choose to *accommodate* rather than challenge existing practices • Has an overwhelming sense of responsibility; finds decision making daunting
Stage 2: Being (4–5 months)	Searching Examining Doubting Questioning Revealing	• Begins a *search* for meaning in the role—asking "why" rather than "what" or "how" • Has increasing comfort with the role, relationships, responsibilities, and knowledge, which allows time to *examine* the workplace • Demonstrates a growing identity—asks *Who am I as a nurse?* that may feed *self-doubt* • Shows advanced thinking that motivates *questioning*; incongruence within the system is *revealed* and may be disturbing—engages in "bigger picture" thinking
Stage 3: Knowing (3–5 months)	Separating Recovering Exploring Critiquing Accepting	• Is exhausted from prior two stages, which can feed discouragement or disillusionment; *separates* from work in an attempt to *recover* energy and gain some perspective • Begins to think about the future; *explores* career possibilities • *Critiques* his or her work, colleagues, and profession, which is part of identity development • *Accepts* what he or she can while seeking to change what is considered untenable; seeks stability

From Boychuk Duchscher, J. (2008). A process of becoming the stages of new nursing graduate professional role transition. *Journal of Continuing Education in Nursing*, 39(10), 441–450.

awareness of the divergence between their professional "self" and the enactment of that self in their new role motivates a relative withdrawal of NGNs from their surroundings. The primary task for NGNs at this stage is to make sense of their role as a nurse relative to other health care providers and to find a balance between their personal and professional lives.

Stage 3, the final stage of transition for NGNs during the initial 12 months of their careers, is focused on achieving a separateness that both distinguishes them from the established practitioners around them and permits them to reunite with their larger community as professionals in their own right. With an increase in both familiarity and comfort in their nursing role, professional responsibilities, and relationships with coworkers, NGNs have the time and energy to begin a deeper exploration and

critique of their professional landscape, making visible the more troubling aspects of their sociocultural and political work environments. If the transition experience to this point has been less than satisfactory for the NGN, he or she may express dissatisfaction with work; this feeling is often fed by a residual exhaustion from prior stages. For some, this is simply a case of adjusting to the work world for the purpose of achieving a sense of job satisfaction. For others, the thought of sacrificing particular professional expectations and aspirations because of perceived inadequacies in the system within which they planned to spend their career can be terminally demotivating. Left unchecked, disenfranchised NGNs may choose to search for alternative avenues of fulfillment (e.g., finding a new job, leaving the country, returning to school, or creating a distinct separation between work and home life).

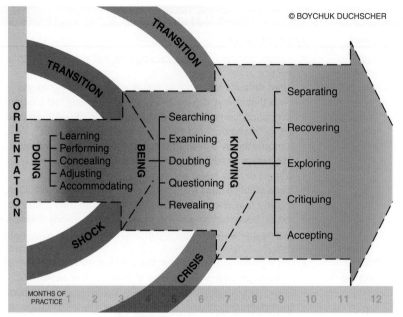

© BOYCHUK DUCHSCHER

Fig. 28.1 Stages of transition model.

From Practicing Nurse to Nurse Leader or Manager

Performing the role of a leadership in nursing or health care (e.g., an educator role) requires an awareness of the complex responsibilities such a position entails. Leading is complex because it involves working with unique (and often very different from each other) individuals at varying stages of professional development, enacting roles that are distinct but synergistic, in a rapidly changing environment that has its own challenges (i.e., fiscal accountability). Examples of the people with whom a leader interacts and the processes involved in each interaction can be found in Table 28.2. In nursing, each of these roles ultimately influences the quality of patient care.

The transition from being a direct care nurse to nurse manager is significant. The nurse moves from leading the clinical work of patient care to leading a group of employees. Clark (2008) noted that "*leadership is not simply granted to individuals and is not about responding passively to events. It is about creating possibilities that were absent before*" (p. 30). McConnell (2008) says that a health care provider who takes on a managerial position is accepting a second occupation: "*The professional who enters [leadership] must wear two hats*" (p. 278). One role is as the professional on technical and clinical matters, and the other is as a generalist responsible for

TABLE 28.2 Leader, Manager, and Follower Roles: the People and Processes Involved

Role	People With Whom Interactions Occur	Processes Involved in the Role
Leader	Persons being led Peers	Listening Encouraging Motivating Organizing Problem solving Developing Supporting
Manager	Persons under leaders' direction Nursing administrators Supervisors Regulatory bodies Faculty	Organizing Planning Budgeting Hiring Evaluating Reporting Disseminating Researching/writing
Follower	Supervisor Peers	Conforming Implementing Contributing Completing assignments Alerting

directing a diverse demographic that itself varies greatly in roles, responsibilities, relationships, and knowledge.

In the evolving contemporary health care environment, the nurse who provides direct care is also expected to function as a leader, assuming the roles of leader, care manager, and team follower in relation to patient care. As *leader*, the direct care nurse recognizes the uniqueness of each patient, planning, implementing, and evaluating clinical progress over time. As a care *manager*, the direct care nurse links the patient and family to resources that optimize clinical outcomes. Health information is translated into a format that the patient can use to make informed decisions about treatment and self-care. Through collaboration with multiple disciplines, the nurse consults and makes referrals as needed, and facilitates continuity of care within the larger system. In the role of *team follower*, the direct care nurse is accountable to a team and a supervisor for completing the work that is assigned. The nurse as a follower must practise within the policies and procedures of the organization and the standards of the profession. Finally, direct care nurses work collaboratively with others, contributing to determining and enacting common organizational and professional goals. In doing so, they are accountable not only to their superiors, but responsible for recognizing that leadership is shared with others in their environment, requiring a collaborative approach to decision making.

Learning the leader, manager, and follower aspects of any new role can be overwhelming. One approach to the complexity of role transition is represented in the acronym *ROLES*, in which each letter represents a component common to all roles.

ROLES: THE ABCS OF UNDERSTANDING ROLES

Acronyms help us retain and organize information. **ROLES** (Box 28.1) is represented in the following way:

R **stands for responsibilities.** What are the specified duties in the position description for the new position? What tasks are to be completed? What decisions must the person in this position make? For example, the job of a nurse manager may involve 24-hour accountability, whereas the job of a staff nurse may involve direct care in a primary care setting. Every position has specific tasks for which the position holder is responsible.

O **stands for opportunities,** which are untapped aspects of one's position. For instance, in the employment

---

BOX 28.1 "ROLES" Acronym

*R*esponsibilities
*O*pportunities
*L*ines of communication
*E*xpectations
*S*upport

---

interview, it may be revealed that previous management did not encourage the staff nurses to participate in continuing education. Or, while touring the unit, one might observe that the family waiting room is in disrepair. Or, in the course of shadowing one of the nurses, it becomes clear that the care delivery routines for the unit could be optimized. These situations represent opportunities for influencing organizational and unit goals.

L **represents lines of communication,** which are at the heart of every nursing role. No matter what position one has, the quality of relationships with supervisors and peers are pivotal to success. Roles are essentially just patterns of structured interaction among people in varying groups, and require that individuals be competent at receiving and sending messages. Being a skillful listener and receiving messages is as important as being skillful at sending them. Skill is required to communicate both the content and the intent of the message effectively. Only through reflective practice can one develop techniques of effective communication.

E **stands for expectations.** Expectations vary depending on one's goals and professional aspirations. Colleagues may expect a new nurse to be on call every weekend or work all major statutory holidays for the first year. New nurses may have specific expectations of their managers related to feedback or promotion, or may respond differently to varying styles of management and leadership. The nursing executive or administrator in transition will likely have expectations about how the nurse managers under their supervision spend their time on the job—even about how much time they spend at work.

Finding out in advance what the explicit and implicit expectations are of the people with whom you are working, and gaining insight into your own leadership style and self-expectations can facilitate a smoother role transition by decreasing role ambiguity (Hardy, 1978). Hardy's seminal work with role theory suggests a strong, positive, relationship between role ambiguity (one type of role stress— a condition in which role demands are conflicting, irri- tating, or impossible to fulfill) and role strain (the sub- jective feeling of discomfort experienced as a result of role stress). The major concepts of role theory are pre- sented in the subsequent Theory Box.

THEORY BOX

Hardy's Role Theory

Theory/Contributor	Key Ideas	Application to Practice
Hardy (1978) is credited with applying role theory to health care providers. A *role* is the expected and actual behaviours associated with a position. Role expectations are the attitudes and behaviours others anticipate that a person in the role will possess or demonstrate.	Role stress is a precursor to role strain. Role stress is associated with low productivity and performance. Role stress and role strain can lead a person to withdraw psychologically from the role. Clear, realistic role expectations can decrease the role stress for someone in a new role (e.g., a new nurse manager).	Clear, realistic role ex- pectations can increase productivity.

From Hardy, M. E. (1978). Role stress and role strain. In Hardy M. E. & Conway M.E. (Eds.), *Role theory: perspectives for health professionals* (pp. 73–109). New York, NY: Appleton-Century-Crofts.

There are also personal expectations related to perfor- mance in a new role. You may have a mental image of an individual in this position, based on prior experi- ences with someone who had assumed the role into which you are transitioning; these images may even have motivated you to move your career in this direc- tion. The process of role transition unfolds as the new employee identifies expectations, recognizes the similarities and differences with preconceptions, and evolves in the roles of leader, manager, and follower within their position.

S **stands for support,** which is closely tied to expec- tations about performance. All roles are shaped to some degree by the support and services others pro- vide. The NGN in an urban acute-care setting often has colleagues readily available when a second opin- ion is needed, whereas the same NGN may feel lost when confronted with clinical issues during a home care visit or when working nights in a rural hospi- tal. The nurse manager who must develop a unit's budget in a health care facility may have no account- ing department to provide a detailed analysis of the facility's prior expenditures. But remember that each role has some support available. When a new posi- tion is being considered, it is important to inquire into the available support, particularly targeted at areas in which the new employee may lack funda-

mental knowledge or skills. When implementing a change in one's nursing role, seek out someone in the organization who can help you identify the skills or knowledge that will be important for success, or even provide the support services that will facilitate your role transition.

ROLE TRANSITION PROCESS

One way to think about the way in which someone tran- sitions to a new role is illustrated in Box 28.2.

STRATEGIES TO PROMOTE ROLE TRANSITION

Becoming a manager or assuming a new role often results in a change in professional identity. Such a trans- formation invokes stress as the person unlearns old roles and learns new ones. Several strategies can help an indi- vidual ease the strain and optimize the process of role transition (Box 28.3).

Strengthen Internal Resources

A key strategy in promoting role transition is to recog- nize and draw on one's own values and beliefs. Behaviour is influenced by values and beliefs. Clark (2008) noted that values and beliefs *"shape how individuals think and*

BOX 28.2 Professional Role Transition Model for the New Nursing Graduate

Unlearning old roles while learning new ones requires an identity adjustment over time. The persons involved must invest themselves in the process, which involves moving through the phases of role preparation, role orientation, role integration, and role stabilization (Boychuk Duchscher, 2012; see Fig. 28.2).

Role Preparation

During this phase of role transition, the individual gets ready to make a major change (assuming that this change is planned and its transition is anticipated). Time is spent exploring and seeking to understand what the new role will entail, the supports available to facilitate the role change, and to whom the incumbent will report and how. Role preparation entails education and socialization to the professional role within postsecondary and/or health care systems. In the case of the newly graduated nurse, time spent in senior clinical placements may serve as the preparatory period. In the case of a new nurse manager or educator, attempts may be made to "preview" the role by spending time working alongside someone who currently assumes that role. Developing accurate role expectations is the primary objective of the preparation phase of role transition, so it is important that the preparatory phase be as realistic and representative as possible. Role discrepancy speaks to the gap between role expectations and role performance, and can cause role frustration, leading to role stress and strain over time. Role discrepancy can ultimately be resolved by changing expectations of role performance or through adaptation to the differences over time, but it is obviously more desirable not to be in this position. If the role is valued and the differences are seen as tenable or amenable, a decision will most likely be made to stay in the role and sort out the discrepancies. This decision requires negotiation and a certain degree of conciliation by all parties.

Role Orientation

Role orientation constitutes a formal employment process whereby the expectations of the role are clearly identified, and the new employee is introduced to the organizational structure within which he or she will be working. Orientation often includes some element of preceptorship (skill, role, or responsibility orientation) as well as mentorship (organizational, cultural, or professional process orientation). The length of time required to orientate to a new role will depend on the individual's existing familiarity with the role, confidence in performing the role in this new context, and degree of role discrepancy revealed during orientation. A new employee who

gradually and progressively assumes the multiple elements of a new role (with planned debriefings and a concerted analysis of the factors contributing to both successes and challenges during the transition) is more likely to become successfully engaged in the new role.

Role Integration

During this phase of role transition, the individual undergoes significant adjustments to his or her perceptions about the role and reconciles discrepancies between the previous understanding of the role and what it is. Feedback and dialogue about the role discrepancies that take place during role integration (the process of adjusting perceptions of one's role and reconciling discrepancies between the previous understanding of the role and what it is) are essential for the individual to realign values that may have become displaced. Failure to undergo this phase may result in role frustration and disillusionment and, ultimately, role disengagement.

Significant to role integration is the consolidation of the individual's sense of accountability and responsibility for the role within the larger work context (unit, centre, or institution). Not uncommonly, skill competence improves during this phase, as does the capacity for independent decision making, judgement, and critical thinking. Tenure in the role has most likely exposed the individual to conflict and crisis, which has equipped him or her with the skills to solve fundamental problems and resolve basic conflicts that arise in the course of the role.

Role Stabilization

Role stabilization occurs as an individual matures in his or her performance of all facets of the role, to the point where he or she internalizes the role, performing it fluidly and with confidence. At this juncture, the individual has learned the behaviours that meet the role expectations, and these behaviours have become second nature. The energy previously expended learning the new role can be redirected toward optimizing the skills required in the role, understanding the gestalt of the role, and critically thinking about the judgements and decisions that are encompassed within the role. The focus shifts from distinction to discernment of role expectations, and energy is now spent accomplishing unit, institutional, or professional goals collaboratively with colleagues. Individuals who have internalized their roles have developed their own unique personal approaches to role performance and role satisfaction and feel valued for their contribution.

Continued

Unexpected Role Transition

Not every transition can be anticipated or predicted. Some changes are unexpected, and the individual must process the end of one way of being or doing before successfully integrating into another. In cases where an employee is terminated, a position is eliminated, or a job description changes dramatically, the response can be shock, disbelief, or possibly grief. In what amounts to a forced role transition, the individual may experience disorientation and confusion to the point of being unable to function. As the shock wears off, the individual may become angered by the change and may direct anger toward those who are perceived as instigating the role change. Conversely, the anger may be directed internally, leading to depres-

sion. If the individual is unable to acknowledge and talk about the loss he or she experienced as a result of the change, the period of grief may be extended or emotional baggage may be created that is carried into the next role. Grieving can eventually resolve into acceptance. Lessons learned from the experience are identified and internalized. A new role is sought, and the cycle begins again.

Health care is in a tumultuous state of affairs. Reorganizations, realignments, restructuring, and downsizing of the workforce are now commonplace. To be successful, work role restructuring must be undertaken with the same sensitivity afforded any significant life change. Role transition takes time, tremendous patience, and understanding.

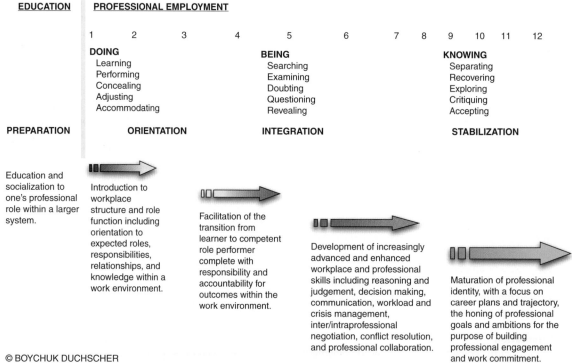

© BOYCHUK DUCHSCHER

Fig. 28.2 Professional role transition for the new nursing graduate.

BOX 28.3 **How to Promote Role Transition**

- Strengthen internal resources (commitment, character, self-respect, and flexibility).
- Assess the organization's resources, culture, and group dynamics.
- Negotiate the role (meet with those to whom you will be reporting and discuss expectations).
- Grow through preceptorship and mentorship (if no formal preceptorship or mentoring process exists, be on the lookout for senior individuals whose

practice you would like to emulate, with whom you can relate either professionally or personally, who express an interest in you, or who seem accepting and embracing of your ideas or approaches to practice).
- Develop role-specific knowledge and skills (determine the primary sets of knowledge and skills that you will be expected to perform with relative frequency and focus on competence in these initially).

see the world, and the meanings they attribute to their experiences, actions and relationships with others" (p. 30). It is important while making any role transition, to not lose sight of what matters to you, reflecting on how that influences both how you lead and want to be led. Work roles or places of work are not equally suited to everyone. One must consider whether personal goals and professional fulfillment can best be achieved through that particular role, within that institution, or under the direction of that supervisor.

Clark (2008) noted that "nurses typically work according to two sets of values; professional values, which are determined by their code of professional conduct, and personal values" (p. 31). If an individual in transition understands his or her own personal values,

these will help frame the way in which that person responds to situations and relationships. An exercise such as writing down short statements of self-belief or posting self-affirmations on the fridge at home, or a wall in your office may be helpful as a visual reminder.

The rapid and constant change that is consistent with health care today dictates the need for flexibility. Successful transition into a new role within the health care system requires the willingness and ability to learn and master new skills, translate information, and adapt behaviour to new situations. The individual making the transition must also temper self-expectations, particularly in the early stages of the change. Understanding transition as a process will help with flexibility.

THEORY BOX

Kramer's Reality Shock/Duchscher's Transition Shock

Theory/Contributor	Key Ideas	Application to Practice
Kramer (1974) is credited with establishing the knowledge behind "reality shock" in her seminal publication *"Reality Shock: Why Nurses Leave Nursing"*. *Reality shock* was coined as the alarming experience of new nursing graduates leaving the safety of a known and relatively protected context (nursing education) and entering the unknown realm of accountable, professional nursing practice. Duchscher (2008, 2009) followed Kramer's work some 4 decades later with a robust theoretical construct that built on Kramer's work, outlining the *Stages of Transition* (Table 28.1) for the newly graduated nurse, along with an experience she coined *"Transition Shock"* (Fig. 28.1), representing the intensity, depth, and breadth of the initial interface between the new practitioner with their professional practice context.	Role change precedes role stress, which can be a precursor to role strain. Role stress is associated with low productivity and performance. Role stress and role strain can lead a person to withdraw psychologically from the role. Knowledge of the impending role change, its ramifications and implications, along with clear, realistic role expectations can decrease the role stress (and even prevent role strain, which speaks to stress over time) for someone in a new role (e.g., a new nurse graduate, a nurse moving from direct care to an educator or manager role).	Knowledge of the Stages of Transition and Transition Shock during the preparatory (undergraduate education or BEFORE the role change), accompanied by clear and realistic expectations of the change, significantly reduce stress, avoid strain and increase both productivity and role fulfillment.

Source: Kramer, M. (1974). *Reality shock: why nurses leave nursing*. St. Louis: C.V. Mosby Company.
Boychuk Duchscher, J. (2008). A process of becoming: the stages of new nursing graduate professional role transition. *Journal of Continuing Education in Nursing*, 39(10), 441–450; Boychuk Duchscher, J. (2009). Transition shock: the initial stage of role adaptation for newly-graduated Registered Nurses. *Journal of Advanced Nursing*, 65(5), 1103–1113.

Assess the Workplace

Taking on a new role is much like being an immigrant in a new country. An immigrant learns how to access the available resources to acclimate to the new environment. Cultural practices of the new country may seem strange or odd. Cultural differences must be analyzed and decisions made about which aspects to adopt. Subtle

differences in communication patterns or group dynamics are also identified. Understanding the nuances of social interactions is often the most difficult aspect of enculturating. The transition is smoother for the immigrant who understands himself or herself, assesses the new environment, and learns how to communicate within their new group.

Navigating a new role requires that the individual learn how to access resources in the work context (e.g., unit, organization). Approaching the workplace as a foreign culture, the nurse can keenly observe the rituals, accepted practices, and patterns of communication within that context. This ongoing assessment facilitates a speedier transition into the new role. Immigrants who spend their energy bemoaning the difficulties of the new country may fail to enjoy the advantages that drew them to the country in the first place. In the same way, the nurse who focuses on the challenges of transition or drawbacks to the workplace may deplete energy required to internalize the new role.

Negotiate the Role

A strategy that is helpful during conflicting role expectations is **role negotiation**. It involves resolving conflicting expectations about personal performance through communication. The ROLES assessment (see Exercise 28.1) may identify areas of significant conflict. Writing down the expectations is the first step in resolving areas of conflict. It is important to review the expectations listed to determine whether they are realistic. Unrealistic expectations strongly held by others may require diplomatic reeducation so that their expectations can become more realistic.

EXERCISE 28.1

Roles Assessment

Assume that you are transitioning to a nurse manager role. Answer these questions about your new role.

Responsibilities

1. From the position description, what are the responsibilities?
2. Is there support for the ongoing learning required during your transition?
3. For what decisions are you responsible, and will you be provided with the time and resources to grow into the role?
4. Consider information about the position that you learned during the interview. Also consider the responsibilities of individuals in similar roles that you have observed. Are there other responsibilities to add to your list?

Opportunities

5. What opportunities for growth and professional development are supported in this workplace?
6. How could your strengths or expertise benefit the individuals in this new workplace?
7. Dream a little (or a lot). If a person who had been a patient on the unit were describing the nursing care to another potential patient, what would you want the first patient to say? Describe the workplace as you want it to be.

Lines of Communication

8. Draw yourself in the middle of a separate piece of paper. Now fill in the people above you and below you with whom you would communicate. Draw lines from you to each person or group. On the line, identify the form of communication.

Expectations

9. This may be the most difficult part to assess. List in short sentences or phrases the expectations you have for yourself and those each person (colleagues or direct supervisors) or group (unit, institution, professional group) may have for you in relation to your new role.

Support

10. What people do you know in the organization who could provide information that you will need to fulfill your roles and responsibilities?
11. What departments provide services that you could access for assistance?

Next Steps

Now compare the lists.

Place a star next to those expectations that are held by more than one person or group. For example, as a *new manager*, you might be expected to handle the budget of a unit in accordance with a vision that is determined by administrators outside your sphere of influence. As a *new nurse*, you might be expected to take a significantly larger workload than was expected of you as a student, while working collaboratively with other scopes of nursing practice, unregulated care providers, and allied health practitioners. As a *new educator*, you may be required to complete multiple unit-based orientations for practice areas outside of your experience or expertise.

Circle those items that could cause conflicts.

Refer to the Strategies to Promote Role Transition section in this chapter on how to resolve these conflicts.

Save your responses to these questions to review in 3 months. You may be surprised how your own perception of your ROLES may change over time.

Grow Through Preceptorship and Mentorship

Although often used interchangeably, the terms preceptorship and mentorship are distinct. Preceptorship is "a period of practical experience and training for a trainee supervised by an expert or specialist in a particular field" (The Ottawa Hospital, n.d.). It is seen as an efficient and effective way to introduce an individual to a new role and its responsibilities (Myrick & Yonge, 2005). Most often used in the context of a student completing a clinical practicum, or a newly graduated nurse making the initial role transition to professional practice, preceptorship focuses on the learning of tasks, skills, and routines necessary to perform one's role efficiently and effectively. Preceptorship is often distinguished from mentorship by its shorter tenure, narrower objectives, and differing supporter characteristics. The attributes of a good preceptor are grounded in a strong practice history relative to the specific role (direct care nurse, nurse manager, or nurse educator). Meanwhile, the attributes of a good mentor are grounded in advanced relational capacity and expertise in the role area, balanced with a strong vision for how the person transitioning can develop and contribute professionally while growing personally through the enactment of the role. Although one individual may serve as both a preceptor and mentor in any given transition-support situation, preceptorship tends to be short lived, terminating once the knowledge and skills required to perform the role have been successfully transferred from preceptor to preceptee.

Mentorship "is a formal supportive relationship between two, or more, health professionals that has the potential to result in professional growth and development for both mentors and mentees" (Ontario Ministry of Health and Long-Term Care, 2014, p. 14). A mentor is there to "pick up the pieces" after the initial transition is complete and when the individual in transition becomes more aware of (and able to think about) the purpose, significance, and relative importance of their work. Mentors are an important component of a nurturing environment that promotes staff retention, serving as a tremendous source of guidance and support for new nurses, nurse managers, and nurse educators in transition, and serving both career and psychosocial support functions. Career support is possible because the mentor has sufficient professional experience and organizational authority to facilitate the career of the mentee. Box 28.4 highlights some key functions of mentors during the role transition of new nursing graduates. The Robert Wood Johnson Nurse Executive Fellows program has identified five core competencies of leaders and mentors: interpersonal and communication effectiveness, risk taking and creativity, self-knowledge and self-renewal, inspiring and leading change, and strategic vision (Center for the Health Professions, 2009).

A mentor often creates opportunities for the mentee to achieve and advance and can provide encouragement and a needed sense of perspective for the mentee that originates out of the mentor's long-standing tenure in the role to which the mentee is transitioning. Mentors offer career guidance and emotional support. Through coaching activities, mentors provide information about how to improve role performance by offering feedback and "in the moment" guidance.

The mentor, as coach, facilitates critical thought, decision making, and judgement that is grounded in extended experience of the role being assumed by the mentee. The interpersonal connection between the mentor and the mentee is critical, as trust and mutual positive regard are required for the relationship to evolve. For this reason, it may be beneficial for mentees to choose their mentors. Mentors may offer counsel to mentees by providing opportunities for mentees to explore personal concerns as filtered through the knowing ear of the mentor. The relational aspects of effective mentorship partnerships or pairings include confidentiality, trust, and respect.

Relationships between mentors and mentees vary because of individual characteristics and the career phase of each. During the early phases of a role transition, a mentee is concerned about competence and a mentor can provide valuable coaching. As the individual advances along the transition continuum, support from a mentor can prepare the individual for career advancement. A mentor nearing the end of his or her work career can find fulfillment in sharing knowledge with others, while equally benefiting from the counsel of a recently retired colleague; and the mentorship cycle continues.

BOX 28.4 Mentoring New Nursing Graduates Through Transition

Role Preparation Phase (Pregraduate)

The relationship is primarily preceptorial in this phase.

Mentor functions:

- Introduce and establish terms of relationship
- Indicate that the responsibility for connection is mutual
- Encourage final practicum in unit to which the student will transition
- Educate the student on role transition stages/transition shock
- Facilitate socialization exercises (i.e., how to engage with other nurses)
- Foster partnerships between the educational institution and workplace
- Develop workplace engagement activities/strategies
- Explore work experiences with the student
- Redirect evaluation to self-appraisal strategies

Role Orientation Phase (1–3 Months Posthire)

The focus is on skill assessment, skill practice for familiarity and performance confidence, and understanding work role expectations.

Mentor functions:

- Facilitate personal (nonworkplace) connection over 1–2 weeks with a focus on encouragement, support, and collegiality
- Assess career intentions (the desired professional trajectory)
- Undertake transition–knowledge framed orientation approaches
- Establish confidential new nurse peer support network
- Seek ongoing (every shift) feedback/performance appraisal by the nurse manager and educator, and the clinical support team

Role Transition Phase (3–6 Months Posthire)

The focus is on progressive (complexity and volume) skill acquisition, time management, and conflict resolution/coping.

Mentor functions:

- Facilitate discussion on professional culture, work relationships

- Ensure that the clinical support team is well versed on transition shock and the stages of transition
- Initiate an interdisciplinary role knowledge sharing program
- Consider supernumerary employment
- Create flexible staffing/scheduling options
- Provide feedback/performance appraisal to move the mentee more toward self-reflection

Role Integration Phase (6–9 Months Posthire)

The focus is on advanced clinical judgement/reasoning/decision making through experiential case study learning and care debriefing.

Mentor functions:

- Facilitate discussion on coping strategies, professional self-care, and big picture thinking about the health care system and its relationship to the workplace
- Ask mentee to consider interinstitutional employment flexibility as career growth option
- Encourage intellectual recovery strategies with a focus on life balance
- Optimize utilization of nursing clinicians and charge nurses

Role Stabilization Phase (10–12 Months Posthire)

The focus is on guiding decisions and experiences through clinical consultation rather than directive approaches.

Mentor functions:

- Use multiple clinical coaches (e.g., other nurse experts)
- Facilitate professional development, practise introspection, and encourage a professional perspective
- Ask the mentee to consider charge nurse orientation toward the 12-month mark
- Facilitate advanced practice rotations (i.e., emergency department/critical care unit rotations)
- Review the career trajectory of the mentee and encourage professional planning
- Encourage the mentee to engage in professional association/workplace committee work

Modified from Boychuk Duchscher, J. (2012). From surviving to thriving: navigating the first year of professional nursing practice. Calgary, AB: Nursing the Future. Retrieved from http://www.nursingthefuture.ca/from_surviving_to_thriving. With permission.

EXERCISE 28.2

Role Transition Self-Assessment

Respond to each item using the following scale. Add up your score.

1 = Strongly disagree
2 = Disagree
3 = Unsure
4 = Agree
5 = Strongly agree

I am aware of the stages of professional role transition.
I am responsible for my own professional development.
I feel confident about my ability to learn the skills I need to be effective in my new role.

I have the support I need to learn the responsibilities expected of me in this new role.

I feel confident in my ability to balance the multiple priorities and activities required of me in this role.

I have the resources to develop a personal network of support.

No magical score indicates your readiness for role transition. If you are unsure in every category, your score will be 6. A score of 25 or above indicates that you are confident that you can master the transition to your new role. If you currently have a mentor, ask that person to respond to each item to analyze your abilities. Compare those responses with your own. Do you have a realistic view of yourself?

CONCLUSION

Professional role transitions—whether they be from nursing student to practicing nurse or practicing nurse to charge nurse, nurse manager, or nurse educator—pose unique challenges. Nurses who make these transitions with minimal discomfort are generally armed with knowledge about transition as a concept, seek out, or are provided with support resources, and understand the need to "ride the wave" of the experience. Although nurses today are better prepared to take on a variety of roles throughout their careers, the breadth and scope of those roles are more challenging. Charge nurses and nurse managers are often responsible for mentoring and coaching new staff even as they themselves transition to

new roles. Facilitating a healthy transition takes time, should be framed on the evidence available about role transition, and requires strategic effort to achieve the best results possible.

Making a successful professional role transition is certainly worth the effort. Learning how to lead a life that is fulfilling, purposeful, and balanced is the intended outcome of role transition. Finding synergy between your work and the level of commitment and integrity you strive for as a professional brings out the best in you and everyone you work with. A sense of role fulfillment and subsequent job satisfaction contributes significantly to the quality of any workplace and directly influences the quality of patient care.

❓ A SOLUTION

The nurse manager could have set up a one-on-one meeting with Claire the day before her first shift, which would have allowed her to gain some familiarization of the unit. The nurse manager could have given Claire a tour around the unit, introduced her to some of the staff (e.g., other nurses, the ward clerk, cleaning personnel). The nurse manager could have shown Claire where to hang her coat, put her lunch, find her mailbox, etc. Doing so would have helped Claire feel less out of place on the first day of work. In addition, the nurse manager could have introduced Claire to the unit educator. On that first shift, Alexis might have met Claire at the entrance to the hospital and walked

with her to the unit. This would have allowed them to have a quick chat so they could get to know each other, making Claire feel a part of the team more quickly. Alexis might have benefited from having an understanding of the stages of transition for NGNs so that she could understand her own needs and maximize opportunities for mentoring and guiding. Lastly, as Claire settles in, it would be beneficial for both the nurse manager and the unit educator to plan to periodically check in with Claire to ensure her successful integration into the unit.

Would this be a suitable approach for you? Why or why not?

■ THE EVIDENCE

Etheridge's (2007) descriptive, longitudinal, phenomenologic study examined the perceptions of recent nursing graduates about learning to make clinical judgements. Semi-structured interviews were conducted to determine the meaning of making clinical nursing judgements. These interviews were conducted on three different dates: within a month after the end of a preceptor experience, 2 to 3 months later, and 8 to 9 months after the first interview.

Major components of learning to think like a nurse included building confidence, accepting responsibility, adapting to changing relationships with others, and thinking more clinically. Discussions with peers were a powerful experience for the individual nurses transitioning to their new role.

✳ NEED TO KNOW NOW

- Be prepared to feel a certain amount of discomfort, anxiety, and loss during role transition. It can be disruptive.
- Keep in mind that professional role transition is a journey that takes place in stages; NGNs and those who support them should understand these stages and target support resources accordingly (see http://www.nursingthefuture.ca/from_surviving_to_thriving for an important resource in supporting NGNs).
- Obtain a complete and detailed position description for the new role.
- Identify critical resources available in the organization to assist with role transition: nurse managers, nurse educators, clinical nurse specialists, preceptors, charge nurses, peers, employee assistance programs.

- Be open to feedback and arrange for it on a regular basis.
- Identify a mentor in the first 1 to 3 months of a new role.
- Attend educational programs that expand your knowledge of the role.
- Recognize that role transition is as personal as it is professional; make sure those on whom you depend for support are aware of the influences this transition is having on your life.
- Be aware of transition shock and the stages of role transition so that you can anticipate stress points during the process and seek help accordingly.

■ CHAPTER CHECKLIST

- Experiencing a role transition yourself or assisting a staff member to successfully integrate into a new role takes time and energy—two scarce resources for nurse managers. Knowing what to expect can optimize advancement through the stages and maximize the outcome while minimizing unnecessary expenditure of energy that can plague individuals going through a professional role transition.
- Role transition is often a process of unlearning old roles while learning new ones.
- The stages of professional role transition for NGNs are doing, being, and knowing.
- Responsibilities, opportunities, lines of communication, expectations, and support (ROLES) are aspects common to all roles. When considering how to effectively navigate (or support others through) a role transition, gather information about each of these aspects.

- Managers are also leaders and followers.
- Unexpected role transitions are particularly challenging and often involve a grieving process.
- Role stress has its roots in discrepancies between role expectations and the reality of role enactment in the "real world".
- Role strain develops when the stressors contributing to a mismatch between expectation and reality go unacknowledged or are insufficiently addressed.
- Role negotiation involves resolving conflicting expecations about personal performance through communication.
- Commitment, character, self-respect, and flexibility are internal resources that can facilitate the process of role transition.
- Preceptors can assist in the understanding and performance of the tasks of a new role, and mentors are there to provide career guidance and emotional support.

■ TIPS FOR ROLE TRANSITIONING

- Anticipate and prepare for transition—remember that it is a normal and healthy process.
- Identify the responsibilities, opportunities, lines of communication, expectations, and support for the new role.
- Understand that a transition involves changing roles, responsibilities, relationships, and knowledge and is

at once physical, emotional, intellectual, sociocultural, and developmental.
- Use both external and internal resources to negotiate a role transition that supports and reinforces your life values and commitments.

Visit the Evolve website for Suggested Readings, Internet Resources, and additional resources related to the content in this chapter: http://evolve.elsevier.com/Canada/Yoder-Wise/leading/.

REFERENCES

Center for the Health Professions. (2009). *RWJ program eligibility*. Retrieved from: http://www.futurehealth.ucsf.edu.

Clark, L. (2008). Clinical leadership: values, beliefs and vision. *Nursing Management, 15*(7), 30–35.

Cooper, H. M. (1989). *The integrative research review: A systematic approach*. Newbury Park: Sage.

Duchscher, J. E. B. (2012). *From surviving to thriving: Navigating the first year of professional nursing practice* (2nd ed.). Calgary, AB: Nursing the Future. Retrieved from: http://www.nursingthefuture.ca/from_surviving_to_thriving.

Hardy, M. E. (1978). Role stress and role strain. In M. E. Hardy, & M. E. Conway (Eds.), *Role theory: Perspectives for health professionals* (pp. 73–109). New York, NY: Appleton-Century-Crofts.

McConnell, C. R. (2008). The health care professional as a manager: Balancing two important roles. *The Health Care Manager, 27*(3), 277–284.

Meleis, A. I. (2010). *Transitions theory: Middle-range and situation-specific theories in nursing research and practice*. New York, NY: Springer.

Menon, S. T. (2002). Toward a model of psychological health empowerment: Implications for health care in multicultural communities. *Nurse Education Today, 22*, 28–39.

Myrick, F., & Yonge, O. (2005). *Nursing preceptorship: Connecting practice and education*. Philadelphia, PA: Lippincott Williams and Wilkins.

Ontario Ministry of Health and Long-Term Care. (2014, May). *Guidelines for participation in the nursing graduate guarantee initiative*. Retrieved from: http://www.healthforceontario.ca/UserFiles/file/Nurse/Inside/ngg-participation-guidelines-jan-2011-en.pdf.

The Ottawa Hospital. (n.d.). (Pain connect—The Ottawa Hospital Pain Clinic (TOHPC) preceptorship. Retrieved from: https://www.ottawahospital.on.ca/wps/portal/Base/TheHospital/ClinicalServices/DeptPgrmCS/Departments/Anesthesiology/ChronicPainUnitTOHPainClinic/Pain-Preceptorship.

29

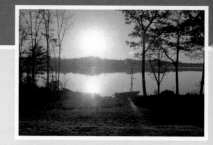

Self-Management: Stress and Time

Krystal Buchanan

This chapter examines the concept of self-management—the ability of individuals to actively gain control of their lives. Through self-management, the professional nurse can effectively engage in work, model powerful persistence, and enjoy daily renewal. Three components of self-management are explored: stress management, time management, and meeting management. Methods for managing stress and organizing time are introduced. Practical exercises and suggestions for stress management and time management are presented that can be used for personal and professional situations to reduce stress and enhance efficiency.

OBJECTIVES

- Define self-management.
- Identify personal and professional stressors.
- Describe physical, mental, and emotional/spiritual strategies to manage stress.
- Understand the nurse manager's role in helping staff manage stress.
- Describe common time wasters.
- Identify time-management techniques that can help manage time more effectively.
- Describe tips for managing meetings effectively.

TERMS TO KNOW

agenda	general adaptation syndrome (GAS)	procrastination
burnout		role stress
coping	information overload	self-management
delegation	overwork	time management
employee assistance program (EAP)	perfectionism	

❓ A CHALLENGE

Maryam feels as if there is never a break from the constant stress in life. Just when Maryam thinks things are becoming easier, another stressful event comes up. Maryam seems to have few stress-free days lately and knows that sustained stress is not good for anyone. Maryam is employed full time at a level-one emergency department and finds that there is ongoing pressure to work overtime to fulfill the unit's staffing requirements. Maryam is also pursuing a Master's degree part-time and has not been able to focus on studying as much as

is required, a source of even more stress. Maryam has a partner and two children that there rarely seems to be time for, and Maryam knows that this is not good for the family. Maryam feels like there is always something to do, is unable to get to the things that are pressing, and has little time to spare. It seems like a never-ending battle.

What do you think you would do if you were Maryam? What are some resources or sources of help Maryam might consider?

INTRODUCTION

What should you do when you have tried your best, but things are not going well? What needs changing, and where do you begin? Self-management is the ability of individuals to actively gain control of their lives. It involves self-directed change to achieve important goals (Stuart & Laraia, 2008). As a nurse leader, your goals will require balancing personal and professional objectives and organizing your time and activities to reach them—and attempting this balance may well be a source of stress. Incorporating interventions for stress management will help a nurse leader understand how thoughts can influence behaviour and mood (McBain et al., 2015). Nurse leaders and managers in the health care setting have a legal and moral obligation to ensure that high quality patient care is provided (Parand et al., 2014). There is positive correlation between overall job satisfaction and quality of care being delivered (Aron, 2015). Compared with other professions, nursing can be highly stressful. How the nurse perceives the stress is a result of personal characteristics and the work environment, including demographic characteristics, working situations, occupational roles, and personal resources (Wu et al., 2010).

Nash (2009) investigated the relationships among nurse manager stress, hardiness, and leadership, and found that nurse managers with higher hardiness had a greater inclination for transformational leadership practices. The presence of hardiness behaviours is positively correlated with good health and performance, and negatively correlated with strain, denial, and avoidance behaviours (Maddi, 2013). To develop stress hardiness, we must actively improve our skills related to stress management, adaptive coping, healthy communication, and problem solving. Research has demonstrated that hardiness can be learned (Maddi, 2013).

The three key strategies for achieving self-management introduced in this chapter—managing and coping with stress, developing effective time management skills, and meeting management—are important ways to do more with fewer resources. Time and stress are somewhat of a "chicken and egg" phenomenon—not enough time contributes to stress, and stress can erode efficiency and thus decrease time on task. The key lies in our ability to manage both time and stress, not only personally but also professionally. The outcome of effective self-management is hardiness and the ability to accomplish professional and personal goals.

UNDERSTANDING STRESS

Nurses have learned about the effects of stress on patients and how to educate patients to manage the consequences of stress. However, very few nurse managers have any sort of formal leadership or managerial training that would prepare them for dealing with multiple sources of stress at the same time (Bailey, 2009). Nurses need to recognize the unique stressors in their professional and personal lives. Everyone experiences stress—the exhilaration of a joyous event, as well as the negative feelings and unpleasant physical symptoms that may be associated with a difficult life situation or even the anticipation of difficulty. Stress is the uncomfortable gap between how we would like our life to be and how it actually is. Although nurses may have knowledge about the effects of stress and may counsel patients on this, nurses are not immune to the effects of stress in their own personal lives. Learning what stress is, its dynamics and sources, and some strategies to manage distress is a part of the personal and professional maturation of each nurse.

Definition of Stress

In this chapter, *stress* is a consequence of or response to an event or stimulus and can be negative (distress) or positive (eustress). Each individual's interpretation determines whether the event is viewed as positive or threatening. In addition, stress management does not necessarily mean stress reduction. It may mean engaging in activities of preventative stress management. Preventative stress management is a philosophy and a set of principles grounded in the health of public and is an important consideration for organizational leaders to consider to operate to their fullest potential and to create an environment that promotes healthy workers and helps prevent the effects of stress spiraling out of control (Campbell et al., 2013). Preventative stress management activities typically exist at every level of most organizations, however effective implementation of these activities is dependent on committed leadership. Stress management is a recognized entry to practice competency for a Registered Nurse in Canada (College of Nurses of Ontario, 2014). Stress management has important implications for the workplace because of its link to low absenteeism rates, improved quality of care, and increased productivity (Limm et al., 2011). While acknowledging that it is challenging, nurses would benefit from learning ways to help transform stress into a tool for achieving their full potential (Guimond-Plourde, 2011).

SOURCES OF JOB STRESS

Job stress can be defined as the physical and emotional responses that arise when job requirements do not match the abilities, resources, or needs of the worker. Work-related stress can lead to poor physical and emotional health and injury. Job stress can motivate us to learn new skills and master our jobs, or it can cause distress, which can lead to exhaustion, feelings of inadequacy, and failure. For example, the stress associated with an interview for a new position can be useful; it may provide you with determination and gives you an "edge" that will help you think quickly and clearly and express your thoughts in ways that will serve to benefit you in the interview process. However, having your car break down on the way to the interview creates distress when you realize that you will be late for the interview. As more is learned about the relationship of stress to physiologic changes, stressors will become even easier to identify. When one looks at job-related stressors, the stressors fall into one of two categories: external sources (working conditions) and internal sources (worker characteristics).

External Sources

Occupational stress in nursing has been well-defined and documented. Nursing is more than just a job, but rather a profession that attracts individuals who put a value on compassion and who want to make a difference. Nurses report actively burning out related to work related stressors, such as schedules, shift work, physical exhaustion, workload, conflict, bullying, challenging patients, rapid advances in technology, and acuity. Patient care, safety, and quality are all affected and may be compromised when stress and fatigue take over the ability of a nurse to prioritize self-care habits and recovery time (Waddill-Goad & Sigma Theta Tau, 2016).

Nursing burnout merits special attention from staff nurses, physicians, managers, and nursing leaders (Bogaert et al., 2010). The nurse practice environment and its connection to stress and burnout is an extremely important leadership and organizational issue (Wolf et al., 2008).

Change

Although the increased stress that results from change takes many forms, two underlying patterns appear to be constant. Often, nurses feel trapped by conflicting expectations. They are expected to provide responsive and compassionate care, to meet patients' needs, and to be accessible and flexible. However, organizations require nurses to be managers of patient care and of systems, and value their contribution to efficiency and cost-effectiveness while simultaneously preserving quality of care. Because in many cases, nurses cannot comply with both expectations, they experience considerable role conflict, frustration, and distress.

Social

Interpersonal relations can buffer stressors or can in themselves become stressors. Outside the work setting, home can be a refuge for overworked or fatigued nurses; however, stresses at home, when severe, can impair work performance and relationships among staff or even result in hostility or violence that may invade the workplace.

Changes in health care delivery systems, as well as the current nursing shortage, have reduced the number of professional nurses, often creating situations of minimally safe staffing levels. Consequently, some nurses lose supportive, collegial relationships that may have been established over many years. Many institutions now depend on supplemental or casual staffing that can create very transient nursing staff. In other situations, nurses are reassigned or they "float" to various patient-care units, which require that they work with unfamiliar staff or in environments where they are less comfortable or confident. Thus they may feel isolated or become unwillingly involved in dysfunctional politics on the unit. When such situations necessitate that nurses work with patients whose requirements for care may be unfamiliar, this can result in further stress related to patient safety concerns.

Persons in management-level positions may also become stressors. Communication may come from the top down, with little opportunity for nurses to actively participate in decisions that affect them directly, or that they may need to implement without proper training or support. Nurses may experience distress from feelings of frustration and helplessness with this lack of opportunity to provide input to decisions. The stress that nurses may experience related to being unable to contribute meaningfully to decisions or to being asked to implement decisions with which they do not agree can also lead to moral distress. Moral distress is a situation when nurses know what they feel is the right thing to do, but are unable to do this because of institutional or managerial constraints (Jameton, 1984). Moral distress is discussed in more detail in Chapter 6.

In addition, disruptive behaviour poses considerable work stress. Disruptive behaviour is any type of unwanted behaviour, such as verbal or physical behaviour that may have adverse outcomes and impact quality care. Effects are not only limited to patient care; the entire health care team can be impacted. Examples of disruptive behaviours can include being impatient, condescending language or tone toward others, intimidation and violence, and sexual violence. Although healthy workplaces include freedom from such behaviour, too many instances occur in health care settings. In addition to being stressful for nurses, such behaviour can disrupt patient safety efforts. Many institutions attempt to improve disruptive behaviour within their team by educating and training staff to enhance communication and collaboration skills and to reduce adverse outcomes.

The Position

Upon entering nursing school, most students expect that caring for patients who are chronically or critically ill and for families who have experienced tragedy will be stressful. The current environment in many health care organizations, however, is more complex and is often characterized by overwork, a situation in which employees are expected to become more productive without additional resources. It is also characterized by the stresses inherent in nursing practice. In some settings, direct care nurses are expected to stay beyond the designated assignment period, often with little or no notice. Some nurse managers experience stress in those situations and resort to threatening behaviours and statements, such as the potential for dismissal or patient abandonment. These situations often escalate when direct care nurses do not believe they can deliver safe care and nurse managers exhaust creative ways to provide adequate coverage.

Role stress is a condition in which role demands are conflicting, irritating, or impossible to fulfill. It is an additional stressor for nurses and is associated with negative consequences for the individual and the organization (Garrosa et al., 2011). Role stress is particularly acute for new graduates, whose lack of clinical experience and organizational skills, combined with new situations and

procedures, may increase feelings of overwhelming stress. Considering the relationship between burnout and turnover in the general nursing population (see the Research Perspective), high burnout of new graduates is particularly alarming in light of the nursing shortage (Laschinger et al., 2009). Nursing the Future Bridge Clubs are available in almost every province and territory to assist new graduate nurses in fostering new and healthy ways to transition to the role of the professional nurse. These clubs were created with the vision of bringing new graduate nurses together to provide the tools to foster healthy transitions. (http://nursingthefuture.ca/bridge_clubs/bridge_club_info). Role transition is also discussed in Chapter 28.

RESEARCH PERSPECTIVE

Resource: Poghosyan, L., Clarke, S. P., Finlayson, M., et al. (2010). Nurse burnout and quality of care: cross-national investigation in six countries. *Research in Nursing and Health*, 33, 288–298.

This study explored the relationship of quality care and nurse burnout with a sample of 53,846 nurses from Canada, the United States, the United Kingdom, Germany, New Zealand, and Japan. Data were collected over a 6-year period using the Maslach Burnout Inventory and a single item reflecting nurse-rated quality of care. Higher levels of nurse burnout were associated with lower quality of care. However, the cross-sectional design and absence of data on processes of care preclude causal interpretations.

Implications for Practice
Reducing nurse burnout is an effective intervention for improving quality of care in hospitals and must be addressed.

Gender Roles

Approximately 92% of the nation's over 300,000 nurses are female (Canadian Nurses Association [CNA], 2017b), and many go home to what are viewed to be traditionally gender-related responsibilities that may include household management, care of children, and aging parents. These additional responsibilities often contribute to the level of stress felt by the nurse. In recent years, a greater emphasis on how work–life balance is defined and can be achieved has become increasingly part of discussions in nursing. Newer generations of professional nurses are more actively advocating for their needs including recognition, flexible work schedules, stability, adequate supervision, and opportunities for professional development (Lavoie-Tremblay et al., 2010).

Internal Sources

Personal stress "triggers" are events or situations that have an effect on specific individuals. A personal trigger might be a specific event, such as the death of a loved one, an automobile accident, losing a job, or getting married. These events are in addition to daily personal stressors, such as working in a noisy environment, job dissatisfaction, or a difficult commute to work. Negative self-talk, pessimistic thinking, self-criticism, and overanalyzing can be significant ongoing stressors. These internal sources of stress may stem, for example, from unrealistic self-beliefs, from having unrealistic expectations, taking things personally, engaging in all-or-nothing thinking, exaggerating, or rigid thinking, perfectionism, or being overly concerned with small details or control of situations (Moustaka & Constantinisis, 2010).

As mentioned earlier in the chapter, an individual's ability to cope with stress has been shown to be influenced by hardiness. Hardiness relates to both attitudes and strategies that facilitate turning stressful situations from potential disasters into opportunities for growth (Maddi, 2013). Whether you are a nurse manager or a staff nurse in the community, long-term care, or acute care setting, strategies and attitudes demonstrating hardiness are invaluable for managing stress in the health care environment. According to Maddi (2013), the three attitudes of hardiness are commitment, control, and challenge. *Commitment* keeps you involved and leads you to make your best effort; when you exert *control*, you see yourself in charge rather than passive; and if you consider change to be a regular part of life, you see it simply as a *challenge* (Bold, 2010).

Lifestyle choices, such as the excessive consumption of caffeine, lack of exercise, poor diet, inadequate sleep and leisure time, and cigarette smoking, may have a direct effect on the individual stress response. In some cases, recognizing that much of the stress an individual has may be self-generated is one step to addressing it and moving toward positive change.

Dynamics of Stress

Stress may result from unrealistic or conflicting expectations, the pace and magnitude of change, human behaviour, individual personality characteristics, the characteristics of the position itself, or the culture of the organization. Other stressors may be unique to certain environments, situations, and persons or groups. Initially, increased stress produces increased performance. However, when stress continues to increase or remains intense, performance decreases. Selye's (1956, 1965) investigations

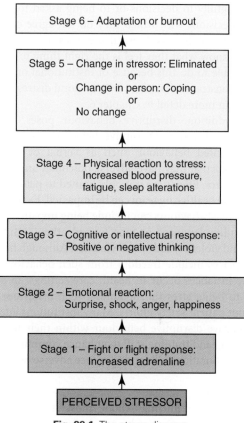

Fig. 29.1 The stress diagram.

of the nature of, and reactions to stress have been very influential in the study of stress. He described the concept of stress and developed the **general adaptation syndrome (GAS)**, which is a theory detailing a predictable multistage response to stress (Fig. 29.1).

More recent investigations of the relationship among the brain, the immune system, and health (psychoneuroimmunology) have generated models that challenge Selye's general adaptation syndrome. Although Selye stated that all people respond with a similar set of hormonal and immune responses to any stress, studies using a response-based orientation indicate that stress is stimulus- and situation-specific, and depends on the individual (Rice, 2013). For example, Roy's (2008) adaptation model is a nursing model that uses stress and stressors as its theoretical underpinning. Roy defines a person as an open, adaptive system constantly interacting with the environment and using coping skills to deal with stressors. Unlike Selye's GAS, Roy's model suggests that each person's ability to deal with stress varies and depends on individual adaptive capacity (Roy, 2008).

TABLE 29.1 Signs of Overstress in Individuals

Physical	Mental	Spiritual/Emotional

• Physical signs of ill health:
 • Increases in flu, colds, accidents
 • Changes in sleeping habits
 • Fatigue
 • Chronic signs of decreased ability to manage stress:
   • Headaches
   • Hypertension
   • Backaches
   • Gastrointestinal problems
 • Unhealthy coping activities:
   • Increased use of substances, such as alcohol or drugs
   • Weight gain or loss
   • Smoking
   • Crying, yelling, blaming
	• Dread going to work every day
	 • Rigid thinking and a desire to go by all the rules in all cases; inability to tolerate any changes
	 • Forgetfulness and anxiety about work to be done; more frequent errors and incidents
	 • Returning home exhausted and unable to participate in enjoyable activities
	 • Confusion about duties and roles
	 • Generalized anxiety
	 • Decrease in concentration
	 • Depression
	 • Anger, irritability, impatience
		• Sense of being a failure; disappointed in work performance
		 • Anger and resentment toward patients, colleagues, and managers
		 • An overall irritable attitude
		 • Lack of positive feelings toward others
		 • Cynicism toward others
		 • Excessive worry, insecurity, lowered self-esteem
		 • Increased family and friend conflict

Critical of stress research using predominantly (83%) male subjects, both human and animal, Taylor et al. (2000) proposed a model of the female stress response, the "tend and befriend," as opposed to the male's "fight or flight" model. The "tend and befriend" response is an estrogen and oxytocin–mediated stress response that is characterized by caring for offspring and befriending those around in times of stress to increase chances of survival (Post, 2010). Women may more often reach out to others during times of stress, whereas men may tend to isolate themselves (Post, 2010). With higher numbers of females in nursing overall, this model may be helpful to understanding some elements of the stress responses nurses tend to experience in health care environments.

Most nurses can easily recognize the origins of stress and its symptoms. For example, a health care employer may make demands on nurses, such as excessive work, that the nurses regard as beyond their capacity to perform. When they are unable to resolve the problem through overwork, with more staff, or by looking at the situation in another way, the nurses may feel threatened or depressed. They may also experience headaches, fatigue, or other physical symptoms. If the stress persists, such symptoms may increase; nurses may attempt to cope by becoming apathetic or by resigning their positions. Table 29.1 outlines physical, mental, and spiritual/emotional signs of overstress in individuals.

There are many physical illnesses that are linked to stress. Studies have found that work-related stressors can lead to migraines, muscle, joint and back pain, hypertension, irritable bowel syndrome, ulcer formation, and immune and endocrine illnesses (Sarafis et al., 2016). In addition, stress can lead to severe life-threatening illnesses, such as heart disease, tachycardias, heart attacks, kidney disease, and cancer (Sarafis et al., 2016).

EXERCISE 29.1 Think back to a particularly stressful time or event in your life. Reflect on how you felt, physically and emotionally? Did you experience any physical symptoms related to unresolved stress? What were some strategies you used to manage the stress, and how well did they work?

Faced with a similarly stressful situation today, would you do anything differently?

STRESS MANAGEMENT

Individuals respond to stress by eliciting coping strategies that are a means of dealing with stress to maintain or achieve well-being. These strategies may be ineffective because of their reliance on methods, such as withdrawal or substance abuse, or they may be effective in helping restore a greater sense of well-being and effectiveness. Some effective strategies are discussed in more detail subsequently.

Stress Prevention

One effective way to deal with stress is to determine and manage its source. Discovering the origin of stress in patient care may be difficult because some environments change so rapidly that the nursing staff are overwhelmed trying to balance bureaucratic rules and limited resources with the demands of vulnerable human beings. When in distress, nurses may need to step back and take time to look at the "big picture." By identifying daily stressors, the nurse can then develop a plan of action for management of the associated stress. This plan may include elimination of the stressor, modification of the stressor, or changing the perception of the stressor using a reframing technique (e.g., viewing mistakes as opportunities for new learning).

The theory of preventive stress management, discussed in Box 29.1, can be used to assess stressors in your nursing practice.

Considering the critical nature of nursing work and the potential for serious injury to others, many of the day-to-day activities of nursing can create workplace stress. Given the stressful nature of nursing, it is wise for the nurse to be alert to signs of stress and to develop lifestyle habits that help reduce stress. Ensuring adequate sleep, eating a balanced diet, engaging in regular exercise, and finding time for family and friends are good stress-buffering habits to develop.

Shirey et al. (2010) studied nurse manager stress and coping experiences using a qualitative methodology with a sample of 21 nurse managers. Their findings suggested that addressing stress, coping, and the complexity of the nurse manager role requires individual and health system strategies. Individual factors (nurse experience), organizational context (organizational culture), and structural elements and systems (span of control, co-manager model, director of nursing empowerment) all influence nurse managers' perceptions of stress and their coping experiences. Minimizing stress for nurse managers can enhance their coping experiences, facilitate good decision making, and improve engagement and retention of nurse managers and staff nurses (Shirey et al., 2010).

LaMontagne and colleagues (2007) reviewed 90 reports on job-stress interventions between 1990 and 2005 and found that they could be divided into three levels of preventive stress management. Primary interventions included techniques for directly managing or changing the stressor; secondary interventions included actions designed to improve individual stress responses (e.g., those that improve individual coping); and tertiary interventions included actions aimed at treating the symptoms of distress (e.g., employee assistance programs [EAPs]). It is important to be aware of the stress that you experience and how you typically manage it. Although dated, this work remains relevant in current context. Analyze your stress experiences by completing Exercise 29.2.

BOX 29.1   Theory of Preventive Stress Management

The theory of preventive stress management (TPSM) is a macro-level theory that is not discipline specific and helps explain or conceptualize potential relationships between stressors, stress responses, and outcomes of stress (Hargrove et al., 2011). In an organization, the stress cycle begins with stressors, moves to the stress response, and then to the outcomes. Stressors can be environmental or self-imposed. The stress response is activated when an individual is exposed to stressors. In terms of outcomes, positive stress responses can lead to eustress, whereas negative stress responses can lead to distress. The stages of an individual's response to stress are illustrated in Fig. 29.1. Stress can originate from role factors, job stressors, and interpersonal demands (Hargrove et al., 2011). The TPSM includes three stages (primary, secondary, and tertiary) to help reduce stressors, moderate the stress response, and reduce the negative impact of distress (Hargrove et al., 2011). Nurse leaders have a responsibility to create and maintain healthy organizations in which nurses can thrive. Good leaders know how to minimize the negative impact of distress and maximize the positive impact of eustress.

Hargrove, M.B., Quick, J.C., Nelson, D.L., et al. (2011). The theory of preventative stress management: a 33-year review and evaluation. *Stress and Health*, 27, 182–193.

EXERCISE 29.2 Identify the stress you most commonly experience and how you usually manage it. Create and complete a reflection at the end of each shift, whether it be a volunteer opportunity, clinical placement, or employment setting. In the reflective exercise, include the date, situation, your response, how you dealt with your response, and the evaluation of the situation. Ask yourself if the stress was good stress (eustress) or bad stress (distress). Review your reflection and note what stressors (e.g., people, technology, values conflict) were the most common. Do you encounter some on a regular basis? If so, try to formulate a plan to conquer the problems. You may need to role play or get continuing education to improve a specific skill. You may need to simply break a task down into smaller pieces or to eliminate interruptions.

Through this exercise, try to identify how you most often react to stress: physically, mentally, or emotionally. Then consider positive strategies that could be used to deal with a similar situation in the future.

Symptom Management

Unpredictable and uncontrollable change, coupled with immense responsibility and little control over the work environment, produces stress for nurses and other health care providers. Consequently, nurses may develop emotional symptoms, such as anxiety, depression, or anger; physical alterations, such as fatigue, headache, and insomnia; mental changes, such as a decrease in concentration and memory; and behavioural changes, such as smoking, drinking, crying, and swearing. The important factor is not the stressor but, rather, how the individual perceives the stressor and what coping mechanisms are available to mediate the hormonal response to the stressor.

Change is inevitable and permeates all areas of health care, sometimes on a daily basis. Knowing how you react to change and how you cope during periods of change can help you build a repertoire of strategies that you can easily apply to reduce your stress during times of change. Exercise 29.3 offers a personal analysis of change.

EXERCISE 29.3 This personal analysis of change exercise can be used when you are considering pursuing a personal or professional change. It helps you analyze your reaction to the planned change.

1. Write down the objective of the change that you want to make.
2. Objectively document the change that you want to pursue, including where the change will happen, when it will happen, and what you have to do to make it happen. Be specific; you have to be able to evaluate the change, so its factors need to be measurable.
3. Write a statement on how confident you are that you will achieve the planned change (on a scale of 1 to 10, with 1 being no confidence and 10 being complete confidence).

As you begin to work toward or implement the change, keep a log of your stress levels in relation to the change. Record any stress-reducing behaviours you engage in to reduce your stress level, including how much your stress level changed afterward. After you complete the change, analyze your log of stress-reducing behaviours and note those that most effectively reduced your stress level.

Multiple "stress-buffering" behaviours can be elicited to reduce the detrimental effects of stress.

The stressor-induced changes in the hormonal and immune systems can be modulated by an individual's behavioural coping response (the immediate response of a person to a threatening situation). Coping responses include leisure activities and taking time for self, decreasing or discontinuing the use of caffeine, positive social support, a strong belief system, a sense of humour, developing realistic expectations, reframing events, regular aerobic exercise, meditation, and use of the relaxation response.

Everyone needs to balance work and leisure in everyday life. Leisure time and stress are inversely proportional. If the time for work is more than 60% of the time awake or if self-time is less than 10% of the time awake, stress levels will increase. Changes should be made to relieve stress, such as decreasing the number of work hours or finding more time for leisure activities. Caffeine is a strong stimulant and, in itself, a stressor. Slowly weaning off caffeine should result in better sleep and more energy. Positive social support can offer validation, encouragement, or advice. By discussing situations with others, one can reduce stress. A great deal of stress may come from our belief systems, which cause stress in two ways. First, behaviours result from them, such as placing work before pleasure. Second, beliefs may also conflict with those of other people, as may happen with patients from different cultures. Articulating beliefs and finding common ground will help reduce anger and stress. Humour is a great stress reducer and laughter a great tension reducer. A common source of stress is unrealistic expectations. Realistic expectations can make life feel more predictable and more manageable. *Reframing* is changing the way you look at things to make you feel better about them or to obtain a different perspective. Recognizing that there are many ways to interpret the same situation, taking the positive view is less stressful. Regular aerobic exercise is a logical method of dissipating the excess energy generated by the stress response.

Mindfulness is a useful strategy for nurses or nursing students to incorporate into their practice and involves being present through a mind-body based approach that helps change the way nurses think and feel about their experiences. Mindfulness is becoming more recognized, and there is increasing exploration of how the practice of mindfulness, along with compassion, can benefit nurses (Brass, 2016). There is a growing body of literature supporting the practice of mindfulness meditation, claiming that it has the potential to reduce stress, anxiety, and burnout, and enhance emotional resilience (Van der Riet et al., 2018).

Meditation to elicit the relaxation response can be beneficial. The benefits of practicing relaxation techniques for up to 20 minutes daily include a feeling of well-being, the ability to learn how tension makes the body feel, and the sense that tension can be controlled. Exercise 29.4 outlines one systematic relaxation technique.

EXERCISE 29.4 This exercise can be used in the middle of a working day, the last thing at night, or at any time you feel tense or anxious. Review the information and strategies of "Meditation: a simple, fast way to reduce stress" at the Mayo Clinic website: http://www.mayoclinic.org/meditation/ART-20045858. Make a short list of steps to take, and put it in your smart phone, personal digital assistant (PDA), or notepad. An alternative exercise to practice mindfulness meditation. This exercise can help put space between your day and how you are reacting to it. Review the information, strategies and practice exercises at the Mindful website: https://www.mindful.org/meditation/mindfulness-getting-started/

Applebaum and colleagues (2010) found a direct relationship between perceived stress and turnover intention. The results of their study indicated that it may not be the stress itself but the physical consequences of stress (missing lunch breaks, physical symptoms, excessive overtime) that cause nurses to leave their job. Similarly, Blake and Robbins (2013) found that a healthy work environment can improve not only patient outcomes but also registered nurse turnover and retention.

Social support in the form of positive work relationships may be an important way to buffer distress and provide a life-enhancing social network ("Understanding the stress," 2011). Although colleagues may form friendships, the workload and the shifting of staff from one unit to another often make it difficult to establish and maintain close relationships with peers. It can also be challenging for the new graduate nurse to develop good working relationships, and therefore effective mentorship is important, along with supportive management. A thorough orientation process provides positive first impressions and assists in the development of good working relationships while decreasing the new nurses' anxiety. When building relationships, it is important to be positive, manage boundaries, avoid gossiping, and continually develop people skills (see Research Perspective later). Nurses in a new position or in an unfamiliar geographic area must anticipate that they will benefit from the security of being part of a group that can furnish emotional support. Without easily accessible family and friends, nurses need to be intentional about seeking new, supportive personal relationships. Positive coping strategies may also make nurses less likely to adopt potentially negative coping strategies, such as withdrawing, lowering their standards of care, and abusing alcohol or other substances.

RESEARCH PERSPECTIVE

Resource: Zangaro, G. A., & Soeken, K. L. (2007). A meta-analysis of studies of nurses' job satisfaction. *Research in Nursing & Health*, 30, 445–458.

This study looked at the strength of the relationship between job satisfaction, autonomy, stress, and collaboration in 31 studies that included 14,567 subjects. Although the findings varied, job satisfaction correlated most strongly with job stress, followed by collaboration and autonomy. These findings have important implications for improving nurses' work environment and although somewhat outdated, this research is still relevant in the current context.

Implications for Practice
Given the current nursing shortage, nurse job satisfaction and employee retention are very important to current health care industry demands for safe, effective, patient-centred, timely, efficient, and equitable care. Nurses and nurse managers in all settings are faced with resource constraints. Identifying and validating nurse perceptions about stress, collaboration, and autonomy facilitate accurate assessment and effective management of staff, turnover rates, and performance.

Burnout

Sometimes individuals cannot manage stress successfully through their own efforts and require assistance. Examples of behaviour related to stress that feels overwhelming appear in Table 29.1. Coping strategies, such as those described previously, may furnish temporary relief or none at all. With this level of distress, one can feel overwhelmed or helpless and may be at a greater risk for mental or physical illness. This constellation of emotions is commonly called *burnout.*

A classic definition of burnout is a "prolonged response to chronic emotional and interpersonal stressors on the job" (Maslach et al., 2000, p. 398). The term "burnout" was first coined in the 1970s by Herbert Freudenberger, an American psychologist who used the term to describe the consequences of severe stress among doctors and nurses. The sources of the stressors may exist in the environment, in the individual, or in the interaction between the individual and the environment. Some stressors, such as employment termination, appear to be universal, whereas other stressors, such as meeting deadlines, are more personal. For example, some nurses thrive on goals and timetables, whereas others feel constrained and frustrated and thereby experience distress. Burnout is not an objective phenomenon as if it were the accumulation of a certain number and type of stressors. How the stressors are perceived and how they are mediated by an individual's ability to adapt are important variables in determining levels of distress.

People's psychologic relationships to their jobs can be considered as a continuum between burnout (negative experience) and job engagement (positive experience). The three interrelated dimensions of this continuum are exhaustion–energy, cynicism–involvement, and inefficacy–efficacy (Maslach & Leiter, 2008). The exhaustion–energy dimension represents the basic individual strain of burnout, including feelings of being overextended and worn out. The cynicism–involvement dimension represents the interpersonal context of burnout, including negative, callous, or excessively detached responses to various aspects of the job. The inefficacy–efficacy dimension represents the self-evaluation component of burnout, including feelings of incompetence and a lack of achievement and productivity in work. The significance of this model is that it clearly places an individual's experience of strain within the social context of the workplace. Research on burnout uses the Maslach Burnout Inventory (Maslach & Jackson, 1981) to assess these three dimensions. Recent research has also turned to an examination of the positive opposite of the three dimensions, or job engagement (Maslach & Leiter, 2008).

New Graduate Nurse Stress

New graduates entering the health care system face many challenges transitioning from the student role to the professional nurse role. Role transition is discussed further in Chapter 28. The influence of the hospital work environments on newly licensed registered nurses' commitment to nursing and intent to leave nursing has been deemed to be important (Unruh & Zhang, 2013). Negative perceptions of the work environment were strong predictors of an intent to leave nursing and that retention of newly licensed registered nurses can be improved through changes in the work environment that seek to reduce stress (Unruh & Zhang, 2013). In another study, 30% of new graduates reported intentions of leaving the profession, mainly as a result of the work environment (Beecroft at al., 2008). When the work environment is positive and offers empowerment, registered nurses are less likely to experience burnout and, therefore more likely to remain in nursing (Wang et al., 2013). It has also been suggested that personal and organizational resources could play a role in protecting new graduate nurses (Spence Laschinger & Fida, 2014). Interventions related to psychologic capital included building self-efficacy, hope, optimism, and resiliency. New graduate nurse transition experience is a key consideration when considering retention and related effective interventions include advocating for effective orientation programs and mentorship opportunities. Being assigned appropriate workloads is also an important factor and has a significant impact on new nurse graduate stress. A supportive environment that fosters growth and development is instrumental at retaining new nurses and decreases the amount of stress that a new nurse has when transitioning into a new role. Given the ongoing nursing shortage in Canada, nurse leaders need to ensure that nursing professional practice environments foster high-quality collegial working relationships to enhance the retention of new graduates.

RESOLUTION OF STRESS

Resolution of stress in its early stages can be accomplished through a variety of techniques. Nurses must be

TABLE 29.2	**Stress-Management Strategies**	
Physical	**Mental**	**Emotional/Spiritual**
• Accept physical limitations • Modify nutrition: moderate carbo-hydrate and protein, high fruits and vegetables, low caffeine and sugar • Exercise: an enjoyable activity 5 times a week for 30 minutes • Make your physical health a priority • Nurture yourself: take time for breaks and lunch • Sleep: get enough in quantity and quality • Relax: use meditation, massage, or yoga	• Learn to say "no"! • Use cognitive restructuring and self-talk • Use imagery • Develop hobbies or activities • Plan vacations • Learn about the system and how problems are handled • Learn communication, conflict resolution, and time-management skills • Take continuing education courses • Learn to delegate	• Use mindfulness and meditation • Seek solace in prayer • Seek professional counselling • Participate in support groups • Participate in networking • Communicate feelings • Identify and acquire a mentor • Ask for feedback and clarification

able to reach a balance of caring for others and caring for self. Table 29.2 summarizes physical, mental, and emotional/spiritual strategies.

Social Support

Peers, and close colleagues can be supportive and help reduce stress by assisting with problem solving and by developing new perspectives. Family, friends, and those in one's social network can provide a safe haven and a "vacation" from sources of stress. Social isolation can, for some people, increase or sustain stress. Social support may allow one to be more playful, to have fun, to laugh, and to vent emotions.

Counselling

Persistent unpleasant feelings, problem behaviour, and helplessness during prolonged stress may suggest the need for assistance from a mental health professional. Examples of problem behaviours include tearfulness or angry outbursts over seemingly minor incidents, major changes in eating or sleeping patterns, frequent unwillingness to go to work, and substance use or abuse. In such cases, the aforementioned coping strategies afford only temporary relief; nurses with this level of distress feel overwhelmed and believe that their well-being cannot be maintained. In these stressful situations, nurses may feel helpless and require professional assistance from an advanced practice psychiatric nurse, clinical psychologist, psychiatrist, or other mental health worker.

In some organizations, EAPs provide free, voluntary, confidential, short-term professional counselling and other services for employees either via in-house staff or by contract with a mental health counsellor. This type of counselling can be effective because the counsellors may already be aware of organizational stressors. Some nurses may have confidentiality concerns when using employer-recommended or employer-provided counselling services. Mental health professionals are bound by their professional standards of confidentiality. Nonetheless, there may be times when it is in the nurse's best interest to sign a release of information, such as when seeking employer accommodation for a certain physical or emotional problem.

Those who seek counselling outside of the workplace may be guided in their selection of mental health professionals by a personal physician, a knowledgeable colleague, their provincial nursing association or college, or by contacting the Canadian Mental Health Association. When the problem underlying the distress is ethical or moral, a trained pastoral counsellor may be helpful in addition to consulting the Canadian Nurses Association Code of Ethics (CNA, 2017a). When private counselling is being arranged, the extended health coverage should be checked to determine mental health benefits and the payment limitations and types of providers eligible for reimbursement.

Leadership and Management

Although social support and counselling can alter how stressors are perceived, time management and effective leadership can modify or remove stressors. Nurse managers have clearly structured formal authority as individuals in most organizations, and managerial groups may be able to influence policy and resource allocation. Nurse managers and leaders can control some environmental stressors on their units. First, nurse managers can examine their own behaviour as a source of stress for others.

In some cases, a controlling or autocratic style of management is appropriate, such as in emergency situations and when working with a large percentage of new and inexperienced employees. For the most part, however, professional nurses need and want the latitude to direct their activities within their sphere of competence. By delegating work, the nurse leader or manager sends the message that the personal integrity and professional competence of the team is trusted. Delegating does not mean abdicating accountability for achieving accepted standards of patient care and agreed-upon outcomes, but rather acknowledging shared accountability.

Assistance with problem solving is another way to reduce environmental stressors. Nurse leaders and managers may provide advice, refer staff to appropriate resources, or mediate conflicts. Often, nurse leaders and managers enable staff to meet the demands of their work more independently by providing time for continuing education and professional meetings to enhance competence and build capacity.

Another way in which nurse leaders can reduce stress is to be supportive of staff. Support of this kind is not the same as, for example, being a friend but rather, it is characterized by helping one's peers and colleagues provide high quality care, develop professionally, and feel valued personally. Leaders and managers can ensure that the expected workload is aligned with nurses' capabilities and resources. They can work to ensure meaningfulness, stimulation, and opportunities for nurses to use their skills. Nurses' roles and responsibilities need to be clearly and publicly defined. For example, work schedules should be posted as far in advance as possible and should be compatible with what is known about patient safety. Encouraging innovation and experimentation, for example, can motivate staff and give them a sense of greater control over their environment. Affirming a good idea or finding resources to study or implement a promising new procedure or proposal by a staff nurse is supportive. In contrast, when staff members struggle with overwork and other stressors, support can be provided by recognizing the condition and helping the nurses avoid such passive coping strategies as feeling helpless or lowering standards of care in favour of active problem solving. Nurse leaders should be sensitive to the distress of the nursing staff and recognize it verbally without becoming counsellors, which may be in conflict with their role. Support may involve making nursing staff aware of resources that provide counselling while being careful to avoid diagnostic labels and to maintain strict confidentiality. When distress relates to the personal life of subordinates, managers and leaders should focus on the effect of such situations on workplace performance—not solely on the events that have produced the stress.

In addition, leaders can enhance the workplace by dealing effectively with their own stressors. Maintaining a sense of perspective as well as a sense of humour is important. Some stressors, in fact, can be ignored or minimized by posing three questions:

1. "Is this event or situation important?" Stressors are not all equally significant. Try not to spend time and energy on minor stressors.
2. "Does this stressor affect me or my unit?" Although some situations that produce distress are institution-wide and need group action, others target specific units or activities. Try not to borrow stressors.
3. "Can I change this situation?" If not, then find a way to cope with it or, if the situation is intolerable, make plans to change positions or employers. This decision may require gaining added credentials that may produce long-term career benefits.

Keeping stressful situations in perspective can enable nurses to conserve their energies to cope with stressful situations that are important, that are within their domain, or that can be changed or modified. Stress management interventions have been studied in relation to nurse leaders. Findings from a randomized control trial, on the effects of a nurse leader mindfulness meditation course for managing stress, demonstrated preliminary effectiveness in reducing self-reported stress symptoms among nurse leaders (Pipe et al., 2009). There is also evidence to suggest that practicing and cultivating mindfulness can assist nurse leaders to relieve stress and feel more in the moment within the workplace setting (Sherman, 2012).

TIME MANAGEMENT

A very close relationship exists between stress management and time management. Time management is one method of stress prevention or reduction. Stress can decrease productivity and lead to poor use of time. Time management can be considered a preventive action to help reduce the elements of stress in a nurse's life.

Most of us have a version of one of two options or approaches to managing time: be organized or "go with the flow." There are only 24 hours in every day, and it is clear that some people make better use of time than others do. *How* people use time makes some people more successful than others. The effective use of time-management skills thus becomes an even more important tool to achieve personal and professional goals. Time management is the appropriate use of tools, techniques, and principles to control time spent on low-priority needs and to ensure that time is invested in activities leading toward achieving desired, high-priority goals. More simply, time management is the ability to spend your time on the things that matter to you and your organization. That goal may also involve delegation. It is important to keep in mind that planning daily time-management strategies takes time. By setting goals and eliminating time stealers, you will have the extra time to accomplish those goals.

Where Does Your Time Go?

Have you ever wasted time? Time, although a cheap commodity, is our most valuable resource. There are some commonly identified time stealers, and individuals must recognize them to guard against them. At the heart of time management is an important shift in focus. Most agree it is better to try to concentrate on results, rather than simply on being busy.

Doing too Much

Do you try to do too much at once? At work, do you have three or four major projects going simultaneously? Are you a member of more than one organizational committee? Do you have to worry about what will be on the table for dinner while you are hanging an intravenous (IV) and planning a staff meeting? Have you ever completed a nursing intervention and realized that your mind was really somewhere else, and you had ignored the patient? If you *think* you have too much to do, you probably do. The first step to trying to resolve this inevitable situation is to be realistic and limit major commitments, and then try to give each activity your full and undivided attention. Sometimes completing one task before starting another is the most efficient method

for getting everything done. Prioritization of goals and activities each day is not easy, but very helpful.

In the nursing profession, however, limiting commitments is not always possible. When you are feeling overwhelmed by the sheer volume of tasks to be completed, take the time to establish priorities for the shift. Decide what must be done versus what would be nice to do. Try not to let yourself get distracted from your priority tasks. It is acknowledged that nursing is a balancing act and that priorities can be constantly changing.

Inability to Say "No"

Sometimes the smallest and simplest words are the most difficult to learn. If you are suffering from overload, you probably have gotten there by not being able to say "no." Learning to say "no" to requests is difficult, and in the process, others may be displeased. If you do not say "no," however, you may end up spending much time on projects that are uninteresting or have no relationship to your personal goals and priorities. When someone asks you to do something, you need to stop and consider the request. Do you want to do the task now or sometime in the future? If not, then say so. If you wish to do the task but simply do not have the time, consider delegation. However, be honest with the requester—if you simply do not have the time, say so as collegially as possible. If you wish to take on the task but at a later date, negotiate. Remember, accepting an assignment you will never be able to complete will likely reflect negatively on you and may affect collegial work relationships.

Procrastination

Do you put off important tasks because they are not enjoyable or because they may be difficult? Do you find excuses for not starting or completing tasks? Are you a procrastinator? By engaging in procrastination, or doing one thing when you should be doing something else, you give up time to complete your task and therefore limit the quality of the work you produce. There are techniques to help deal with procrastination. First, identify the reason for procrastinating. Then make that task your highest priority the next day. Reward yourself after you finish the task. Another technique is to select the least attractive element of the task to do first, and the rest will seem easier.

Some people find that they procrastinate when the task ahead is significant or overwhelming. One solution is to break the task down into manageable pieces and plan rewards for accomplishing each of the smaller tasks. Developing a *program evaluation and review technique* (PERT) chart or a Gantt chart may help in this process. PERT charts were originally developed as tools to assist in complex projects that require a series of activities, some of which must be performed sequentially and others that can be performed in parallel with other activities. Envisioned as a network diagram, a PERT chart (Fig. 29.2) indicates dependent activities that must be completed before a new activity is undertaken. A Gantt chart (Fig. 29.3) consists of a table of project task information and a bar chart that graphically displays the project schedule. This method of tracking project activities in relation to time is often used in planning and project management. Both chart techniques can be used to outline how you will approach a large project. The PERT chart clearly illustrates task dependencies but can be more difficult to interpret than the Gantt chart.

Complaining

Complaining is the act of expressing dissatisfaction ("Complain," 2004). Often, the time people spend complaining about a task or a particular situation is greater than the time needed to complete the task or to deal

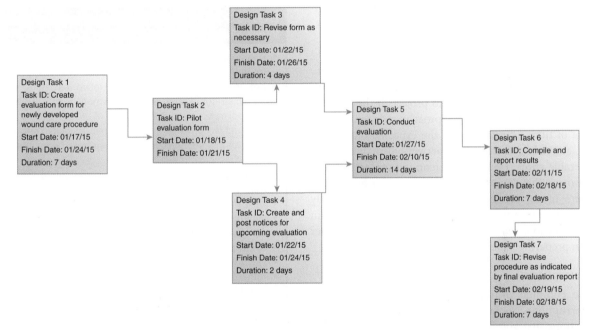

Fig. 29.2 A sample PERT chart.

TASK	ACCOUNTABILITY	JAN	FEB	MAR	APR	MAY	JUNE
1. Conduct literature search	Unit clinical nurse specialist	———————	→				
2. Hold nursing practice committee meeting to review material	Chair, nursing practice committee		X				
3. Create a report for the medical staff	Chair, nursing practice committee			———————	→		
4. Disseminate findings to nursing and medical staff	Chair, nursing practice committee					———————	→

Fig. 29.3 A sample Gantt chart.

with the issue. If you find yourself complaining repeatedly about something, stop and ask yourself what the ideal solution would be and then take the risk to act on it. If the complaint is related to another person, either take the time to talk with the person and get the problem out in the open or write a letter to the person discussing your point of view (even if you do not mail it). If you find yourself complaining about something within the workplace, rethink the problem, generate some possible solutions, and then talk to your manager. Look for solutions that are simple or that may be "outside the box." Talk to your manager and be prepared to discuss solutions, not simply your dissatisfaction or annoyance. In this way, your manager will see you as interested in contributing to the goals of the organization.

Perfectionism

Perfectionism is the uncompromising pursuit of perfection ("Perfectionism," 2004). Some perfectionists have a hard time completing tasks and projects if they are not yet perfect. A perfectionist approach tends to consume a lot of time, especially when the expected outcome is not attainable. Overcoming perfectionism takes considerable effort. However, overcoming perfection does not mean that you should do less than your best. Being aware of perfectionism means that you occasionally need to give yourself permission to do slightly less than a perfect job, such as buying a takeout dinner rather than preparing a four-course meal after a day at work.

Interruptions

One common distraction from priority activities is interruptions. Some interruptions are integral to the positions that you hold, but others can be controlled. A home care nurse with a large caseload can expect to be paged at any time. More commonly, however, are the numerous small interruptions by individuals who want just a "minute of your time" and take 10 minutes getting to the point. Box 29.2 identifies some strategies to prevent and control interruptions. The two keys to dealing with interruptions are to resume "doing it now" so that an interruption does not destroy your schedule, and to maintain the attitude that whatever the interruption, it is a part of your responsibility. When you make a conscious decision not to worry about the things you cannot control, you have more energy to maintain a positive perspective and to move projects forward.

EXERCISE 29.5 Think of an example of a clinical situation in which an unexpected interruption or distraction in the workplace would affect the quality of care a nurse is providing (e.g., an emergency with another patient, a cancelled or unscheduled patient procedure, or an unexpected absence leaving the nursing unit suddenly short-staffed). Describe how you would respond to being in this type of situation. Reflect on how this could affect the work environment and patient experiences. How could the use of mindfulness benefit you in a situation like this?

BOX 29.2 Tips to Avoid Interruptions and Work More Effectively

- Ask people to put their comments in writing—do not let them catch you "on the run."
- Let the office or unit administrative assistant or administrator know what information you need immediately.
- Conduct a conversation in the hall to help keep it short or in a separate room to keep from being interrupted.
- Do paper work away from your computer to maximize time spent on task.
- Be comfortable saying "no."
- When involved in a long procedure or home visit, ask someone else to cover your other responsibilities.
- Break projects into small, manageable pieces.
- Get yourself organized.
- Minimize interruptions—for example, allow voice mail to pick up the phone or shut the door.
- Set a specific time each day to read and respond to e-mails.
- Keep your work surface clear. Have available only those documents needed for the task at hand.
- Keep your manager informed of your goals.
- Plan to accomplish high-priority or difficult tasks early in the day.
- Develop a plan for the day and stick to it. Remember to schedule in some time for interruptions.
- Schedule time to meet regularly throughout the shift with staff members for whom you are responsible.
- Recognize that crises and interruptions are part of the position.
- Be cognizant of your personal time-waster habits and try to avoid them.

Disorganization

One of the most serious time wasters of all is disorganization. Organization can be a great time saver. Remember that the guiding principle is that organization is a process rather than the product. You can spend so much time organizing that you will never get to the task at hand (procrastination). Organization can be a challenge for new graduate nurses and seasoned nurses in a new environment and for anyone whose environment or work situation is constantly changing. Commonly cited organizing guidelines and tips include eliminating clutter, keeping everything in its place, and doing similar tasks together. With that in mind, however, there are also claims that those in disorderly environments (e.g., working in a messy office) were more likely to be able to think creatively and produce stimulating new ideas as compared with those in more orderly environments (Vohs et al., 2013).

Too Much Information

The newest time waster to evolve is data proliferation. The technology within our workplace forces us to receive huge amounts of data and to transform these data into useful information. The computer workstation, once touted as a time-saving device, has become the driving force behind care delivery. Nurses can view the computer either as a stress-producing slave driver or as a simple tool to assist them in their daily activities.

Information overload, or "data smog," is a state of stress brought about by the reception of too much information, too fast, and too often and not having adequate information-processing skills. Information literacy is a self-directed independent ability to access information efficiently and evaluate its quality, as well as manage and organize the information, while understanding the implications of doing so (Belcik, 2007). In the information age, information literacy skills are imperative for reducing stress and improving productivity (Badke, 2010). Gaining a new appreciation of information is important. Information is simply a tool to use to plan action or make decisions. By learning what information is important, you can learn to use it to your advantage.

Time-Management Concepts

Table 29.3 presents a classification scheme for time-management techniques. The unifying theme is that each activity undertaken should lead to goal attainment and that goal should be the number-one priority at that time.

Goal Setting and Plan Development

The first steps in time management are goal setting and developing a plan to reach those goals. Set goals that are reasonable and achievable. Do not expect to reach long-term goals overnight—*long term* means just that. Give yourself time to meet the goals. Determine many short-term goals to reach the long-term goal, giving you a frequent sense of goal achievement. Give yourself flexibility. If the path you chose last year is no longer appropriate, change it. Write your goals, date the entry, keep it handy, and refer to it often to give yourself a progress report.

Setting Priorities

Once the goals are known, priorities are set. They may, however, shift throughout a given period in terms of goal attainment. For example, working on a budget may take precedence at certain times of the year, whereas new staff orientation is a high priority at other times.

TABLE 29.3	Classification of Time-Management Techniques	
Technique	**Purpose**	**Actions**
Organization	Designed to promote efficiency and productivity	Organize and systematize things, tasks, and people. Use basic time-management skills.
Keep focused on goals	Focuses on goal achievement	Assemble a prioritized "to do" list daily, based on goals.
Tool usage	Uses the right tool for planning and preparation	Use tools, such as a smart phone. Use organizational tools to organize patient load and tasks
Time-management plan	Helps to refocus, to gain control, and to use information	Develop a personal time-management plan appropriately.

Knowing what your goals and priorities are helps shape the "to do" list. In any nursing work setting, you must be aware of your personal goals and current priorities. How you organize work may depend on other things as well, such as geographic considerations, patient acuity, or other priorities.

A particular strategy to assist in prioritization suggests that people generally focus on those things that are important and urgent. By placing the elements of importance and urgency in a grid (Fig. 29.4), all activities can be classified as shown (Covey et al., 1994).

Typically, we tend to focus on those items in cell A because they are both important and urgent and therefore command our attention. Making shift assignments is an A task because it is an important and urgent part of allocating work in a manner that is fair and practical, while also matching patients to staffing competencies to ensure safe and effective patient care. Conversely, if something is neither important nor urgent (cell D), it may be considered a waste of time, at least in terms of personal goals. An example of a D activity might be reading "junk" e-mail. Even if something is urgent but not important (cell C), it contributes minimally to productivity and goal achievement. An example of a C activity might be responding to a memo that has a specific time line but is not important to goal attainment. The real key to setting priorities is to attend to the B tasks, those that are important but not urgent. Examples of B activities are reviewing the organization's strategic plan or participating on organizational committees.

Organization

A number of simple routines for organization can save many minutes over a day and enhance your efficiency. Organization can be a challenge for new nurse graduates as nursing is no longer the task-orientated profession it once was. Organizational skills take time to develop and thinking, whereas acting can pose a challenge to many new graduates. Time management and organization takes time to develop and requires practice and skill. A new nurse can start focusing on organization skills,

while in school, before entering a clinical placement setting. Keeping a workspace neat or arranging things in an orderly fashion may be a powerful time-management tool. Rather than a system of "pile management," use "file management." Keep in mind the following organizing tips:

- Plan where things should go: your desk or your flash drive.
- Keep a clean workspace.
- Create a "to do" folder.
- Create a "to be filed" folder for any papers.
- Schedule time to work your way through the folders.
- Determine your priority goals for the next day and have the materials ready to work on when you start the next morning.

Time Tools

Sometimes, the real problem is that the events of the day become the driving force, rather than a planned schedule. Days may become so tightly scheduled that any little interruption can become a crisis. If you do not plan the day, you may be responding to events rather than prioritized goals. If you think you are a reactor rather than a proactive time user, use a time log to list work-related activities for several days. You may not be able to plan well because you really do not have a good estimate of how long a particular activity actually takes or you do not know how many activities can be accomplished in a given time frame.

As the nurse's role in care management becomes more complex, the need for organizational tools increases. Tracking the care of groups of patients, either as the member of a care team or in a leadership capacity, can be overwhelming. Each nurse should devise a method for tracking care and organizing time, as well as delegating and monitoring care provided by others. Although some nurses depend on a shift flowsheet or a Kardex system, others have the benefit of computerized information tracking systems. Handheld computer devices, such as PDAs, smartphones, or barcode scanners for medication administration serve as methods to track information and increase safety and efficiency. However, the issue of patient confidentiality cannot be ignored when entering data into a mobile device that you take home at the end of your shift. Chapter 7 provides further discussion about how technologies are used in the health care environment.

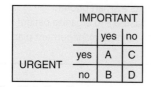

Fig. 29.4 Classification of priorities.

Managing Information

The first step in managing information is to critically assess the source. Once you have identified the sources of your data, you have a better idea of how to deal with the information and whether the information is trustworthy.

By developing information-receiving skills, you can quickly interpret the data and convert them to useful information, discarding unneeded data. Initially, you should reduce or eliminate that which is useless. Delete the e-mail, or toss the memo in the garbage. Next, monitor the information flow and decide what to do with incoming data. Find and focus on the most important pieces, and then quickly narrow down the specific details you need. Identify resources that are most helpful, and have them readily available. Be able to build the "big picture" from the masses of data you receive. Finally, recognize when you have enough information to act.

Once you have mastered the receiving end of information, concentrate on information-sending skills. Remember, information you receive is simply another person's data. Try to keep your outflow short; make it a synthesis of the information. Finally, select the most appropriate mode of communication for your message from the technology available. You may be sending your information in written (memo or report) or verbal (face-to-face or presentation) form or via telephone, voice mail, e-mail, text, Twitter, or fax. Remember, the most important skill is to know when you have said enough. Exercise 29.6 will help you consider how you have dealt with information.

> **EXERCISE 29.6** Think of the last time you were in a clinical area. How often did you record the same piece of data (e.g., a finding in your assessment of the patient)? Remember to include all steps, from your jotting down notes on a piece of paper or entering data into the computer to the final report of the day. What information-processing tools could help to decrease the number of steps?

Delegating

Delegation involves achieving performance of care outcomes for which you are accountable and responsible by sharing activities with other individuals who have the appropriate authority to accomplish the work. It is a critical component of self-management for nurse managers and care managers. Appropriate delegation not only increases time efficiency but also serves as a means

of reducing stress. Delegation is discussed in depth in Chapter 27, but it is also appropriate to discuss it briefly as a time-management strategy. Delegation works only when the delegator trusts the delegatee to accomplish the task and to report findings back to the delegator. The delegator wastes time if he or she checks and redoes everything someone else has done. Delegation requires empowerment of the delegatee to accomplish the task. If the nurse does not delegate appropriately, with clear expectations, the delegatee will constantly ask for assistance or direction. Delegation can be a means of reducing stress if used appropriately. However, if the nurse does not understand delegation and does not use it appropriately, it can be a major source of stress as the nurse assumes accountability and responsibility for care administered by others.

MEETING MANAGEMENT

Meeting management is a key time-management strategy. Even nurses who may not have extensive management responsibilities can benefit from learning to make the most of meetings, either as the leader or a group member. Often, students are placed into groups to complete projects, and these groups require ongoing meetings and management. It is recommended that there be clear roles within the group to manage important tasks and achieve outcomes, for example, a group leader or facilitator, a note taker, and a time keeper.

Managing Meetings

Meetings serve various purposes, ranging from creating social networks to setting formal policy. Wodak and colleagues (2011) investigated the impact of leaders' communication strategies on the consensus-building process in meetings. They identified five discursive strategies that meeting chairs employed to drive decision making: bonding, encouraging, directing, modulating, and recommitting. During bonding, the leader uses the term *we* rather than *I* to cultivate group identity and promote consensus and shared decision making. Encouraging stimulates the participation of members to explore new ideas and develop synthesis with existing ideas related to the current topic. Directing occurs after encouraging and is used to bring about closure and resolution by reducing the equivocality of ideas that have been discussed. Modulating allows the leader to achieve a balance between encouraging and directing. Lastly, recommitting moves the group from a consensual understanding of the issue toward a commitment to action (Wodak et al., 2011). Critical findings from this research indicate that the meeting chair influences the outcome of the meetings in both negative and positive ways and that the specific meeting context mediates participation and the ability of the chair to control interactions within the committee (Wodak et al., 2011). Nurse leaders who embrace these techniques can make meetings more productive with tangible outcomes, leaving all members feeling a sense of empowerment and accomplishment. This can also be true for nursing students working in a group setting while attempting to achieve a similar goal. Group meetings need to be productive to be able to meet the desired outcomes.

Tips for Managing Meetings Effectively

Consider if the meeting is necessary. For example, a phone call, posted notice, e-mail, or brief "huddle" (a short, check-in meeting) might suffice. If the right people are not available, rescheduling may be a good option.

Scheduling meetings right before lunch or at the end of the day might mean that participants will have an incentive to stick to the schedule. Set a start time and a stop time, and always aim to start on schedule. Avoid meetings lasting longer than necessary. Select an appropriate setting in which the participants are not readily accessible to interruptions. If necessary, plan the seating arrangement to prevent inappropriate behaviours, such as whispering or other interruptions. If the group meets over a period of time, have group members set group norms for conduct and behaviour. Often group norms can be outlined in a group contract to hold members accountable within the group in regard to their assigned tasks.

Distribute an agenda. Whenever possible, provide a written agenda to each member in advance of the meeting. Group members can discuss the agenda for the meeting before the meeting and all agree to the goals for the meeting. Attach all needed preparation reading to the agenda. The more advanced the reading or preparation that is required, the earlier members should receive agendas. Different types of agendas can be used for different purposes:

- *Structured agendas:* If a topic is particularly controversial, consider setting a rule that requires any negative comment to be preceded by a positive one.
- *Timed agendas:* Consider setting a specific amount of time to be dedicated to each item on the agenda. If

you stick to the schedule, discussion will stay focused and you will be more likely to make it through the agenda. However, setting realistic times is critical to the success of this strategy.
- *Action agendas:* Consider submitting an agenda with a description of the needed or desired actions, such as review proposals, approve minutes, or establish outcomes.

Keep the group on task. Use rules of order to facilitate meetings. Robert's Rules of Order (Robert, 2017) may seem overly structured; however, this structure is particularly helpful when diversity of opinion is likely or important. Specifically, these rules help the person chairing the meeting by setting limits on discussion and using a specific order of priorities to effectively deal with concerns or in-depth discussions.

Keep minutes, and distribute them to participants. Minutes of meetings provide a record for reference if needed and convey contents to persons unable to attend.

Participants must also prepare for meetings. Reviewing the agenda or requesting one in advance if not provided, reviewing preparatory materials, and thinking through agenda items are ways that group members may assist in accomplishing the meeting goals. Meeting participants should be on time for all meetings or communicate that they will be late or unable to attend. Participants should be prepared to leave on time as well. When a meeting is poorly chaired, a committee member could volunteer to ensure that the meeting agendas and minutes are distributed. It is important to recognize that some people deliberately avoid preparing agendas and distributing minutes in an attempt to control the meeting. Exercise 29.7 will help you understand the importance of well-run meetings.

EXERCISE 29.7 Have you ever sat in a meeting and wondered why you were there? Perhaps the purpose of the meeting, where the meeting was heading, or even who was in charge was unclear to you. Do the members often engage in lengthy discussion off the main topic of discussion?

Write down the three things about meetings you have attended that were most annoying, and then analyze how they could have been handled better. If you are a nursing student, think about a meeting you attended while working on a group project and answer the same questions noted above. An example may include a clinical preparedness meeting or a meeting for a group project.

CONCLUSION

Self-management is a means to achieve work–life balance, as well as a way of life to achieve personal goals within self-imposed priorities and deadlines. Time management is clock-oriented, and stress management is the control of external and internal stressors.

To achieve a balance in life and minimize stressors, nurses must learn to sit back and see their own personal "big picture" and examine their personal and professional goals. Personal priorities also must be established. Stressors and coping strategies need to be identified and used. By developing these techniques, nurses can gain a sense of control and become far better nurses in the process.

? A SOLUTION

Maryam sought advice from co-workers, their manager, and a counsellor on how to better handle stress, and as a result, feels that the stress experienced can be better handled. Maryam takes better care of self than before by getting more sleep, trying to eat a more balanced diet, exercising at least every other day; and trying not to procrastinate too much.

Maryam's partner is very supportive, and Maryam takes yoga classes with another good friend. Maryam leaves the building to go out for lunch when work is becoming too stressful. Meditating for 20 minutes each day also helps tremendously. Probably the most important thing Maryam has learned to do is to be *present* in the moment. For example, when spending time with their children or partner, Maryam does not

fixate on what is happening at work or next week's schedule. Maryam has come to realize that how stress is handled is essential, that it is not the stress per se that can cause problems; it is also one's reaction to the stress that is a key consideration. Because of this realization, Maryam has worked to consciously reframe to focus on one thing at a time. Doing so has helped reduce stress levels and increase productivity because Maryam is fully engaged in the task at hand. After completing a personal analysis of change exercise, Maryam was able to create a list of stress-reduction strategies for different types of stressful events and keeps this list on a mobile device.

Would this be a suitable approach for you? Why or why not?

▋ THE EVIDENCE

Bogaert et al. (2010) investigated the impact of unit-level practice environment factors and burnout on nurse-assessed quality of care. A total of 546 staff nurses from four acute care hospitals were surveyed during the study, and the data were analyzed using a two-level random intercept model. The Nursing Work Index–Revised instrument was used to measure nurse

practice environment dimensions, and the Maslach Burnout Inventory was used to measure burnout dimensions. The study found that emotional exhaustion is linked to job satisfaction, nurse turnover intentions, and assessed quality of care. The study concluded that widespread burnout merits special attention from all health care providers.

✴ NEED TO KNOW NOW

- Choose to practice in a workplace environment that works best for you. Consider the working environment, your own practice needs, and the availability of resources to support your development.

- Be alert to stress levels and your own stress responses and how they affect your work and your personal life.
- Create a list of stress management interventions that are most helpful to you.
- Work to master information management skills.

▋ CHAPTER CHECKLIST

Stress management and time management are two strategies for self-management. Balancing stress means caring for your emotional/spiritual, physical, and

mental health needs. Delegating effectively, acquiring good information literacy skills, using schedules and calendars and other planners, using time-management principles, and managing meetings are key strategies to be integrated into the nurse leader role. By accomplishing self-management, managers, leaders, and followers will find themselves in control of work time and stressors, as well as more confident in achieving both personal and work-related goals. Effective leaders are responsible for creating an environment conducive to an excellent followership style (Gibbons & Bryant, 2013).

Stress and overwork are inherent in the nursing profession, and nurses can adapt and cope with stress and time pressures by learning effective ways to care for themselves and to manage time. By assessing and reducing specific stressors and time wasters, nurses can thrive in the health care challenges before them. Increasing skills in coping, organization, delegation, and effective time management is vital for effective leadership. A nurse manager who can be a role model and support staff in turbulent times is a true leader.

- Self-management includes stress management, time management, and meeting management.
- Time management includes using tools and strategies to ensure that priority goals are achieved.
- Signs of excess stress must be heeded to prevent burnout or chronic health problems.
- Strategies to reduce stress include physical, mental, and emotional approaches.
- Strategies to improve time management include identification of potential time wasters, use of time-management strategies, and appropriate delegation.
- Strategies to improve meeting management include effective organization, following an agenda, and using rules of order to facilitate the meeting.

TIPS FOR SELF-MANAGEMENT

- Know what your high-priority goals are, and use them to filter decisions.
- Know your personal response to stress and self-evaluate frequently.
- Make your health a priority and use strategies that keep yourself in control.
- Use organizational systems that meet your needs.
- Simplify where and when you are able.
- Refocus on your priorities whenever you begin to feel overwhelmed.
- Do not be afraid to ask for help or assistance.

Visit the Evolve website for Suggested Readings, Internet Resources, and additional resources related to the content in this chapter: http://evolve.elsevier.com/Canada/Yoder-Wise/leading/

REFERENCES

Applebaum, D., Fowler, S., Fiedler, N., et al. (2010). The impact of environmental factors on nursing stress, job satisfaction and turnover intention. *Journal of Nursing Administration, 40*(7/8), 323–328.

Aron, S. (2015). *Relationship between nurses' job satisfaction and quality of healthcare they deliver. All Theses, Dissertations, and Other Capstone Projects.* Paper 506. Retrieved from: https://cornerstone.lib.mnsu.edu/cgi/viewcontent.cgi?article=1505&context=etds.

Badke, W. (2010). Why information literacy is invisible. *Communications in Information Literacy, 4*(2), 129–141.

Bailey, J. (2009). The challenge for today's nurse managers: How to be fiscally competent & efficient while nurturing the workforce and sustaining self. *Spinal Cord Injury, 29*(1), 25–28.

Beecroft, P. C., Dorey, F., & Wenten, M. (2008). Turnover intention in new graduate nurses: A multivariate analysis. *Journal of Advanced Nursing, 62*(1), 41–52.

Belcik, K. (2007). *Information literacy: A pre-requisite to evidence-based nursing. Paper presented at the 18th International Nursing Research Congress Focusing on Evidence-Based Practice* Vienna, Austria.

Blake, N., & Robbins, W. (2013). Health work environments and staff nurse retention: The relationship between communication, collaboration, and leadership in the pediatric intensive care unit. *Nursing Administration Quarterly, 37*(4), 356–370.

Bogaert, P., Clarke, S., Roelant, E., et al. (2010). Impacts of unit-level nurse practice environment and burnout on nurse reported outcomes: A multilevel model approach. *Journal of Clinical Nursing, 19,* 1664–1674.

Bold, K. (2010). Stressing the positive. *ZotZine, 3*(2). Retrieved from: http://zotzine.uci.edu/v03/2010_10/maddi.php.

Brass, E. (2016). How mindfulness can benefit nursing practice. *Nursing Times, 112*(18). Retrieved from: https://www.nursingtimes.net/roles/mental-health-nurses/how-mindfulness-can-benefit-nursing-practice/7004433.article.

Campbell Quick, J., Wright, T., Adkins, J., Nelson, D., & Quick, D. (2013). *Preventative stress management in organizations* (2nd ed.). Washington DC: APA.

Canadian Nurses Association. (2017a). *Code of ethics for registered nurses*. Ottawa, ON: Author. Retrieved from: https://www.cna-aiic.ca/~/media/cna/page-content/pdf-en/code-of-ethics-2017-edition-secure-interactive.

Canadian Nurses Association. (2017b). *Workforce profile of registered nurses in Canada*. Ottawa, ON: Author.

College of Nurses of Ontario. (2014). *Entry-to-Practice Competencies for Registered Nurses*. Retrieved from: https://www.cno.org/globalassets/docs/reg/41037_entrytopractic_final.pdf.

Complain. (2004). In K. Barber (Ed.), *Canadian Oxford Dictionary* (2nd ed). Don Mills, ON: Oxford University Press.

Covey, S. R., Merrill, A. R., & Merrill, R. R. (1994). *First things first: To love, to learn, to leave a legacy*. New York, NY: Simon & Schuster.

Garrosa, E., Moreno-Jimenez, B., Rodriguez-Munoz, A., et al. (2011). Role stress and personal resources in nursing: A cross-sectional study of burnout and engagement. *International Journal of Nursing Studies, 48*, 479–489.

Gibbons, A., & Bryant, D. (2013). Followership: The forgotten part of leadership. *Casebook, 21*(2), 12–13.

Guimond-Plourde, R. (2011). Stress care: Turning failure into triumph. *Canadian Nurse, 107*(1), 16–17.

Hargrove, M. B., Quick, J. C., Nelson, D. L., et al. (2011). The theory of preventative stress management: a 33-year review and evaluation. *Stress and Health, 27*, 182–193.

Jameton, A. (1984). Dilemmas of moral distress: Moral responsibility and nursing practice. *AWHONN's Clinical Issues in Perinatalogy and Women's Health Nursing, 4*(4), 542–555.

LaMontagne, A. D., Keegel, T., Louie, A. M., et al. (2007). A systematic review of the job stress intervention evaluation literature: 1990–2005. *International Journal of Occupational and Environmental Health, 13*(3), 268–280.

Laschinger, H. K. S., Finegan, J., & Wilk, P. (2009). New graduate burnout: The impact of professional practice environment, workplace civility and empowerment. *Nursing Economic$, 27*(6), 377–383.

Lavoie-Tremblay, M., Leclerc, E., Marchionni, C., et al. (2010). The needs and expectations of generation Y nurses in the workplace. *Journal for Nurses in Staff Development, 26*, 2–8.

Limm, H., Gundel, H., Heinmuller, M., et al. (2011). Stress management interventions in the workplace improve stress reactivity: A randomised controlled trial. *Occupational and Environmental Medicine, 68*, 126–133.

Maddi, S. (2013). *Hardiness: Turning stressful circumstances into resilient growth*. New York, NY: Springer.

McBain, H., Mulligan, K., & Newman, S. (2015). Nonpharmacologic pain management. *Rheumatology, 1*(1). (6th ed.), 1(1). Retrieved from: https://doi.org/10.1016/B978-0-323-09138-1.00050-4.

Maslach, C., & Jackson, S. E. (1981). *Maslach Burnout Inventory manual*. Palo Alto, CA: Consulting Psychologists Press.

Maslach, C., & Leiter, M. (2008). Early predictors of job burnout and engagement. *Journal of Applied Psychology, 93*, 498–512.

Maslach, C., Schaufeli, W., & Leiter, M. (2000). Job burnout. *Annual Review of Psychology, 52*, 397–422.

Moustaka, A., & Constantinidis, T. (2010). Sources and effects of work-related stress in nursing. *Health Science Journal, 4*(4).

Nash, S. (2009). *Stress, hardiness and leadership style: an examination of factors that foster nurse manager survival in the healthcare environment (Unpublished master's thesis)*. San Diego, CA: San Diego State University. Retrieved from: http://www.leadershipchallenge.com/Research-section-Others-Research-Detail/abstract-nash--stress-hardiness-and-leadership-style.aspx.

Parand, A., Dopson, S., Renz, A., & Vincent, C. (2014). The role of hospital managers and patient safety: A systemic review. *BMJ Open, 4*(9) e005055.

Perfectionism. (2004). In K. Barber (Ed.), *Canadian Oxford Dictionary* (2nd ed). Don Mills, ON: Oxford University Press.

Pipe, T. B., Bortz, J. J., Dueck, A., et al. (2009). Nurse leader mindfulness meditation program for stress management: A randomized controlled trial. *Journal of Nursing Administration, 39*, 130–137.

Poghosyan, L., Clarke, S. P., Finlayson, M., et al. (2010). Nurse burnout and quality of care: Cross-national investigation in six countries. *Research in Nursing and Health, 33*, 288–298.

Post, G. (2010). *Tend and befriend behavior in women. Women's Issues*. Retrieved from: http://www.goodtherapy.org/blog/women-stress-social-relationships-psychology/.

Rice, V. (2013). *Handbook of stress, coping and health* (2nd ed.). Washington, DC: Sage.

Robert, H. (2017). *Robert's rules of order: The original manual for assembly rules, business etiquette and conduct*. New York, NY: Clydesdale Press.

Roy, C. (2008). *The Roy adaptation model* (3rd ed.). Upper Saddle River, NJ: Pearson-Prentice Hall.

Sarafis, P., Rousaki, E., Tsounis, A., et al. (2016). The impact of occupational stress on nurses' caring behaviors and their health related to quality of life. *BMC Nursing, 15*(56).

Selye, H. (1956). *The stress of life*. New York, NY: McGraw-Hill.

Selye, H. (1965). The stress syndrome. *American Journal of Nursing, 65*(3), 97–99.

Sherman, R. (2010). *Cultivating mindfulness in nursing leadership*. Retrieved from: https://www.emergingrnleader.com/mindfulnursingleadership/.

Shirey, M., McDaniel, A., Ebright, P., et al. (2010). Understanding nurse manager stress and work complexity. *Journal of Nursing Administration*, 40(2), 82–91.

Spence Laschinger, H., & Fida, R. (2014). New nurse burnout and workplace wellbeing: The influence of authentic leadership and psychological capital. *Burnout Research*, 1(1), 19–28.

Stuart, G. W., & Laraia, M. T. (2008). *Self-modification assistance*. In G. M. Bulechek, & H.K. (Eds.), *Nursing interventions classificiations* (5th ed., pp. 644–645). St. Louis, MO: Mosby.

Taylor, S. E., Klein, L. C., Lewis, B. P., et al. (2000). Biobehavioral responses to stress in females: Tend-and-befriend, not fight-or-flight. *Psychological Review*, 107, 411–429.

Understanding the stress response. *Harvard Mental Health Letter*, 27(9), (2011), 4–6. Retrieved from: http://www.health.harvard.edu.

Unruh, L., & Zhang, N. (2013). The role of work environment in keeping newly licensed RNs in nursing: A questionnaire survey. *International Journal of Nursing Studies*, 50(12), 1678–1688.

Van der Riet, P., Lovett-Jones, T., & Aquino-Russell, C. (2018). The effectiveness of mindfulness for nurses and nursing students: An integrated literature review. *Nurse Educator Today*, 65(1).

Vohs, K. D., Redden, J. D., & Rahinel, R. (2013). Physical order produces healthy choices, generosity, and conventionality, whereas disorder produces creativity. *Psychological Science*, 24(9), 1860–1867.

Waddill-Goad, S., & Sigma Theta Tau, I. (2016). *Nurse burnout: Combating stress in nursing*. Indianapolis, IN: Sigma Theta Tau International.

Wang, X., Kunaviktikul, W., & Wichaikhum, O. A. (2013). Work empowerment and burnout among registered nurses in two tertiary general hospitals. *Journal of Clinical Nursing*, 22(19–20), 2896–2903.

Wodak, R., Kwon, W., & Clarke, I. (2011). Getting people on board: Discursive leadership for consensus building in team meetings. *Discourse Society*, 22, 592.

Wolf, G., Triolo, P., & Ponte, P. (2008). Magnet recognition program: The next generation. *Journal of Nursing Administration*, 38, 200–204.

Wu, H., Chi, T. S., Chen, L., et al. (2010). Occupational stress among hospital nurses: Cross-sectional survey. *Journal of Advanced Nursing*, 66, 627–634.

Zangaro, G. A., & Soeken, K. L. (2007). A meta-analysis of studies of nurse's job satisfaction. *Research in Nursing & Health*, 30, 445–458.

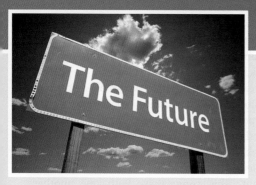

30

Thriving for the Future

Sandra Regan

Contemplating the future of nursing allows nurses, across the career continuum, to explore how the changes they will face can be maximized to benefit the profession and the public. This chapter presents the key leadership skills of visioning and forecasting. Projections for the future and their implications for nursing are also discussed.

OBJECTIVES

- Value the need to think about the future while meeting current expectations.
- Describe the six leadership strengths that will be essential in the future.

- Ponder two or three projections for the future and what they mean to the practice of nursing.
- Determine three projections for the future that have implications for individual nursing practice and nurse leadership.

TERMS TO KNOW

chaos

complexity compression

shared vision

vision

? A CHALLENGE

Janice, a student in the last year of their undergraduate nursing program, is beginning to plan their career in nursing. They know that health care is changing to meet the complex needs of the population and that nurses have an important role in leading change to meet these needs. Janice is reflecting on what practice setting they would most like to work in, which roles they might work toward, and how they can be involved in the profession. Janice wonders what the future will bring.

What do you think you would do to better understand your future and that of nursing if you were Janice?

INTRODUCTION

Leading and managing in nursing are a consistent challenge. Even nurses who say they do not want to lead or manage find that new demands call for continuous leadership and increased self-management skills. More important, the work of the future is being accomplished in teams, with people working together to achieve a vision.

The first part of the twenty-first century brought new challenges and opportunities, some for which society was well prepared and others for which it struggled for some time. Think, for example, about concerns regarding the new millennium with the change to year 2000, or *Y2K* as it was called. There were predictions that computers could shut down everywhere because they might not be able to recognize that the number *2000* was a new century. Endless hours were spent in testing and fixing computers worldwide so that when the clock struck midnight throughout the world, people would still have computer access. We are an increasingly global community, and events occurring thousands of kilometres away might be felt locally. Consider the impact of the 2004 Indian Ocean earthquake and subsequent tsunami, or the more recent hurricanes in Puerto Rico. How did these disasters affect you and your community? The global health community responded and was instrumental in leading humanitarian efforts in these and other disaster events. Canadians have also experienced recent challenges, such as the fires in Fort McMurray and the train derailment in Lac-Mégantic, Quebec. Consider how the SARS (Severe Acute Respiratory Syndrome) outbreak of 2003 or concerns about avian flu in 2009 have influenced health care delivery in your province and nationally. Pandemic plans have been implemented, infection control practices changed in hospitals, and the public health system was revitalized. Clearly, past events have shaped the present, and the present will influence the future. What role will you have in influencing health care, today and tomorrow?

For nurses to lead in health care, a number of present challenges need to be addressed. These include an aging nursing workforce, a current nurse shortage that is projected to worsen in the next decade, a shortage of nursing faculty to teach the next generations of nurses, and a lack of succession planning for future nurse leaders in administrative positions. In addition to these issues, societal issues, such those related to current economies and changing population demographics, will influence health service delivery. As Sister Elizabeth Davis noted:

> We're in a new place; we're not on the edge of the old place. We're not pushing the envelope; we're in a totally new envelope. So the rules have changed. Every fundamental premise of the old way of thinking no longer applies (as cited in Villeneuve & MacDonald, 2006, p. 3).

LEADERSHIP DEMANDS FOR THE FUTURE

Nurse administrators and leaders consistently report that the characteristic they are most seeking in tomorrow's professional nurse is leadership. In probing what that means, we often find themes that relate to nursing activities that have serendipitous outcomes. Nurses shape the public's view of the profession, the organizations in which they work, and health care in general. Nurses influence interdisciplinary views of what it is to be a professional, and they create expectations for the profession's potential. All of these examples form some of the leadership potential that exists for the future.

If we think about the world as a loose web, we know that every element has the potential to influence every other element. This connectivity with one another, whether among those within our profession or within a team, means that we influence others all of the time, just as others influence us. This influence moulds our practices and beliefs as we move health care forward and changes how we influence others subsequently. Thus even positions without formal leadership titles contain an element of leadership, and we must all be prepared and willing to lead whenever the need arises. In their book *The Starfish and the Spider*, Brafman and Beckstrom (2006) liken this type of decentralized leadership to the starfish and centralized leadership to the spider. A starfish has no head and its major organs exist in each arm, so if one arm is damaged or removed, the starfish can grow a new arm and will continue to thrive (which is what happens in a decentralized organization with members who take on leadership roles as needed). By contrast, if you remove the leg of a spider, it is crippled; if you remove its head, it dies (which is what happens in a centralized organization when the main leader is no longer in charge).

EXERCISE 30.1 Using the analogies of the starfish (decentralized) and the spider (centralized), analyze two or three community or health care organizations with which you are familiar including if you wish, your own school of nursing. If the leader left, what do you think would happen to the organization? Would it flourish or diminish? And why?

LEADERSHIP STRENGTHS FOR THE FUTURE

When Lipman-Blumen (2000) proposed her six strengths of connective leaders, she may have had no idea how important these strengths would be for the future (Box 30.1). Any one of these strengths is valuable to an organization or an individual, but in combination, they make a leader invaluable. A nurse leader's ethical political savvy can be based on the *Code of Ethics for*

BOX 30.1	Six Leadership Strengths for the Future

Ethical political savvy: knowing how to effect change and use resources from an ethical, altruistic perspective

Authenticity and accountability: being committed to the group rather than self, which leads to credibility; being open in decisions

Politics of commonalities: ensuring an environment that allows as many stakeholders as possible to achieve at least a part of their respective agendas

Thinking long term, acting short term: committing to what is best for the future and acting in the present to move toward that goal, including developing the future leadership to succeed current leaders

Leadership through expectation: encouraging others through expectations rather than through micromanagement

Quest for meaning: leaving a legacy by guiding others

From Lipman-Blumen, J. (2000). The age of connective leadership. *Leader to Leader,* 17 (Summer), 39–45. Copyright © 2000 the Drucker Foundation.

Registered Nurses (Canadian Nurses Association [CNA], 2017) and provincial or territorial nursing professional standards. Basing our actions on ethical principles to affect the political system that influences the availability of health care (and other) resources allows us to demonstrate the trust the public places in us. Most of us have capitalized on our authenticity and accountability to demonstrate our concern for others, whether through collective action, crying with families, or listening carefully to what our colleagues and patients say.

Because nursing work is relational, nursing leadership styles have been the focus of studies, particularly by Canadian nurse researchers. A growing body of literature suggests that leaders who are transformational, resonant, supportive, and considerate influence patient, nurse, and organizational outcomes (Cummings et al., 2010; Wong et al., 2013). Leadership styles that are relational in nature (rather than task oriented) promote and facilitate change, which is important to realizing a future vision.

When we are faced with the pressures of providing care to patients versus changing the system, we often remain focused on the individual patient, thus losing the opportunity to change an issue for many patients. To be effective in the future, we must embrace the opportunities to think longer term so that more people are affected by our actions. Perhaps, because of our history of being attentive to the details, we may need to challenge ourselves to develop broader leadership skills. Moving from micromanaging to focusing on setting expectations for those who are accountable to us, may feel uncomfortable at first. However, that movement reinforces our ability to deal with longer-term issues. In addition, the quest for meaning suggests that our actions today create the foundation on which future leaders will build. Thus if we fail to capitalize on today's opportunities, we are diminishing the place at which future leaders will start their leadership careers.

It is incumbent on nurses to raise expectations about what comprises good, safe, quality, patient-centred care and how nurses in leadership roles contribute to those expectations. Developing one's ability to lead occurs over time, but the key is that the foundation be present. Our foundation begins with our concern for and advocacy of patient care. That foundation is fairly well engrained in professional nurses' beliefs. The movement from focusing on the nurse–patient relationship to the "big picture" of nursing (politics and public or health policy activities) may take several years but is rewarding nonetheless. What we do in our professional lives is the legacy we leave for future generations.

LITERATURE PERSPECTIVE

Resource: Snethen, J. A. (2018). Emerging leaders in practice: identifying and developing them. *Nursing Outlook,* 66, 1–2.

The author draws on research suggesting that future nurse leaders can be fostered by creating a space for "career curiosity". Traits of those who exhibit career curiosity include embracing learning, being curious, and promoting new ideas. Experienced leaders can assist emerging leaders, particularly millennials, by creating a work environment that encourages exploration and innovation, support flexibility in location of practice and in staffing, and recognize and appreciate the expertise that emerging leaders bring, such as in the use of technology and social media.

Implications for Practice

Creating a culture that encourages career curiosity can be an important path to leadership. How will you, whether an established leader or an emerging leader, promote career curiosity?

> **EXERCISE 30.2** Using the six strengths cited in Box 30.1, write a description of what you believe your leadership strengths to be. Provide as much detail as possible so that the description helps you see your best strengths. What competencies have you gained—or will you focus on developing—in your nursing education program that align with the six strengths?

Nurses who seek leadership opportunities will find that many are available—in the employment setting, in professional associations, and in voluntary community organizations. Balancing multiple demands in an era of rapid changes and new expectations can be challenging. Merely being employed is no longer sufficient; an individual must be *employable*. This suggests that we must constantly be focused on competence, on learning, on what the future holds, and on what patients want and need. Failure to do so will make us unemployable and will make the profession undesirable. To be valued in the future, we need to know what the future might encompass.

VISIONING

Whether you are a leader, a manager, a follower or a student, the ability to visualize in your mind what the ideal future is becomes a critical strategy. A vision is the articulated goals to which an individual, group, or an organization aspires. No matter how we engage in this visioning activity, we must be open and honest about what we think. Creating our own circle of advisors or brain trusts (those who do not necessarily think as we do, but who are creative thinkers) allows us to test ideas so that we enhance our own thinking and performance to higher levels.

This chapter is designed to share some views about the future so that you can think about them in relation to what it means to lead and manage, and your role in shaping the future and your own career within that future (see Chapter 31). This "thinking about" the future, like visions, is further enriched through sharing in open dialogue with colleagues.

> **EXERCISE 30.3** Select a group of three or four peers and brainstorm what you think the future of nursing will be. Consider how technology will affect nursing; consider where our primary place of service will be and how we will deliver care. Think about the changes in society and the political pressures for effective health care and what those might mean for nursing. Think about how you would reform health care. Create a list of ideas to share with others.

Although no one knows the future for certain, many entities engage in formal predictions. These predictions arise from structured groups, such as the World Future Society (http://www.wfs.org), regular trend reports, and books. Although not everyone is a futurist, each of us needs to be aware of trends. Thinking about the future should be mind expanding; it is the most nonstereotypical thinking you can do. In everyday practice, you can ask yourself and others "what if" questions. We take for granted that certain practices have remained unchanged. Yet, technology and creative thinkers and investigators prove us wrong on a regular basis. Our challenge is to think about the future in a way that does not necessarily rely on history and yet builds on today.

Because the future is about teams and collaborative work, many implications exist for nursing. Skills related to working with others and facilitating their work, as well as reaching decisions about practice and the workplace, will be crucial.

SHARED VISION

The concept of shared vision suggests that two or more people endorse a particular view. How society and we view the world as individuals is always evolving. Consider stability and chaos (a condition of disorder or confusion) as the opposite ends of a continuum. Moving in some way between those two ends suggests that we live in a constant state of disequilibrium in which we strive toward stability while recognizing that we experience chaos. In times of great stability, society makes little progress (but life probably seems serene). In times of great chaos, by contrast, society may transform itself (and life may seem uncontrollable). Thus it is even more important to think about projections for the future to have a sense of the direction we are heading on the continuum (see figure below).

Stability ←————————————————→ Chaos

Society

Consider the idea of a shared vision of health care. As we continue to move from "traditional" practices to evidence-informed ones and from a heavy focus on tertiary (hospital-based) care to one that includes community (including the home) and primary health care, we can assume that we might experience more chaos. The comfort of the known is gone; rather, practices are evaluated on a regular basis and changes are incorporated so that we are all doing the latest "best" for patients. In our efforts to do the best we can, as soon as we can, we have experienced the phenomenon of complexity compression. In essence, this term refers to the intensity of increasing functions and expectations without a change in resources, including time. This compression can be distracting or useful. Krichbaum et al. (2007) studied nurses' experiences of complexity compression and identified common themes. For example, when nurses experienced rapid changes in practice (e.g., through the introduction of new technology) without the supports to learn, or were given additional responsibilities without additional time, they expressed concern about patient safety. The authors suggested that nurses were frustrated with not being included in decisions about changes that affect their practice. They emphasized the importance of nurse involvement in decisions and control over their practice. Krichbaum et al. (2011) have gone on to develop a tool to measure factors that contribute to complexity compression in nurses. As changes occur in health care, it is important for nurse leaders, managers, and followers to be aware of the factors that can impede or support involvement in creating the shared vision.

Our ability to retrieve, analyze, and evaluate information influences our currency with practice expectations. We seem to value the need for a shared vision, which includes the idea of operating from a rich data-based approach. To be able to achieve a shared vision, however, we also need to hone our skills in projecting for the future so we know where practice is headed, we need to consider how we interact with our patients, and we need to consider how quickly we can elevate all nursing practitioners to a satisfactory level of working with an evidence-informed practice approach. Still relevant today, Kouzes and Posner (2009)* indicated how leaders can help create a shared vision:

> As counterintuitive as it might seem, then, the best way to lead people into the future is to connect with them deeply in the present. The only visions that take hold are shared visions—and you will create them only when you listen very, very closely to others, appreciate their hopes, and attend to their needs.

*Reprinted by permission of Harvard Business Review. Excerpt. From "To lead, create a shared vision" by Kouzes, J.K., & Posner, B.Z., Vol. January/2009. Copyright ©2009 by Harvard Business Publishing; all rights reserved.

> The best leaders are able to bring their people into the future because they engage in the oldest form of research: They observe the human condition. (pp. 20–21)

PROJECTIONS FOR THE FUTURE

If you watch future reports on television or read *The Trend Letter* or *The Futurist* (The World Society publication) or books, such as *The World Is Flat 3.0: a Brief History of the Twenty-First Century* (Friedman, 2007) or *Hot, Flat, and Crowded* (Friedman, 2008), you will find comparable themes about the future. The following are some forecasts for the future that will affect nursing; it is possible to ask "What if" questions about each.

Knowledge and Technology Influences

- Knowledge will change dramatically, requiring that we all be dedicated learners.
- Knowledge will evolve from the intensity of the current information evolution, so that we will access content with meaning and applicability for our work.
- Leaders will continue to require the best evidence available to inform decisions.
- Technology will continue to revolutionize health care; use of social media and "apps" will be ubiquitous.
- A power shift will occur toward health care because of the intensity of the developing knowledge and its use in making cost-effective decisions about care; technology will enhance the patient focus including patient-centred care and patient safety.
- Every person will have an electronic health record that will be used by all members of the team across sectors.

Economic Influences

- The health care system will have to change to remain financially sustainable.
- Department and grocery stores will be either very small or huge; people will shop "online."
- Macromarketing (targeting masses) will be out; micromarketing (targeting specific populations) will be in.

Global Trends

- The world will be seen increasingly as a continuum without borders that prevent trade and inventions, including those related to health care.
- Increasing diversity will result in the following:
  - More people who are older than younger
  - A mobile population with people moving to different parts of the country or the world
  - People will have a greater need for speaking two or three languages
- There will be increased violence and, simultaneously, an increased expectation for civility.
- Climate change will affect the social determinants of health.

Health Trends

- More older adults living longer will require innovations in health and social care.
- More people will be living with chronic diseases.
- More people will be overweight and consequently experience various related diseases.
- Bioengineering will make possible interventions that currently do not exist.
- As genetics allows us to know more about how an individual would respond to treatment, a shift toward eliminating the current disparities is more likely.
- Emphasis on health promotion and disease prevention rather than "illness care" will redirect health care efforts.

Work Trends

- Job security will be out; career options will be in.
- Competition will be out; cooperation will be in.
- Work will be sporadic and potentially precarious.
- Work will be accomplished by teams.
- Everyone will need to be a leader.

Canadian Nurses Association's 20/20 Vision

Villeneuve and MacDonald (2006) conducted an extensive "visioning" consultation for the CNA to provide a starting place for discussions about nursing's role in shaping the Canadian health care system of the future. *Toward 20/20: Visions for Nursing* describes several "preferred futures" and various scenarios. For example, the authors suggested that patient-led care will increase; nurses will assist patients to navigate the system and coordinate care; a significant shift will occur to community-based care (see the Research Perspective) as opposed to hospital-based care; and care delivered by interprofessional teams will integrate a variety of health care workers, including assistive and support workers and those providing complementary and alternative health services. At the core of these envisioned changes is "nurses leading." The authors observed: "Nurses can be at the forefront of the coming changes, setting the agenda to create a health care system that truly serves and reflects the priorities of Canadians. But no one will appoint them to the task" (Villeneuve & MacDonald, 2006, p. 3).

In 2011, the CNA (2012) established the National Expert Commission to identify ways to meet the future health needs of Canadians. The Commission spoke with the public, nurses, policy-makers, and other health professionals. Their consultation identified

---

RESEARCH PERSPECTIVE

Resource: Schofield, R., Ganann, R., Brooks, S., et al. (2011). Community health nursing vision for 2020: Shaping the future. *Western Journal of Nursing Research*, 33(8), 1047–1068.

The authors conducted a qualitative study to understand priority issues currently facing Canadian community health nurses related to education, practice, research, administration, and policy. The aim of the study was to develop a national vision for community health nursing to shape the future of the profession moving toward the year 2020. Focus groups and key informant interviews were conducted with 35 community health nurses across Canada. Five key themes were identified: community health nursing in crisis now, a flawed health care system, responding to the public, vision for the future, and community health nurses as solution makers. Study participants identified a number of key strategies, including developing a common definition and vision of community health nursing, collaborating on an aggressive plan to shift to a primary health care system, developing a comprehensive social marketing strategy, refocusing basic baccalaureate education, enhancing the capacity of community health researchers and knowledge in community health nursing, and establishing a community health nursing centre of excellence.

Implications for Practice

The nursing profession needs to continually look to the future to ensure its relevance and maintain its ability to respond to the changing context. Visioning exercises can be useful strategies to reflect on a preferred future and strategically plan to achieve it.

key priorities for health care transformation including focusing on primary health care for all; address the social determinants of health; addressing needs of vulnerable and marginalized people and communities; integrate health in all policies; ensure safe and quality care; ensuring health care providers are well-prepared to practice in the health care system of the future; and enhanced and appropriate use of technology. CNA has developed a video that discusses nursing's role in achieving these priorities called A Nursing Call to Action.

> **EXERCISE 30.4** Review the list of projections for the future, the CNA's priorities, and some of the preferred futures and scenarios in *Towards 20/20: Visions for Nursing* and consider how each might affect how you envision your career. Make a note of one or two phrases that are the top implications. Look at the list of projections again, and evaluate each of the items to determine which ones you believe will be most important to you. Rank in order the top five. Compare your list with those of two or three colleagues and offer your rationale for your selection. After you hear their viewpoints, consider whether you would change your own rankings.

NURSING: PREPARING FOR THE FUTURE

A number of issues will influence nursing's direction in the future. For example, consider the following questions:

- How will shared governance and interprofessional collaboration change the role of staff nurse and enhance patient care?
- How will increased public accountability of health care providers and health care services change nursing practices?
- How will changes to the practice environment affect nurse recruitment and retention?
- Will we have a dramatically richer set of evidence to describe the difference nurses make in patient care and health promotion and disease prevention?
- How will continuing competence and quality assurance be measured in the future?
- How will health care emerge over the next several years as a desirable place to work and as a source of help for health-related needs?

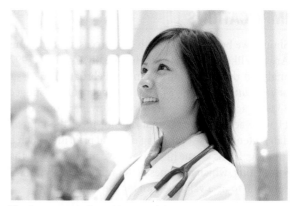
The future explodes with potential.

- Will nurses be paid by a salary, or will their economic worth be reflected in what they are paid?
- How can we achieve a diverse profession?
- What can health care organizations learn from other sectors and vice versa?
- Will increasing concern about terrorism, pandemics, and trade and mobility agreements affect the flow of nurses across borders?

How does nursing prepare itself for the future? One way is through how we prepare the future nursing workforce, and nursing education programs play a very important role. The nursing profession has identified that the knowledge, skills, attitudes, and judgement required to meet the demands of the health care system, today and in the future, are gained through baccalaureate education. All Canadian provinces and territories (with the exception of Quebec) require a baccalaureate education as the entry to the profession for registered nurses. This ensures that new registered nurses have the competencies required to navigate the complexity of health care and actively participate as advocates for change. Baccalaureate degrees are now also offered in psychiatric nursing, although not required for entry to practice, and practical nursing diploma programs are increasingly more comprehensive and lengthier than in the past. All point to the importance of enhanced and responsive nursing education to support the future of nursing. See Chapters 28 and 31 regarding the increasing focus on student and new graduate nurse self-development and management of their careers.

IMPLICATIONS

Should we be concerned with the forecasts for nursing? Are they likely to come true? Historically, Cornish (1997) analyzed the predictions from the February 1967 issue of *The Futurist*. Of the 34 forecasts that could be judged, 23 were accurate and 11 were not. However, some of the 11 were accurate trends that did not meet the targeted date, often because of shifting national priorities, such as funding. If this is true historically, we might assume that forecasting, which becomes better refined each year, will continue to be a valuable tool for the future.

CONCLUSION

Numerous changes will occur throughout our lifetimes. It is only a matter of time before we say (if we have not already), "When I was young." Our description might be of something that today is considered fairly advanced. For those who want to thrive, the future forecasts are like the gold ring on the merry-go-round. If you risk and reach far enough, you can grasp it! Lead on. The future is now!

❓ A SOLUTION

Janice, like most students, is asking important questions, searching for meaning, and beginning the process of shaping their future as a nurse. They can use tools gained from this textbook and this chapter to reflect on and identify their role as a leader and follower in nursing and health care, examine trends that will influence nursing and health care, and look toward a future that they can help to shape. New graduate nurses often take on a follower role initially but, because of the competencies gained in their undergraduate nursing program, they often have the most "up-to-date" information and competencies that can help them lead evidence-informed practice

initiatives. Their exposure to practice experiences from acute care to community settings, their knowledge of health promotion, and their exposure to interprofessional collaboration means they are well-prepared for changes in practice. Over the course of their career in nursing, Janice will apply the competencies gained in their educational program and in practice to lead in a variety of settings and with different populations. They have the tools to thrive in the future.

Would this be a suitable approach for you? Why or why not?

✳ NEED TO KNOW NOW

- Ask "what if" when challenged by a problem in your work.

- Use the changes you have seen in health care in the past 6 months as a reminder that the future will be different from the past.

CHAPTER CHECKLIST

This chapter addresses the need to think about the future and what that means for current practice. Involvement by all nurses is needed to keep the profession relevant to the constantly emerging future.

- Six leadership strengths are needed for the future:
- Ethical political savvy
- Authenticity and accountability

- Politics of commonalities
- Thinking long term, acting short term
- Leadership through expectation
- Quest for meaning
- Shared visions are important.
- Numerous projections for the future can shape what our individual and collective practices will be.

◼ TIPS FOR THE FUTURE

- At least monthly, read literature external to nursing and health care. Then ponder whether what you have read has implications for nursing.
- Talk with people outside of nursing about their view of the world and what is happening in their discipline.

- Be aware of current events—political, social, cultural, technologic—that will shape the future.

Visit the Evolve website for Suggested Readings, Internet Resources, and additional resources related to the content in this chapter: http://evolve.elsevier.com/Canada/Yoder-Wise/leading/

REFERENCES

Brafman, O., & Beckstrom, R. A. (2006). *The starfish and the spider: The unstoppable power of leaderless organizations.* New York, NY: Penguin.

Canadian Nurses Association. (2017). *Code of Ethics for Registered Nurses (2017 edition).* Toronto, ON: Author. Retrieved from https://www.cna-aiic.ca/html/en/Code-of-Ethics-2017-Edition/files/assets/basic-html/page-3.html.

Canadian Nurses Association. (2012). *A Nursing Call to Action.* Retrieved from https://www.cna-aiic.ca/-/media/cna/files/en/nec_report_e.pdf?la=en&hash=3659EA41A22369AF14FFD057284414B264FD58E0.

Cornish, E. (1997). The Futurist forecasts 30 years later. *The Futurist, 31,* 45–48 (January/February).

Cummings, G. G., MacGregor, T., Davey, M., et al. (2010). Leadership styles and outcome patterns for the nursing workforce and work environment: A systematic review. *International Journal of Nursing Studies, 47*(4), 363–385.

Friedman, T. L. (2007). *The world is flat 3.0: A brief history of the twenty-first century.* New York, NY: Farrar, Straus & Giroux.

Friedman, T. L. (2008). *Hot, flat, and crowded: Why we need a green revolution and how it can renew America.* New York, NY: Farrar, Straus & Giroux.

Krichbaum, K., Diemert, C., Jacox, L., et al. (2007). Complexity compression: Nurses under fire. *Nursing Forum, 42*(2), 86–94.

Krichbaum, K., Peden-McAlpine, C., Diemert, C., Koenic, P., Mueller, C., & Savik, K. (2011). Designing a measure of complexity compression in registered nurses. *Western Journal of Nursing Research, 33*(1), 7–25.

Lipman-Blumen, J. (2000). The age of connective leadership. *Leader to Leader, 17*(Summer), 39–45.

Schofield, R., Ganann, R., Brooks, S., et al. (2011). Community health nursing vision for 2020: Shaping the future. *Western Journal of Nursing Research, 33*(8), 1047–1068.

Snethen, J. A. (2018). Emerging leaders in practice: Identifying and developing them. *Nursing Outlook, 66,* 1–2.

Villeneuve, M., & MacDonald, J. (2006). *Toward 20/20: Visions for Nursing.* Ottawa: ON: Canadian Nurses Association. Retrieved from http://www.cna-nurses.ca/CNA/documents/pdf/publications/Toward-2020-e.pdf.

Wong, C. A., Cummings, G. G., & Ducharme, L. (2013). The relationship between nursing leadership and patient outcomes: A systematic review update. *Journal of Nursing Management, 21,* 709–724.

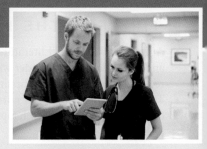

31

Leading and Managing Your Career

Janice I. Waddell, Mary Wheeler

Students' nursing career begins the first day of their program and meaningful engagement in their nursing education will enhance their capacity as individuals and a collective to influence the quality of health care for individuals, families and communities. In doing so, students grow as nursing leaders. The goal of this chapter is twofold: (1) to foster each student's ability to shape their engagement in their nursing education to achieve their unique career goals, and (2) approach their learning with intention and personal commitment. To this end, an evidence-informed career planning and development model is presented to provide students with a process to develop the skill and capacity to lead and manage their own career, at each stage of their nursing program —and as they move to the next phase of their nursing journey. Engagement in each phase of the career planning and development process will provide students with the opportunity to reflect on their hopes for their career, their current strengths, and areas for development in relation to their desired career and how they can take charge of their career development, regardless of whether they are at the beginning, middle, or end of their nursing education program. Each chapter of this textbook offers rich and relevant information and perspectives to inform students' understanding of nursing leadership and management within the Canadian context, serving as a comprehensive resource for their own professional development as nurse leaders and managers.

Finally, students and faculty members can access a comprehensive, multimodal online career planning and development program, It's Your Career: Take Charge: Career Planning and Development (CPD) Guide (https://careeraction. blog.ryerson.ca/), to refer to as an adjunct to this chapter, and upon graduation.

OBJECTIVES

- Describe the five stages of career continuum.
- Describe the concepts of leadership and management within the context of their own career planning and development.
- Describe the Donner-Wheeler Career Planning and Development Model (Donner-Wheeler Model) adapted for student nurses.
- Engage in all elements of the Donner-Wheeler Model to shape their unique engagement in their nursing curriculum.

- Discuss the evidence that supports the efficacy of curriculum-based career planning and development model in fostering career resilience for student and new graduate nurses.
- Describe how to find a mentor to support their career planning and development activities.

TERMS TO KNOW

career management skills
career plan
career planning and development
career resilience

Donner-and Wheeler Career
    Planning and Development
    Model
environmental scan

marketing
mentorship
self-assessment
visioning

❓ A CHALLENGE

Hazel is at the beginning of their third year as a BScN nursing student. In high school, they were drawn to nursing. Hazel knows they made the right decision, loves their program, and is passionate about their clinical placements so far in both community health and acute care. Hazel's practicum experiences have introduced them to the concepts of mental health, family centred care, and equity, diversity, and inclusion. Through conversations with their preceptors and faculty members, Hazel has developed a strong interest in pediatric nursing because of the strong emphasis on family centred care and the opportunity to work with an interprofessional team in the care of children across developmental stages and their families. However, Hazel has discovered that there is no guarantee that they will have a practicum placement in a pediatric centre because of a high student demand for this area of focus. In fact, Hazel was informed that their 3rd year practicum would be located in a complex long-term care facility. Without the opportunity of a practicum in a

pediatric setting Hazel is not sure how they can position themselves to get job in a children's health care setting after graduation and worries that their dream will not become a reality.

Hazel is also committed to further developing their leadership abilities so that they can have an impact, not only on the care of children and families but also within the nursing profession. Hazel is an active member of their nursing course union and the Canadian Nurses' Student Association (CNSA) but is not sure that they have what it takes to secure a leadership role in CNSA. Although they were one of the student leaders in residence, Hazel is not sure that experience would be enough to position them to be successful in a more professional leadership role.

How can Hazel engage in their nursing curriculum, school, and professional community in ways that will help them in the quest to be a pediatric nurse and to continue to develop their leadership skills?

INTRODUCTION

The number of career options and paths within nursing is staggering. Some of these options are the "traditional" and highly valued roles nurses have performed for years—providing direct care to patients, leading teams or organizations, teaching, researching, providing public health or school health services, or working in an occupational field. Other options have emerged over the past decade, and new options continue to emerge. For example, current career choices include working with philanthropic organizations or insurance companies, working as a pharmaceutical company representative, assessing disability claims for government agencies, providing counselling, and taking on a political role. However, with career choices come challenges: how best to build a career, which education best serves the role, which experiences best prepare nurses for a specific field or role, and what new activities and roles need to be developed. Because a career extends over a lifetime, making choices can redirect a nurse's future. Some options build primarily on experience and others on education and experience; all, however, require that nurses engage in self-reflection, actively shape their education and overall professional development in ways that advance their capacity to meet evolving challenges

in health care. How nurses reach their career goals depends on knowing themselves, the context in which they learn and work, the goals they set, and how they manage their career development.

WHAT IS A CAREER?

A career is more than a job. A career is often described as one's chosen profession, path, or course of life work. The work we do and the roles we play both inside and outside our workplaces are all part of one's career. In today's world, the term *career* is seen as a continuous process of learning and development. Activities that contribute to pursuing and developing a rewarding career can include education, employment, work experience, community activities, volunteer work, and leisure activities.

Typically, careers can be described as passing through five stages. The first stage, *learning*, is an individual's introduction to a profession. It begins with the first learning experience and, if the learner is in a nursing program, it is primarily concerned with learning how to "become" a nurse, so your nursing career began the first day you started your nursing program! The second stage, the *entry* phase, begins when newly graduated nurses select their first workplace. It is when they explore their various employment options keeping in mind their career goals and/or the areas of practice they found were rewarding and a good fit with the strengths they developed over the course of their program. In the third stage, the *commitment* phase, early career nurses clarify identifying their likes and dislikes in terms of their professional practice options, location, and overall work–life balance. In the fourth stage, the *consolidation* phase, nurses become comfortable with their chosen career path and with their relationship between the personal and the professional dimensions of their career. This latter stage is distinguished by an individual's dedication to career, commitment to ongoing and continuous learning, and focus on making a contribution to the nursing profession, to health care and to society. In the fifth or *withdrawal* stage, nurses prepare for either taking on a new role in nursing and going back to the learning stage, or retirement where they begin to think about what might come after nursing.

Regardless of the stage one may be at in their career, career planning is a continuous process of visioning, self-assessment, and goal setting. It offers individuals the means to respond to both short- and long-term changes in their profession and in the health care system. The professional competencies required to engage in career planning, including a focus on leadership and management, are the same as those needed in their daily practice as part of planning and delivering quality patient care. Just as you develop care plans with and for your patients/clients, so too must you learn to design career plans for yourself.

There is no question that the twenty-first century brings a time of accelerated change, increased stress and life at a hastened pace. Nursing students enter a health care system that holds diverse and exciting opportunities for professional practice, and the number of career options and paths can be overwhelming. As you move through your academic and professional nursing career, your professional needs change, and your goals and plans evolve. Career planning is both important and useful at every stage of your academic and professional career. It is a dynamic process that changes and adapts to changes in you and in the world in which you live, learn, and work; it also requires reflective thought, insight, and intention. In this chapter, and the text more broadly, you will find a vast resource of information, scholarship, perspectives, and tips to help inform your career planning as a student and leader—but the one most important to your career development is *you*.

LEADING AND MANAGING YOUR CAREER

The Canadian Nurses Association (CNA) acknowledges that all nurses are leaders, including new students, new graduate nurses, and staff nurses. CNA describes the attributes of a nurse leader as being: an advocate for quality care, a collaborator, an articulate communicator, a mentor, a risk taker, a role model, and a visionary (CNA, 2017).

You may not envision yourself in a formal leadership position, but you still must lead yourself, which involves incorporating your identity as a leader into your sense of who you are and what you do. Every day we use leadership and management skills to navigate our world, whatever hat we are wearing—be it student, employee, volunteer, or other (Donner & Wheeler, 2009). You need these same skills to lead and manage your career so you will have a career in nursing by design not by drift. Let's take a closer look at these two concepts and skillsets.

Leadership is a way of being and exists independently of job title. Leaders are those individuals who are recognized by their peers and colleagues as visionaries who believe that others know what they want to do, are prepared to let them do it, and who act when the opportunity presents itself. Just think of some words that are used to describe effective leadership: self-awareness, visionary, risk taking, motivating, enabling, and inspiring. *Leading* your career requires that you create a vision of who and what you wish to be. Your vision allows you to "imagine what is possible, provides a purpose and insight as to what you need to achieve your dream" (Waddell et al., 2009, p. 6). Regardless of whether your vision focuses on a specific focus of nursing practice, a leadership position or a way of being, it serves as an inspiration and motivating guide for your involvement in your nursing education and your career.

> *"Vision without action is merely a dream. Action without vision just passes the time. Vision with action can change the world".*
>
> *(Joel Barker [n.d])*

You demonstrate leadership when you volunteer to join committees seeking student membership, for example your student body organization, committees within your school of nursing or academic institution, your professional association or within your personal community. You are a leader when you engage with student colleagues and faculty and work collaboratively to develop the structures and processes that will enable students at all levels of their education to grow and develop and be the best they can and want to be. And you are a leader when you mentor or coach student colleagues who are in earlier years of their nursing program, who are wanting to develop, enhance, and sustain their leadership skills within their educational experience. Your capacity to demonstrate leadership did not begin when you were admitted to your school of nursing; you came to your program with attitudes, skills, and behaviours and, if you are intentional in how you engage in curricular and extracurricular activities, you will have endless opportunities to build and lead your unique nursing career (see Chapter 32, *Nursing Students as Leaders* for exemplars of how nursing students have engaged in professional activities to build their leadership knowledge, attitudes and competencies).

Management in relation to your career requires that you take action in relation to your career vision, by making decisions and engaging in activities that enable you to achieve your vision. Setting goals and engaging in activities that allow you to progress toward your vision requires dedication and effective management. The same skills you use to organize your time and resources to achieve success in your academic work are also needed to make your career vision come to life.

Words used to describe management include problem-solving, decision-making, planning, delegation, communication, and time management. These words speak to the "how" of accomplishing the activities in which you need to engage to achieve the desired outcomes. For example, you might have an inspiring vision for your career but you also need knowledge and skills to actualize that vision. Just as you came to your program with leadership attitudes, skills, and behaviours, so did you bring your experience and attributes in the area of managing important elements of your life and work,

Chapters 1 and 3 of this text offer you valuable guidance as to the competencies required for effective leadership and management. Chapter 32 illustrates how your vision can guide your engagement in leadership and management activities and initiatives within your program and professional communities. Through your enhanced understanding of what is required to be effective leaders and managers, and your thoughtful and intentional involvement in your program and community, you will advance your own competencies in relation to both nursing leadership and management.

Furthermore, the leadership and management skills and attributes you use to develop and work toward your career vision are highly transferrable, typically acquired through a combination of education and life experience, and can be applied to a broad range of professional settings and situations.

THE DONNER-WHEELER CAREER PLANNING AND DEVELOPMENT MODEL (DONNER-WHEELER MODEL)

Career planning and development is a process. Iterative rather than linear, it requires individuals to understand the environment in which they live, learn, and work, assess their own strengths and limitations and validate that assessment, articulate their personal career vision, and develop a plan that will guide their activities now, and for the future, that is realistic for them, and then market themselves to help achieve that plan. Career planning and development is something you engage in as part of your everyday life as a student and as you transition into the role of registered nurse. Using a career planning and development model will guide your efforts to grow and develop as a professional and to begin to envision and work toward your unique nursing career throughout your academic program. The Donner-Wheeler Model presented in this chapter has been used to support the career planning development activities of undergraduate and graduate nursing students for over a decade and has been endorsed by the Canadian Nursing Students' Association (CNSA, 2018). It is also the only career planning and development model that has been tested through a rigorous research process for efficacy in supporting students' development of *career resilience* and self-efficacy within their nursing curriculum and 12-months postgraduation (see Research Perspectives box for the outcomes of this research).

The five phases of the Donner-Wheeler Model (Donner & Wheeler, 2009) are described in Fig. 31.1. Although you can begin at any phase, we have found over the years that students find it helpful to first create their career vision. Box 31.1 provides a guide to creating your vision as does the It's Your Career: Take Charge CPD Guide (https://careeraction.blog.ryerson.ca/). Use that vision to guide your self-assessment, which in turn helps you to identify your strengths and areas for development in relation to your ability to

RESEARCH PERSPECTIVE

Resource: Waddell, J., Spalding, K., Navarro, J., Caniza-res, G., Connell, M., Jancar, S., Stinson, J. & Watson, C. (2015). Integrating a career planning and development program into the baccalaureate nursing curriculum: part I. Impact on students' career resilience. *International Journal of Nursing Education Scholarship*, 24(1), 163–173; Waddell, J., Spalding, K., Navarro, J., Canizares, G., & Jancar, S. (2015). Integrating a career planning and development program into the baccalaureate nursing curriculum: part II. Outcomes for new graduate nurses 12 months post-graduation. *International Journal of Nursing Education Scholarship,* 24(1), 175–182.

Waddell et al. 2009 conducted a longitudinal, mixed-methods study of a curriculum-based career planning and development (CPD) program to determine the program's effects on participating students and new graduate nurses. Quantitative and qualitative study findings demonstrated the benefit of integrating career planning and development (aimed at enhancing career resilience) throughout all years of an undergraduate nursing curriculum. Across the program years, intervention group participants, through the facilitated use of the Donner-Wheeler Model (CPD), described being internally focused, self-directed, goal oriented, and confident in their ability to shape their academic experiences to help them achieve their career goals—all attributes associated with career resilience. Furthermore, students in the CPD intervention group reported higher career resilience at graduation than those in the control group.

Based on student findings, the authors concluded that, "situating the CPD process within participants' program years prompted them to consider how they could shape their work within each term to help them respond to their self-assessment and achieve their goals. Envisioning their ideal career motivated them to be creative and to dream" (Waddell et al., 2015, p. 167)

In contrast, control group participants reported experiences less illustrative of career resilience in that they indicated that they relied on others to help shape their career path and indicated they were less able to independently create their own career plan. They also indicated that their sense of uncertainty about their ability to engage in career planning was consistent across all years of their nursing program.

Implications for Practice

Results from both the student and new graduate nurse participants suggest that students at all stages of their academic preparation should be encouraged to engage in career planning and development. Imbedding CPD as a core element of undergraduate nursing education would offer students the opportunity to develop career self-management attitudes and skills, which in turn would engage them more meaningfully in their academic programs and foster a sense of career resilience, as they make the transition from student to registered nurse. Professional development for nurse educators to prepare them to fulfill the role of career mentors/coaches would foster a culture of career support for students across years of their program and as they begin their professional practice career.

"live" your vision now and as you progress in your program. The self-assessment process also gives you direction to look at opportunities and strategize as to how to shape your engagement in your curriculum to help you progress toward your unique vision. Even if your vision changes as you progress in your program—which is often the case for undergraduate nursing students—your strengths are transferable, and you can continue to build your knowledge, skills, and your professional values.

Attending to your professional and personal development within the context of your nursing program requires reflection as well as planning. The Donner-Wheeler Model offers an approach whereby you can get the most out of yourself, your nursing program, extracurricular activities, and your growing career. The

career planning process is really about the development of a life skill, one that you can apply in your professional life as a nursing student and registered nurse and in your personal life as well. Our professional and personal lives are intertwined. As one makes plans and develops in their personal life, the choices they make can influence their professional life and vice versa. It is all about values and self-awareness; what is important to you at various stages of your personal life should inform the decisions you make in your professional life, if you are to have a career that Fredric Hudson describes as a " a life expression of how a person wants to be in the world."

The following is a general overview of the model, and then a discussion of how you can apply this model to your role as a student.

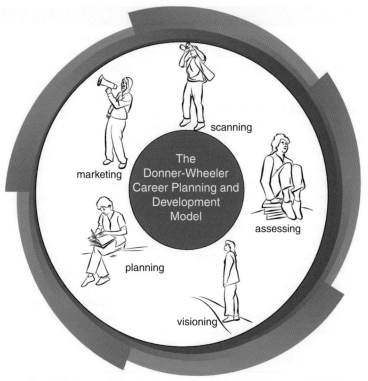

Fig. 31.1 Donner-Wheeler Career Planning and Development Model

VISIONING—WHAT DO I REALLY WANT TO BE DOING?

Your vision is your dream for your career. Who do you wish to be as a nurse? What do you wish to be doing? In what kind of workplace do you want to begin your career? What do you want for yourself and from your colleagues? To prepare you to practice as a registered nurse, your nursing curriculum includes many required courses and practice experiences aimed at helping you to develop core professional knowledge and competencies. Waddell et al. (2009) suggest that developing a career vision will help you to capitalize on your classroom and practice placement experiences in intentional and meaningful ways. Your vision can also help you to recognize and take advantage of an opportunity when it occurs. You can situate your vision to be at the time of graduation, or as an early career nurse. Your vision then guides your engagement in your curriculum, school, academic organization, and external communities in ways that are important to you and that help you to develop in areas that will foster your capacity to

actualize that vision. Furthermore, your program offers you continuous opportunities for new learning and growth so your vision may change frequently as you progress in your studies or it may remain consistent over time. Take time to revisit your vision at the beginning and end of each term of your program and revise/update it as necessary. See Box 31.1 for a guide to help you create your career vision. Write your current career vision down in as much detail as possible, and keep it in an electronic file or someplace where you can refer to it and reflect upon it on an ongoing basis. Your vision will be the foundation for your ongoing self-assessment, your scanning, and the continuous development of your career plan.

ASSESSING—WHO AM I? HOW DO OTHERS SEE ME?

Once you have completed your career vision, you are ready to begin your self-assessment. Just as your vision may shift and change over time, so will your self-assessment expand over time. A self-assessment is about

BOX 31.1   Visioning

You can access, It's Your Career: Take Charge CPD Guide (https://careeraction.blog.ryerson.ca/) visioning video for a guided career visioning exercise, or write your responses to each of the subsequent questions.

Questions to Guide Your Reflective Career Vision

- Imagine that you are leaving home to go to your perfect job in your perfect career. Before you head off for the day, turn and look at your home and reflect on who and what in your home allows you to go to work with such positive anticipation? Tuck that information away as you may need to draw on it, as you move through your day.
- As you make your way to this wonderful job, what are you most looking forward to as you begin your day?
- You are approaching the area in which you work—how would you describe it to someone who does not know you? Is it a building, a community, an office, a shared area, or somewhere you have never been but have always wanted to be?
- When you enter where your work is located, you are about to turn a corner, but before you make the turn, you hear a colleague of yours who is providing a bit of an orientation to a new person and just happens to

be describing you. Your colleague speaks of what the new person can expect from you as a colleague—what you contribute to the success of the work of those with whom you work, who you are as an individual, your strengths, and what makes you unique. You are delighted with what you hear and, just as you think your colleague has finished describing you, he/she uses a term or a word to describe you that surprises you—and you are humbled to know that your colleague has chosen such a descriptor. What descriptor has your colleague used that offers such a sense of pride?

- As you make your way through the day reflect on what your colleagues offer to you that allows you to be the best that you can be.
- What does your place of work provide you with that fosters your ability to use your strengths and build areas that you wish to further develop?
- It is time to go home—what are you most looking forward to as you end your day?

Keep this vision in mind as you review each of the chapters in the textbook and identify which leadership/management concepts/roles resonate with your vision

---

looking inside yourself. You would not consider developing a care plan without a thorough assessment, and so it does not make sense to develop your own career plan without a thorough self-assessment. With your unique career vision as your guide, reflect on the question "Who am I?" What are your professional and personal values, your knowledge, skills, your interests, and your accomplishments? Values are a set of beliefs, the principles, and ideals that guide and give meaning to our lives, our decisions, and our work. Knowledge is what we have learned through formal and informal education, and through work and life experiences. Skills are the abilities and behaviours we use to produce results—what we do, and interests are those things we like doing. An accomplishment is created when you go beyond what is expected; you have identified a challenge, applied a specific approach, and had a successful outcome. Which of your values, strengths, knowledge/skills, and accomplishments would allow you to "live" your career vision now? What are key areas for development that would enhance your ability to actualize your vision? Your self-assessment includes those values, knowledge, skills, interests, and accomplishments that you bring to your nursing

program and that you have strengthened and developed as a nursing student. With your self-assessment always in mind, you can engage in your courses to meet your unique needs for growth, in areas you have identified for development, and enrichment of those that you have identified as your strengths.

As with your career vision, the self-assessment process is not a one-time activity. At the end of each academic term, take the time to revisit your vision and reflect on what you have learned, the areas in which you have strengthened your development in areas of knowledge and practice competencies, the values that have guided your work, new professional values you have realized, and the accomplishments of which you are most proud.

"How do others see me?" is the critical next question. Careful career planning requires feedback, both formal and informal, from faculty, mentors, student colleagues, friends, and family. It involves listening and accepting positive feedback, acknowledging those areas where change is needed, and seeking advice about new knowledge and skills that you may require and how to develop them. When you seek feedback on elements of your

---

BOX 31.2 Self-Assessment

You may also refer to the It's Your Career: Take Charge CPD guide (https://careeraction.blog.ryerson.ca/) to complete your self-assessment.

Reflecting on Your Vision: Questions to Guide Your Self-Assessment

- What are the key values you hold that stand out in your vision?
- What are your key beliefs that are evident in your vision?
- What descriptor used by your colleague surprised you, and why?
- If you were able to "live" your vision tomorrow, what do you know are your key strengths that you hold, as you actualize your vision?
- What are areas that you wish/need to further develop to actualize your vision?

As you read each chapter in the textbook, reflect on how your areas of strengths align with different leadership and management roles, functions, responsibilities, and attributes. Add to your areas for development as you learn more about what is required for effective leadership and management behaviours/attitudes and impact. Chapter 32 provides exemplars of student leadership that you can use to help you identify strengths you might not have identified and areas of development that you may wish to add to your assessment, particularly as they relate to your career vision and, more specifically, to developing competencies in nursing leadership and management. If you are early in your program and have difficulty identifying your general areas of strength, you can begin with a more formal resource, such as the Clifton Strengths assessment (http://www.strengthsquest.com/help/general/142454/cliftonstrengths-assessment.aspx) or StrengthFinders 2.0 (http://strengths.gallup.com/110659/Homepage.aspx), both of which may provide you with some insight as to your personal strengths.

---

self-assessment in relation to your career vision, share your vision as well so that those who are serving as your "reality check", also know where you are wishing to go and who you are hoping to become. "Using your self-assessment to guide your participation in your curriculum will give you the confidence to find or create meaning in your current and future learning experiences" (Waddell et al., 2009, p. 25) (Box 31.2).

SCANNING—WHAT ARE THE CURRENT REALITIES AND FUTURE TRENDS?

An environmental scan is about looking outside yourself and into the world. With your current career vision and self-assessment in hand, you are ready to seek further information, to identify possible opportunities to build your career within your program and in the future.

We observe, learn about, and assess the world around us through reading, talking with others, and continuing our education, and through exposing ourselves not only to information and ideas from and about nursing and health care, but from other disciplines as well. Chapters and 2 and 10 are good places to start your scan, as they provide you with an overview of the Canadian Health Care System and Nursing in Canada. Your program offers you structured opportunities to gain an understanding of the current realities and possibilities in the health care system and the work environment, as well as the future global, national, and local trends inside and outside health care and within your profession. You also have faculty, preceptors, mentors, and student colleagues "at the ready" to help you become better informed, learn to see the world through differing perspectives, and to identify opportunities that align with your current and evolving vision of your career. All chapters of this textbook provide an "at your fingertips" scanning resource for current leadership and management theories, roles, expectations, and opportunities that may align with your career vision, self-assessment, and career planning activities.

As with your vision and self-assessment, your scan is a work in progress and can span many areas. For example, you can begin your scan by examining your curriculum (including elective courses) and the areas of expertise of the faculty and instructors within your academic setting to determine the courses and faculty/instructors with a focus on key areas within your career vision. Scanning your environment on an ongoing basis will ensure that your vision is responsive to your hopes, and dreams, as well as to the environment in which you hope to "live" that vision (Box 31.3).

PLANNING—HOW CAN I ACHIEVE MY CAREER GOALS?

A strategic career plan is a blueprint for action. Similar to a care plan, it consists of the identification of goals,

---

BOX 31.3 Scanning

You may also refer to the It's Your Career: Take Charge CPD Guide (https://careeraction.blog.ryerson.ca/) to help you with your environmental scan

Reflecting on Your Vision and Your Self-Assessment

- What opportunities are there available that would help me progress toward my career vision and help me grow in relation to my areas for development?
  - At my school?
  - At my academic organization?
  - At my placement?
  - In my community?
  - Other?
- What do I need to be aware of?
  - Important nursing, health, and social issues
  - Significant issues specific to the focus of my vision and self-assessment
  - Other?
- Who and what are my resources/supports?
  - My curriculum (course readings/assignments/placement opportunities
  - Faculty and staff members
  - Institutional career centre
  - Preceptors
  - Mentor(s)
  - Student colleagues
  - Professional organizations (CNSA, institutional student organizations, provincial and national professional organizations) community organizations

---

BOX 31.4 Finding a Mentor

Reflecting on Your Vision, Self-Assessment and Scan

- Who are possible mentors (person &/or professional role)?
  - At my school?
  - At my academic organization?
  - At my placement?
  - In my community?
  - Other?
- Why do I think they would be a good mentor(s)?
  - Area of expertise aligns with my vision
  - Admire their work
  - They are strong in areas I need to develop
  - Style and personality
  - Their connections
  - Other?

"How do I achieve my goals?" A strategic career plan is like a map outlining a series of specific goal-directed activities that, over time, will guide you to your destination, and is more effective when it is broken down into specific, manageable action steps. Do not forget to use your curricular and extracurricular activities, as well as your faculty and mentor(s) to help you work toward your goals. Refer to It's Your Career: Take Charge CPD Guide (https://careeraction.blog.ryerson.ca/) for further guidance regarding developing your career plan (Box 31.4). Also refer to Chapter 32 for exemplars of nursing student career plans.

MARKETING—HOW CAN I BEST MARKET MYSELF?

Marketing involves the ability to identify your professional and personal qualities, attributes, and expertise, so that you can effectively communicate what you have to offer and why you are the best person for the role you are seeking. Your work in developing a career vision and your self-assessment are foundational to your marketing. Marketing yourself is facilitated by making yourself visible, establishing a network, acquiring a mentor, and developing your written and verbal communication skills.

Throughout their daily interactions, individuals have many opportunities to present themselves to—and to influence—others. In fact, you began marketing yourself the day you began your nursing program. As we do this,

action steps, resources, timelines, and evaluation of success. By creating a career plan, you begin to move and to make decisions. As with your vision and self-assessment, it is important to write down your plan. Without a written version, it is easy to forget steps or fall out of sequence with the things that need to be achieved. A written plan also makes it much easier to continually review, reflect, refine, and reevaluate both your goals and your progress.

To begin, you need to set career goals. You may choose a combination of short-term and long-term goals to transform your career vision into a reality. Your goals will also be guided by your self-assessment, particularly your identified areas for development. Whatever goal you set, it should be realistic, desirable, and motivating. Once you have identified and written down your goals, you are ready to answer the question,

BOX 31.5 Social Media

How you engage online can have consequences, both positive and negative.

Research shows that a large percentage of employers use social networking sites to screen job applicants. Imagine for a moment you are one of these employers screening your online presence, what would they see? What digital footprint have you left for them to find? What is public facing?

Try signing out of your accounts on each of the social media websites and see what others see of your public profiles. If you are not happy with what you find, see what changes you can make to your profile to make it more private, or more public. Consider adding more public facing content that you feel better reflects the message you want to give employers.

Do a web search on yourself, what comes up? Is it even you? Could it be misleading to a potential employer about what you want them to know about you. Similar to social media, consider adding content if possible that is in line with what you want to be seen. If there is a large amount of content not related to you and that could be perceived as very negative, you may want to seek advice from others on how you can deal with that.

---

we create a certain image and send a particular message about who we are. In fact, you are your own best marketer, so before you begin to use all the other marketing tools and strategies available, consider the "product" that is you. Being successful in marketing ourselves is having the confidence in who we are and in what we want to do and projecting that to others.

You market yourself on paper through your resumé and cover letter, curriculum vitae (CV), business cards, and publications; in person through interviews, making presentations, acting as a mentor, and through your online communication (e.g., e-mail and text messages), profiles in your professional and social networks. See Boxes 31.5 and 31.6 for tips to consider in social media and e-mail communication.

A mentor can assist you with your marketing strategies. Many academic settings have a career centre or faculty advisors/coaches that you can access for assistance with developing a range of professional marketing strategies including resumé writing, interviewing, and within both professional and social media. Refer to the It's Your Career: Take Charge CPD (https://careeraction.blog.ryerson.ca/) guide for marketing tips and exemplars of professional marketing for examples of year- and program-specific examples of resumés/CV, interview tips, online marketing strategies, and worksheets).

Keep in mind that you also market yourself in your everyday communication with your peers, faculty members, staff, preceptors, and clients. In addition to the suggestions included in Boxes 31.5 and 31.6, you can refer to tips for online marketing in the It's your Career: Take Charge CPD guide (https://careeraction.blog.ryerson.ca/).

What if graduate education is needed for you to actualize your career vision?

You may have had a longstanding desire to pursue graduate studies following completion of your undergraduate nursing program, or your career vision may highlight graduate education as a requisite to actualizing your vision. In either case, there are important questions for you to consider, data to gather, people to speak with, and decisions to make so that you can engage in your graduate program and as a registered nurse in ways that position you for success in gaining entry to the right graduate program for you. The Donner-Wheeler Model will help you to reflect on questions, such as how to find the right graduate program that aligns with your interests and needs, the types of questions you should be asking and who you should be seeking to respond to your questions, and how to position yourself for success in securing entry into the program of your choice.

A strategic career plan devoted specifically to the pursuit of graduate studies will help you move from the idea to an action plan. Begin by reflecting on why you want to embark on graduate studies and on your specific goals related to graduate work. Knowing what is important to you right now and blending that with your long-term goal for your nursing career guides you as you research the options.

(Waddell, 2005, p. 30)

For further discussion regarding how to choose the graduate program that best fits your need, refer to the article by Waddell (2005) included in the reference list for this chapter.

LITERATURE PERSPECTIVE

Resource: Sultana, R.G. (2012) Learning career management skills in Europe: a critical review. *Journal of Education and Work* 25 (2), 225–248.

This paper focused on the lifelong acquisition of career management skills (CMS) and how these skills are promoted and developed through career guidance in education and labour markets across a number of countries. Two surveys were completed by delegates from 14 countries. Together, the surveys focused on the definition of CMS, how, when, and by whom CMS was taught in education and employment services, how CMS is fostered within specific groups. The definition that evolved from these surveys was, "career management skills refer to a whole range of competencies which provide structured ways for individuals and groups to gather, analyze, synthesize and organize self, educational and occupational information, as well as the skills to make and implement decisions and transitions" (p. 229). The authors noted that, in essence, CMS helps people to develop resources and competencies to better manage their "life course" (p. 229). CMS programs, included in the education system, include themes that the Canadian Blueprint for Life/Work Designs Framework (Jarvis, 2003) groups into the three categories (personal management, exploring learning and work, and work/life building). These categories reflect the ability to understand oneself in making decisions about education and career paths, as well as self-efficacy. The rationale for promoting CMS within curricula is to help students to become confident and competent in planning and managing their education, as well as enhancing the capacity for students and new graduates to be successful in a changing world of work. The importance of context in CMS education, both in terms of the location of educational institutions and the labour market, is emphasized, as is the importance of curricular frameworks in the development of CMS. Survey data and analyses also indicated that is a need for evidence to support that CMS education does indeed improve employability, particularly during transitions, for example, that experienced by students as they move from student to registered nurses. The need for teachers to be trained to develop and implement CMS programs is also recommended. The author also emphasizes that students often come to their education programs with employment and other experiences and, as such, have developed insights, knowledge, skills, and attitudes, which foreground their ability to be confident in what they know and to build on their strengths and areas of development through ongoing self-reflection.

Implications for Practice

Survey findings from this study reinforce the value of developing CMS knowledge and competencies for students to develop the capacity to actively and strategically engage in their education, and make informed decisions, both within their curricula and as they transition to the workplace. The efficacy of such education is enhanced through the use of a framework and by educators who are qualified to develop and implement career education. When these elements are in place and are responsive to the context in which they are situated, students have the opportunity to develop confidence and competence in making and implementing informed, relevant, and meaningful career decisions.

CONCLUSION

Now you have an understanding of the role and importance of career planning and development in shaping your engagement throughout your nursing education and how the Donner-Wheeler Model can guide your career planning, at all at stages of your academic and professional practice career. Regularly evaluating how your career planning activities are working for you will help you determine which phases of the model need more attention, updating, or consultation and support. The chapters in this book are valuable resources to help you to achieve your career goals. As previously noted, Chapter 32 is an excellent resource for exemplars of nursing students who have engaged in career planning and development within their nursing program to build their capacity as leaders and managers.

BOX 31.6 Ten Tips for E-Mails

1. **Think before you type:** Avoid being too casual in your communication. Take the time to organize your thoughts, decide the purpose of the communication, then be clear and polite. Check your e-mail again before sending. In situations requiring particular care, it may be useful to ask a trusted colleague to read the note for tone before you send it.

2. **Use a precise subject line:** The subject line reinforces your message and helps the receiver manage your request.

3. **Use a greeting and closing:** Avoid being too casual. Use formal greetings like "Dear Dr. Grant" or "Dear Sarah" and formal closings like "Sincerely," or "Regards," for communications outside of your organization. Even when communicating within your organization, use greetings like "Hello Jim," and closings that are more casual but do not imply overfamiliarity.

4. **Use standard punctuation, capitalization, spelling, and grammatical form:** Your work may look sloppy and your message may be misunderstood or ignored if difficult to read. Using good paragraph structure helps readability. When you change ideas, change paragraphs; one-sentence paragraphs are acceptable in e-mails.

5. **Avoid using words in all capital letters:** Words written in ALL CAPS are considered "yelled" in e-mail etiquette and should not be part of business communication.

6. **Copy only those necessary:** Most people now receive too many e-mails, so include only those necessary in any recipient list. Doing so will help ensure that your e-mail is preserved as important to read and not simply viewed as creating unnecessary work for others.

7. **Use "reply all" judiciously:** E-mail has created additional workload for almost all who use it, so be sure that those included in any communication *must* be included before using the "reply all" option.

8. **Never include confidential or embarrassing information:** E-mails can too easily be forwarded, with or without intent, and can be permanently stored.

9. **Avoid fancy fonts and formatting:** Not all fonts, formatting, or backgrounds are easily recognized by other systems or after an e-mail transmission. Avoid hard-to-read coloured or fancy fonts, background patterns, and pictures.

10. **If another form of communication is better suited or saves time, use it:** E-mail is not always the best form of communication. Know its limitations and disadvantages.

From Gaertner-Johnston, L. (n.d.). Email etiquette: 25 quick rules. Retrieved from http://www.syntaxtraining.com/PDF/Rules_of_Email_Etiquette.pdf.

A SOLUTION

How can Hazel engage in their nursing curriculum, school and professional community in ways that will help them in the quest to be a pediatric nurse and to continue to develop their leadership skills?

To further engage in their nursing curriculum, school, and professional communities to further develop her pediatric practice competencies Hazel should consider:

- developing their unique career vision related to pediatric nursing practice
- explore the nursing practice competencies for pediatric nursing practice
- explore the nursing practice competencies for complex long term care nursing practice
- compare the competencies required for pediatric and long term care practice
- determine what are common competencies for both areas of nursing practice
- completing a self-assessment guided by their vision and what they have discovered in their scan of nursing competencies for both pediatric and long term care practice
- based on their vision and self-assessment, determine who can serve as their reality check and why they have identified this/these individuals
- the scope of Hazel's plan can include:
  - to further knowledge base of nursing practice competencies required for both areas of practice

- possibilities for a mentor(s) who could inform and support the career vision and shaping engagement in the program to position for success in relation to her vision
- develop career plan for coming year (focus on competency development responsive to the vision)

To further engage in their nursing curriculum, school, and professional communities, to further develop leadership skills Hazel should consider:

- developing a second career vision specific to their desire to further enhance the leadership
- based on their vision, complete a comprehensive leadership focused self-assessment
- based on their vision and self-assessment, meet with the school CNSA representative to discuss options for engagement in more formal leadership activities within the school

For both practice and leadership visions/assessment/plans, Hazel may also speak with a mentor/faculty advisor for guidance and feedback.

Would this be a suitable plan for you? Why or why not? Reflecting on this scenario, consider other strategies that Hazel may employ to assist them in participating in their program, to help them develop key competencies responsive to their nursing practice goals, and their wish to expand their leadership experience and strengths.

THE EVIDENCE

Waddell et al. (2009) reported that the curriculum-based CPD intervention continued to have a positive impact on intervention participants, 12-months postgraduation, who reported attitudes and behaviours consistent with ongoing career resilience. For example, graduates reported that they felt able to respond positively to their work environments, adapt to ever-changing workplaces, and to engage in self-directed opportunities for professional growth and development. Furthermore, intervention participants reported continued use of the CPD model, particularly the career visioning, to engage in ongoing development of their personal career goals and plans.

In contrast, the authors reported that findings from the control group suggested that this group of new graduates sought external support and described a primary focus on achieving clinical competence within their current role. The authors suggested that with a singular focus on the here and now, "NGNs without a strong sense of career resilience may be more vulnerable to the challenges and stress that typify the transition from student to registered nurse" (Waddell et al., 2015, p. 180).

✳ NEED TO KNOW NOW

- Your current vision for your career
- Your strengths and areas for development in relation to your vision
- Who you will choose to provide your reality check
- What to include in your environmental scan
- Your plan for building on your strengths and advancing in your areas for improvement
- Who and what can help you to go forward with your plan
- Ideas for effective marketing

CHAPTER CHECKLIST

- Use of the Donner-Wheeler Career Planning and Development Model, presented in this chapter, fosters students' ability to take advantage of meaningful and career enhancing experiences within their classrooms, nursing programs, and both academic and practice settings.
- Developing the knowledge and skills necessary for career resilience is a process that students can engage in as early as the first year of their nursing program.
- Developing career resilience, through active engagement in career planning and development, allows students to build their careers in meaningful ways—beginning in the first year of their academic program.
- Students can use their dreams, their academic and practice environments, self-knowledge, and intentional planning to achieve their career goals within and across the roles of practitioners, leaders, and managers.
- Effective marketing is a key professional competence

TIPS FOR LEADING AND MANAGING YOUR CAREERS

- **Tip One: Know your why**—your purpose for being—and then be passionate about what you do and demonstrate it every day. That is what leadership is all about. Ask yourself "Why did I choose nursing, why am I here?" In answering these questions, you will develop a clearly articulated purpose, then embrace and commit to your career in nursing.
- **Tip Two: Keep your dream alive**! Your career vision is the dream that will sustain you and keep you moving forward. Over the span of your academic and professional career, you will have dreams that at times may feel unachievable. Do not give up. Keep your vision updated, use your program and resources strategically, stay connected to your network, and keep scanning the environment for opportunities that will help you to "live" your vision.
- **Tip Three: If you think opportunity may be behind the door, open it.** Your success rests on active career management at all stages of your career and the ability to adapt to your environment. Often, we look at the success of others and wonder how they got there, and why we have not yet arrived at where we wish to be.

What makes the difference, is the ability to recognize opportunity, have confidence in your own potential, and be able to communicate your career vision and what you have to offer. Self-awareness, situational awareness, and self-confidence can be developed and must be nurtured. It is what gives us the courage to take risks and be truly open to opportunities.

- **Tip Four: To realize your dream, you need to learn from both success and failure.** Always remember to acknowledge and celebrate your successes and accomplishments, both big and small. Find opportunities that maximize your strengths and limit the probability of failure. If you are turned down for an opportunity, take the time to ask why you were unsuccessful. Do not fear failure—embrace it—we can learn a lot from our failures, as much as our successes.

- **Tip Five: Ensure you have good supports in place.** Surround yourself with individuals who can encourage you along your career journey. Tap into faculty, mentors, student colleagues, and family, those that are positive influencers who can listen, ask good questions, and provide feedback, especially when you feel uncertain about taking a risk. Make your needs known. The more you reach out and articulate what you need, the easier it is for others to help you.

Visit the Evolve website for Suggested Readings, Internet Resources, and additional resources related to the content in this chapter: http://evolve.elsevier.com/Canada/Yoder-Wise/leading/.

REFERENCES

Barker, Joel. (n.d.) Retrieved from: https://www.brainyquote.com/quotes/joel_a_barker_158200.

Canadian Nurses Association (CAN). (2018). *Leadership*. Retrieved from: https://www.cna-aiic.ca/en/nursing-practice/the-practice-of-nursing/health-human-resources/leadership.

Donner, G., & Wheeler, M. (2009). *Taking control of your career: A handbook for health professionals*. Toronto: Elsevier.

Sultana, R. G. (2012). *Learning career management skills in europe: a critical review*.

Waddell, J., Donner, G. J., & Wheeler, M. (2009). *Building your nursing career: A guide for students* (3rd ed.). Toronto: Elsevier.

Waddell, J., Donner, G. J., & Wheeler, M. (2011). *Building your nursing career: A guide for students* (3rd ed.).

Retrieved from: http://cnsa.ca/publication/building-your-nursing-career-3rd-edition-a-guide-for-students.

Waddell, J., Spalding, K., Navarro, J., Canizares, G., & Jancar, S. (2015). Integrating a career planning and development program into the baccalaureate nursing curriculum: Part II. Outcomes for new graduate nurses 12 months post-graduation. *International Journal of Nursing Education Scholarship, 24*(1), 175–182.

Waddell, J., Spalding, K., Navarro, J., Canizares, G., Connell, M., Jancar, S., et al. (2015). Integrating a career planning and development program into the baccalaureate nursing curriculum: Part I. Impact on students' career resilience. *International Journal of Nursing Education Scholarship, 24*(1), 163–173.

Waddell, J. (2005). Choosing the right graduate program. *Canadian Nurse, 101*(5), 30–31.

32

Nursing Students as Leaders

Annita Velasque Moreira, BA, BScN, Ryerson University
Genevieve Armstrong, RN, BScN, MN; Ryerson University

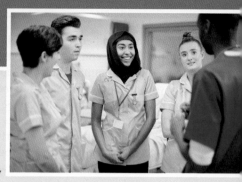

Nursing school can provide students with many relevant opportunities to develop their leadership skills. Students can become engaged in their own career planning, take a leadership role within their academic community, get involved in research projects and participate in professional practice initiatives. In this chapter, we explore student leadership through the lens of four domains: Career Planning and Development, Academic Community, Research Engagement and Professional Practice. As nursing students and recent alumni, we have reflected on our own experiences and have shared our personal trajectories with you through the stories of three students in our case scenarios. Each student's trajectories will evolve throughout the chapter, as we tell the story of how they intentionally enhanced their leadership capacity within the identified domains. In each section, we propose exercises to help you think about your own leadership knowledge and competencies and how they can be applied to your academic trajectory.

OBJECTIVES

- Describe the four domains of Career Planning and Development, Academic Community, Research Engagement, and Professional Practice.
- Identify leadership strategies students can build upon and apply in the four interrelated domains.
- Examine how leadership can be developed and actualized by students through critical analysis of three student case scenarios.

- Demonstrate how students can assume a variety of leadership roles in their undergraduate nursing programs and as new graduate nurses.
- Describe different trajectories and experiences in student leadership engagement through real life narratives.

TERMS TO KNOW

academic community
advocacy
career planning and development

interprofessional collaboration
network
professional practice

research engagement
student leadership
student-led initiatives

❓ A CHALLENGE

Angela, Toby, and Shaneika are nursing students in different stages of a 4-year Baccalaureate Nursing Degree Program. They are all interested in developing their leadership skills and would like to engage with their academic communities. They each face individual challenges in achieving their goals. Angela is in their second year of the program and is interested in taking on leadership roles. However, they are insecure about their ability to balance new responsibilities with their academic commitments. Toby has been involved

in formal leadership roles, however, would like to take a step down. They are unsure how to transition from a formal student leadership role to engagement in informal student-led initiatives. Shaneika is starting their first nursing job after graduation, and simply doesn't know how to start engaging with leadership within their organization. They feel unprepared because they are a novice nurse and lack previous leadership experience. Follow the journeys of Angela, Toby, and Shaneika throughout the chapter (Box 32.1).

INTRODUCTION

Nursing leadership has the potential to promote great change, from improving the lives of individual patients to advancing the quality of health care systems. Nursing students should be introduced early on to the possibilities that leadership can bring to their academic and professional careers. In this chapter, we introduce four domains of student leadership in nursing. The domains are areas in which we believe students have the greatest potential to grow as leaders and foster skills that they will carry into their nursing practice upon graduation. Read on to learn about the four domains of student leadership: Career Planning and Development, Academic Community, Research Engagement, and Professional Practice.

BOX 32.1   Case Scenarios

Meet Angela, Toby, and Shaneika. They are nursing students and new graduates who are at different stages of their leadership journeys! We acknowledge there are different structures of nursing curricula across Canada. The following case scenarios refer to a 4-year bachelor's degree in nursing. However, the experiences described are applicable to all nursing students in any type of nursing program.

Second Year Nursing Student—Angela

Angela is in their second year of a bachelor's degree in Nursing at a university in a large city. Their first year was a period of adaptation to the new demands of being an undergraduate student. Now they feel ready to explore extracurricular activities and opportunities outside of the classroom. After completing a course in nursing research, they realize they are interested in pursuing a position as a research assistant. Angela is also interested in student advocacy and is considering applying to a position with the Canadian Nursing Students' Association (CNSA) chapter at their school. They are concerned that taking on too many responsibilities could become a challenge, however they are enthusiastic about engaging with their school community and developing their leadership skills.

Challenge: Angela is ready to take on leadership roles but is insecure about their ability to balance new responsibilities with their academic commitments.

Reflective exercise:

(1) Angela feels ready to take on new challenges but is hesitant to sign up for too many responsibilities. Have you ever felt like that?

(2) What strategies could Angela employ to feel comfortable adding commitments to their schedule?

Fourth Year Nursing Student—Toby

Toby is a fourth-year undergraduate nursing student in their final semester at a university in a mid-size city. They have been involved as a formal student leader with the CNSA chapter in their school for the past 2 years. Now in their fourth year, they wish to pursue their own student-led initiatives. However, they are unsure if they can do that without a formal leadership role. Among other initiatives, Toby is interested in creating a research interest group at their school.

Challenge: Toby is no longer interested in a formal student leadership role, however they would still like to engage in student-led initiatives. They are not sure how to make this happen, once they are no longer with the CNSA.

Reflective exercise:

(1) Have you ever considered the differences between formal and informal leadership roles?

(2) Who could Toby speak to about beginning their own student-led initiative?

New Graduate Nurse—Shaneika

Shaneika recently graduated from an undergraduate nursing program at a university located in an urban setting. As a novice nurse, they are enthusiastic about contributing to nursing outside of their everyday work. However, they feel intimidated to become active in leadership roles and activities given their limited nursing experience. They were not involved in leadership-related initiatives as a student but were able to take lead of their career and obtain a competitive public health nurse position. They are interested in joining committees within and external to their department.

Challenge: Shaneika is keen to participate in leadership activities but does not know how to and where they should start. They feel unprepared because they are a novice nurse and lack previous leadership experience.

Reflective exercise:

(1) Do you feel unprepared to become engaged in leadership?

(2) What knowledge and skills can Shaneika bring to future leadership activities based upon their previous clinical and academic experiences?

Career Planning and Development

As described in by Waddell and Wheeler in Chapter 31, career planning and development is an iterative process that students may use to develop leadership skills and can assist them in achieving their career goals. Student leadership requires skills that encompass creating a vision, knowing where to go and how to get there, identifying common goals, developing plans, establishing collaborative relationships, and being aware of the strengths and weaknesses of oneself and others. The career planning and development process can help students not only to take leadership of their own careers but also to better lead others. This process may also help student leaders to build and establish a nursing network, foster their professional development, and help in successfully searching for student leadership opportunities.

A longitudinal study conducted by Waddell et al. (2015) examined the impact of the Donner-Wheeler Career Planning and Development (CPD) Model adapted for students and new graduate nurses on career resilience among undergraduate nursing students. Participants in the intervention group self-reported higher career resilience and decision-making self-efficacy than participants in the control group. At 12-months postgraduation, participants were able to seek and build effective and reciprocal relationships with their peers, colleagues, and mentors; use a strategic and proactive approach to their career; and actively seek out professional development activities (Waddell et al., 2015). Overall, results of this study provided evidence that curriculum can positively enhance a student's academic experience, which in turn may lead to a satisfying and fulfilling nursing career.

In the preceding chapter, you were introduced to the Donner-Wheeler Career Planning and Development Model. In this chapter, we will employ this particular model to illustrate how each phase can guide your unique growth as a student leader across all years of your nursing program.

Academic Community

Students, faculty, and staff are all important members of the nursing academic community, all of whom work toward the same goal of creating the next generation of nurses. Students are a vital part of this community. They share unique challenges and experiences throughout their academic journey. Through leadership in the school of nursing, students have an opportunity to learn how to contribute meaningfully to their community. They can engage in various activities, such as being a part of official student groups, organizing events, and leading advocacy endeavours. Students leaders also play important roles in advancing nursing education, by influencing schools to respond to ever-changing nursing work environments. Students who take on leadership roles and/or participate in leadership activities at school will learn valuable lessons in communication, advocacy, conflict management, collaboration, and team dynamics, which can be carried into their nursing careers.

Research Engagement

Students' participation in research has become more important than ever. Nursing practice is heavily weighted upon evidence-informed practice, therefore it is critical for students not only to understand the research process but also to engage in and with research. Engaging in research does not end upon completing a nursing research course. It is a continual process in one's nursing career. Nurses in all areas take part in research. By participating in research, students cultivate strong interpersonal skills, advance critical thinking competencies, and better understand the research process. These skills may all contribute to becoming an effective student leader.

Students can develop leadership skills through research engagement in a multitude of ways. Taking on research assistant positions and participating as a student representative on their university's research ethics board are some of them. Coyne and colleagues (2018) described a comprehensive approach to undergraduate nursing students' research experiences. Their study highlighted the impact of three university initiatives that positively influenced undergraduate nursing students. They increased their knowledge of nursing research and learned the importance of applying research to their practice. Participants highly valued their nursing research course and, 1 year after graduation, indicated that they planned to pursue further education (Coyne et al., 2018). Research engagement can not only enhance student's leadership skills but can positively impact their overall academic experience.

Professional Practice

In the clinical and professional practice environment, students learn and shape what kind of nurse they wish to become. It is also where they have the opportunity to get involved in leadership and develop leadership skills, including teamwork, interprofessional collaboration, and advocacy. Pepin and colleagues (2011) identified five learning stages of clinical nursing leadership for students. The first stage is being aware of leadership in nursing, which is the goal of this book.

Next, students must apply leadership to their routine professional practice (Pepin et al., 2011). They can do so by participating in professional development initiatives, taking the lead in learning opportunities, modelling effective followership, and advocating for various groups, including patients. In professional practice, students are also exposed to current issues in health care, and learn about the context in which they will practice as nurses in the future. This knowledge is fundamental to becoming effective nurse leaders upon graduation.

LEADERSHIP DOMAIN: CAREER PLANNING AND DEVELOPMENT

Given the complexities and challenges of an ever-changing health care system, competitive job markets, and fiscal constraints, it is important for you to begin the career planning and development process as soon you begin your nursing program. Engaging in career planning and development will help in achieving your personal career and leadership related goals. You can also apply the process of the Donner Wheeler CPD Model with a dedicated focus on your unique leadership development through finding, creating, and engaging in leadership initiatives in your school, academic, and professional communities. This process is explained subsequently.

Scanning

Conduct environmental scans of your academic and clinical placement environments to learn about the leadership opportunities available. Scanning is a great way to examine who and what is out there, and it will better equip you to capitalize on leadership opportunities when they arise. Your academic and clinical environments can be scanned in numerous ways. Here are a few tips.

Connect with your peers and faculty within and external to your nursing program. You will learn what programs, interest groups, committees, councils, initiatives, and student-related activities are happening and about what you are interested in joining. Speak to your preceptors or mentors about student leadership and different ways you may become engaged in your

clinical placements or in the community. Seek information online through organizational websites and formal student groups, such as the Canadian Nurses Student Association (CNSA).

Scanning is a life-long skill that will continue to be useful not only during your academic career but also when you work as a registered nurse.

> **EXERCISE 32.1** When conducting an environmental scan, reflect upon the following questions:
> 1. What kind of leadership opportunities and positions are available in your academic and clinical placement settings?
> 2. Who could you speak to about student leadership opportunities?
> 3. What attributes and skills do you require to lead?
> 4. How can you engage in student leadership without being in a formal leadership position?

Assessing

Continually assessing your personal strengths and areas for development is essential to student leadership. Being self-aware of these aspects can help you maximize your personal strengths and explore strategies to further develop and grow.

Student leadership also entails the ability to assess the strengths and weaknesses of your peers, and examine ways in which teamwork and collaboration can be fully realized. This is just as important as being aware of your own. Knowing what someone does best comes in handy when leading a team, as you can allocate work to capitalize on what your team members are best at. It is a great motivational booster for the team, and it helps you to achieve your collective goals more easily.

You should also assess your personal values and beliefs. That way, you will be able to focus on and build your capacity to establish better rapport and trusting relationships with your peers and others. Being able to work effectively within a team and having strong interpersonal skills are all essential to student leadership.

Conduct a self-assessment by finding a quiet space and engage in reflective practice. Be honest about yourself and write down your personal strengths and areas for development. Seek verbal or written feedback from your peers, faculty, friends, and family. As you continue to professionally develop and grow, you will conduct self-assessments regularly throughout your academic and nursing career. Why not start practicing now? Refer to Chapter 31 for a more in-depth look into the career planning process.

EXERCISE 32.2 When conducting a self-assessment, consider the following questions:

1. What are your personal values and beliefs about leadership?
2. What knowledge, traits, and skills related to leadership do you have?
3. What are your strengths?
4. What are your areas for development?
5. What would your peers, faculty, friends, and family say about your ability to lead?
6. What knowledge, skills, and attributes do you need to become the leader you envision?

Visioning

Let your imagination take you for a ride! Visioning is taking a blank canvas and painting a picture of how you envision yourself as a leader. It allows you to reflect upon different styles of leadership, leadership roles and activities, and nurse leaders.

Imagining and creating a vision will help you to identify the type of leader you wish to become. Find a quiet space, let your imagination run wild, and write down your vision. It will continually evolve and develop as you progress through your academic trajectory and learn more about yourself. Visit the *It's Your Career: Take Charge* online program for a guided visioning exercise.

EXERCISE 32.3 When creating your vision reflect upon the following questions:

1. Who are nursing leaders, nurses, and peers that inspire you, and what qualities and attributes do they exhibit?
2. Who do you aspire to be like?
3. What kind of leader do you envision yourself to be?
4. What types of extracurricular activities would you be interested in participating in?
5. Who do you want to lead, and how can you lead them?
6. What issues and challenges are you interested in making a difference in?
7. How would you like to contribute to your academic community?

Planning

Once you create a vision, you need to develop a strategic plan to help guide you in achieving your leadership goals. Your plan should include your short- and long-terms goals, the types of leadership activities you would like to engage in, resources you may use, timelines, and indicators of success.

Short-terms goals are those you would like to achieve in the next 3 to 6 months. Perhaps, you are interested in peer mentoring new undergraduate nurses within the next few months. Long-terms goals are those you would like to attain throughout your academic trajectory. Maybe you are thinking of running for presidency for the CNSA during the final year of your nursing program. Short-term goals can also be stepping stones to achieving your long-terms goals. To become president of the CNSA, you may have to strategically plan short-term goals that may help you to become a favourable candidate.

Keep in mind, your strategic plan may and will most likely change over time. That's okay! Be flexible. Flexibility is also key to being an effective student leader as things may not necessarily go as planned. For an example of a strategic plan see Table 32.1.

EXERCISE 32.4 When developing your strategic plan, consider the following questions:

1. What are your short- and long-term goals?
2. Are there any particular leadership roles you are interested in?
3. What types of leadership related activities would you like to participate in?
4. What resources do you need to achieve your goals?
5. When would you like to achieve your goals by?
6. How do you know you have achieved your goals?

Marketing

Marketing yourself is an integral part of career planning and development. If you wish to engage in student leadership you need to be able to articulate and demonstrate your knowledge, skills, and vision. You should also be able to convince your peers and others of what makes you a good and effective leader. Strategies you can take include establishing a nursing network, seeking out a mentor or coach, developing a resumé, and taking workshops to improve public speaking skills. See Chapter 31 for resources on marketing.

TABLE 32.1 Example of Strategic Plan

Short-Term Goal	Resources	Deadline	Indicator of Success
To learn about leadership opportunities within the School of Nursing	• Peers • Faculty • School of Nursing website • Student organization website (CNSA)	1 month	I will be able to describe different leadership opportunities within the School of Nursing

Establish a Nursing Network

Attend and participate in social and academic events within your school. Keep attuned to your university e-mail for upcoming events, workshops, and opportunities. Go to events prepared. Bring your business card with you, and get to know your faculty and peers. Find out what their nursing interests are, what type of leadership activities they may be involved in. Develop a 2-minute speech that best summarizes you. By having an established nursing network, you will start building your credibility.

> **EXERCISE 32.5** If you met a nursing leader who inspired you, what would you ask them?

Take Advantage of Social Media

Social media can work for or against you. The good news is, it is entirely under your control. Take advantage of this by making sure that all your social media channels reflect your desired professional image. For example, be mindful of what you post, who is able to view it, and review your privacy settings. Although it is not mandatory, social media can be a great platform to market yourself professionally. Create a professional blog, join LinkedIn, or use twitter to share professional content.

> **EXERCISE 32.6** If you use social media, do you know what your privacy settings are? Have you ever googled your name? Do you read any nursing blogs that inspire you?

Find a Mentor

A mentor is someone you look up to, inspires you, and guides and supports you in your academic trajectory and beyond. It may be a faculty member, preceptor, clinical instructor, new graduate from your program, or a peer. Before looking for a mentor, think about what you would like in a mentor. What leadership traits and qualities should they possess? What are their nursing interests, and do they align with yours? What knowledge and expertise do they hold? What kind of student leadership activities are they involved in? Do your research. Faculty members will often have an online biography on the university website. Some academic settings have peer mentorship programs. Speak with preceptors who inspired you. Having a mentor can be highly beneficial so begin your search now!

> **EXERCISE 32.7** Think about nurses who have inspired you. Would you consider asking them to become your mentor?

Highlight Student Leadership in Your Resumé

When developing your resumé, highlight your knowledge, skills, and experience that are relevant to student leadership. For example, identify student leadership activities you were or are involved in and describe what role you played. Perhaps you helped organize a workshop at your school, or you were an active member on a committee. Emphasize this in your resume. Describe what makes you a good student leader. Skills that you should focus on include your ability to develop relationships with others and work interprofessionally, your capacity to solve problems and deal with conflict, presentation and public speaking skills, and program planning and evaluation. You can find great examples of year specific resumes, cover letters, online marketing, and other strategies in the It's Your Career: Take Charge online program.

> **EXERCISE 32.8** Write down the knowledge, skills, and experience related to student leadership that you have gained over the course of your academic trajectory. What makes you unique? What makes you a good student leader?

Professional Development

Participating in professional development activities, such as workshops and educational training, can contribute to the development of your leadership skills. Consider learning about the following topics: leadership principles, emotional intelligence, interprofessional collaboration, conflict management, building your credibility, and program planning and evaluation.

Developing skills in these areas will help you become an effective student leader. You can learn about different professional development activities by visiting organizational websites, such as those of your nursing school, the CNSA, your course union, and your provincial, territorial, or national professional nursing association. Ask your peers, professors, clinical instructors, or preceptors about events and workshops that they have participated in on topics that may be of interest to you. Look for online modules on student leadership. Stay in the know! Subscribe to your school's and professional nursing organization's newsletter and join their electronic mailing list.

Searching for Leadership Opportunities

Take initiative and learn about the different student leadership activities that are happening both within your academic setting and in the community. You can do this by speaking with your faculty, peers, preceptors, and clinical instructors. Even asking a faculty member a simple question, such as, "What kind of student leadership activities are you aware of in our school?" can open new doors. Pay attention to flyers that are posted on bulletin boards in your school. You can find lots of information about diverse activities and initiatives that are happening. Be informed of different ways you can be involved in nursing through your provincial professional nursing and formal student organizations. For example, there may be interesting committees and councils to join. Speak to your peers who have been or are on a committee to learn more about their roles, experiences, and the application process. Perhaps you are interested in an initiative that you learned about during one of your clinical placements, talk to your preceptor about ways you can contribute and be involved. Not only would you be contributing to the unit and organization, you will also be building your nursing network outside of your academic setting. Double bonus! As you know, you can also find plenty of information online.

Next, see how Angela, Toby, and Shaneika used career planning and development to address their individual leadership challenges (Box 32.2).

LEADERSHIP DOMAIN: ACADEMIC COMMUNITY

Students are a vital part of the nursing school community, which makes their contributions ever more important. Student leadership within the school of nursing can take many shapes and influence different aspects of the academic environment. Here are some of ideas on how you can become involved!

Participating in An Official Student Leadership Group

The most common way of getting involved as a student is by joining a leadership group, such as your local CNSA chapter, or the nursing students' union (NSU). Groups like these are attuned to students' needs and have an important role in advocacy within the school of nursing. They also organize educational and social events that foster a sense of community among students.

> **EXERCISE 32.9** Are you aware of student leadership groups within your school of nursing? Do you know what they do? Do you know any students who are a part of a leadership group? Explore how you can get involved!

There are usually two ways to join student leadership groups: elections and applications. Both processes require that you explain your rationale for joining. A position as a student leader is a chance to contribute toward improvements in your school. Think about what inspires you to apply, what issues you see, and what solutions you would like to propose. Talk to other students to get to know their needs. Ask for their input on potential changes, projects, and events. This assessment should inform your leadership platform.

Know the scope and limitations of the role to which you are applying. Make sure that your platform is realistic, and that you will actually have the power to influence the changes you propose. That being said, know that your role as a student leader is to challenge the way things have always been done. Do not be afraid of thinking outside the box.

BOX 32.2 Case Scenarios

Second Year Student—Angela

Angela is interested in becoming a research assistant (RA) and a member of the CNSA. They completed an environmental scan by speaking with their research professor about potential RA opportunities and with CNSA leaders. They received advice about how to seek out RA opportunities and how to become actively involved in the CNSA. Angela asked their peers specifically about how they maintained balance between competing priorities. They also conducted a self-assessment and examined their areas of strengths and development to help them identify how they could effectively contribute to the CNSA and RA roles. They developed a strategic plan and carried out different marketing strategies. They created a LinkedIn profile, conducted a Google search of their name and managed any undesirable content, and changed privacy settings in their social media accounts. Understanding the importance of networking, Angela decided to attend a few CNSA events.

Fourth Year Student—Toby

Toby is aware that they would like to start a student-led initiative by creating a research interest group. They scanned their environment and developed a strategic plan to carry out their leadership goal. Toby spoke with the research chair of their school and learned about available funding for student-led research initiatives. They then connected with their peers to see if there would be any interest in the initiative. Along with 10 other students, they wrote a proposal and were successful in obtaining funding. They used social media to promote their interest group and started the activities. They plan to send out a survey to evaluate how the initiative contributed to their peers' academic experience.

New Graduate Nurse—Shaneika

Shaneika wants to feel better prepared to take on a leadership role in their new job. They decided to look for professional development workshops that could help them gain new skills. They conducted an online search and found a leadership module from their provincial nursing association. Through the module, they were able to plan their next steps. Shaneika then talked to their manager and verbalized their interest in leadership. They learned there would be an opportunity to be part of the Tuberculosis quality improvement committee and the public health unit's nursing practice council in the next few months. In the meantime, Shaneika is planning to continue their professional development. They also decided to start a blog to share their experiences as a new nurse and create a marketing venue for their career.

Running for a position will involve following the rules of your local chapter. It is possible that you will need to gather support for your candidature from other students by collecting signatures. Campaigning commonly runs for 1 to 2 weeks. Most student candidates will use a mix of social media, posters around the university, e-mail, and class presentations to make themselves known. Convincing students to actually vote can be a challenge in and of itself. It requires ensuring that your peers, faculty, and university staff members are aware of who you are to gather support for the solutions and projects you wish to implement. However, the effort you put into this step is worthwhile once you are elected.

Often student leadership groups will have some roles that do not require being elected. These positions can be filled through applications. This means submitting a resume and cover letter, and participating in interviews, just like you would in a job application process. Be ready to talk about your platform, to discuss how much time you can invest in the group, and your motivations for joining. Also prepare some stories that demonstrate how you can work well within a team. Groups often want to make sure new associates will collaborate with all members.

Once you are part of the leadership team, you must be available to meet periodically, and also to contribute toward the group's projects, not only your own. Get to know everyone and their roles. Effective teams are those whose members know and appreciate each other. Gather support for your own projects by supporting your teammates with their initiatives. Continue to listen to the students in the program, as they should always be the focus of your contributions. Be sure that this experience will teach you immensely about team dynamics, politics, collaboration, and advocacy.

Advocating for Yourself and Others

Being a leader should not require a formal leadership role. You can become involved in stand-alone advocacy initiatives, such as requesting improvements in clinical placements, pushing for curriculum changes, or for the creation of new work-study positions. Such opportunities to get involved usually come from talking to your peers at school and realizing you face common issues or have similar interests. Go beyond just talking about it by getting to know what processes are in place in your school. For example, is there a specific form you should fill out if you want to file a complaint? There could be funding available for advocacy groups, or a certain procedure you can follow to schedule a meeting with the Dean to discuss an issue. Learn about these procedures by talking to faculty and administrative staff and put a plan in place.

Whenever acting as an informal leader, there are some important tips to keep in mind:

1. *Be collaborative:* Remember your goal is to reach a resolution, and for that you need to gather support. Keep arguments factual and use good conflict management skills. Trust that if there is a real issue, the school is interested in finding a solution. Remember you and the school are on the same team. They should always be regarded as allies.

2. *Do not go at it alone:* Leaders need followers and vice versa. It is not enough to be the only student affected or interested in advocating for a solution. Seek support from peers who may accompany you to a meeting with faculty. Identify students who are strongly involved in making a change for the better. Bring as many people as you can with you to demonstrate the impact of the issues and solutions you are advocating for.

3. *Value teamwork:* Success usually is the outcome of a group's collective efforts. Connect a group of students who are invested in an initiative and treat the issue at hand as you would a group assignment. Schedule meetings, divide tasks, develop a plan, and identify common goals. The work does not have to be labour intensive, but it should always be intentional.

4. *Get support from a faculty member:* There are always professors interested in students' initiatives. They can be crucial to bringing your team's agenda forward to faculty meetings, advise you about who is the best person(s) to share information with and when, and to bounce off ideas about your goals.

5. *Change takes time:* As important and interesting as advocacy initiatives may be, they usually require extra effort and time investment from students. It may be that your timeline will need to be extended,

or that the project needs to be postponed to the following academic year. Furthermore, change requires readiness and patience. Some ideas might need more time to be accepted. Be ready for that.

> **EXERCISE 32.10** Who could you speak to in your school regarding a problem or concern? Do you know the names of the school director or chair, program advisor or associate director, or dean?

Organizing a Student-led Event or Initiative

Students are diverse and have multiple interests. The school cannot possibly cater to all of them. Hence, the importance of student-led initiatives is to fulfill students' needs that may not be provided by the university. You can contribute to the community by organizing an event, such as a workshop on a specific topic. You can form nursing interest groups, such as a street nursing group. You can also contribute by helping out with events being organized by the student leadership groups. Do not be shy! You do not need to be part of any official group or association to organize an event. Any student can and should consider putting one together.

> **EXERCISE 32.11** Have you ever considered organizing a workshop or event in your school? Do you know about the funding options your school offers to such student-led initiatives? Who could you speak to at your school about organizing your event?

Start by asking your friends and peers about their interests. Ask what kinds of events they would like to attend. No matter how big or small your event or initiative is, some things are always important:

1. *Make sure there is real interest:* Conduct an informal poll to gauge students' interest in your event. Maybe you need to adjust your initial idea to better suit their needs. This is also a good way to let people know something is coming down the pipe.

2. *Get help from a team of students:* You cannot single-handedly organize an event. Do not even try it! Find people who are excited with the idea and who you can rely on. Discover what each person does best and let them take responsibility for it.

3. *Market the event way in advance:* Students are busy people, as you know it. Give them enough time to plan for your event. At least 2 weeks, but preferably

4. Identify ways to market the event multiple times to the same groups, by using different mediums, such as social media, class presentations, posters, and one-to-one invitations.

4. *Have a sign-up system:* When people sign-up, they have a chance to put the event on their calendar, or at least take a mental note of it. It is more likely that they will show up. However, know that not everyone will. You can usually register about 10% more people than you have space for.

5. *Find an accessible and appropriate venue and time:* Keep it on campus as much as possible. Students will try to avoid commuting whenever they can. Also look into class times and clinical days. This will directly impact their capacity to attend and the success of your event.

6. *Food brings people in:* If you can offer a meal, great. However, even potato chips and cookies will attract more people to your event. Look into possible sponsorships from local restaurants, or even from the university's cafeteria vendors.

7. *Be professional and appreciative of guest speakers:* They are just as important as the students who are in attendance. Make sure they have all the information they need. This can include a briefing of what the event is about, how many people will attend, and what they are expected to present. They should have a phone number to get in touch on the day of the event, in case they need help finding the venue or need to cancel. A thank-you card signed by the event's team, with a small gift is always a great way to show gratitude for their time. If they like the experience, they are much more likely to come again.

8. *Evaluate the impact of your event:* Always send an evaluation survey. This is a great way to know how your event performed, and if it met students' needs and expectations. It is also very important to give feedback to sponsors and guest speakers. Hold on to the results and go back to them when planning your next event.

Attending Town Halls and Community Meetings

Nursing schools usually offer opportunities for students to speak directly to their administration through town halls or other kinds of community assembly. Unfortunately, they may be poorly attended for many reasons. Some students may believe their concerns will be dismissed, others may feel insecure about showing up and making themselves known. Some students may not even notice the invitations in their mailbox.

> **EXERCISE 32.12** Do you know if your school organizes periodic community meetings or town halls? Have you ever been to one? When is the next meeting going to take place?

Regardless of how popular such meetings are, the school is opening up a communication channel that you can capitalize on. For that, take note of the following:

1. *Give positive feedback:* Start off by acknowledging what the school has done well. It shows that you come from a balanced position, not just an oppositional stance. Faculty and staff will be much more receptive to your critiques after that.

2. *Do not stop with the issues:* Come prepared with possible solutions. Take some time before the meeting to consider what the school could do, and how students could contribute toward a common resolution. This should be your main focus. Speak and obtain feedback from your peers when proposing a solution!

3. *Respect other students' participation:* Community meetings are an open forum for all who wish to speak. Be mindful that other students also deserve time to voice their concerns. If you feel like your concerns cannot be fully addressed then, ask for an individual follow-up meeting.

4. *Support each other:* Listen to others and contribute to the points they are making when you can. Maybe they are voicing a situation that you have also encountered. Do not hesitate to chime in and support them.

5. *Invite more students:* Let your friends and peers know you will be attending the meeting. Spread the word! More people present means the school must listen more carefully.

Collaborating With Students from Other Disciplines in University-Wide Initiatives

Health care is increasingly interprofessional. As future nurses, students should feel comfortable working with those from other disciplines. You can seek out opportunities to collaborate within your faculty but also on a broader level. Examples include being part of the university's student union, participating in academic committees, and volunteering on university-wide events. You can also look for peer mentorship positions, help others with academic tutoring, and be a part of a student support team.

Most universities have an international students' office which may be interested in engaging noninternational students in mentorship or support to newcomers. Finally, universities usually have multidisciplinary committees, such as the senate, that bring students from various programs together to make decisions that will have university-wide effects.

> **EXERCISE 32.13** Do you know of any opportunities to work with students from other disciplines in your university? Do you know people from other programs and what they are up to?

Interdisciplinary initiatives are always valuable opportunities to learn about fields outside of nursing. Most likely you will work or collaborate with people from any number of professions once you are a nurse. The university is a safe and exciting space to get to know their roles and scopes of practice. Take these as chances to learn about the following.

- What are the issues and solutions their profession is working with?
- How can nursing collaborate with their professional realm?
- How can their profession influence nursing's mandate?
- What kind of projects could involve both disciplines outside of university boundaries?
- Which social determinants of health does their field of work touch upon?

Advocating for Nursing Education

Nursing education must continually evolve to match the needs of an evolving job market. The transformation of the profession continues at great speed, with increasing scopes of practice, new professional opportunities, and patient's changing needs. Nursing students work toward their degree for 4 years, during which many changes can be implemented in the work environment. Students can be attuned to such changes and advocate for new educational methods and content, to best prepare them for what lies ahead.

> **EXERCISE 32.14** How has the nursing profession changed in the last year? What are the trends you can foresee in the next few years? How can your university best help you prepare to be an effective member of an evolving health care team?

You can have a lasting impact in your school when advocating for changes that advance nursing education. Suggesting the implementation of new ways of learning, asking for more simulation and laboratory time, making recommendations for new or revised curriculum, or collaborating on academic success initiatives can lead to long-term benefits for all students. Consider the following when advocating for nursing education:

1. *Work with faculty:* Find a professor who is open to new ideas in education and who is receptive to students' input. Work with them to find ways to implement potential changes. They can help mature your ideas and connect you to other staff who have the power to implement them.
2. *Discuss impact:* When proposing a new idea to the school, focus on how this change will impact learning and success for students. This shows you are thinking of the big picture, and not only about the here and now. If it is an idea that has been implemented elsewhere, highlight how the initiative has been successful.
3. *It is about everyone:* Schools like to be consistent and fair with students. Your proposed change must be relevant to most if not all students in your program or year. When the school realizes you are advocating for all and not just for an individual exception, they may be more open to listening.
4. *Offer to help with implementation:* Stick with the school after your suggestions are accepted. It could become an opportunity for you to participate in the process and learn from it. Maybe the school needs to talk to more students, whom you can help recruit. Maybe they open volunteer or work-study positions to increase open laboratory hours, and you could be the first to take a spot. It is an ongoing process!

Continue reading to learn how Angela, Toby, and Shaneika engaged with their own academic communities and further developed their leadership skills (Box 32.3).

LEADERSHIP DOMAIN: RESEARCH ENGAGEMENT

Often students do not think about research outside of their academic requirements. Being able to identify a problem, critically examine a situation, develop, implement, and evaluate strategies to address an issue are all research-related skills that are transferable to student

BOX 32.3 Case Scenarios

Second Year Student—Angela

After receiving advice from their peers, Angela volunteered to help with the orientation of first year nursing students which was an event led by the CNSA. Staying cognizant of their interest in an RA position, they decided to not take a formal student leadership role. Angela also learned about a current issue in the school regarding the lack of affordable textbooks and, along with some of their peers, advocated on behalf of their fellow students with a positive outcome.

Fourth Year Student—Toby

Toby has already contributed to the academic community through their formal leadership role with the CNSA. However, since they have started the research interest group, the feedback they have received from peers has been positive. Since the group has been meeting periodically, they have discussed potential changes to their school's curriculum, to emphasize research. They decide to advocate for such changes and devise a plan.

New Graduate Nurse—Shaneika

As Shaneika prepares to join the TB Quality Improvement Committee and Nursing Practice Council, they reflect back to their nursing school and volunteer experiences. Shaneika realizes they have many transferable leadership skills they can apply to the work of the committee and council. Some of the skills that they identified include interprofessional collaboration, program planning and evaluation, and how to navigate complex situations.

student, you can contribute to the development of new nursing knowledge by participating in research studies. You will learn about the research process from a participant perspective. This can be particularly helpful if you are interested in student leadership roles, such as a Research Assistant (RA) position or student representative role on a Research Ethics Board (REB). It will broaden your knowledge and understanding of research, and you will be contributing to the nursing profession in a positive way!

> **EXERCISE 32.15** What research studies are currently being conducted at your school? How can you find out more information?

To learn more about how you can participate in research studies, consider the following:

1. *Speak to your professors:* Sometimes students find speaking with their professors intimidating. Do not be shy. Take initiative, get to know your professors and learn about the different research studies that are being conducted at your school.
2. *Pay attention to bulletin boards:* In general, you will find research study recruitment postings on bulletin boards around your school. Take a minute and see if there are any research studies that are of interest to you. A recruitment posting will often include information about any participant requirements and who to contact should you be interested in joining.
3. *Online recruitment:* Sometimes researchers will recruit participants through different avenues online. This may include social media platforms, discussion boards, e-mail, and web pages. As students, you have many competing priorities on your plate, but take some time to do your homework and learn about potential research study opportunities.

Taking on Research Assistant Positions

Faculty who conduct research often hire research assistants (RA) to help with various project activities. This can include anything from a literature review, participant recruitment, conducting interviews, to manuscript development. As an RA, you will also be actively participating in team meetings and presenting at academic conferences. Learning how to work within a team, critically appraising literature, writing a manuscript for publication, and increasing your overall knowledge about the research process are some of the many benefits of

leadership. Presenting to groups and public speaking, manuscript and grant writing, and working within a team are other skills that you can also develop through research engagement. Being involved in research can be an exciting and unique experience because you can contribute to the development of new nursing knowledge. Pretty neat! Engaging in research does not end in your academic trajectory and will continue to be important throughout your nursing career. Get ahead of the game and engage in research now. Here are a few tips as to how you can become involved.

Participating in Research Studies

New nursing knowledge is always being developed and is important for the advancement of health care, clinical practice, nursing education, and profession. As a becoming an RA. These are all skills that can help you become a good and effective student leader.

> **EXERCISE 32.16** What areas of nursing practice and research are you interested in? What kind of research studies are being conducted by professors in your school? Do they match your nursing interests? What specific student leadership skills are you looking to gain from an RA position?

Seek out an RA position by doing the following:

1. *Get in the know*: Visit your school of nursing website, and learn about the different research activities and projects that are currently taking place in your school. Usually you can learn about a faculty member's research foci by reviewing their online biography.
2. *Network*: Speak to your professors about available and/or upcoming RA opportunities. Let them know you are interested and offer to forward your resumé.
3. *Connect with your peers*: Perhaps some of your peers have been or are RAs. Talk to them to learn about the role and how they were able to successfully obtain a position.
4. *Search for job postings*: Visit the careers page on your university's website. This is where you will find job postings for RA positions.

Joining the Research Ethics Board

REBs review, approve, monitor, and provide ethical consultations on all research studies that are being conducted involving human participants. All universities have an REB. An REB may comprise of a chair, ethicist, faculty, students, and community members. You can take on a formal student leadership role by joining your university's REB. As a student representative, you will attend meetings and be actively involved in the review and approval of research projects and related decision-making processes. This can help you develop leadership skills related to interprofessional collaboration, conflict resolution, public speaking, and nursing research ethics. It can also broaden your professional network.

> **EXERCISE 32.17** Are you familiar with your university's REB? Who can you speak to about joining? What skills related to student leadership would you like to develop? How can you contribute as a student representative in a meaningful way?

Here are some tips to help you find out how you can join your university's REB.

1. *Learn about your university's REB:* Visit the REB's webpage on your university's website. Find out who is on the REB and how many student representatives they have. Perhaps there may be a member from the School of Nursing. If yes, connect with them. Review their terms of reference if available.
2. *Review the requirements and application process:* To join an REB, you may have to meet certain requirements and criteria (e.g., completed a research course, minimum grade point average). There may also be an application process. Find out more information by visiting the REB's webpage or by contacting the REB about your interest in joining.
3. *Connect with student representatives:* Student representatives can give you insider perspectives of what your role would be on the REB. Contact them and ask to arrange an in-person meeting or phone conversation. This way, you can obtain detailed information about what they do and what their role entails.
4. *Review and update your resume:* Highlight what makes you a good candidate to become a student representative. Indicate what research-related activities and courses you have taken. Maybe you worked as an RA, participated in research studies or completed quantitative and qualitative research courses. Show the REB why they should choose you!

Applying Research to Practice

It is all about the evidence! More than ever before, evidence-informed practice has become important for nursing. Students use evidence too. When writing papers or preparing scholarly presentations, you have to seek out relevant literature. During clinical placements, you use guidelines and/or organizational policies and procedures to inform your nursing practice. These are all different ways of applying research to practice. Evidence comes in many shapes and forms. It may be scholarly literature, grey literature, and/or anecdotal. Applying research is also essential to student leadership. Such roles and activities require the ability to find and apply relevant information to help guide your actions as a leader.

> **EXERCISE 32.18** You are a member of the CNSA and are organizing a student tutoring session. How do you inform any decisions that are made in planning the session? Where and how do you obtain information?

Practice! Practice! Practice! Consider the following approaches to help you further develop this skill:

1. *Learn how to conduct a literature review:* Universities offer library services that may include workshops on how to conduct a literature search. This can help you become familiar with different search databases and effective approaches in finding relevant literature.

2. *Use your clinical placement time:* Become familiar with the organization's and unit's policies and procedures. Review relevant best practice guidelines. Apply this evidence when providing nursing care to patients and families.

3. *Consider different types of evidence:* Besides scholarly literature, there are different types of evidence. Grey literature includes materials external to traditional academic settings, such as governments and organizations. Some examples include government documents and organizational annual reports. Anecdotal evidence also counts. For example, when you ask a patient to rate their pain on a scale of 1 to 10, that is considered anecdotal evidence. Your nursing intervention for managing the patient's pain, would be based upon how the patient rates and describes their level of pain.

Joining a Nursing Research Interest Group

A nursing research interest group consists of nurses who are interested in the conduction, promotion, and use of nursing research. The group may examine current issues and trends in nursing research, provide opportunities for grants, and access to research resources for nurses. Joining a nursing research interest group can help you develop student leadership skills, such as public speaking, presenting, grant and manuscript writing, and resource development. You will also become more engaged with the research process. Often these groups include student representation.

> **EXERCISE 32.19** Are you aware of any nursing research interest groups? What knowledge and skills would you bring to the group? What student leadership skills would you like to focus and develop on by joining a group?

Here are some tips to get you started in joining a research interest group:

1. *Begin your search:* Look for different nursing research interest groups that exist. You can do this by simply googling. Your provincial professional nursing organization (e.g., Registered Nurses Association of Ontario) may have a nursing research interest group.

2. *Network:* Perhaps you may know professors and/or peers that may already be part of a nursing research interest group. Connect with them to learn more about their role and the work of the group. Usually a group is led by a chair. Contact the chair to obtain further information about the group and to discuss your potential interest in joining.

3. *Create your own:* If you cannot find a group to join, consider creating your own group. This can simply be a group of five or 10 nursing students who want to read and discuss research on a regular basis. It can be a fun way to learn from your peers and also a chance to lead by creating the opportunity for other students to become more engaged in research.

Follow Angela, Toby, and Shaneika as they integrate leadership into their research activities (Box 32.4).

LEADERSHIP DOMAIN: PROFESSIONAL PRACTICE

Most nursing students are engaged in clinical practice from the beginning of their program. Being at the hospital, clinic, or community primarily serves the goal of applying nursing skills. However, clinical practicums are also a great opportunity to learn about, and be engaged in, leadership. You will learn by observing leaders in your unit, advocating for your assigned patients, engaging in professional development initiatives, and much more. We will look at some of the ways to engage in leadership in your professional practice environments.

Attending Professional Development Workshops and Presentations

Teaching hospitals and clinics often grant professional development opportunities to students. These are learning sessions that emphasize specific aspects of professional practice, such as communicating with bereaved family members, reading electrocardiogram (ECG) strips, or developing wound care skills. We would go as far as to say you should attend as many of these sessions as possible. They are extremely informative, in a way that is difficult to accomplish in your regular classes. This is because the group in attendance usually includes experienced professionals, who enrich the discussions and provide an empirical perspective.

BOX 32.4   Case Scenarios

Second Year Student—Angela

Angela successfully completed their nursing research course and discovered that they enjoy writing research assignments and feel competent in reading scientific literature. Angela also spoke with their friend Havana, who is currently working as an RA, to learn more about their role and how they successfully obtained a position. Their research professor contacted them about an open opportunity with another faculty's team. Angela prepared their resume and crossed their fingers as they hit send.

Fourth Year Student—Toby

Toby and their peers conducted a literature review of different educational approaches to teaching research to nursing students. This helped them craft a strong advocacy proposal, which reflected the need for a more research focused curriculum at their school. They argued that nursing is moving increasingly to an evidence-informed approach to practice, and that students should have this skill upon graduation. On top of simply reading research for their courses, they asked that the school promote knowledge translation workshops, and increase RA positions for undergraduate students. Toby and their group scheduled a meeting with the Dean of Nursing and will present their proposal next week.

New Graduate Nurse—Shaneika

Shaneika applies for and successfully obtains positions on both the TB Quality Improvement Committee and the Nursing Practice Council. As they begin their work in both groups, they realize that their RA experience is becoming handy. For example, the TB Quality Improvement Committee is currently working on a quality project that looks at the improvement of documentation processes. As an RA, Shaneika had to develop a documentation process to keep track of all decisions that were made regarding the research project. They are now bringing that experience to help the committee to achieve their goals.

EXERCISE 32.20 Do you know if your clinical placement agency offers professional development sessions? Have you been to any? Are there any upcoming sessions in the next few weeks that you could attend?

Participating in professional development sessions is an important aspect of clinical leadership. Leaders must have the knowledge to support their team in performing their work to the best of their abilities. Every clinical setting has its go-to nurse, someone who has increasing knowledge and clinical judgement to be a resource in many different situations. This nurse was also a student like you. What sets them apart is their willingness to continue learning and improve their clinical skills, to the point where they are comfortable helping others achieve the same. When attending a professional practice workshop or presentation, consider the following tips:

1. *Prepare:* When you sign up for a workshop, take 5 minutes to think about how the information you will learn can help you in your current clinical environment. For example, if you are attending a presentation on the latest wound care techniques, consider what is the most common type of wound you see in your unit. This will help you focus your attention on relevant aspects of the presentation.

2. *Avoid zoning out:* Put the smartphone away. Resist the urge to search the web for random bits of information during the session. Write down what you want to research further and get it off your mind. Be present, as this is an opportunity that will not repeat itself. You can miss important information that cannot be reassessed later on.

3. *Be professional:* This is not a lecture, but a professional presentation. Show interest in what the presenter and other participants have to say. Respect their time by being punctual. Introduce yourself as a nursing student, not simply by your name.

4. *Raise your hand:* No matter how simple, it is always a good idea to ask a question during the Q&A period. This is a unique opportunity to ask someone with a lot of experience about something that is pertinent to your clinical environment. If speaking publicly is not your cup of tea, send questions through e-mail afterwards.

5. *Networking:* Providers from different units and health care disciplines attend professional development sessions. Take this opportunity to meet new people, talk about their field, and make professional connections. Do not forget to keep a business card on you at all times. You never know who you are going to meet!

Embracing Learning Opportunities

There is so much to be learned in the clinical setting. However, students may feel shy to take learning opportunities, especially in the first few years of the program.

They do not want to make mistakes in front of others or are afraid of hurting a patient. However, leadership involves taking initiative. When your instructor asks who wants to take off staples from an incision, raise your hand. When your preceptor asks if you would like to learn how to insert an intravenous (IV) catheter, say yes. Everything has a first time, and nursing is a very practical profession. By taking the lead, you will also be inspiring your peers to be proactive.

EXERCISE 32.21 What learning opportunities have you taken in your clinical setting recently? What skills would you like to learn, and could you ask your preceptor for such opportunities? How can you be well prepared for when these chances arise?

Make the most out of each learning opportunity by considering the following:

1. *Come prepared:* Do your readings and be as ready as possible to apply the knowledge you gained in class. Be very confident in your theoretical and technical information so that you can apply them to the best of your ability and maintain high quality of care.

2. *It is okay to feel inadequate:* As much as you may know all the theory behind a certain nursing skill, you may feel inadequate once you are actually applying it. Furthermore, no books can prepare you for talking to patients and making them feel comfortable in your presence. These skills take experience. So, embrace the feelings of inadequacy so that you can come out on the other end as a great nurse.

3. *Ask good questions:* Enjoy the opportunity to learn about nursing practice and go beyond the theory. Avoid questions you can easily find in a textbook. Instead, focus on questions such as how to interact with your patient when performing a painful procedure, or what to do in unusual cases where the patient does not present as expected.

4. *Advocate for mentorship:* Some settings are less welcoming to students. Nurses on your unit may not be willing to teach. This should not mean you and your classmates do not get any learning opportunities. Discuss the situation and possible solutions with your preceptor, or with the unit's nurse educator. If there is no one, talk to the charge nurse. If that does not work, consider bringing it to your school faculty or staff.

Becoming an Effective Follower

Nursing students know what it means to be a follower, especially in the clinical practice environment. Not only are you the most junior provider, but you often literally follow your preceptor around. However, students are not the only ones who must follow. Experienced nurses and other providers are followers in many situations. Thus achieving effective followership skills will only enhance your professional development. These skills and attitudes include being a collaborative team member, giving helpful feedback, and taking initiative.

EXERCISE 32.22 When was the last time you supported the team in your unit? Have you contributed to an important team goal at your placement yet? What seems to be the biggest challenge the team faces, and how could you help them overcome it?

Being a follower is not the same as being a quiet subordinate. Great followers are creative, observant, and responsive to their leader's and team's needs. You also demonstrate leadership by modelling good followership skills to your fellow nursing students in the clinical placement. Do not underestimate what you can accomplish as a follower. A few suggestions to be a great follower include:

1. *Have the courage to contribute your ideas:* Students enter placement with a fresh set of eyes and great ideas come from observing your environment. Look around your placement. Certainly, you will find ways to make things easier for the team. You could inspire new ways of doing things that will last long after you have completed your placement.

2. *Master the learner role:* Effective followers are masters of their role and the skills that come with it. As a student, your role is to be an effective learner. For that, focus on three main skills: asking great questions, always saying "yes" to a learning opportunity, and deliberately filling your knowledge gaps as they become apparent to you.

3. *Speak up:* Effective followers are critical thinkers. They do not simply follow orders. Think about why and how you should follow your preceptor's orders. Be mindful of your scope of practice, your knowledge, and the ethical considerations. If something is not how it should be, speak up about it in a professional manner. This means being factual and respectful of others' opinions, actively listening, and communicating clearly.

4. *Communicate:* Followers must know what is required of them, and what their contributions are. To accomplish this, communicate constantly. Do not hesitate to ask for feedback and clarification. Also, offer feedback and information to your team and preceptor to keep the work moving forward.

5. *Remember your value as a follower:* All of us play both the follower and the leader roles at some point of our careers, sometimes even on the same day. You can be the nurse manager on your floor in the morning and sit as a member of a committee in the afternoon. Take advantage of the opportunities you have as a student to learn how to be a great team player both as a follower and as a leader.

Advocating for Nursing

Canadian health care is an amazing powerhouse, but it also has its challenges. Nurses are essential to this system. We know a lot about the daily challenges faced at the frontlines, long before we reach graduation. Nurses must have a place at the table if the solutions to such challenges are to be coherent and effective. Nursing is evolving continually as a profession, and this includes increasing involvement in policy making. As a student, consider this added role you will have when you are a registered nurse and how can you be prepared to make a positive contribution.

> **EXERCISE 32.23** Are there any opportunities to become involved in policy and population-wide initiatives in your school? Are there any nursing interest groups or associations that do work on big-picture issues in health care? Do you know what they do? Could you help them in any way?

Advocating for nursing does not need to be restricted to your professional or school activities. In fact, it should mostly happen in the environments external to nursing. Consider the following tips:

1. *Interprofessionality and intersectionality:* Whenever you work with or meet a health care professional from a different discipline, chat about how nursing is connected to their work. The same can be done when meeting professionals from other sectors, such as law, education, housing, transportation, and so on. You could learn a lot about their field while also discussing social determinants of health. It is a way of spreading the word about the role of nurses and our large impact on society.

2. *Think about where nurses should be:* Hopefully your school has opened your mind to what nurses can actually do nowadays. We should not be constricted to the hospital setting. In fact, there are many places where nurses should be, but are not yet. For example, not all schools have a nurse. Nurses could have a big impact on promoting healthy childhood development if they were placed in all public schools.

3. *You are an ambassador:* A common experience for nursing students is being regarded as somewhat experts in health care as soon as university begins. Suddenly, your family and friends are asking you about their health concerns, even though you know you probably cannot help just yet. The reality is that nursing is a highly regarded, trusted profession. We are resources to people around us. Consider this whenever you are interacting with others. As an ambassador of the profession, your actions speak to how the public regards nurses in general. If it sounds like a big responsibility, it is because it is. Be mindful of it.

Advocating for Patients and Families

Especially during the early years of the program, nursing students are assigned a reduced number of patients during clinical placements. That means you have time to spend getting to know the people you are caring for. You also have time to advocate for those who are unable to do so, and to empower those who can advocate for themselves.

> **EXERCISE 32.24** How have you used downtime in your clinical placement? Have you spent time getting to know the patients you care for? Have you identified situations where they need someone to advocate for them? Have you been that person yet?

You should enjoy the extra time at clinical to learn about your patient and find out how you can help them beyond physical care. Do they know how to navigate the clinic or hospital environment? Do they have unanswered questions about their condition or treatment? Can they understand the instructions to care for themselves upon discharge?

To be an informed and effective advocate for your patients and their families, consider these suggestions:

1. *Get to know your patient:* A patient will spend most of their day with their assigned nurse. Doctors,

physiotherapists, respiratory therapists, and social workers come and go. The nurse, or nursing student, is the one constantly at the bedside. Take advantage of that, and get to really know your patient.

2. *Think social determinants of health:* Remember the socio-environmental model of health care, and think about what is impacting your patient and possibly creating barriers to health. Be knowledgeable of the different community resources that may be available.

3. *Listen carefully:* Stop assuming you know what your patient needs. Ask them, and then listen to their response carefully and critically. Understand where they are coming from. Confirm what they know about what is happening to them. Explore how can you work with what they know to help improve their situation.

4. *Look at the bigger picture:* Navigating the health care system can be daunting and overwhelming for patients. Learn about the processes in place at your practice setting and think of how they can be impacting the care your patient is receiving. Know how to help your patient to navigate the system.

5. *Some things just cannot be fixed:* As health care providers, we usually wish we could help everyone and every situation. Unfortunately, this is not the case. Not everything is fixable in health care. However, if anything, rest assured that even being a kind listener can improve how your patient or their family feels about their situation. Take the time.

Learn about how Angela, Toby, and Shaneika further developed their leadership skills through engagement in professional practice (Box 32.5).

CONCLUSION

As a student, it might not feel like leadership is at the top of your priority list. However, we would like for you to remember that you are about to enter a profession that is central to the Canadian health care system. Nurses make up one of the largest groups in health care, and this will likely continue in the coming decades. As such, nurses should be taking up larger and stronger policy and leadership roles, and collectively creating change for the better. Investing time and effort to develop your own leadership skills will be a worthwhile exercise not only for your own career but for society at large. We hope you take the plunge!

BOX 32.5   Case Scenarios

Second Year Student—Angela

Angela soon got great news: they were chosen for the RA position they had applied for. They started working with a professor, doing literature reviews, organizing team meetings, and keeping minutes. This work made them realize research is another exciting professional practice environment for nurses. Angela decided to get training on a research software, so that they could move on to data analysis in their RA role. They have also been learning a lot from the other RAs who have been part of the project for longer. They follow their lead in meeting the professor's expectations. Even though they are still the newbie, they often contribute their ideas during team meetings.

Fourth Year Student—Toby

Toby is consolidating at a long-term care facility and becomes aware of many existing challenges, including a Personal Support Workers (PSW) shortage. They find that this impacts patient care as patients are not being turned every 3 hours as recommended by best practice guidelines. They use the same strategies and skills applied in their experience in advocating for changes in the school research curriculum and conduct a literature review. Toby learns about how other long-term care facilities have solved this issue and shares their findings with the health care team. Through their initiative, Toby successfully advocates for organizational changes that improve patient care.

New Graduate Nurse—Shaneika

Given the experiences Shaneika has gained through their work on the TB Quality Improvement Committee and Nursing Practice Council, their manager promotes them to a Health Promotion Specialist Role for 3 months. They are nervous, excited, and anxious about the role, however they embrace this new opportunity. They ask for formal mentorship from their colleague who was previously in the role to learn about strategies they should take to be successful. Shaneika also signed up for a professional development workshop on writing policies and procedures because this will be a large focus of their role.

? A SOLUTION

Angela, Toby, and Shaneika all used the four domains of career planning and development, academic community, research engagement, and professional practice to address their individual and unique challenges in student leadership.

Angela discovered strategies to find balance between research, leadership engagement, and academic commitments. After conducting a self-assessment, they were able to prioritize their research interest while also staying engaged in ad-hoc student-led and advocacy initiatives.

Toby realized that they could still engage in leadership without holding a formal position. They discovered that they could remain engaged by starting their own initiative, a research interest group with the support of peers.

Shaneika took charge of their professional development by taking online courses and preparing for future opportunities. Meanwhile, they made sure to demonstrate their interest in leadership within their organization. That way they were ready to take on a leadership role when it became available.

Would these solutions be suitable plans for you? Why or why not?

✸ NEED TO KNOW NOW

- What leadership means to you, as a nursing student.
- Where do you stand within the four student leadership domains: career planning and development, academic community, research engagement, and professional practice.
- What are the leadership opportunities available to you in your school, community, and professional practice placement?
- What actions are you going to take to help you achieve your leadership goals?

▐ CHAPTER CHECKLIST

- Career planning and development is a process that can be strategically used to achieve all of your student leadership goals. Develop your vision, continually identify your strengths and areas of development, plan, network, find a mentor, and market yourself as an effective leader.
- Your community is fertile ground for leadership development. Engage with student groups, take on formal roles, or start your own initiatives with the help of your peers. Start activities that will enrich other students' experiences. This will not only help to develop your leadership skills but also make your own student journey much more meaningful and enjoyable.
- Contribute to nursing scholarship through formal and informal research activities, such a starting your own research interest group, joining your school's research ethics board, becoming a research assistant, or participating in research studies. You will develop leadership skills including working interprofessionally, speaking publicly, and using evidence to inform your practice and initiatives.
- Leading within your professional environment can range from small actions, such as volunteering to try new nursing skills, participating in professional development workshops, and advocating for patients. Resist the comfort of quietly going through your clinical placement. Taking the lead will create a much more significant learning experience. Do not let the opportunity pass you by. You will need those skills once you are a new graduate nurse.

TIPS TO ENGAGE IN STUDENT LEADERSHIP

Career Planning

- Use the Career Planning and Development Model to help you be engaged in student leadership.
- Find a mentor.
- Strategically search for leadership opportunities.

Academic Community

- Participate in official leadership groups, such as the Canadian Nursing Students' Association.
- Organize student-led initiatives and events.
- Attend Town Halls and other community meetings.

Research Engagement

- Take Research Assistant and other research-related positions.
- Join your university's Research Ethics Board.
- Participate in research studies.

Professional Practice

- Attend professional development workshops and presentations.
- Embrace learning opportunities.
- Advocate for nursing, patients, and families.

Visit the Evolve website for Suggested Readings, Internet Resources, and additional resources related to the content in this chapter: http://evolve.elsevier.com/Canada/Yoder-Wise/leading/

REFERENCES

Coyne, B. M., Kennedy, C., Self, A., & Bullock, L. (2018). A comprehensive approach to undergraduate nursing students' research experiences. *Journal of Nursing Education*, *57*(1), 58–62.

Pepin, J., Dubois, S., Girard, F., Tardif, J., & Ha, L. (2011). A cognitive learning model of clinical nursing leadership. *Nurse Education Today*, *31*(3), 268–273.

Waddell, J., Spalding, K., Canizares, G., Navarro, J., Connell, M., Jancar, S., et al. (2015). Integrating a career planning and development program into the baccalaureate nursing curriculum: part I. Impact on students' career resilience. *International Journal of Nursing Education Scholarship*, *12*(1), 163–173.

Waddell, J., Spalding, K., Navarro, J., Jancar, S., & Canizares, G. (2015). Integrating a career planning and development program into the baccalaureate nursing curriculum. Part II. Outcomes for new graduate nurses 12 months post-graduation. *International Journal of Nursing Education Scholarship*, *12*(1), 175–182.

GLOSSARY

A

absenteeism The rate at which an individual misses work on an unplanned basis. (Ch. 25)

academic community The body of people who compose the community at your university or school, including students, faculty, and supporting staff. (Ch. 32)

accommodating An approach to conflict resolution in which people neglect their own needs, goals, and concerns (unassertive) while trying to satisfy those of others (cooperative). (Ch. 24)

accountability The obligation to account for one's actions. (Ch. 27)

active listening Focusing completely on the speaker and listening without judgement to the essence of the conversation; an active listener should be able to repeat most of the speaker's intended meaning. (Ch. 20)

adverse event An event that results in unintended harm to the patient and is related to the care and services provided to the patient rather than to the patient's underlying condition. (Ch. 5)

advocacy Acting to support a cause or an interest; it is often embedded in nursing codes of ethics. (Ch. 21, 32)

agenda A written list of items to be covered in a meeting and the related materials that meeting participants should read beforehand or bring along. Types of agendas include structured agendas, timed agendas, and action agendas. (Ch. 29)

appreciative inquiry (AI) An attribute associated with how we question and problem solve; it focuses on identifying what is working well and building on those strengths. (Ch. 1)

artificial intelligence Computers and machines with simulated intelligence to think or act person-like (Ch. 13)

authentic leadership Leadership where leaders are constantly realigning their actions to match their values and moral convictions. (Ch. 1)

autonomy Personal freedom and the right to choose what will happen to one's own person. (Ch. 6)

availability bias The tendency for people to base their judgement on a preceding and memorable event that is readily recalled rather than complete information on the present situation. (Ch. 8)

average daily census (ADC) Average number of patients cared for per day in the unit for the reporting period. (Ch. 16)

average length of stay (ALOS) Average number of days that a patient remained in an occupied bed. (Ch. 16)

avoidance An approach to conflict resolution that is very unassertive and uncooperative because people who avoid neither pursue their own needs, goals, or concerns immediately nor assist others to pursue theirs. (Ch. 24)

B

barcode medication administration Medication administration which requires that the medication and a patient identifier like a wristband both have a barcode present and are scanned to verify accuracy. (Ch. 13)

battery When someone intentionally touches another without consent. (Ch. 7)

benchmarking The process of comparing best practices, processes, or systems with the practice, process, or system under review. (Ch. 22)

beneficence The principle that states that the actions one takes should "do good." (Ch. 6)

bioethics A division of applied ethics rooted in biological research and medicine and increasingly concerned with questions related to health care; its major principles are autonomy, justice, beneficence, and nonmaleficence. (Ch. 6)

budget A detailed financial plan for carrying out the activities an organization wants to accomplish for a certain period. (Ch. 14)

budgeting process An ongoing activity in which plans are made and revenues and expenditures are managed to meet or exceed the goals of the plan. (Ch. 14)

bullying A practice closely related to lateral or horizontal violence, but a real or perceived power differential between the instigator and recipient must be present in bullying. (Chs. 24, 26)

bureaucracy Characterized by formality, low autonomy, a hierarchy of authority, an environment of rules, division of labour, specialization, centralization, and control. (Ch. 10)

burnout A prolonged response to chronic emotional and interpersonal stressors on the job. (Ch. 29)

C

Canada Health Act The Canada Health Act (CHA or the Act) is Canada's federal legislation for publicly funded health care insurance. (Chs. 1, 9)

capital budget A budget that reflects expenses related to the purchase of major capital items, such as equipment and physical plant. (Ch. 14)

career management skills A range of skills that allow individuals to make and implement individualized career decisions. (Ch. 31)

career plan Includes the goals, activities, timelines and resources individuals will need to achieve their career goals and overall vision. (Ch. 31)

career planning and development An iterative process of assessing one's strengths, interests, and values and goal setting. (Chs. 31, 32)

career resilience The capacity and confidence to develop and use professional knowledge, skills, and attitudes to create a career that is personally meaningful, productive, and satisfying. (Ch. 31)

case management model A model of delivering patient care based on patient outcomes and cost containment. Components of case management are a case manager, clinical pathways/critical pathways, and unit-based managed care. (Ch. 15)

case manager A master's degree–prepared clinical nurse specialist who coordinates patient care from preadmission through discharge. (Ch. 15)

case method A model of nursing care delivery in which one nurse provides total care for a patient during an entire work period. (Ch. 15)

case mix groups (CMGs) A patient classification system used to group the types of inpatients a hospital treats. (Ch. 14)

chain of command The hierarchy depicted in vertical dimensions of organizational charts. (Ch. 10)

change theory A methodology to systematically transform existing conditions to a more equitable and just situation. (Ch. 19)

chaos A condition of disorder or confusion. (Ch. 30)

charge nurse A registered nurse responsible for delegating and coordinating patient care and staff on a specific unit. (Ch. 15)

chemical dependency A psychophysiologic state in which an individual requires a substance, such as medications or alcohol, to prevent the onset of symptoms of abstinence. (Ch. 25)

circle of care The individuals and institutions directly connected to an individual's health care. (Ch. 7)

clinical decision support systems (CDSSs) Interactive computer programs designed to assist health care providers with decision-making tasks by mimicking the inductive or deductive reasoning of a human expert. (Ch. 13)

clinical information system Electronic system in which health professionals obtain and document clinical information. (Ch. 13)

clinical nurse leader (CNL) A highly skilled Master's degree–prepared nurse who has completed advanced studies in clinical care with a focus on the improvement of quality outcomes for specific patient populations at the point of care. (Ch. 15)

clinical pathway A patient-focused document that describes the clinical standards, necessary interventions, and expected outcomes for the patient at each stage of the treatment process or hospital stay. (Ch. 15)

clinical practice guidelines Systematically developed statements of practice that assist practitioners and patients in making appropriate clinical decisions. (Ch. 23)

coaching A process in which a manager helps others learn, think critically, and grow through communications about performance. (Ch. 17)

coalitions Groups of individuals or organizations that join together temporarily around a common goal. (Ch. 12)

code of ethics A statement of a set of values that help guide nurses in ethical practice. (Chs. 5, 6)

collaborating A group of people working together to achieve a common goal. (Ch. 24)

collaboration A complex, voluntary, and dynamic process with underlying concepts of power, interdependency, sharing, partnership, and process. (Chs. 19, 27)

collaborative practice An interprofessional process for communication and decision making that enables the separate and shared knowledge and skills of the care providers to synergistically influence the client/patient care provided. (Chs. 5, 27)

collective action Activities that are undertaken by a group of people who have common interests or goals. (Ch. 21)

collective agreements A special type of employer–employee contract that governs employment arrangements including wages, benefit entitlement, job protection, and employee rights. (Ch. 7)

collective bargaining A mechanism for negotiating a labour contract between the employer and representatives of the employees. (Ch. 21)

colonization unjustified action of European settlers to invade, dominate, occupy and establish control over Indigenous peoples, land, and resources. (Ch. 4)

common law Laws that have been derived from the system of courts that operate in Canada and are commonly referred to as "judge made." (Ch. 7)

compassionate care Demonstrating empathy, sympathy and humanness during care to another. (Ch. 13)

competing An approach to conflict resolution in which people pursue their own needs and goals at the expense of others. (Ch. 24)

complexity compression The intensity of increasing functions and expectations without a change in resources, including time. (Ch. 30)

complexity science The study of complex systems, including how they are related, sustained, and able to self-organize, as well as how outcomes emerge. (Ch. 1)

compromising An approach to conflict resolution that involves both assertiveness and cooperation on the part of everyone and requires maturity and confidence. (Ch. 24)

computerized provider order entry Physicians and other health professionals who are able to write orders enter these into a computer system. (Ch. 13)

confidentiality The promise to hold in private any information provided and to prevent the release of information to those who are unauthorized. (Chs. 6, 7)

confirmation bias The tendency for people to seek information that reaffirms past experience and to discount information that contradicts past judgements. (Ch. 8)

conflict Two or more competing responses to a single event. (Ch. 20) Also, a disagreement in values or beliefs within oneself or between people that causes harm or has the potential to cause harm. (Ch. 24)

congruence an alignment of one's real and ideal self, resulting in a greater ability to be authentic and self-actualize/thrive in one's life roles. (Chs. 24, 25)

coping The immediate response of a person to a threatening situation. (Ch. 29)

cost The amount spent on something. (Ch. 14)

cost centre An organizational unit for which costs can be identified and managed. (Chs. 14, 16)

creative decision making The generation of new and imaginative ideas that are critical for problem solving. (Ch. 8)

critical thinking The intellectually disciplined process of actively and skillfully conceptualizing, applying, analyzing, synthesizing, and/or evaluating information gathered from, or generated by, observation, experience, reflection, reasoning, or communication, as a guide to belief and action. (Ch. 8)

cross-culturalism Mediating between or among cultures. (Ch.11)

cultural competence The process of integrating values, beliefs, and attitudes different from one's own perspective to render effective nursing care. (Ch.11)

cultural diversity The variation between people in terms of a range of factors, such as ethnicity, national origin, race, gender, ability, age, physical characteristics, religion, values, beliefs, sexual orientation, socioeconomic class, or life experiences. (Ch.11)

cultural humility ongoing process of self-awareness, learning and openness to respect the cultural identity and experiences of a person or group as a foundation for trust, while noting the impact of personal biases and systemic discrimination including power and privilege. (Ch. 4)

cultural imposition The tendency of an individual or group to impose their values, beliefs, and practices on another culture for varied reasons. (Ch.11)

cultural marginality Situations and feelings of passive betweenness when people exist between two different cultures and do not yet perceive themselves as centrally belonging to either one. (Ch.11)

cultural safety The effect of respecting cultural identity and establishing trust that results in improved health outcomes, with services and workplaces that are safe, respectful and free of discrimination. (Chs. 4, 5, 11)

cultural sensitivity The capacity to recognize that people from cultures other than our own are individuals who share similarities and differences. (Ch.11)

culture Shared patterns of learned behaviours and values transmitted over time, and that distinguish the members of one group from another. (Ch.11)

D

decision bias An error in judgement, when relevant information is omitted. (Ch. 8)

decision making A process that chooses a preferred option or a course of actions from among a set of alternatives on the basis of given criteria or strategies. (Ch. 8)

decolonization Ongoing process to redress effects of colonization, respect Indigenous ways of knowing and uphold human rights in accordance with the United Nations Declaration of Rights for Indigenous People, with critical awareness and conscientious righteous reforms in Eurocentric dominant society. (Ch. 4)

deficit-based approach Focus on needs, challenges and problems with risk of residual effect to create a negative bias. (Ch. 4)

delegation Achieving performance of care outcomes for which you are accountable and responsible by sharing activities with other individuals who have the appropriate authority to accomplish the work. (Chs. 27, 29)

differentiated nursing practice A model of clinical nursing practice that recognizes the difference in each nurse's level of education, expected clinical skills or competencies, job descriptions, pay scales, and participation in decision making. (Ch. 15)

diffusion of innovations The process by which an idea is spread through a culture. (Ch. 23)

direct care hours Paid time used for the care of patients. (Ch. 16)

disease management A model of care that coordinates health care interventions and communication for those individuals whose self-care needs are significant. (Ch. 15)

Donner-and-Wheeler Career Planning and Development Model A model and process that assists student and registered nurses to build their careers in a meaningful way. The Model is comprised of 5 phases. (Ch. 31)

dualism An "either/or" way of conceptualizing reality in terms of two opposing sides or parts (right or wrong, yes or no), limiting the broad spectrum of possibilities that exists between. (Ch. 20)

duty of care The obligations that nurses have toward others, to treat them in ways that in keeping with specific outlined standards and expectations. This term may refer to duties aligned with professional standards, ethical obligations or legal requirements. (Ch. 7)

E

electronic health record (EHR) A complete health record under the custodianship of a health care provider(s) that holds all relevant health information about a person from a particular organization or system. (Ch. 13)

electronic medical record (EMR) A health record under the custodianship of a health care provider(s) that holds relevant health information about a person and is often referred to in primary care environments. (Ch. 13)

electronic medication administration record Electronic version of the medication administration record. (Ch. 13)

emancipatory Relates to liberation and freedom; to be free from restrictions or restraints. (Ch. 19)

emotional intelligence (EI) The ability to know one's own and others' feelings and emotions. (Ch. 1)

employee assistance program (EAP) A program designed to provide counselling and other services for employees through either in-house staff or by contract with a mental health counsellor. (Ch. 29)

empowerment The process of exercising one's own power; also the process by which we facilitate the participation of others in decision making and taking action so they are free to exercise power. (Chs. 12, 17)

environmental assessment An assessment carried out to understand the specific internal and external forces that influence the health care setting. (Ch. 18)

environmental scan Scanning the environment involves looking around you with the goal of identifying how the immediate and surrounding environment can help you to work toward your vision of your ideal career. (Ch. 31)

equity Fair and just access to resources so all people may reach their full potential. (Ch. 4)

ethical dilemma A situation in which equally compelling reasons exist for and against two or more possible courses of action, and when choosing one course of action means that something else is let go. (Ch. 6)

ethics A branch of philosophy that deals with what is right and wrong. (Ch. 6)

ethnocentrism The belief that one's own ways are the best, most superior, or preferred ways to act, believe, or behave. (Ch.11)

evidence-based practice The integration of the best research evidence with clinical expertise and the patient's unique values and circumstances in making decisions about the care of individual patients. (Ch. 23)

evidence-informed decision making A process of gathering and translating all forms of knowledge to make the best-informed decision when delivering health care. (Ch. 23)

evidence-informed practice A systematic approach to clinical decision making that provides the most consistent and best possible care to patients. It integrates current research findings that define best practices, clinical expertise, and patient values to optimize patient outcomes as well as their quality of life. It also involves acknowledging and considering the myriad factors beyond evidence, such as local indigenous knowledge, cultural and religious norms, and clinical judgement. (Ch. 23)

expected outcomes See *Patient outcomes*. (Ch. 15)

expenditures Money spent on goods and services. (Ch. 14)

F

factor evaluation system A patient classification system that gives each task, thought process, and patient care activity a time or rating. These indicators are then summed to determine the hours of direct care required, or they are weighted for each patient. (Ch. 16)

fallacies Beliefs that appear to be correct but are found to be false when examined by logical reasoning rules. (Ch. 8)

fiduciary duty This refers to the legal or ethical obligation of many professionals, including for example nurses, doctors and lawyers, to act in the best interests of another person (e.g., a patient) and to put their own best interests aside, as part of a relationship involving trust and good faith. (Ch. 6)

First Nations General term describing the original inhabitants of Canada who speak 50 unique languages and represent over 600 distinct Indigenous nations who now live in urban and rural settings including Reserve lands; this population includes status (registered with the federal government) and nonstatus (replaces the racial government term "Indian"). (Ch. 4)

fixed costs Costs that do not change as the volume of patients changes. (Ch. 14)

fixed full-time equivalent (FTE) A full-time equivalent position that does not fluctuate based on patient care demands. (Ch. 16)

flat organizational structure A structure characterized by the decentralization of decision making to the level of personnel carrying out the work. (Ch. 10)

followership Engaging with others who are leading or managing by contributing to the work that needs to be done. (Ch. 1)

forecast The process of making decisions about the future based on multiple sources of data. (Ch. 16)

foreseeability The concept that certain events may reasonably be expected to cause specific consequences; an element of negligence and malpractice. (Ch. 7)

full-time equivalent (FTE) An employee who works full-time, typically 37.5 hours per week (1950 hours per year). (Chs. 14, 16)

functional nursing A model for providing patient care in which each regulated and unregulated member of the care team performs specific tasks for a large group of patients. (Ch. 15)

functional structure Arrangement of departments and services by specialty. (Ch. 10)

G

general adaptation syndrome (GAS) A theory by Hans Selye that details a predictable multistage response to stress. (Ch. 29)

goal setting The process of developing, negotiating, and formalizing the targets or objectives of an organization. (Ch. 18)

grievance An allegation, usually by an individual (employee), but sometimes by the union or management, of misinterpretation or misapplication of a collective bargaining agreement or of traditional work practices. (Ch. 25)

group A number of individuals assembled together or who have some unifying relationship. (Ch. 20)

group invulnerability The perception of group members that the group cannot be wrong, which can lead the group to make overly optimistic or overly risky decisions. (Ch. 8)

group polarization The tendency for groups to make decisions that are more extreme (risky or conservative) than the privately held beliefs of individual group members. (Ch. 8)

groupthink A phenomenon in which group members are so concerned with avoiding conflict and supporting their leader and other members that important facts, concerns, and differing views are not raised that might indicate an alternative decision. (Ch. 8)

H

halo effect A type of cognitive bias where our perception of one personality trait influences how we view a person's entire personality. (Ch. 17)

hardware Physical technology and devices. (Ch. 13)

harmful event An unintended outcome of care that could be prevented with evidence-informed practices and identified and treated in the same hospital stay. (Ch. 5)

health equity The absence of unfair or unjust differences in life circumstances and access to resources so that all persons have fair opportunities to achieve their full health potential to the extent possible. (Ch. 21)

health information technologies Technologies used in health-related environments, often containing information about a patient. (Ch. 13)

healthy work environment A practice setting that maximizes the health and well-being of nurses, quality patient outcomes, and organizational and system performance. (Ch. 3)

heuristics Educated guesses or "rules of thumb" based on experience and general knowledge about how things work, as opposed to specific information about the situation at hand. (Ch. 8)

hierarchy Chain of command that connotes lines of authority and responsibility. (Ch. 10)

high-reliability organization Organizations that operate in complex, high hazard domains for extended periods without serious accidents or catastrophic failures. (Ch. 22)

hindsight bias The tendency for people to overestimate their ability to predict an event after the fact. (Ch. 8)

horizontal violence An act of aggression that is perpetuated by one colleague toward another colleague. (Ch. 26)

hospital-acquired conditions Hospital-acquired conditions (HACs) and infections are medical conditions or complications that were not present when a patient was admitted to the hospital but develop as a result of errors or accidents in the hospital. (Ch. 22)

hospital information system Electronic system in which health professionals obtain and document clinical information. (Ch. 13)

hybrid organizational structure A structure that has characteristics of several types of organizational structures. (Ch. 10)

I

incivility A wide range of behaviours from ignoring, to rolling one's eyes, to yelling, and eventually to personal attacks, both physical and psychologic. (Ch. 26)

Indian Act federal legislation authorizing the Canadian government to impose control and regulate day-to-day lives of Indigenous peoples. (Ch. 4)

Indigenous Collective term for those who self-identify as First Nations, Inuit and Métis, with distinct languages, cultures, social systems, traditions, ceremonies, health practices and interrelated connection with community and the land (replaces the government term "Aboriginal"). (Ch. 4)

Indigenous Nursing Leadership respectful engagement with Indigenous Nursing Knowledges to guide authentic relational leadership in education, standards, politics and research from a collective stance that respects holism and interconnection of self, family, community and nation within structural and ecological systems. (Ch. 4)

indirect care hours Paid time used for other required unit activities, such as staff meetings or continuing education. (Ch. 16)

influence The process of using power—from the punitive power of coercion to the interactive power of collaboration. (Ch. 12)

informatics The use of technology and information systems to support improvements in patient care and health care administration. (Chs. 3,13)

information overload A state of stress brought about by the reception of too much information, too fast, and too often and not having adequate information-processing skills. (Ch. 29)

informed consent Authorization to undergo a proposed treatment by a patient who has fully understood and weighed the risks of that treatment. (Ch. 7)

interactional justice The perceived fairness of the quality of interactions by people who are affected by decisions and subsequent outcomes. (Ch. 3)

interdisciplinary team A team that comprises members from different clinical disciplines who have specialized knowledge, skills, and abilities. (Ch. 20)

interpersonal conflict Conflict that occurs between and among patients, family members, nurses, physicians, and members of other departments. (Chs. 24, 26)

interprofessional collaboration The process of working collaboratively with interdisciplinary team members. (Ch. 32)

interprofessional team A team that comprises different health care disciplines working together toward common goals to meet the needs of a patient population. Team members divide the work based on their scope of practice; they share information to support one another's work and coordinate processes and interventions to provide a number of services and programs. (Chs. 20, 27)

intrapersonal conflict Conflict that occurs within a person when confronted with the need to think or act in a way that seems at odds with one's sense of self. (Ch. 24)

intraprofessional team Health care professionals collaborating as a team who are from the same profession. For example, an RN, an RPN and NP who are facilitating a patient's transition from in-hospital psychiatric care to home. Or, an RN and 3 LPNs providing care to patients in a residential care home. (Ch. 27)

intuition A gut feeling; the subconscious integration of all the experiences, conditioning, and knowledge of a lifetime. (Ch. 8)

Inuit distinct Indigenous population with languages including Inuktut and local dialects who reside mainly over 50 arctic communities in Inuit Nunangat, with a smaller population in urban areas; this population includes status (registered with the federal government) and nonstatus. (Ch. 4)

J

justice The principle that everyone should be treated equally and fairly. (Ch. 6)

K

knowledge translation (KT) A dynamic and iterative process that includes synthesis, dissemination, exchange, and ethically sound application of knowledge to improve people's health, provide more effective health care services and products, and strengthen the health care system. (Ch. 23)

L

labour cost per unit of service A measure that compares budgeted salary costs per budgeted volume of service (productivity target) with actual salary costs per actual volume of service (productivity performance). (Ch. 16)

lateral violence Psychologic harassment evidenced by verbal abuse, intimidation, exclusion, unfair assignments, denial of access to opportunities, and withholding of information. (Ch. 26)

leader A person who sets a direction, develops a vision, and communicates the new direction to staff. (Ch. 3)

leadership The process of engaging and influencing others (Ch. 1). Also, the use of personal traits to constructively and ethically influence patients, families, and staff through a process in which clinical and organizational outcomes are achieved through collective efforts; the process of influencing others. (Ch. 2, 4, 19)

leadership framework A set of practices or competencies that provide a structure from which to develop leadership knowledge and skills. (Ch. 2)

leadership styles A particular leader's ways of imparting a vision and strategies about leadership which enable success. (Ch. 2)

liability One's responsibility for his or her own conduct; an obligation or duty to be performed; responsibility for an action or outcome. (Ch. 7)

licensure A right granted that gives the licensee permission to do something that he or she could not legally do absent of such permission; the minimum form of credentialing, providing baseline expectations for those in a particular field without identifying or obligating the practitioner to function in a professional manner as defined by the profession itself. (Ch. 7)

line function A function that involves direct responsibility for accomplishing the objectives of a nursing department, service, or unit. (Ch. 10)

lobbying Seeking to influence. (Ch. 12)

M

malpractice Failure of a professional person to act in accordance with the prevalent professional standards or failure to foresee potential consequences that a professional person, having the necessary skills and expertise to act in a professional manner, should foresee. (Ch. 7)

management Ensuring that the job gets done and providing people with the necessary resources to get the job done. The activities needed to plan, organize, motivate, and control the human and material resources required to achieve outcomes consistent with the organization's mission and purpose. (Ch. 1)

manager A person who addresses complex issues by planning, budgeting, and setting target goals. (Ch. 3)

mandatory overtime The expectation that staff will stay on duty after their shift ends to fill staffing vacancies. (Ch. 16)

marketing Marketing means being able to communicate effectively, and with confidence, your career vision, your strengths, interests and goals. (Ch. 31)

matrix structure An organizational structure influenced by dual authority, such as product line and discipline. (Ch. 10)

measurement A step to improve health care quality, using systematic approaches to quantify performance. (Ch. 22)

mediation A process using a trained third party to assist with conflict resolution. (Ch. 24)

Medical assistance in dying In Canada, medical assistance in dying (referred to as "MAiD") is option to end one's life with the assistance of a medical doctor or nurse practitioner. This option is available to patients with grievous and incurable illnesses or medical conditions who meet all legal eligibility criteria and in the context of outlined legal processes. (Ch. 7)

mentorship A formal supportive relationship between two, or more, health professionals that has the potential to result in professional growth and development for both mentors and mentees. (Ch. 28, 31)

metaanalysis A tool, resulting from the culmination of disparate but similar data points, used to further test significance of a divergent outcome. (Ch. 23)

Métis Distinct Indigenous population of mixed First Nations and European ancestry with languages including Michif who reside mainly in urban communities across Canada with a smaller population in constitutionally protected Métis Settlements across northern Alberta. (Ch. 4)

mindfulness Being aware and present in the moment. (Ch. 1)

mission Statement of an organization's reason for being. (Ch. 10)

moral agency Moral agency refers to the ability for a person, called a moral agent, to make moral judgements and in doing so, discern between what is considered to be right and wrong and to be held accountable for their actions. (Ch. 6)

moral distress Moral distress is the feeling that one knows what they consider is the right thing to do, but is unable to carry out that decision or action, because of constraints outside of the person, for example, institutional or organizational constraints. Moral distress usually occurs within the context of a situation that is deemed to have a moral dimension. (Ch. 6)

moral residue Moral residue occurs when a moral agent experiences morally distressing situations repeatedly and over time. This residue represents the remnants that remain with the person who experiences unresolved moral distress, and may have a lasting and damaging effect on one's view of self and others. (Ch. 6)

moral resilience This is the ability of a person to sustain their moral integrity, even in the face of morally challenging situations, moral distress, and other adversity. (Ch. 6)

moral uncertainty Feeling indecisive or unclear about a moral problem, while at the same time feeling uneasy or uncomfortable. (Ch. 6)

multiculturalism A society characterized by ethnic or cultural heterogeneity; it is an important part of Canadian identity that is recognized in the *Canadian Charter of Rights and Freedoms*. (Ch.11)

N

natural law A higher law that applies to all human beings and thus should override a human-made law. (Ch. 7)

near miss A clinical situation that resulted in no harm but highlights an imminent problem that must be corrected. (Ch. 22)

negligence Failure to exercise the degree of care that a person of ordinary prudence, based on the reasonable standard, would exercise under the same or similar circumstances. (Ch. 7)

negotiation Conferring with others to bring about a settlement of differences. (Ch. 24)

network The result of identifying, valuing, and maintaining relationships with a system of individuals who are sources of information, advice, and support. (Ch. 12)

networking Connecting and fostering relationships with other students and professionals within your field or area of interest. (Ch. 32)

never events Errors in medical care that are clearly identifiable, preventable, and serious in their consequences for patients and that indicate a real problem in the safety and credibility of a health care facility. (Ch. 22)

nominal group technique A technique that involves asking individual group members to respond to questions posed by a moderator and then asking participants to evaluate and prioritize the ideas of all group members. (Ch. 8)

nonmaleficence The principle that states that the actions one takes should "do no harm." (Ch. 6)

nonproductive hours Paid time that is not worked, such as vacation, statutory holidays, orientation, education, and sick time. (Chs. 14, 16)

nonpunitive discipline A disciplinary measure, usually verbal, describing existing standards and goals to which the parties agreed; pay is not withheld, and the employee agrees either to adhere to the standards in the future or to be terminated. (Ch. 25)

norms Expectations about behaviours and the ways things *should* be done, typically within social groups. (Ch. 6)

nurse outcomes The result of nursing work, including staff vacancy rate, nurse satisfaction, staff turnover rate, retention rate, and nurse burnout rate. (Ch. 16)

nursing care delivery model The method used to provide care to patients. (Ch. 15)

nursing case management The process of a nurse coordinating health care by planning, facilitating, and evaluating interventions across levels of care to achieve measurable cost and quality outcomes. (Ch. 15)

nursing governance The methodology or system by which a department of nursing controls and directs the formulation and administration of nursing policy. (Ch. 21)

nursing informatics The convergence of nursing science, information science and computer science. (Ch. 13)

nursing informatics competencies The knowledge, skills and judgment specific to nursing informatics. (Ch. 13)

nursing leadership Leadership of a group or individual within the nursing profession. (Ch. 13)

nursing practice The nursing practice refers to the activities RNs are authorized, educated and competent to perform. (Ch. 22)

nursing practice act Legislation that creates nursing regulatory authorities or regulatory bodies. (Ch. 7)

nursing productivity A formula-driven calculation that represents the ratio of required staff hours to actual provided staff hours. (Ch. 16)

nursing professional practice council A formal committee of nurses in a health care setting that identifies, reviews, and addresses issues that influence nursing professional practice. (Ch. 21)

nursing-sensitive outcomes Patient outcomes that are sensitive to nursing practice or interventions. (Chs. 5, 22)

O

operating budget The financial plan for the day-to-day activities of the organization. (Ch. 14)

opportunity cost Defined as providing service X is the amount of service Y that is not provided because resources are used to provide service X rather than service Y. (Ch. 14)

optimizing decision Selecting the ideal solution or option to achieve goals. (Ch. 8)

organization A business structure designed to support specific business goals and processes; or a group of individuals working together to achieve a common purpose. (Ch. 10)

organizational chart A graphical representation of work units and reporting relationships. (Ch. 10)

organizational conflict Conflict that arises when discord exists about policies and procedures, personnel codes of conduct, or accepted norms of behaviour and patterns of communication. (Ch. 24)

organizational culture The implicit knowledge or values and beliefs within the organization that reflect the norms and traditions of the organization. (Chs. 3, 10, 21)

organizational structure How work is divided in an organization; it delineates points of authority, responsibility, accountability and nondecision-making support. (Ch. 10)

organizational theory The systematic analysis of how organizations and their component parts act and interact. (Ch. 10)

outcome criteria The result of patient goals that are expected to be achieved through a combination of nursing and medical interventions. (Ch. 15)

outcomes The overall end results of an action, plan, or direction. (Ch. 2)

overtime Time in excess of the standard amount per day. (Ch. 16)

overwork A situation in which employees are expected to become more productive without additional resources. (Ch. 29)

P

participatory Allows people to be involved in and have a voice in activities that concern or interest them. (Ch. 19)

partnership model A method of providing patient care when a registered nurse is paired with another nurse

(e.g., a technical assistant) to provide total care to a number of patients. (Ch. 15)

patient allocation a nursing care model where one RN is responsible for the total care of an assigned number of patients. (Ch.15)

patient- or client-centred care An approach in which the patient is viewed as a whole person; it is not just about delivering services and involves advocacy, empowerment, and respecting the patient's autonomy, voice, self-determination, and participation in decision making. It includes patients and their family members in the design and delivery of health care at all levels. (Ch. 5)

patient engagement Providers and patients (and their families) working collaboratively together to improve health and health care processes. (Ch. 13)

patient-focused care model A team-based approach to care incorporating principles of patient-centred care with the goals of: (1) improving patient satisfaction and other patient outcomes, (2) improving worker job satisfaction, and (3) increasing efficiencies and decreasing costs. (Ch. 15)

patient outcomes The result of patient goals that are achieved through a combination of medical and nursing interventions with patient participation. (Chs. 15, 16, 22)

patient safety The absence of preventable harm to a patient during the process of health care. (Chs. 5, 13, 22)

percentage of occupancy The patient census divided by the number of beds in the unit. (Ch. 16)

perfectionism The uncompromising pursuit of perfection. (Ch. 29)

performance review Individual evaluations of work performance and behaviour. (Ch. 17)

personal liability A person's responsibility at law for his or her own actions. (Ch. 7)

philosophy Values and beliefs regarding the nature of work derived from a mission and the rights and responsibilities of people involved. (Ch. 10)

policy A specifically designated statement to guide decisions and actions. (Ch. 12)

policy process The process of developing, implementing, and evaluating policy on the basis of the best evidence available. (Ch. 12)

politics The use of power to influence, persuade, or otherwise change—it is the art of understanding relationships between groups in society and using that understanding to achieve particular outcomes. (Ch. 12)

position description A statement of the role and responsibilities of a specific position in an organization. It also describes the scope and duties of the work assignment, as well as to whom the individual reports. (Ch. 17)

power The ability to get things done, to mobilize resources, to get and use whatever it is that a person needs for the goals he or she is attempting to meet. (Chs. 12, 19)

preceptorship A period of practical experience and training for a trainee supervised by an expert or specialist in a particular field. (Ch. 28)

price The rate that health care providers set for the services they deliver. (Ch. 14)

primary care The first point of entry in the Canadian health care system and deals with the majority of health issues. (Ch. 9)

primary health care (PHC) A community-based health care service philosophy that is focused on illness prevention, health promotion, treatment, rehabilitation, and identification of people at-risk. (Ch. 9)

primary nurse The registered nurse who is responsible for planning and delivering care to a consistent group of patients. Typically, the primary care nurse works with a team to deliver care. (Ch. 15)

primary nursing A model for organizing patient care delivery in which one nurse functions autonomously as the patient's primary nurse throughout the hospital stay. (Ch. 15)

privacy The right of the individual to determine when, how, and to what extent he or she will release personal information. (Ch. 7)

private funding All nongovernment funded health care services. This would include funding of health care services directly from individuals (sometimes referred to as "out of pocket" expenses), such as home care nursing services or from third party insurance companies, such as physiotherapy in private clinics. (Ch. 9)

problem solving A comprehensive, sequential, cognitive process used to solve a problem by reducing the difference between current and desired conditions. (Ch. 8)

process improvement (PI) The proactive task of identifying, analyzing and improving upon existing processes within an organization for optimization, efficiency or meeting of quality standards. It often involves a systematic approach which follows a specific methodology (i.e., PDSA, Lean, Six Sigma). (Ch. 22)

procrastination Doing one thing when you should be doing something else. (Ch. 29)

productive hours Paid time that is worked. (Chs. 14, 16)

productivity The ratio of outputs to inputs; that is, productivity equals output/input. (Ch. 14)

professional association An alliance of practitioners within a profession that provides members with opportunities to meet leaders in the field, hone their own leadership skills, participate in policy formation, continue specialized education, and shape the future of the profession. (Ch. 21)

professional standard An authoritative statement that sets out the legal and professional basis of nursing practice. (Ch. 5)

progressive discipline A step-by-step process of increasing disciplinary measures, usually beginning with a verbal warning, followed by a written warning, suspension, allowing the employee to return with conditions, and termination (if necessary). (Ch. 25)

prototype evaluation system A patient classification system that classifies patients into broad categories and uses these categories to predict patient care needs. (Ch. 16)

professional governance A structure wherein nursing focused committees/councils consult and collaborate with each other to determine the most effective processes and actions to ensure quality patient care and outcomes. (Ch. 21)

professional practice The actions and activities developed by nursing students and nurses within their professional environments. (Ch. 32)

prudence trap The tendency for people to be too cautious and avoid risks that may be justified. (Ch. 8)

public funding Funding of health care services by government. (Ch. 9)

public policy A course of action that is anchored in a set of values regarding appropriate public goals and a set of beliefs about the best way of achieving those goals. (Ch. 12)

Q

quality improvement (QI) An ongoing process of innovation, error prevention, and staff development that is used by organizations that adopt the quality management philosophy. (Ch. 22)

quality indicators Measurable elements of quality that specify the focus of evaluation and documentation. (Ch. 3)

quality management (QM) The philosophy of a health care culture that emphasizes patient satisfaction, innovation, and employee involvement. (Ch. 22)

quality practice environment Anywhere a client receives health care. It provides organizational structures and resources that put the client, their families and caregivers at the forefront of their health care needs. It ensures safe, compassionate, competent and ethical care and is a basic human right. (Ch. 3)

R

randomized controlled trial (RCT) A study involving at least two groups where study participants are randomly assigned to either the control group or the intervention group to test a treatment's effectiveness. The gold standard in RCT is the double-blind study, where participants and those who are evaluating the outcomes do not know who has received a particular treatment. (Ch. 23)

reconciliation Ongoing healing process of historic injustice to constructively restore relations and equity between Indigenous and non-Indigenous Canadians based on the United Nations Declaration of Rights for Indigenous People. (Ch. 4)

redesign A process of analyzing tasks to improve efficiency (e.g., identifying the most efficient flow of supplies to a nursing unit). (Ch. 10)

reengineering A total overhaul of an organizational structure. It is a radical reorganization of the totality of an organization's structure and work processes. (Ch. 10)

regulatory body A body that controls who can be licensed, the types of actions that are regulated or reserved to nurses, and scope of practice; set out educational and examination requirements for registration and continuing competency requirements; and establish governing bodies and processes for monitoring professional conduct and acting on misconduct. (Ch. 7)

relational The authentic meaning connection between and among people. (Ch. 19)

relational ethics An ethical approach that focuses on the ethical action that takes place in relationships. Its core elements are engaged interactions, mutual respect, embodied knowledge, uncertainty and vulnerability, and interdependent environment. (Ch. 6)

research The diligent, systematic inquiry or investigation to validate and refine existing knowledge and generate new knowledge. (Ch. 23)

research engagement Formal and informal research activities in which students actively participate in. (Ch. 32)

research utilization The process of synthesizing, disseminating, and using research-generated knowledge to influence or change existing practices. (Ch. 23)

restructuring Fundamental changes to an organization to achieve greater efficiency or profit. (Ch. 10)

resilience The capacity to bounce back and grow through adversity. (Ch. 1)

revenue Money received for providing goods or services. (Ch. 14)

risk management The systematic identification, assessment, and prioritization of risks and the development and implementation of strategies to reduce adverse events and liability associated with these risks. (Chs. 7, 22)

robotics A wide array of technology that may be used to complete human-like tasks or functions. (Ch. 13)

role ambiguity A situation in which individuals do not have a clear understanding of what is expected of their performance or how they will be evaluated. (Ch. 17)

role clarity When an individual understands his or her own role and that of others and applies this understanding while performing the role, communicating within the role, collaborating with others, and delivering care. (Chs. 17, 27)

role conflict A condition in which individuals understand the role but are unwilling or unable to meet the requirements. (Ch. 17)

role discrepancy The gap between role expectations and role performance. (Ch. 28)

role expectations The attitudes and behaviours others anticipate that a person in the role will possess or demonstrate. (Ch. 28)

role integration The process of adjusting perceptions of one's role and reconciling discrepancies between the previous understanding of the role and what it is. (Ch. 28)

role negotiation Resolving conflicting expectations about personal performance through communication. (Ch. 28)

role orientation A formal employment process whereby the expectations of the role are clearly identified and the new employee is introduced to the organizational structure within which he or she will be working. (Ch. 28)

role preparation Education and socialization to the professional role within postsecondary and/or health care systems. (Ch. 28)

role stabilization When an individual matures in his or her performance of all facets of the role, to the point where he or she internalizes the role, performing it fluidly and with confidence. (Ch. 28)

role strain The subjective feeling of discomfort experienced as a result of role stress; it may be reflected by: (1) withdrawal from interaction, (2) reduced involvement with colleagues and the organization, (3) decreased commitment to the mission and the team, and (4) job dissatisfaction. (Chs. 25, 28)

role stress A condition in which role demands are conflicting, irritating, or impossible to fulfill. (Chs. 25, 28, 29)

role theory A framework used to understand how individuals perform within organizations. (Chs. 3, 17)

role transition The process of moving from a role that is familiar (e.g., nursing student) to one that is unfamiliar (e.g., novice professional nurse). (Ch. 28)

root-cause analysis A deeper review of an incident and the sequence of events that led to it with the goals of identifying and addressing the underlying causes to reduce the likelihood of reoccurrence. (Ch. 22)

S

satisficing decision Selecting an option that is acceptable but not necessarily the best option. (Satisfy + suffice = satisfice.) (Ch. 8)

scheduling The implementation of the staffing plan by assigning unit personnel to work specific hours and days of the week. (Ch. 16)

self-assessment The self-assessment helps you identify your interests, values, strengths, areas for development and then to link them to your career vision and environmental scan to plan your active engagement in your curriculum. (Ch. 31)

self-compassion Having unconditional positive regard toward one's self. (Ch. 24)

self-management The ability of individuals to actively gain control of their lives; components include stress management, time management, meeting management, and the ability to delegate. (Ch. 29)

sentinel event A serious, unexpected occurrence involving death or physical or psychologic harm, such as inpatient suicide, infant abduction, or wrong-site surgery. (Ch. 22)

service-line structure A type of structure in which the functions necessary to produce a specific service or product are brought together into an integrated organizational unit under the control of a single manager or executive. (Ch. 10)

shared governance A flat type of organizational structure with decentralized decision making. It is also described as a democratic, an egalitarian, and a dynamic process resulting from shared decision making and accountability. (Chs. 10, 21)

shared vision When two or more people endorse a particular view; it also describes concurrence on what the desired state in the future will be. (Ch. 30)

situational leadership The premise is that no single "best" leadership style exists, but rather that effective leaders and managers adapt their behaviours based on the situation. (Ch. 3)

six thinking hats A decision-making tool that can be used by groups to look at problems laterally from six different perspectives. (Ch. 8)

S.M.A.R.T. objectives The key attributes of effective objectives; that is, objectives are *S*pecific, *M*easurable, *A*greed on (or some use the word *A*chievable), *R*ealistic, and *T*ime bound. (Ch. 18)

social determinants of health The conditions in which people are born, live, and work; these conditions are shaped by economics, social policies, and politics. (Ch. 1, 9)

social dominance A hierarchical orientation to the world. Those coming from a socially dominant orientation oriented are motivated by a group that wields power over others. When motivated by a hierarchical/power over orientation, we are more likely to pursue self-interests over group interests. As a result, if work environments are largely coloured by socially dominant behaviour, there is often a lack of empathy for co-workers (making exclusion and scrutiny of those with less status more palatable), a lack of desire to help co-workers (unless it bolsters status), and a high degree of hostility (horizontal violence) if the hierarchy is challenged. (Ch. 24)

social justice The fair distribution of society's benefits, responsibilities, and consequences for all. (Chs. 4, 6, 19)

software The computer programs that are used. (Ch. 13)

span of control The number of individuals a supervisor manages. For budgetary reasons, span of control is often a major focus for organizational restructuring. (Ch. 10)

staff function Function that assists those in line positions in accomplishing primary objectives. (Ch. 10)

staff mix The proportion of regulated nurses and unregulated care providers in a specific setting. (Ch. 15)

staffing Planning for recruiting, hiring, deploying, and retaining qualified human resources to meet the needs of a group of patients. (Ch. 16)

staffing plan The conceptual approach of accomplishing the work to be done on a given unit. (Ch. 16)

stakeholders Individuals, groups, or organizations that are influenced by an issue or invested in policy related to an issue. (Ch. 12)

standards An established norm that can be applied for both technical and clinical reasons. (Ch. 13)

statute A rule/regulation created by elected legislative bodies. (Ch. 7)

steadfastness The ability of a person to be consistent, and firm in their approach to morally complex situations. Someone who consistently acts in a way that is consistent with their values, even when difficult, is felt to demonstrate steadfastness. (Ch. 6)

strategic planning A process by which the guiding members of the organization envision their future and develop the necessary and appropriate procedures and operations to actualize that future. (Ch. 18)

strengths-based leadership The notion that people are more productive when they build on their strengths rather than focusing on addressing their weaknesses. (Ch. 1)

student leadership The engagement of students in leadership actions that inspire and gather support from peers and others within the academic community. (Ch. 32)

student-led initiatives Activities that are internal and/or external to an academic setting which are primarily led by students. (Ch. 32)

subculture A group within a main culture that differs from the main culture with respect to core values, goals, and relationships, including approaches to issues and conflicts. (Ch. 21)

SWOT analysis A study of an organization's internal strengths and weaknesses, as well as its external opportunities and threats. (Chs. 8, 18)

synergy A phenomenon in which teamwork produces extraordinary results that could not have been achieved by any one individual. (Ch. 20)

Synergy Model A model of care delivery adopted by the American Association of Critical-Care Nurses that matches the needs and characteristics of the patient with the competencies of the nurse. (Ch. 15)

system A group or organization working together as a unified whole. (Ch. 10)

systems theory An approach to consider how various independent parts interact to form a unified whole or to disrupt a unified whole; the construct related to the operation of the whole process or entity. (Ch. 10)

T

team A number of individuals who work closely together toward a common purpose and are accountable to one another. (Ch. 20)

team dynamics The way team members interact and react to changing circumstances. (Ch. 8)

team nursing A small group of regulated and unregulated personnel, with a team leader, responsible for providing patient care to a group of patients. (Ch. 15)

technology adoption The characteristics and frequency of use of technology by health professionals and/or patients. (Ch. 13)

telehealth The use of telecommunications and information technologies for the provision of health care to individuals at a distance and the transmission of information to provide that care; involves use of two-way interactive video conferencing, high-speed telephone lines, fiber-optic cable, and satellite transmissions. (Ch. 13)

terminology A word used to represent a concept or set of concepts. (Ch. 13)

time management The appropriate use of tools, techniques, and principles to control time spent on low-priority needs and to ensure that time is invested in activities leading toward achieving desired, high-priority goals. (Ch. 29)

tort A civil wrong or injury, not related to a contract, for which a court will provide a remedy (usually monetary damages). (Ch. 7)

total patient care See *Case method.* (Ch. 15)

toxic workplace An organization in which people feel devalued or dehumanized and in which disruptive behaviour often flourishes. (Ch. 26)

transactional leadership The act of using rewards and punishments as part of daily oversight of employees in seeking to get the group to accomplish a task. (Ch. 1)

transculturalism Bridging significant differences in cultural practices. (Ch.11)

transformational leadership A process whereby leaders and followers set higher goals and work together to achieve them. It involves leadership that encourages followers to follow the leader's style and change their interests into a group interest with concern for a broader goal. (Ch. 1)

Transforming Care at the Bedside (TCAB) An initiative focused on redesigning the work environment and work processes of nurses to improve care for patients. (Ch. 15)

U

union An organization that undertakes collective action on issues, such as nurses' working conditions, salaries, and benefits. (Ch. 21)

unit of service A measure of the work being produced by the organization; for example, patient days, clinic or home visits, hours of service, admissions, deliveries, or treatments. (Chs. 14, 16)

unregulated care providers (UCPs) Unregulated caregivers who perform a variety of nursing tasks. (Chs. 15, 27)

utilization The quantity or volume of services provided. (Ch. 14)

V

variable costs Costs that vary in direct proportion to patient volume or acuity. (Ch. 14)

variable full-time equivalent (FTE) A full-time equivalent position that depends on the demand for care, and is typically a staff position. (Ch. 16)

variance The difference between the projected budget and the actual performance for a particular account. Also, a deviation from the normal path. (Chs. 14, 15)

variance analysis The process of determining differences between projected and actual costs. (Ch. 14)

variance report A report defining the difference between the actual and projected staffing or budgeting. (Ch. 16)

vision The articulated goals to which an individual, group, or an organization aspires. (Chs. 10, 30)

visioning Creating a vision for your ideal career describes where you want to go in your career and how you wish to build and enact your role as a nursing student and registered nurse. (Ch. 31)

W

whistle-blowing Exposing negligence, abuses or dangers, professional misconduct, or incompetence that exists in the organization. (Ch. 21)

workflow A set of tasks or process and their order to accomplish an outcome. (Ch. 13)

workload The amount of work distributed to a person or unit for a given time period. (Ch. 16)

workplace advocacy An umbrella term that encompasses advocacy activities within the practice setting. (Ch. 21)

Note: Page numbers followed by "f" indicate figures, "b" indicate boxes, and "t" indicate tables.